Core Topics in Transesophageal Echocardiography

Core Topics in Transesophageal Echocardiography

Edited by

Robert Feneck

John Kneeshaw

Marco Ranucci

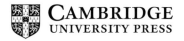

CAMBRIDGE UNIVERSITY PRESS
Cambridge, New York, Melbourne, Madrid, Cape Town, Singapore,
São Paulo, Delhi, Dubai, Tokyo, Mexico City

Cambridge University Press
The Edinburgh Building, Cambridge CB2 8RU, UK

Published in the United States of America by
Cambridge University Press, New York

www.cambridge.org
Information on this title: www.cambridge.org/9780521731614
© Cambridge University Press 2010

First published 2010
3rd printing 2011

Printed in the United Kingdom at the University Press, Cambridge

*A catalog record for this publication is available from the
British Library*

Library of Congress Cataloging in Publication data

Core topics in transesophageal echocardiography / edited by Robert O.
Feneck, John Kneeshaw, Marco Ranucci.
     p. ; cm.
Includes bibliographical references and index.
ISBN 978-0-521-73161-4 (pbk.)
1. Transesophageal echocardiography. I. Feneck, Robert O., 1950–
II. Kneeshaw, John. III. Ranucci, Marco. IV. Title.
[DNLM: 1. Echocardiography, Transesophageal – methods. 2. Heart
Diseases – ultrasonography. WG 141.5.E2 C797 2010]

RC683.5.T83C67 2010
616.1′207543–dc22   2009046624

ISBN 978-0-521-73161-4 hardback

Contents

Contents

Contributors

Sean Bennett
Consultant Anaesthetist
Castle Hill Hospital
Hull, UK

Dominique Bettex
Assistant Professor, Chief of Cardiac Anaesthesia
Department of Anesthesia
University Hospital Zurich
Zurich, Switzerland

Gianfranco Butera
Consultant, Department of Pediatric Cardiology
IRCCS Policlinico San Donato
San Donato Milanese (Milan), Italy

Mario Carminati
Director of the Department of Pediatric Cardiology
IRCCS Policlinico San Donato
San Donato Milanese (Milan), Italy

Serenella Castelvecchio
Consultant
Department of Cardiothoracic Anesthesia and
Intensive Care
IRCCS Policlinico San Donato
San Donato Milanese (Milan), Italy

John B. Chambers
Consultant Cardiologist
Cardiothoracic Centre
Guy's and St Thomas' Hospitals
London, UK

Pierre-Guy Chassot
Assistant Professor, Chief of Cardiac Anaesthesia
Department of Anaesthesia
University Hospital Lausanne (CHUV)
Lausanne, Switzerland

Massimo Chessa
Consultant
Department of Pediatric Cardiology and Adult
Congenital Heart Disease

IRCCS Policlinico San Donato
San Donato Milanese (Milan), Italy

Marisa Di Donato
Research Consultant
Department of Adult Cardiac Surgery
IRCCS Policlinico San Donato
San Donato Milanese (Milan), Italy

Joerg Ender
Professor or Anaesthesia
Department of Anaesthesiology and Intensive Care
Medicine II
Heart Center, University of Leipzig
Leipzig, Germany

Joachim Erb
Consultant Anaestheiologist
University Clinic of Anaesthesiology and Intensive
Care Medicine
Charité Universitätsmedizin Berlin
Berlin, Germany

Robert Feneck
Consultant Anaesthetist
Department of Anaesthesia
St Thomas' Hospital
London, UK

Fabio Guarracino
Director of Cardiothoracic Anaesthesia and Intensive
Care Medicine
Cardiothoracic Department
Azienda Ospedaliera Universitaria
Pisana
Pisa, Italy

John Kneeshaw
Consultant in Cardiothoracic Anaesthesia and
Intensive Care
Papworth Hospital
Cambridge, UK

Luca Lorini
Director of Anaesthesia and Intensive Care
Department
Azienda Ospedali Riuniti Bergamo
Bergamo, Italy

Chirojit Mukherjee
Consultant
Department of Anaesthesiology and Intensive Care
Medicine II
Heart Center, University of Leipzig
Leipzig, Germany

Diana Negura
Consultant
Department of Pediatric Cardiology
IRCCS Policlinico San Donato
San Donato Milanese (Milan), Italy

Alexander Ng
Consultant Anaesthetist
Heart and Lung Centre
Royal Wolverhampton Hospitals NHS Trust
Wolverhampton, UK

Alison Parnell
Cardiac Fellow/Specialist Registrar Anaesthesia
Glenfield Hospital
Leicester, UK

Alfredo Pazzaglia
Consultant
Department of Cardiothoracic–Vascular Anesthesia
and Intensive Care
IRCCS Policlinico San Donato
San Donato Milanese (Milan), Italy

Luciane Piazza
Consultant
Department of Pediatric Cardiology
IRCCS Policlinico San Donato
San Donato Milanese (Milan), Italy

Marco Ranucci
Director of Clinical Research
Department of Cardiothoracic–Vascular Anaesthesia
and Intensive Care
IRCCS Policlinico San Donato
San Donato Milanese (Milan), Italy

Erik Sloth
Consultant in Cardiothoracic Anaesthesiology
Department of Anaesthesiology and Intensive Care
Aarhus University Hospital – Skejby Sygehus
Aarhus, Denmark

Justiaan Swanevelder
Consultant Anaesthetist
Department of Cardiac Anaesthesia
Glenfield Hospital
Leicester, UK

Heinz D. Tschernich
Clinical Department of Cardiothoracic and Vascular
Anaesthesia and Intensive Medicine
Medical University of Vienna
Vienna, Austria

Kamen Valchanov
Consultant in Cardiothoracic Anaesthesia and
Intensive Care
Papworth Hospital
Cambridge, UK

Andrzej Wielogorski
Consultant Anaesthetist
Department of Anaesthesia
St Thomas' Hospital
London, UK

Patrick Wouters
Professor and Chairman
Department of Anaesthesia
University of Ghent
Ghent, Belgium

Preface

There has been a substantial increase in the use of transesophageal echocardiography (TEE) in the last 10 years. Much of this has been due to the increase in perioperative echocardiography in patients undergoing cardiac and major non-cardiac surgery, and in intensive care. Knowledge and skills in echocardiography are now part of the fundamental training of not only cardiologists but also cardiac anesthesiologists and intensivists, and indeed are commonly acquired by all specialists who care for patients undergoing cardiac surgery.

This book is the result of a frequently asked question, 'Which book would you recommend that will cover the necessary topics required for the accreditation exams, but will also help the reader in daily TEE practice?'

The first section covers topics that are essential reading for those who require a basic grounding in TEE for both their clinical practice and preparation for accreditation exams. The second section covers practical issues which will be relevant to the more experienced practitioner. These include mitral valve repair, transcatheter procedures such as septal defect closure and aortic valve surgery, and off-pump cardiac surgery. These are relevant to specialists from either a cardiology or an anesthesiology background. The speed with which new technology is made available to TEE suggests that the chapters on 3D imaging, myocardial velocity imaging, and speckle tracking will constitute a valuable introduction to these techniques.

The contributing authors are not only experts in TEE but also have a long and proven track record in education and training in echocardiography. We are grateful to them all for their excellent and timely contributions.

It is said that a picture is worth a thousand words. In echocardiography, that is a conservative estimate! We are therefore grateful to the publishers for agreeing to make available video files that provide examples of information referred to in the text. We believe this will be of substantial value to the reader, experts and novices alike.

Finally, we would like to thank the publishers for their patience and perseverance, and for their faith in our ability to deliver the finished article.

Addendum to Chapter 1: updated indications for perioperative TEE

Robert Feneck, John Kneeshaw, Marco Ranucci

The evidence supporting the indications for perioperative TEE has evolved over time. The lack of randomized controlled trials and meta-analyses has previously justified a cautious approach. The earlier North American guidelines referred to in Chapter 1 identified separate classes of indications, including recommendations on those conditions where TEE is recommended for use, and on those where it is not (see Table 1.2) [1]. Previously published European Guidelines made no mention of separate indications for perioperative echocardiography [2].

Very recently, guidelines and recommendations for the use of perioperative TEE from North America and Europe have been updated [3,4]. Both groups have produced similar recommendations, which differ from previously published guidelines in some important respects. We believe that these new recommendations are sufficiently important to justify this addendum.

The new guidelines from North America make a number of recommendations, as shown in Table 1. Most strikingly, they recommend that "for adult patients without contraindications, TEE should be used in all open heart (e.g., valvular procedures) and thoracic aortic surgical procedures, and should be considered in CABG surgeries as well."

In addition to a survey of the literature, these authors took opinion from expert consultants and experienced practitioners. Of the 58 experts, 96% agreed with the proposition that "TEE should be used for *all* cardiac and thoracic aortic surgical patients." For the small number who disagreed, CABG surgery in patients with normal ventricular function, and surgery to the descending thoracic aorta were notable exceptions. When considered as a whole, these new guidelines were assessed by a sample of the responding experts as being in accordance with their current practice, and therefore not requiring any change in practice on their part.

In these circumstances, contraindications to perioperative TEE became even more important, and the new North American guidelines have given some thought to this issue also (Table 1). Apart from previous esophageal surgery, the authors found little consensus on absolute contraindications, although the document correctly highlights the concept of "relative risk" and makes recommendations accordingly.

Recommendations from the European Association of Echocardiography are, at the time of writing, still in press and must therefore be considered as provisional. They state that "TEE should be used in adult patients undergoing cardiac surgery or surgery to the thoracic aorta under general anaesthesia, in particular in valve repair procedures."

Table 1. Indications and contraindications for perioperative TEE [3]

Indications: recommendations

1. For adult patients without contraindications, TEE should be used in all open heart (e.g., valvular procedures) and thoracic aortic surgical procedures, and should be considered in CABG surgeries as well.

2. For patients undergoing transcatheter intracardiac procedures, TEE may be used.

3. In non-cardiac surgery, TEE may be used when the nature of the planned surgery or the patient's known or suspected cardiovascular pathology might result in severe hemodynamic, pulmonary, or neurologic compromise. If equipment and expertise are available, TEE should be used when unexplained life-threatening circulatory instability persists despite corrective therapy.

4. For critical care patients, TEE should be used when diagnostic information that is expected to alter management cannot be obtained by TTE or other modalities in a timely manner.

Contraindications: recommendations

1. TEE may be used for patients with oral, esophageal, or gastric disease, if the expected benefit outweighs the potential risk, and provided the appropriate precautions are applied. These precautions may include: considering other imaging modalities (e.g., epicardial echocardiography), obtaining a gastroenterology consultation, using a smaller probe, limiting the examination, avoiding unnecessary probe manipulation, and employing the most experienced operator.

The authors noted that these recommendations are dependent on the fact that "there is appropriate technology available, and that those charged with undertaking TEE have the knowledge and skills appropriate to the task."

In non-cardiac surgery, the authors recommend that TEE "may be used in patients undergoing specific types of major surgery where its value has been repeatedly documented," including "neurosurgery at risk from venous thromboembolism, liver transplantation, lung transplantation and major vascular surgery, including vascular trauma." It may also be used in "patients undergoing major non-cardiac surgery in whom severe or life-threatening haemodynamic disturbance is either present or threatened," and "patients who are at a high cardiac risk, including severe cardiac valve disease, severe coronary heart disease or heart failure."

In critical care the authors recommend that TEE may be used "in the patient in whom severe or life threatening haemodynamic disturbance is present and unresponsive to treatment, or in patients in whom new or ongoing cardiac disease is suspected and who are not adequately assessed by transthoracic imaging or other diagnostic tests."

These new recommendations represent a significant enhancement of the role of perioperative TEE, particularly in adult cardiac surgery. Given these recommendations, it is clear that a perioperative TEE service should be available in every adult cardiac surgery unit, and that training in TEE should be regarded as an essential part of the training of the modern cardiac anesthesiologist.

References

1. Cheitlin MD, Armstrong WF, Aurigemma GP, *et al.* ACC/AHA/ASE 2003 guideline update for the clinical application of echocardiography: summary article. A report of the American College of Cardiology/American Heart Association Task Force on Practice Guidelines (ACC/AHA/ASE Committee to Update the 1997 Guidelines for the Clinical Application of Echocardiography). *Circulation* 2003; **108**: 1146–62.

2. Flachskampf FA, Decoodt P, Fraser AG, *et al.* Working Group on Echocardiography of the European Society of Cardiology. Guidelines from the Working Group. Recommendations for performing transesophageal echocardiography. *Eur J Echocardiogr* 2001; **2**: 8–21.

3. Thys DM, Abel MD, Brooker RF, *et al.* Practice guidelines for perioperative transesophageal echocardiography: an updated report by the American Society of Anesthesiologists and the Society of Cardiovascular Anesthesiologists Task Force on Transesophageal Echocardiography. *Anesthesiology* 2010.

4. Flachskampf FA, Badano L, Daniel WG, *et al.* for the European Association of Echocardiography. Recommendations for transoesophageal echocardiography: update 2010. *Eur J Echocardiogr* 2010; in press.

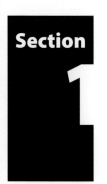

Fundamentals of transesophageal echocardiography

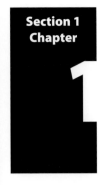

Introduction: indications, training, and accreditation in transesophageal echocardiography

Robert Feneck, Marco Ranucci

History and development of TEE

Transesophageal echocardiography (TEE) is a relatively recent development in imaging. The major innovations in TEE have all occurred since 1970. Early workers had both Doppler [1,2] and M-mode technology [3] available for use via the esophageal route, but the most significant development was the rigid, mechanical, two-dimensional, echocardiographic transesophageal endoscope in 1977 [4]. The initial device was a mechanical rotating transducer mounted on a rigid endoscope. This was replaced by a flexible endoscope, and linear and sector phased array technology was further incorporated.

Initially, transducers ranging from 10 MHz to 2.25 MHz were used, although the highest-frequency transducers were developed for gastrointestinal rather than cardiac imaging. In the early 1980s, following further technological developments, the value of TEE was established both as an outpatient diagnostic tool and for intraoperative monitoring of left ventricular function and air embolism. Further development was accelerated in the later 1980s by two separate events: the reporting of the value of TEE in establishing the diagnosis of aortic dissection [5,6], and the development of a high-resolution transesophageal probe with pulsed and color-flow Doppler technology.

This specification has formed the basis for the current standardized TEE probe, i.e. a flexible endoscope without optics or suction, 5 MHz transducer, 8–11 mm diameter adult endoscope with a 100 cm shaft length, four-way movable tip, and pulsed-wave and color-flow Doppler technology. Other more recent developments include a smaller endoscopic shaft with a diameter as small as 4 mm, variable-frequency transducers ranging from 3.5 to 7 MHz, omniplane transducers capable of viewing the heart from a wide variety of angles, and continuous-wave Doppler technology. Most recently, tissue Doppler imaging has become standard on most TEE systems, and three-dimensional

(3D) imaging. 'Live' 3D and further 3D technologies are becoming routinely incorporated [7].

Despite its relatively short history, TEE has become a well-established imaging modality. It has enabled the more accurate diagnosis of complex lesions in cardiology, and its use in the perioperative setting has had a marked impact on the development of cardiac anesthesia and surgery.

Indications for TEE examination

The indications for TEE examination in Europe were first published on behalf of the Working Group of the European Society of Cardiology in 2001 [8].

The authors' intention was to briefly describe the minimal requirements for a complete TEE examination. The primary indications for TEE stated by the authors were to identify sources of embolism, and to evaluate infective endocarditis, aortic aneurysm and aortic dissection, mitral regurgitation, and prosthetic valves (Table 1.1). However, the authors also noted that the indications for TEE were constantly increasing, and that frequently TEE was undertaken in circumstances where transthoracic echo had failed to provide sufficient information in an individual patient.

In contrast, perioperative TEE is undertaken as a stand-alone procedure, although there is a high likelihood that many patients will have received a preoperative transthoracic (TTE) examination at some point.

The first report on the indications for perioperative TEE was published in 1996 by the American Society of Anesthesiologists (ASA) and the Society of Cardiovascular Anesthesiologists (SCA) [9]. In these guidelines, the authors addressed the indications for TEE based on the level of evidence supporting their use, and also the proficiency of those carrying out the examination. Category I indications were supported by the strongest level of evidence or expert opinion, Category II indications were supported by lesser

3

Core Topics in Transesophageal Echocardiography, ed. Robert Feneck, John Kneeshaw, and Marco Ranucci.
Published by Cambridge University Press. © Cambridge University Press 2010.

Table 1.1. Principal TEE indications: essential views and structures in specific clinical conditions [8]

1. Source of embolism

- Left ventricular apex or aneurysm (transgastric and low transesophageal two-chamber views)
- Aortic and mitral valve
- Ascending and descending aorta, aortic arch
- Left atrial appendage (including pulsed-wave Doppler exam); note spontaneous contrast
- Left atrial body including interatrial septum; note spontaneous contrast
- Fossa ovalis/foramen ovale/atrial septal defect/atrial septal aneurysm; contrast + Valsalva

2. Infective endocarditis

- Mitral valve in multiple cross-sections
- Aortic valve in long- and short-axis views; para-aortic tissue (in particular, short-axis views of aortic valve and aortic root) to rule out abscess
- Tricuspid valve in transgastric views, low esophageal view, and right ventricular inflow–outflow view
- Pacemaker, central intravenous lines, aortic grafts, Eustachian valve, pulmonary valve in longitudinal right atrial views and high basal short-axis view of the right heart (inflow–outflow view of the right ventricle)

3. Aortic dissection, aortic aneurysm

- Ascending aorta in long-axis and short-axis views, maximal diameter; note flap or intramural hematoma, para-aortic fluid
- Descending aorta in long- and short-axis views; note maximal diameter, flap, intramural hematoma, para-aortic fluid
- Aortic arch; note maximal diameter, flap, intramural hematoma, para-aortic fluid
- Aortic valve (regurgitation, annular diameter, number of cusps)
- Relation of dissection membrane to coronary ostia
- Pericardial effusion, pleural effusion
- Entry/re-entry sites of dissection (use color Doppler)
- Spontaneous contrast or thrombus formation in false lumen (use color Doppler to characterize flow/absence of flow in false lumen)

4. Mitral regurgitation

- Mitral anatomy (transgastric basal short-axis view, multiple lower transesophageal views); emphasis on detection of mechanism and origin of regurgitation (detection and mapping of prolapse/flail to leaflets and scallops, papillary muscle and chordal integrity, vegetations, paraprosthetic leaks)
- Left atrial color Doppler mapping with emphasis on jet width and proximal convergence zone
- Left upper pulmonary, and, if eccentric jet present, also right upper pulmonary venous pulsed Doppler
- Note systolic or mean blood pressure!

5. Prosthetic valve evaluation

- Morphological and/or Doppler evidence of obstruction (reduced opening/mobility of cusps/disks/leaflets and elevated velocities by CWD)
- Morphological and Doppler evidence of regurgitation, with mapping of the origin of regurgitation to specific sites (transprosthetic, paraprosthetic); presence of dehiscence
- Presence of morphological changes in the prosthetic structure: calcification, perforation of bioprostheses, absence of occluder
- Presence of additional paraprosthetic structures (vegetation/thrombus/pannus, suture material, strand, abscess, pseudoaneurysm, fistula)

evidence or expert consensus, and Category III indications had little scientific or expert support. The Category III level may have been in part due to the absence of evidence, rather than the presence of evidence refuting any claim to benefit or value. As with the European consensus, which was published a few years later [8], the indications referred to clinical problems, which may be multiple in some patients.

In 1997 the American College of Cardiology (ACC) and the American Heart Association (AHA) published guidelines for the clinical application of echocardiography [10]. These guidelines referred to the overall indications for echocardiography, rather than addressing the relative merits of transthoracic and transesophageal studies. The guidelines were updated in 2003 [11], and that publication included a new and in-depth analysis of the indications for intra-operative echocardiography. These recommendations are shown in Table 1.2.

Once again the levels of evidence were stratified, although on this occasion the indications were divided into Classes I, IIa, IIb, and III, as follows:

- Class I – conditions for which there is evidence and/or general agreement that a given procedure or treatment is useful and effective

- Class II – conditions for which there is conflicting evidence and/or a divergence of opinion about the usefulness/efficacy of a procedure or treatment
  - IIa – weight of evidence/opinion is in favor of usefulness/efficacy
  - IIb – usefulness/efficacy is less well established by evidence/opinion
- Class III – conditions for which there is evidence and/or general agreement that the procedure/treatment is not useful/effective and in some cases may be harmful

Taking into account the original 1996 literature and the newer literature considered in the update, the authors identified a total of 706 publications that have contributed to this recent evidence base on intraoperative TEE.

Table 1.2. Indications for intraoperative TEE [11]

Class I

1. Evaluation of acute, persistent, and life-threatening hemodynamic disturbances in which ventricular function and its determinants are uncertain and have not responded to treatment

2. Surgical repair of valvular lesions, hypertrophic obstructive cardiomyopathy, and aortic dissection with possible aortic valve involvement

3. Evaluation of complex valve replacements requiring homografts or coronary reimplantation, such as the Ross procedure

4. Surgical repair of most congenital heart lesions that require cardiopulmonary bypass

5. Surgical intervention for endocarditis when preoperative testing was inadequate or extension to perivalvular tissue is suspected

6. Placement of intracardiac devices and monitoring of their position during port-access and other cardiac surgical interventions

7. Evaluation of pericardial window procedures in patients with posterior or loculated pericardial effusions

Class IIa

1. Surgical procedures in patients at increased risk of myocardial ischemia, myocardial infarction, or hemodynamic disturbances

2. Evaluation of valve replacement, aortic atheromatous disease, the Maze procedure, cardiac aneurysm repair, removal of cardiac tumors, intracardiac thrombectomy, and pulmonary embolectomy

3. Detection of air emboli during cardiotomy, heart transplant operations, and upright neurosurgical procedures

Class IIb

1. Evaluation of suspected cardiac trauma, repair of acute thoracic aortic dissection without valvular involvement, and anastomotic sites during heart and/or lung transplantation

2. Evaluation of regional myocardial function during and after off-pump coronary artery bypass graft procedures

3. Evaluation of pericardiectomy, pericardial effusions, and pericardial surgery

4. Evaluation of myocardial perfusion, coronary anatomy, or graft patency

5. Dobutamine stress testing to detect inducible demand ischemia or to predict functional changes after myocardial revascularization

6. Assessment of residual duct flow after interruption of patent ductus arteriosus

Class III

1. Surgical repair of uncomplicated secundum atrial septal defect

Table 1.3. New intraoperative TEE findings in two large series of patients

New finding	Mishra *et al.* [13]	Click *et al.* [14]
Mitral regurgitation	0.4%	—
Aortic regurgitation	0.2%	—
Tricuspid regurgitation	0.3%	—
Overall different valve pathology	1.0%	7.5%
Left ventricular thrombi	0.6%	1.1%
Ventricular septal defect	0.05%	—
Ascending/descending aorta pathology	0.7%	—
New ischemic areas	1.6%	—
Patent foramen ovale	—	3.1%
Overall	4%	15%

Given that some of the conditions considered are pathophysiological states, for example the risk of ischemia and/or myocardial infarction, rather than specific diagnoses, it could be argued that the 10 indications identified as being worthy of Class I and Class IIa cover the majority of cardiac surgery in adults and pediatrics. Thus, unless there are specific contraindications to TEE, many centers view the intraoperative use of TEE as a routine procedure with potential value in all cardiac surgery patients.

Notwithstanding the clear authority of these guidelines, it is pertinent to consider some of the evidence base for their conclusions.

Savage *et al.* [12] demonstrated that in high-risk coronary patients the routine use of intraoperative TEE resulted in major changes in surgery in 33% of the patients, and in major changes in the hemodynamic management in 51% of the patients. Mishra *et al.* [13] examined 5025 patients, including 3660 coronary bypass (CABG) surgeries and 1365 valve surgeries. Routine TEE examination before cardiopulmonary bypass (CPB) led to a major change in surgical planning in 5% of the coronary cases and in 3.5% of the valve cases. Following CPB, hemodynamic interventions were introduced on the basis of the TEE-derived information in 26% of the CABG patients and in 10.5% of the valve patients.

Click *et al.* [14] reported unexpected findings before CPB in 15% of the patients undergoing routine TEE during cardiac surgery. In 95% of these cases, these new findings resulted in major changes in the planned surgery. In the same series, 4% of the patients required major changes in surgery including a second run on CPB, or complex hemodynamic management after CPB (Table 1.3). Schmidlin *et al.* [15] reported a series of 2296 cardiac operations with the routine use of TEE: 9.6% of the patients received additional surgery and 49% required changes in the hemodynamic management based on TEE assessment and monitoring.

Studies on the intraoperative management of patients undergoing valve replacement have shown that TEE contributes frequently to intraoperative decision making and assessment, and on occasion to a substantial alteration in the surgical plan [16,17]. Similar findings have been shown in patients undergoing mitral valve repair [18–22]. Intraoperative TEE has been found to be useful in locating the size and source of air embolization following withdrawal of cardiopulmonary bypass [23], and in stratifying the risk of embolization from aortic atheroma in cardiac surgery patients [24].

The incidence of new intraoperative findings during a TEE examination has been identified as a reason for routine TEE examination during cardiac surgery, but also as a cause for concern. Clearly, a full preoperative examination and work-up should remove the possibility of unexpected and new findings on intraoperative TEE examination. However, the demonstration of new information is a common finding in many series of patients, and from major institutions. This does not necessarily imply an inadequate preoperative study, but may be due to the higher definition of a TEE examination in patients with poor transthoracic acoustic windows, the non-routine use of preoperative TEE in the majority of institutions, and recent changes that may have occurred in the clinical status of the patient.

Routine intraoperative use of TEE has been shown to lead to an improvement in both surgical and anesthetic management, which presumably is translated into better and more consistent outcomes for patients. However, for TEE to be routinely available during cardiac surgery there needs to be both adequate equipment and sufficient trained operators, both of which may be a major limitation to the provision of a comprehensive service. In this situation, the perioperative TEE service may need to be limited to Class I indications.

However, even in those circumstances where a comprehensive intraoperative TEE service is available, patients should have their primary echocardiographic evaluation before surgery, not during it. Whilst it is doubtless useful to be able to check the preoperative findings, in particular intraoperative TEE should not replace preoperative assessment of a valve lesion by transthoracic echocardiography or catheterization. Intraoperative transesophageal echocardiography can confirm the preoperative diagnosis, provide additional

details that may guide the surgical procedure, and help to guide management of hemodynamics. It remains the best means of immediately assessing the technical results of the surgical procedure in the operating room [25].

Training and accreditation in TEE

The use of TEE as a diagnostic tool in the echo lab, and as a diagnostic and monitoring tool during and after cardiac or other major operations, has increased significantly. As a result, patient benefit is maximized not only by expert consensus on indications for the procedure, but also by the proficiency and training of the echocardiographer. Both of the early documents on guidelines for practice make it clear that training and continuing education, practice, and update is necessary for an effective service [8,9].

The AHA/ACC updated guidelines published in 2003 [26] contain recommendations for the cognitive and technical skills required for competence in TEE (Table 1.4), cognitive and technical skills needed

Table 1.4. Cognitive and technical skills required for competence in TEE [26]

Cognitive skills

- Basic knowledge outlined in Tables 2 [Basic cognitive skills required for competence in echocardiography] and 4 [Cognitive skills required for competence in adult TEE]
- Knowledge of the appropriate indications, contraindications, and risks of TEE
- Understanding of the differential diagnostic considerations in each clinical case
- Knowledge of infection control measures and electrical safety issues related to the use of TEE
- Understanding of conscious sedation, including the actions, side effects, and risks of sedative drugs, and cardiorespiratory monitoring
- Knowledge of normal cardiovascular anatomy, as visualized tomographically by TEE
- Knowledge of alterations in cardiovascular anatomy that result from acquired and congenital heart diseases and of their appearance on TEE
- Understanding of component techniques for transthoracic echocardiography and for TEE, including when to use these methods to investigate specific clinical questions
- Ability to distinguish adequate from inadequate echocardiographic data, and to distinguish an adequate from an inadequate TEE examination
- Knowledge of other cardiovascular diagnostic methods for correlation with TEE findings
- Ability to communicate examination results to the patient, other healthcare professionals, and medical record

Technical skills

- Proficiency in using conscious sedation safely and effectively
- Proficiency in performing a complete transthoracic echocardiographic examination, using all echocardiographic modalities relevant to the case
- Proficiency in safely passing the TEE transducer into the esophagus and stomach, and in adjusting probe position to obtain the necessary tomographic images and Doppler data
- Proficiency in operating correctly the ultrasonographic instrument, including all controls affecting the quality of the data displayed
- Proficiency in recognizing abnormalities of cardiac structure and function as detected from the transesophageal and transgastric windows, in distinguishing normal from abnormal findings, and in recognizing artifacts

to perform perioperative echocardiography at a basic (Table 1.5) and advanced (Table 1.6) level, as well as training and performance maintenance requirements in both laboratory and perioperative settings (Table 1.7). For echocardiographers in the laboratory, recent publications have outlined the requirements for accreditation of echo labs under the auspices of the European Society of Cardiology (ESC) and the European Association of Echocardiography (EAE) [27], and also recommendations for the standardization of performance, digital storage, and reporting of echocardiographic studies as it relates to transthoracic echocardiography [28]. Whilst not exact in every detail, many of these recommendations would be appropriate to TEE studies also, particularly when the TEE study is a comprehensive perioperative study.

Anesthesiologists have become increasingly involved in perioperative echocardiography, for a number of reasons. First, the anesthesiologist's constant intraoperative presence means that instead of performing a "snapshot" preoperative study, there is no constraint to performing serial studies, extending from the preoperative to the postoperative period. Second, the use of TEE as a monitoring as well as a diagnostic tool has allowed us to benefit from a wealth of hemodynamic and other information to aid the patient's perioperative management.

Initially, apart from those anesthesiologists with formal training in cardiology, training in TEE was variable and frequently poorly structured. Attempts

Table 1.5. Cognitive and technical skills needed to perform perioperative echocardiography at a basic level [26]

Cognitive skills

- Basic knowledge outlined in Table 2 [Basic cognitive skills required for competence in echocardiography]
- Knowledge of the equipment handling, infection control, and electrical safety recommendations associated with the use of TEE
- Knowledge of the indications and the absolute and relative contraindications to the use of TEE
- General knowledge of appropriate alternative diagnostic modalities, especially transthoracic and epicardial echocardiography
- Knowledge of the normal cardiovascular anatomy as visualized by TEE
- Knowledge of commonly encountered blood flow velocity profiles as measured by Doppler echocardiography
- Detailed knowledge of the echocardiographic presentations of myocardial ischemia and infarction
- Detailed knowledge of the echocardiographic presentations of normal and abnormal ventricular function
- Detailed knowledge of the physiology and TEE presentation of air embolization
- Knowledge of native valvular anatomy and function, as displayed by TEE
- Knowledge of the major TEE manifestations of valve lesions and of the TEE techniques available for assessing lesion severity
- Knowledge of the principal TEE manifestations of cardiac masses, thrombi, and emboli; cardiomyopathies; pericardial effusions and lesions of the great vessels

Technical skills

- Ability to operate the ultrasound machine, including controls affecting the quality of the displayed data
- Ability to perform a TEE probe insertion safely in the anesthetized, intubated patient
- Ability to perform a basic TEE examination
- Ability to recognize major echocardiographic changes associated with myocardial ischemia and infarction
- Ability to detect qualitative changes in ventricular function and hemodynamic status
- Ability to recognize echocardiographic manifestations of air embolization
- Ability to visualize cardiac valves in multiple views and recognize gross valvular lesions and dysfunction
- Ability to recognize large intracardiac masses and thrombi
- Ability to detect large pericardial effusions
- Ability to recognize common artifacts and pitfalls in TEE examinations
- Ability to communicate the results of a TEE examination to patients and other healthcare professionals and to summarize these results cogently in the medical record

Table 1.6. Skills necessary to perform perioperative echocardiography at the advanced level [26]

Cognitive skills

- All the cognitive skills defined for the basic level
- Knowledge of the principles and methodology of quantitative echocardiography
- Detailed knowledge of native valvular anatomy and function. Knowledge of prosthetic valvular structure and function. Detailed knowledge of the echocardiographic manifestations of valve lesions and dysfunction
- Knowledge of the echocardiographic manifestations of congenital heart disease (CHD)
- Detailed knowledge of echocardiographic manifestations of pathologic conditions of the heart and great vessels (such as cardiac aneurysms, hypertrophic cardiomyopathy, endocarditis, intracardiac masses, cardioembolic sources, aortic aneurysms and dissections, pericardial disorders, and post-surgical changes)
- Detailed knowledge of other cardiovascular diagnostic methods for correlation with TEE findings

Technical skills

- All the technical skills defined for the basic level
- Ability to perform a complete TEE examination
- Ability to quantify subtle echocardiographic changes associated with myocardial ischemia and infarction
- Ability to utilize TEE to quantify ventricular function and hemodynamics
- Ability to utilize TEE to evaluate and quantify the function of all cardiac valves including prosthetic valves (e.g. measurement of pressure gradients and valve areas, regurgitant jet area, effective regurgitant orifice area). Ability to assess surgical intervention on cardiac valvular function
- Ability to utilize TEE to evaluate congenital heart lesions. Ability to assess surgical intervention in CHD
- Ability to detect and assess the functional consequences of pathologic conditions of the heart and great vessels (such as cardiac aneurysms, hypertrophic cardiomyopathy, endocarditis, intracardiac masses, cardioembolic sources, aortic aneurysms and dissections, and pericardial disorders). Ability to evaluate surgical intervention in these conditions if applicable
- Ability to monitor placement and function of mechanical circulatory assistance devices

Table 1.7. Numbers of examinations and other key training recommendations for basic and advanced perioperative echocardiography [26]

	Basic	Advanced
Minimum number of examinations	150	300
Minimum number personally performed	50	150
Program director qualifications	Advanced perioperative echocardiography training	Advanced perioperative echocardiography training plus at least 150 additional perioperative TEE examinations
Program qualifications	Wide variety of perioperative applications of echocardiography	Full spectrum of perioperative applications of echocardiography

were made to improve this, and the first educational programmes in the USA consisted of a combination of cardiology tutorials, self-learning, participation in echo courses, and residency in echo-labs and operating rooms [29,30]. Subsequently, a joint effort of the ASA and SCA produced a common pathway leading to practice guidelines for perioperative transesophageal echocardiograpy [9].

In 1999, the American Society of Echocardiography (ASE) and the SCA jointly published guidelines for performing a comprehensive intraoperative TEE study [31], and the guidelines for training in perioperative echocardiography were published by the same group in 2002 [32]. Two levels of practice were defined: basic and advanced, with different theoretical and practical requirements for each. A written examination administered by the National Board of Echocardiography has been in place since 1996 for those seeking to demonstrate skills and knowledge through an accreditation process.

Table 1.8. European accreditation in TEE: European Association of Echocardiography (EAE) and European Association of Cardiothoracic Anaesthesiologists (EACTA)

Step 1

A written exam held twice a year

This exam consists of multiple choice questions (MCQ, single best answer format) divided into two sections:

- Reporting related to TEE videos displayed on screen

- Theory

To be successful, a candidate *must pass both sections of the written exam* (reporting and theory) at the same time

Step 2

A practical assessment to be completed within 12 months of passing the written examination

TEE accreditation in Europe

In Europe, the problem of training and accreditation in perioperative TEE has been addressed, during the last decade, by the EAE, which is a formal association of the ESC, and the European Association of Cardiothoracic Anaesthesiologists (EACTA). Both groups have worked toward a common process of accreditation and examination in TEE applicable to both cardiologists and anesthesiologists, and indeed any others who may wish to demonstrate skills and knowledge in TEE. The process of accreditation and examination in adult TEE was finally established in 2004, and the first accreditation examination was held in 2005.

In Europe, accreditation in TEE is obtained in two parts. First, the written exam is a compulsory part of the accreditation. Second, a practical assessment must be completed within a fixed time period, currently within 12 months of passing the written examination. The details of the current process are identified in Table 1.8. Prospective candidates can obtain updated information on the accreditation process from the websites of EAE (www.escardio.org/comunities/EAE) and EACTA (www.eacta.org). The performance of the EAE accreditation exams has recently been reviewed [33].

Accreditation is run as a service and is not a compulsory or regulatory certificate of competence or excellence. It is available to sonographers and doctors of all disciplines. In common with similar groups elsewhere, the goals of accreditation are to protect patients from undergoing transesophageal echocardiographic examinations performed by unqualified persons and to set a European standard for competency and excellence, which is expected to be recognized more widely. Accredited echocardiographers are expected to be able to perform and report routine transesophageal echocardiographic studies unsupervised, but whilst European accreditation is designed to test the competency of an individual to be able to perform, interpret, and report routine transesophageal echocardiographic studies unsupervised, the right to report and sign clinical studies in individual countries will be defined by national laws and regulations.

Conclusion

Transesophageal echocardiography has undergone remarkable progress in a very short space of time. This progress has been evident on a number of fronts. The technology has improved immeasurably, and continues to do so apace. This has facilitated the widespread use of TEE, and so has encouraged the establishment of practice recommendations and guidelines. Following on from this, assessments of personal proficiency and the proficiency of laboratories, including quality assurance and digital storage recommendations have followed.

References

1. Side CG, Gosling RG. Non-surgical assessment of cardiac function. *Nature* 1971; **232**: 335–6.

2. Daigle RE, Miller CW, Histand MB, McLeod FD, Hokanson DE. Nontraumatic aortic blood flow sensing by use of an ultrasound esophageal probe. *J Appl Physiol* 1975; **38**: 1153–60.

3. Frazin L, Talano JV, Stephanides L, *et al.* Esophageal echocardiography. *Circulation* 1976; **54**: 102–8.

4. Hisanaga K, Hisanaga A, Nagata K, Yoshida S. A new transesophageal real-time two-dimensional echocardiographic system using a flexible tube and its clinical application. *Proc Jpn Soc Ultrason Med* 1977; **32**: 43–4.

5. Erbel R, Börner N, Stellar D, *et al.* Detection of aortic dissection by transoesophageal echocardiography. *Br Heart J* 1987; **58**: 45–51.

6. Erbel R, Engberding R, Daniel W, *et al.* Echocardiography in diagnosis of aortic dissection. *Lancet* 1989; **1**: 457–61.

7. Sugeng L, Shernan SK, Salgo IS, *et al.* Live 3-dimensional transesophageal echocardiography initial experience using the fully-sampled matrix array probe. *J Am Coll Cardiol* 2008; **52**: 446–9.

8. Flachskampf FA, Decoodt P, Fraser AG, *et al.* Working Group on Echocardiography of the European Society of Cardiology. Guidelines from the Working Group. Recommendations for performing transesophageal echocardiography. *Eur J Echocardiogr* 2001; **2**: 8–21.

9. Practice guidelines for perioperative transesophageal echocardiography. A report by the American Society of Anesthesiologists and the Society of Cardiovascular Anesthesiologists Task Force on Transesophageal Echocardiography. *Anesthesiology* 1996; **84**: 986–1006.

10. Cheitlin MD, Alpert JS, Armstrong WF, *et al.* ACC/AHA Guidelines for the Clinical Application of Echocardiography. A report of the American College of Cardiology/American Heart Association Task Force on Practice Guidelines (Committee on Clinical Application of Echocardiography). Developed in collaboration with the American Society of Echocardiography. *Circulation* 1997; **95**: 1686–744.

11. Cheitlin MD, Armstrong WF, Aurigemma GP, *et al.* ACC/AHA/ASE 2003 guideline update for the clinical application of echocardiography: summary article. A report of the American College of Cardiology/American Heart Association Task Force on Practice Guidelines (ACC/AHA/ASE Committee to Update the 1997 Guidelines for the Clinical Application of Echocardiography). *Circulation* 2003; **108**: 1146–62.

12. Savage RM, Lytle BW, Aronson S, *et al.* Intraoperative echocardiography is indicated in high-risk coronary artery bypass grafting. *Ann Thorac Surg* 1997; **64**: 368–74.

13. Mishra M, Chauhan R, Sharma KK, *et al.* Real-time intraoperative transesophageal echocardiography – how useful? Experience of 5,016 cases. *J Cardiothorac Vasc Anesth* 1998; **12**: 625–32.

14. Click R, Abel M, Schaff HV. Intraoperative transesophageal echocardiography: 5-year prospective review of impact on surgical management. *Mayo Clin Proc* 2000; **75**: 241–7.

15. Schmidlin D, Bettex D, Bernard E, *et al.* Transoesophageal echocardiography in cardiac and vascular surgery: implications and observer variability. *Br J Anaesth* 2001; **86**: 497–505.

16. Nowrangi SK, Connolly HM, Freeman WK, Click RL. Impact of intraoperative transoesophageal echocardiography among patients undergoing aortic valve replacement for aortic stenosis. *J Am Soc Echocardiogr* 2001; **14**: 863–6.

17. Ionescu AA, West RR, Proudman C, Butchart EG, Fraser AG. Prospective study of routine perioperative transesophageal echocardiography for elective valve replacement: clinical impact and cost saving implications. *J Am Soc Echocardiog* 2001; **14**: 659–67.

18. Morehead AJ, Firstenberg MS, Shiota T, *et al.* Intraoperative echocardiographic detection of regurgitant jets after valve replacement. *Ann Thorac Surg* 2000; **69**: 135–9.

19. O'Rourke DJ, Palac RT, Malenka DJ, *et al.* Outcome of mild periprosthetic regurgitation detected by intraoperative transesophageal echocardiography. *J Am Coll Cardiol* 2001; **38**: 163–6.

20. Kawano H, Mizoguchi T, Aoyagi S. Intraoperative transoesophageal echocardiography for evaluation of mitral valve repair. *J Heart Valve Dis* 1999; **8**: 287–93.

21. Saiki Y, Kasegawa H, Kawase M, Osada H, Ootaki E. Intraoperative TEE during mitral valve repair: does it predict early and late postoperative mitral valve dysfunction? *Ann Thorac Surg* 1998; **66**: 1277–81.

22. Grewal KS, Malkowski MJ, Piracha AR *et al.* Effect of general anesthesia on the severity of mitral regurgitation by transesophageal echocardiography. *Am J Cardiol* 2000; **85**: 199–203.

23. Tingleff J, Joyce FS, Pettersson G. Intraoperative echocardiographic study of air embolism during cardiac operations. *Ann Thorac Surg* 1995; **60**: 673–7.

24. Choudhary SK, Bhan A, Sharma R, *et al.* Aortic atherosclerosis and perioperative stroke in patients undergoing coronary artery bypass: role of intra-operative transesophageal echocardiography. *Int J Cardiol* 1997; **67**: 31–8.

25. Bonow RO, Carabello BA, Chatterjee K, *et al.* 2008 Focused update incorporated into the ACC/AHA 2006 guidelines for the management of patients with valvular heart disease: a report of the American College of Cardiology/American Heart Association Task Force on Practice Guidelines. *Circulation* 2008; **118**: e523–661.

26. Quiñones MA, Douglas PS, Foster E, *et al.* American College of Cardiology/American Heart Association clinical competence statement on echocardiography: a report of the American College of Cardiology/American Heart Association/American College of Physicians–American Society of Internal Medicine Task Force on Clinical Competence. *Circulation* 2003; **107**: 1068–89.

27. Nihoyannopoulos P, Fox K, Fraser A, Pinto F. EAE laboratory standards and accreditation. *Eur J Echocardiogr* 2007; **8**: 80–7.

28. Evangelista A, Flachskampf F, Lancellotti P, *et al.* European Association of Echocardiography. European Association of Echocardiography recommendations for standardization of performance, digital storage and reporting of echocardiographic studies. *Eur J Echocardiogr* 2008; **9**: 438–48.

29. Cahalan MK, Foster E. Training in transesophageal echocardiography: in the lab or in the job? *Anesth Analg* 1995; **81**: 217–18.

30. Savage RM, Licina MG, Koch CG, *et al.* Educational program for intraoperative transesophageal echocardiography. *Anesth Analg* 1995; **81**: 399–403.

31. Shanewise JS, Cheung AT, Aronson S, *et al.* ASE/SCA guidelines for performing a comprehensive intraoperative multiplane transesophageal echocardiography examination: recommendations of the ASE Council for intraoperative echocardiography and the SCA Task Force for certification in perioperative transesophageal echocardiography. *Anesth Analg* 1999; **89**: 870–84.

32. Cahalan MK, Abel M, Goldman M, *et al.* American Society of Echocardiography and Society of Cardiovascular Anesthesiologists task force guidelines for training in perioperative echocardiography. *Anesth Analg* 2002; **94**: 1384–8.

33. Fox K, Popescu BA, Janiszewski S, *et al.* Report on the European Association of Echocardiography Accreditations in Echocardiography: December 2003–September 2006. *Eur J Echocardiogr* 2007; **8**: 74–9.

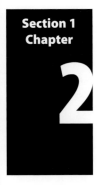

2

Basic principles of physics in echocardiographic imaging and Doppler techniques

Joachim Erb

Introduction

Modern-day ultrasound equipment harnesses complex high-end technology and enormous computing power in order to enable the various forms of imaging and Doppler techniques. Although computerized programmes, presets, and other factors help in making the use of the echocardiographic equipment a relatively straightforward task, a basic understanding of ultrasound physics and engineering is essential if we are to acquire adequate information and interpret it correctly. Furthermore, although it seems that the heart can virtually be seen on the screen, the image which is presented to us is the result of a very complex transformation of reflected sound signals into a mosaic of pixels in various shades of gray. The better our understanding of the physical principles determining the echocardiographic information, the better will be the interpretation of the clinical information. It is especially important to recognize the limitations of the technology in order to ensure that image information is not based on artifacts and thus wrongly interpreted. Therefore, this chapter will provide a basic understanding of the most important physical principles and an introduction into the basics of ultrasound techniques. For a more detailed description the reader is referred to the further reading recommendations at the end of the chapter.

Ultrasound physics

Sound waves

Sound is traveling mechanical energy. It propagates through any medium by causing oscillations in molecules, thereby creating a cycle of high pressure (compression) and low pressure (rarefaction) (Fig. 2.1). A sound wave is therefore an alternating series of cycles with compressions and rarefactions that are characterized by:

- cycle length (wavelength λ [mm])

- frequency (frequency f [Hz])
- energy (amplitude [dB])
- speed (propagation velocity c [m/s]) in the respective medium

The relationship of these parameters is described by the wave equation:

$$c = \lambda \times f \tag{2.1}$$

Audible sound frequencies for the human ear range between 20 and 20 000 Hz. Ultrasound is defined as frequencies above 20 000 Hz. Cardiac sonography uses ultrasound frequencies between 1 and 10 MHz (1 MHz = 10^6 Hz). The resulting wavelengths are in the range between 0.1 and 1.5 mm, and can be calculated using the wave equation:

$$\lambda = c / f \, [\lambda = 1.54 / f \, (\text{in MHz})] \tag{2.2}$$

The propagation velocity of ultrasound depends on the medium through which it is traveling; velocity increases with the density of the medium (Table 2.1).

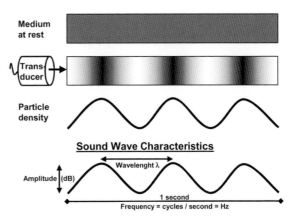

Figure 2.1. Sound passing through any medium causes areas of compression (dark) and rarefaction (white). The change in particle density over time is equivalent to a sine wave. The frequency describes the number of cycles per second, the wavelength is the length of one cycle, and the amplitude describing the extent of compression and rarefaction expresses the energy of the wave.

13

Core Topics in Transesophageal Echocardiography, ed. Robert Feneck, John Kneeshaw, and Marco Ranucci.
Published by Cambridge University Press. © Cambridge University Press 2010.

Table 2.1 Propagation velocity (V) of ultrasound in different media

Medium	Air	Lung	Fat	Water	Blood	Muscle	Bone
V (m/s)	330	600	1450	1450	1560	1580	4080

As can be seen, the propagation velocities in soft tissue (fat, muscle) and body fluids (water, blood) are in a close range. Therefore, the propagation velocity of ultrasound in soft tissue, for example in the heart, is assumed to be fairly constant at 1540 m/s [1–3].

Ultrasound and tissue interaction

Ultrasound cannot propagate through tissues without interference, but is influenced by various modes of interaction with those tissues. This both facilitates and limits its use for echocardiography. Four forms of interaction are discussed below, namely reflection, refraction, scattering, and attenuation (Fig. 2.2).

Reflection

Ultrasound is partially or totally reflected at organ boundaries and tissue interfaces. The amount of reflected ultrasound energy depends on the difference in acoustic impedance Z between tissues [4]. Acoustic impedance is defined as the product of tissue density σ and propagation velocity c:

$$Z = \sigma \times c \qquad (2.3)$$

The greater the difference in acoustic impedance across a tissue boundary, the more ultrasound energy will be reflected. This is expressed in the reflection coefficient.

Tissue boundaries with a smooth surface and a lateral dimension greater than the ultrasound wavelength used, which will be in the range of 1 mm, act as specular reflectors. This means that ultrasound is reflected as light is reflected in a mirror. The law determining incidence and reflection is as follows:

$$\text{angle of incidence } \theta_i = \text{angle of reflection } \theta_r \quad (2.4)$$

Therefore, although the ratio of reflected ultrasound energy is defined by the difference in impedance at a given interface, the amount of reflected energy received back at the transducer depends on the intercept angle and the resulting angle of reflection. The maximal amount of reflected ultrasound energy can only be received if the transmitted ultrasound beam hits the tissue boundary at a perpendicular angle (90°). In contrast, the less perpendicular the ultrasound beam/

tissue interface, the less reflected ultrasound will reach the transducer. This may result in poor image quality or even echo "dropout," where the transducer is blind to tissue interfaces because of near-parallel alignment of ultrasound beam and tissue boundary (Fig. 2.2).

Refraction

Ultrasound waves are refracted on their passage between tissues of only slightly different acoustic impedance, which means they are deflected from their initial straight path in a manner comparable to the refraction of light through optical lenses. The relationship between the angle of incidence θ_i and the angle of refraction θ_t is proportional to the propagation velocities c in the neighbouring tissues:

$$\sin\theta_i \,/\, \sin\theta_t = c_1 \,/\, c_2 \qquad (2.5)$$

where c_1 and c_2 are the propagation velocities in tissue 1 and tissue 2.

Refraction may improve image quality if it is consciously used for acoustic focusing in a transmitter. During imaging, unplanned and unrecognized refraction of ultrasound on its way through the tissue is the source of ultrasound imaging artifacts, the most prominent being the double-image artefact (Fig. 2.2).

Scattering

If the ultrasound wave hits a very irregular, rugged border or small objects with a lateral dimension less than one wavelength, the ultrasound is not reflected, but scattered. Its energy is diffused in all directions. Only a small amount reaches the transducer, which accounts for the fact that the energy of a scattered signal (40–60 dB) is 100–1000 times less than that of a reflected signal. Scattering occurs in the myocardium itself (which explains why the signal of the myocardium is weak compared to the reflection at the endocardial and epicardial borders), at anatomical edges, and at blood cells. This important observation forms the basis of Doppler echocardiography (Fig. 2.2).

Waveform distortion

Ultrasound waves with a high-pressure amplitude, that is ultrasound emitted from the transducer with relatively high energy, change their sinusoidal shape when traveling through tissue. In addition to the emitted frequency (f_0), called fundamental frequency, multiples of this frequency are generated which have double $(2\,f_0)$ or triple $(3\,f_0)$ the original frequency. Analogous to music, where we hear this phenomenon

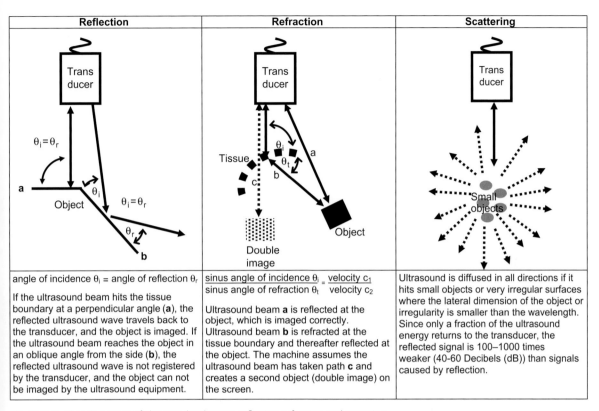

Reflection	Refraction	Scattering
angle of incidence θ_i = angle of reflection θ_r	$\dfrac{\text{sinus angle of incidence } \theta_i}{\text{sinus angle of refraction } \theta_t} = \dfrac{\text{velocity } c_1}{\text{velocity } c_2}$	Ultrasound is diffused in all directions if it hits small objects or very irregular surfaces where the lateral dimension of the object or irregularity is smaller than the wavelength. Since only a fraction of the ultrasound energy returns to the transducer, the reflected signal is 100–1000 times weaker (40–60 Decibels (dB)) than signals caused by reflection.
If the ultrasound beam hits the tissue boundary at a perpendicular angle (**a**), the reflected ultrasound wave travels back to the transducer, and the object is imaged. If the ultrasound beam reaches the object in an oblique angle from the side (**b**), the reflected ultrasound wave is not registered by the transducer, and the object can not be imaged by the ultrasound equipment.	Ultrasound beam **a** is reflected at the object, which is imaged correctly. Ultrasound beam **b** is refracted at the tissue boundary and thereafter reflected at the object. The machine assumes the ultrasound beam has taken path **c** and creates a second object (double image) on the screen.	

Figure 2.2. The interactions of ultrasound with tissue: reflection, refraction, and scattering.

when a tone is played one octave higher by doubling its frequency, the fundamental frequency is called the first harmonic, and the next multiples become the second harmonic, third harmonic, etc. For example, if the fundamental frequency is 2 MHz (first harmonic), the second harmonic displays a frequency of 4 MHz and the third harmonic 6 MHz. Waveform distortion into harmonic frequencies is the basis for the harmonic imaging mode, as explained later in this chapter [5].

Attenuation

As ultrasound propagates through any medium by causing oscillations in molecules, frictional forces occur which absorb a part of the kinetic energy by transformation into heat, similar to tissue heated in a microwave oven. The deeper the ultrasound beam travels into the tissue, the more energy it will lose, and the weaker the reflected and scattered ultrasound signals registered at the transducer will be. Another mechanism leading to attenuation of the ultrasound beam is scattering. Furthermore, waveform distortion by creation of harmonics contributes to attenuation, as energy is transferred into higher frequencies showing higher attenuation. Overall attenuation is

expressed in the "half-power-distance" – that is, the distance at which ultrasound energy is reduced by half when an ultrasound beam travels in a specific medium. As attenuation is frequency-dependent, the "half-power-distance" will decrease with increasing frequency [6,7].

Penetration depth and image resolution

Ideally, we would like to have an ultrasound image that gives us the highest resolution possible, expressed in a high pixel density, on a wide and deeply penetrating imaging sector. Unfortunately, we cannot optimize both parameters simultaneously, as they have a reciprocal relationship:

$$\text{Penetration depth} \Leftrightarrow \text{Image resolution} \qquad (2.6)$$

Penetration depth

Optimal imaging is limited to a depth of penetration of approximately 200 wavelengths, although images can be obtained at greater depths with special equipment. Thus longer wavelengths will penetrate further than shorter wavelengths. For clinical purposes, the result is that the wavelength must be adapted to the

Table 2.2 Wavelength, penetration depth, and image resolution resulting from transducer frequencies in the range 2.5–7.5 MHz, usually selectable with current TEE probes

Transducer frequency	2.5 MHz	5.0 MHz	7.5 MHz
Resulting wavelength (c = 1540 m/s)	0.616 mm	0.308 mm	0.205 mm
Penetration depth (at 200 wavelengths)	12.3 cm	6.2 cm	4.1 cm
Image resolution (2 wavelengths)	1.2 mm	0.6 mm	0.4 mm

distance between the transducer and the object of interest to be imaged. This will be reached by adjusting the image frequency to the examination conditions (remember, $\lambda = c/f$). Table 2.2 shows some examples.

Image resolution

The key parameter for image resolution is the wavelength. Image resolution cannot be greater than one wavelength. This means that the minimal distance between two points has to be at least one wavelength in order for them to be recognized and imaged as two separate points. Objects closer to each other than this will be recognized and imaged as one object only. The determinant for image resolution, wavelength, can be modified by changing the emitted ultrasound frequency (remember, $\lambda = c/f$). Therefore, the higher the ultrasound frequency used, the better the maximal image resolution obtainable (Table 2.2).

Since we are viewing a three-dimensional space with a two-dimensional imaging modality, image resolution is also dependent on the dimension in relation to the ultrasound beam, as well as a number of other technical aspects (Table 2.3, Fig. 2.3). Three types of image resolution have to be considered:

Axial resolution

If two objects are insonated by one ultrasound beam and reflect energy back to the transducer, their distance will be calculated by the ultrasound equipment using the time delay of the returned signals, with the distance being expressed as the number of wavelengths fitting between these objects. Axial resolution is the most precise resolution and is obtained along the length of the ultrasound beam, where the smallest measurable distance equals one wavelength. All quantitative measurements should therefore be made in axial alignment, where the object boundaries are perpendicular to the ultrasound beam (Fig. 2.3).

Lateral resolution

If two objects are hit by neighbouring ultrasound beams, the precision of the measurement is mostly dependent on the beam width. As the beam is narrow close to the transducer and widens with penetration depth, lateral resolution decreases with imaging depth. Close to the transducer and in the area of maximum focus, lateral resolution will be in the range of 2–3 wavelengths and is comparable to the axial resolution. This means that point targets will be imaged as such. At greater depths, ultrasound beams widen and overlap, leading to the effect that several point targets are hit by one beam, therefore being depicted as lines on the image, accounting for the diffuse image in the far field [8]. Measurements using the lateral resolution should be avoided, and, if necessary, should only be taken in the near field or focus region. Lateral resolution can be optimized by placing the focus at the level of interest.

Elevational resolution

Although not obvious on the two-dimensional image screen, the emitted ultrasound beam is always three-dimensional. The tomographic image is a summation

Table 2.3 Adjustable and fixed constructional parameters determining the three types of image resolution

		Axial resolution	Lateral resolution	Elevational resolution
Adjustable parameters	Increase transducer frequency	+	+	(+)
	Optimal focus setting	0	+	+
	Short pulse length	+	0	0
Constructional parameters	Transducer bandwidth	×	×	(×)
	Transducer aperture	0	×	(×)
	Side lobes and grating lobes	0	×	×

+ = improvement; × = determinant; 0 = no influence.

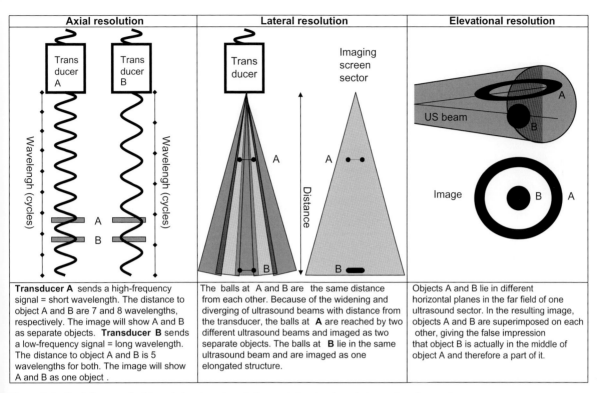

Axial resolution	Lateral resolution	Elevational resolution
Transducer A sends a high-frequency signal = short wavelength. The distance to object A and B are 7 and 8 wavelengths, respectively. The image will show A and B as separate objects. **Transducer B** sends a low-frequency signal = long wavelength. The distance to object A and B is 5 wavelengths for both. The image will show A and B as one object .	The balls at A and B are the same distance from each other. Because of the widening and diverging of ultrasound beams with distance from the transducer, the balls at **A** are reached by two different ultrasound beams and imaged as two separate objects. The balls at **B** lie in the same ultrasound beam and are imaged as one elongated structure.	Objects A and B lie in different horizontal planes in the far field of one ultrasound sector. In the resulting image, objects A and B are superimposed on each other, giving the false impression that object B is actually in the middle of object A and therefore a part of it.

Figure 2.3. The influence of axial resolution, lateral resolution, and elevational resolution on imaging results.

of the entire information contained in a tomographic cut having a slice thickness which ranges between 3 and 10 mm depending on the distance from the transducer, with the slice thickness increasing with distance. This leads to decreased image quality in the far field and is of special significance if signals from strong reflectors at the border of the slice are projected into central structures on the two-dimensional imaging screen.

Ultrasound technology

Piezoelectricity

At the heart of an ultrasound transducer are the piezoelectric crystals. These are made from quartz or ceramic material, being polarized particles and having the property of spatial orientation if an electric voltage is applied across them. If the voltage applied is different to the natural electrical orientation of the particles, their reorientation leads to a change in crystal configuration, measurable as an expansion of the crystal. After discontinuing the voltage, the crystal will return to its natural configuration. If an alternating electrical voltage is applied, the crystals undergo an enduring sequence of configuration change, causing oscillations which are transmitted as mechanical energy in the form of ultrasound waves into the surrounding materials or tissues. Thus the piezoelectric crystals act as a transmitter of ultrasound waves. Conversely, if an ultrasound wave compresses the piezoelectric crystal, its deformation will lead to a configuration change of the crystal resulting in a periodical change of its natural electrical polarization, whereby electrical energy is produced. In this way, the piezoelectric crystal acts as a receiver of ultrasound waves (Fig. 2.4).

The piezoelectric crystal therefore acts as a converter between electrical and mechanical energy and serves both as transmitter and receiver of ultrasound waves. In its practical application, a short electrical impulse will cause a brief oscillation of the piezoelectric crystal, which will generate a brief ultrasound burst. Thereafter, the piezoelectric crystal will be switched to receive mode, and incoming reflected ultrasound waves will be registered by the resulting electrical impulse. The number of cycles contained in a burst determines the pulse length, with a very brief ultrasound burst (i.e. short pulse length) improving axial resolution. Pulse length will decrease with an increase in ultrasound frequency.

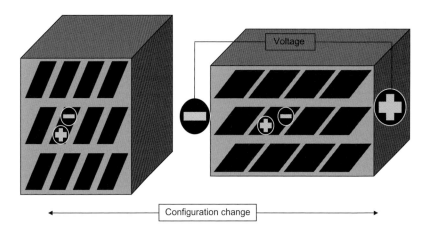

Figure 2.4. A piezoelectric crystal is made of polarized particles. If a voltage is applied, the orientation of the particles towards the voltage will lead to a change in crystal configuration. Similarly, if the crystal is mechanically deformed, this will lead to a polarization change, causing electrical energy to be released.

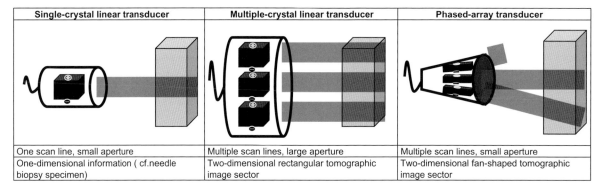

Single-crystal linear transducer	Multiple-crystal linear transducer	Phased-array transducer
One scan line, small aperture	Multiple scan lines, large aperture	Multiple scan lines, small aperture
One-dimensional information (cf.needle biopsy specimen)	Two-dimensional rectangular tomographic image sector	Two-dimensional fan-shaped tomographic image sector

Figure 2.5. With a single-crystal linear transducer, information in space has to be gathered by moving the scan line across the object. With a multiple-crystal linear or phased-array transducer, three-dimensional information is gathered by moving the tomographic plane across the object. For echocardiographic imaging, a small aperture is necessary for the transthoracic as well as the transesophageal approach.

Transducers

In general, transducers are made by putting one or more piezoelectric crystals into a case with damping material, an aperture, and a specially designed acoustic lens. The simplest type of transducer is the linear transducer holding a single piezoelectric crystal. This sends out an ultrasound beam along a single line, and the information contained in the reflected ultrasound signal is comparable to a needle biopsy specimen. Combining multiple piezoelectric crystals into a linear transducer sending out multiple parallel ultrasound beams creates a tomographic imaging plane, but results in a large transducer aperture which will require a large imaging window. Phased-array transducers send out multiple ultrasound beams originating from a central point and diverging in a fan-shaped fashion. This creates a fan-shaped tomographic imaging plane, but allows for a small transducer aperture that requires only a small imaging window [9]. These phased-array sector scanners are routinely used in transthoracic and transesophageal probes (Fig. 2.5).

Ultrasound beam

It is important to consider that the three-dimensional ultrasound beam is not an ideal, linear beam, but has a cylindrical near zone and a cone-shaped far field (Fig. 2.6). As the calculations in Figure 2.6 show, a larger aperture and a small wavelength will decrease beam divergence. Modern transducers work with an adjustable focus. This allows the user to position the narrowest part of the ultrasound beam at the distance from the transducer upon which the investigator wishes to focus. This has the advantage of optimizing lateral and elevational resolution in this area. As a result, image quality will be best in the focus zone and decrease beyond the focal area [9,10].

While the main ultrasound energy travels along the previously described ultrasound beam, fractions

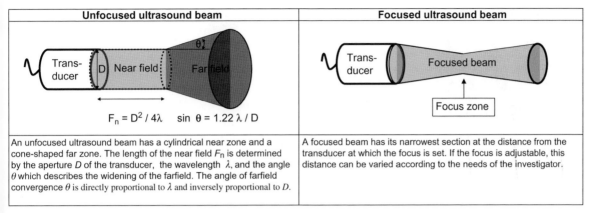

Unfocused ultrasound beam	Focused ultrasound beam
 $$F_n = D^2 / 4\lambda \qquad \sin \theta = 1.22 \, \lambda / D$$	 Focus zone
An unfocused ultrasound beam has a cylindrical near zone and a cone-shaped far zone. The length of the near field F_n is determined by the aperture D of the transducer, the wavelength λ, and the angle θ which describes the widening of the farfield. The angle of farfield convergence θ is directly proportional to λ and inversely proportional to D.	A focused beam has its narrowest section at the distance from the transducer at which the focus is set. If the focus is adjustable, this distance can be varied according to the needs of the investigator.

Figure 2.6. Ultrasound beam geometry of an unfocused and a focused beam.

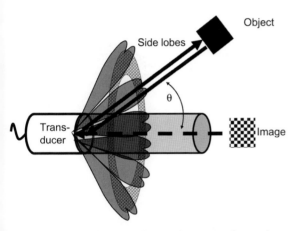

Figure 2.7. Side lobes are ultrasound energy radiating three-dimensionally off the main beam with an angle θ. If the low energy of the side lobe hits an object acting as a specular reflector while no objects are found in the main beam, the reflected energy can be higher than energy reflected from the main beam. As this is not recognized by the equipment, the reflected signal is assumed to be a reflection from the main beam. Therefore the image is malpositioned. This is the basis for double images and side-lobe images.

of ultrasound energy are dispersed laterally from the main beam, with an emission angle θ that can be calculated by $\sin \theta = 1.22 \, \lambda/D$. These three-dimensional ultrasound waves are called side lobes, and can be best compared with the weak halos of light emerging laterally from the main light beam of a car headlight. As the emitted ultrasound energy in a side lobe is low, the potentially reflected ultrasound signal will also be low compared to signal energy reflected from the main beam. As this is true for all beams in an imaging sector, reflections from side-lobe energy usually create an insignificant amount of background noise which can be filtered out.

Of interest is the situation where little signal energy is reflected from the main beam, but the side-lobe energy causes specular reflection from a highly echogenic structure. In this situation, the energy of the reflected signal originating from the side lobe is higher than the energy of signals reflected back from the main beam and is not filtered out. As the equipment has no way to recognize the incoming signal as originating from the side beam, it attributes its origin to the main beam, thereby creating an imaging artifact (Fig. 2.7).

Imaging modes

The same basic principle underlies all echo applications. It is that a short pulse of sound or ultrasound is sent out in a known direction at a known time. If the sound wave hits an object, it is reflected back to the source, which may then be able to detect its reflection. When the reflected signal is received, the time delay between transmitting and receiving is registered. The product of traveling time and sound velocity in the respective medium gives the "to and fro" distance the sound has traveled, half of which is the distance between transmitter/receiver and object. The knowledge of direction and distance allows the location of the object to be calculated, and the energy of the returned signal gives information about the size of the object. This cycle of sending and receiving is repeated in short intervals to update the information frequently.

Amplitude mode (A-mode)

The first application of cardiac ultrasound used a linear single-crystal transducer. Short pulses of ultrasound are sent out along one ultrasound beam. Objects reflect short pulses of ultrasound energy, which are displayed on an oscilloscope screen. The position of the signal spikes on the x-axis of the

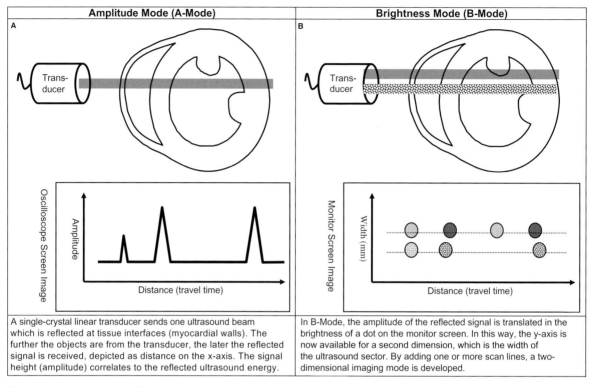

Amplitude Mode (A-Mode)	Brightness Mode (B-Mode)
A single-crystal linear transducer sends one ultrasound beam which is reflected at tissue interfaces (myocardial walls). The further the objects are from the transducer, the later the reflected signal is received, depicted as distance on the x-axis. The signal height (amplitude) correlates to the reflected ultrasound energy.	In B-Mode, the amplitude of the reflected signal is translated in the brightness of a dot on the monitor screen. In this way, the y-axis is now available for a second dimension, which is the width of the ultrasound sector. By adding one or more scan lines, a two-dimensional imaging mode is developed.

Figure 2.8. The development from amplitude mode (A-mode) as a one-dimensional imaging process to brightness mode (B-mode), allowing two-dimensional imaging.

display marks the distance of objects from the transducer and each other, while the height or amplitude of the spikes gives information about the energy of the returning ultrasound signal. Repeated and rapid cycles of transmission and receiving show a moving structure as a spike moving along the x-axis of the oscilloscope screen [11]. A-mode allows for high temporal resolution of information collected on a single beam, comparable to a needle biopsy (Fig. 2.8A).

Brightness mode (B-mode)

In order to use transducers which send out multiple scan lines, the mode in which the information is displayed was adapted. This development is known as the B-mode, where the amplitude of the reflected signal is no longer coded by the height of the signal spike. Instead, the reflected signal is imaged as a spot on the screen, the brightness of which resembles the amount of reflected ultrasound energy, using various shades on a gray scale. Therefore, the brighter a spot marked on the screen, the more ultrasound energy has been reflected to the transducer from the respective tissue interface (Fig. 2.8B).

Two-dimensional (2D) echocardiography

In order to create a tomographic two-dimensional image, a sector scanner in B-mode electronically sweeps across a plane, sending out and receiving ultrasound beams in a fan-shaped fashion [12] (Fig. 2.9). All of the information received from the reflected ultrasound signals is translated to gray-scale pixels and imaged on the screen (Fig. 2.10). As the cycle length to collect the information along one ultrasound beam is constant for a given imaging depth, the time to collect all the information for one tomographic image is proportional to the number of scan lines used. The more scan lines are used, the wider the imaging sector will be, but the longer it will take to generate one image, and the less often this image can be updated. On the other hand, if fewer scan lines are used, image generation will take less time, allowing the image to be updated much more often. Again, we find a reciprocal relationship:

temporal resolution ⇔ spatial image resolution (2.7)

For example, with a imaging depth r of 20 cm and a imaging sector width using 128 scan lines, image

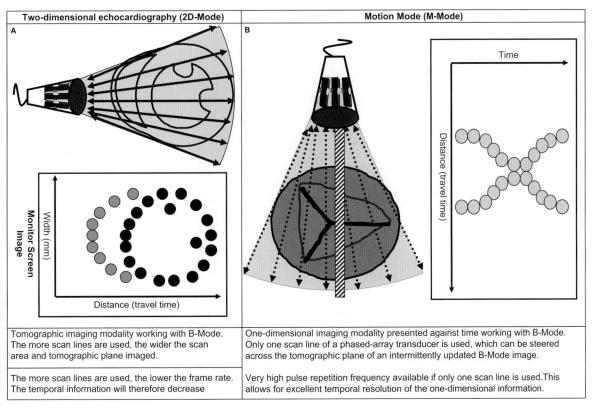

Two-dimensional echocardiography (2D-Mode)	Motion Mode (M-Mode)
Tomographic imaging modality working with B-Mode. The more scan lines are used, the wider the scan area and tomographic plane imaged.	One-dimensional imaging modality presented against time working with B-Mode. Only one scan line of a phased-array transducer is used, which can be steered across the tomographic plane of an intermittently updated B-Mode image.
The more scan lines are used, the lower the frame rate. The temporal information will therefore decrease	Very high pulse repetition frequency available if only one scan line is used. This allows for excellent temporal resolution of the one-dimensional information.

Figure 2.9. 2D-mode and M-mode are both B-mode imaging processes but focus on two contrary qualities: while 2D-mode (A) offers high spatial resolution, M-mode (B) allows high temporal resolution.

acquisition will need about 33 ms, thus allowing a frame rate of 30 images per second. Frame rate could be doubled either by decreasing imaging depth to $r = 10$ cm or by narrowing the imaging sector width to 64 scan lines. A combination of both would quadruple the temporal resolution.

Motion mode (M-mode)

The above-mentioned method to improve temporal resolution will often be insufficient to allow adequate description of really fast and complex moving structures, for example heart valves. In this case, it is possible to switch to only one scan line in the transducer array, along which cycles of transmission and receiving will now follow each other with a high repetition frequency (up to 2000 times per second). On the image screen, the B-mode information of the single scan line will be plotted on the y-axis against time on the x-axis. This M-mode is ideal for imaging rapid cardiac motion. In order to allow orientation, a small 2D-image showing the position of the selected single M-mode scan line is displayed simultaneously with a low frame rate (Figs. 2.9, 2.11, 2.12).

Tissue harmonic imaging (THI)

Waveform distortion in tissues creates multiples of the fundamental frequency sent out by a transducer, as described earlier. THI sends out the first harmonic (for example a fundamental frequency of 1.8 MHz), but uses the detection of the second harmonic (3.6 MHz) in the reflected ultrasound beam to create the image. This is indicated in the display. Although the second harmonic signal is a weaker signal than the fundamental signal, it is virtually devoid of artifacts, as clutter, side lobes, scattering, and reverberation are generated at the first harmonic. Devoid of acoustic noise, THI generates better contrast enhancement and border delineation. As the beam width narrows with higher frequency, THI displays better lateral resolution. However, this is at the cost of decreased penetration, because of the higher frequency [13]. THI, initially used in transthoracic echocardiography, is now also available with transesophageal echo probes.

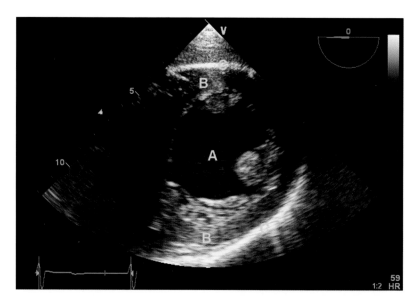

Figure 2.10. 2D echocardiographic image showing a transgastric mid-papillary short-axis view of the left ventricle. Dark zones mark areas from which minimal or no ultrasound energy is reflected, for example the ventricular cavities (A). From the myocardium itself, low signal intensity is reflected mainly by scattering (B). Bright pixels mark tissue interfaces from which high ultrasound energy is reflected, for example from the pericardium acting as a specular reflector (C).

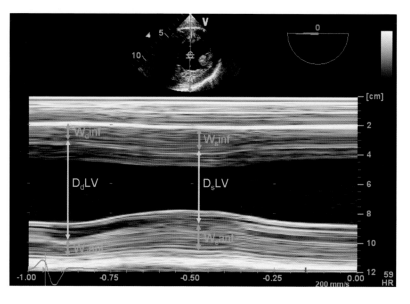

Figure 2.11. Representation of 2D-mode (above) and M-mode (below) of a transgastric short-cut view of the left ventricle. The cursor line in the 2D-mode image shows the position of the M-mode scan line running from the transducer cutting through the inferior wall (I), the cavity (C), and the anterior wall (A), helping orientation. In the M-mode image, the changes in wall thickness and cavity diameters over time during systole and diastole are presented. $W_d$inf, diastolic wall thickness of inferior wall; $W_s$inf, systolic wall thickness of inferior wall; $W_d$ant, diastolic wall thickness of anterior wall; $W_s$ant, systolic wall thickness of anterior wall; D_dLV, diastolic left ventricular diameter; D_sLV, systolic left ventricular diameter.

Three-dimensional (3D) echocardiography

Conventional two-dimensional (2D) echocardiography creates tomographic images of three-dimensional tissues and organs, and it relies upon the echocardiographer to create a mental 3D image of the structure examined from a series of 2D images. This requires sound anatomical knowledge and considerable experience, and the result will differ between individuals. Furthermore, the measurement of volumes relies on complex formulae of varying precision. Three-dimensional echocardiography may solve many of these problems.

Initial systems acquire a large series of 2D images in order to reconstruct 3D images. For image acquisition, the 2D imaging sector has to be automatically rotated or swept through the anatomical structure in small steps. With a steadily positioned transducer, this is relatively easy to accomplish with static structures. In echocardiography, it requires that 2D image acquisition is electrocardiographically triggered. Other motion effects are eliminated, for example translation as a result of respiratory movement. Since the collection of the volume information takes at least as many heartbeats as the number of 2D slices selected for 3D

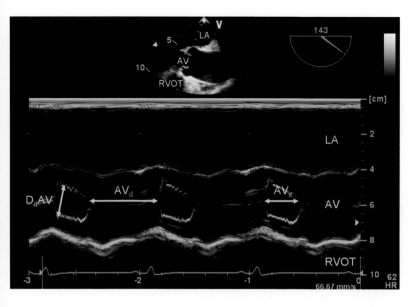

Figure 2.12. Representation of 2D-mode (above) and M-mode (below) of a mid-esophageal long-axis cut through the aortic valve. The cursor line in the 2D-mode image shows the position of the M-mode scan line running from the transducer cutting through the left atrium (LA), the aortic valve (AV), and the right ventricular outflow tract (RVOT), helping orientation. In the M-mode image, the opening and closing of the aortic valve leaflets during systole and diastole are presented. AV_d, aortic valve closing time in diastole; AV_s, aortic valve opening time in systole; D_sAV, systolic separation distance of aortic valve leaflets.

generation, acquisition of the necessary 2D planes takes in the order of minutes. Using a large amount of computing capacity, all the information of the individual 2D images is transformed into points in a three-dimensional volume. Although comprised within one 3D image, the single pieces of information are drawn not from one, but from many heart cycles, making these reconstructed images prone to artifacts. Furthermore, dynamic processes extending beyond one heart cycle cannot be captured. Image resolution and temporal resolution are in principle dependent on the single 2D images, but suffer from motion artifacts.

The result displayed is a freely movable 3D image which can be cut along virtual planes, a process known as rendering. Multiple planes can be displayed at once in addition to a 3D axis display allowing orientation (multiplanar reformatting). Alternative display modes are surface rendering, where the contour of a surface, for example a fetal face in obstetric ultrasound, is automatically displayed, or volume rendering, showing projection images of 3D volumes.

4D echocardiography – real-time 3D echocardiography

The recent major development of 3D echocardiography is based on the technological advance in miniaturization and transducer design consequent on the creation of the volumetric 2D array transducers. Instead of sweeping a beam across a scan plane, the surface of one single large crystal is cut into several thousand squares, each functioning as a single element in emitting and receiving sound [14]. Therefore thousands of ultrasound beams simultaneously penetrate into and are reflected from a volume of tissue, the size of it depending on scan-line density and frame rate. The initial frame rate was around 20 volumes per second, but this is increasing with new developments. Live moving 3D displays are now possible with this technique, which has accordingly been named 4D echocardiography or real-time 3D echocardiography.

For real-time 3D echocardiography, current systems are able to provide a so-called reduced volume comprising a sector volume of about 30° × 60° with some ability to provide 3D information of color-flow Doppler. Also available in real time is a pyramidal 30° × 30° zoom volume for high resolution. For a full volume of about 90° × 90°, four consecutive reduced volumes are combined into one image, the quality of which is thus dependent on artifacts through motion and rhythm changes, and color-flow mapping is not routinely possible. As every alternate heartbeat is imaged, the full volume acquisition takes around eight cardiac cycles to acquire [15]. As described earlier, spatial and temporal resolution depend mainly on transducer technique and processing power, but are at the moment far lower than with 2D systems. However, with new systems under development offering full volume acquisition in one beat, the challenge of improving time and spatial resolution of 4D echocardiography, including 3D color-flow Doppler, may be met [16].

Instrumentation controls and settings

When converting a received ultrasound signal into a gray-scale pixel on the imaging screen, the signal undergoes a process of multiple and complex transformations, called pre- and post-processing. In principle, each of these steps can be adjusted to influence the image result. As this requires a full understanding of a complex and detailed process, selectable presets with defined processing settings are usually available for the respective imaging requirements and modality. Nevertheless, the user needs to be familiar with the following important controls, which have to be optimized repeatedly during each study in order to achieve optimal results:

- **Imaging depth and sector width**. Allow just enough imaging depth and sector width to fit the structure of interest on the screen. Increasing imaging depth and/or sector width helps orientation, but decreases pulse repetition frequency and frame rate, thereby decreasing temporal resolution.
- **Ultrasound frequency**. Adjust the ultrasound frequency to the required imaging depth. Remember that low ultrasound frequency improves penetration but resolution decreases.
- **Gain**. This control regulates the amplitude of the displayed signals on the screen. The more gain is selected, the brighter the points will appear on the screen. Too low gain settings will hide information, as will gain settings that are too high. Optimal settings should display areas without significant ultrasound reflection (e.g. blood-filled spaces) as nearly black. Time gain and lateral gain settings allow gain adjustments in selected areas on the imaging screen.
- **Gray scale or contrast**. the different returning signal amplitudes generate a multitude of shades of gray from dark to bright. While theoretically the widest range of the gray scale will present the most detailed information, the human eye is usually not able to detect such subtle differences. According to user preference this graduation between dark and light areas can be adjusted such that greater differences are easier to detect.
- **Focus**. Remember that the ultrasound beam is three-dimensional, and that optimal resolution can only be achieved at the focus level.
- **Power output**. Higher ultrasound output will result in more energy in the reflected signal, but will also increase noise.

Doppler echocardiography

Doppler principle

If a source of sound moves towards the listener, the sound frequency increases. If a source of sound moves away from the listener, the sound frequency decreases. This phenomenon, which we encounter daily for example in traffic, where the engine sound of an approaching vehicle increases its pitch and decreases again when moving away (Fig. 2.13), was mathematically described in 1842 by Christian Doppler, an Austrian physicist. This so-called Doppler principle also applies to the reflection of sound. If sound is reflected by moving objects, the frequency of the reflected sound is changed. The difference between the emitted frequency and the received frequency is described by the term *Doppler shift*:

$$\text{Doppler shift } (f_d) = \text{received frequency } (f_r) - \text{transmitted frequency } (f_0). \quad (2.8)$$

With the object moving towards the transducer, the frequency is increasing (positive Doppler shift), while with the object moving away from the transducer, the frequency is decreasing (negative Doppler shift) (Fig. 2.14). In echocardiography, Doppler shift is caused by the velocity of blood cells as well as myocardium and heart valves. As Doppler echocardiography normally focuses on the reflection of the ultrasound signal by fast-moving blood cells, low-pass filters

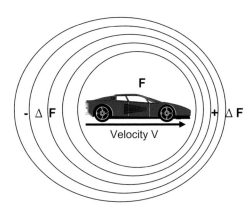

Figure 2.13. Doppler effect: the car is emitting sound with the frequency *f* while moving with the velocity *V* in the direction of the arrow. In the direction of motion, the sequence of sound waves will be compressed, resulting in a higher sound frequency (sound pitch) perceived by any listener the car is approaching. Against the direction of motion, the sequence of sound waves will be rarefied, resulting in a lower sound frequency perceived by any listener from whom the car is moving away.

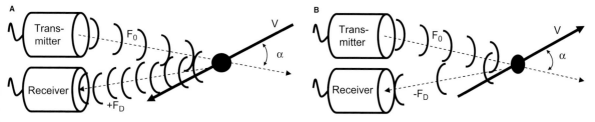

Figure 2.14. If sound is reflected by an object moving towards the sound source (A), the emitted frequency f_0 is increased depending on the velocity V and the insonation angle a. This is called a positive Doppler shift $(+f_D)$. If the object is moving away from the sound source (B), the resulting Doppler shift will be negative $(-f_D)$.

Table 2.4. Intercept angles and resulting measurement errors in blood flow velocity. According to the Doppler equation , the measured Doppler shift is directly proportional to the cosine of the intercept angle a. Therefore any deviation from absolute parallel alignment between blood flow direction and ultrasound beam direction will lead to a smaller Doppler shift recorded and an underestimation of the velocity causing the Doppler shift. Intercept angles above 20° cannot be tolerated, as they will lead to a measurement error greater than 6%

Angle a	0°	10°	20°	30°	45°	60°	90°
Cosine a	1	0.98	0.94	0.87	0.71	0.5	0
Error in V	0	−2%	−6%	−13%	−29%	−50%	No results

are used to remove the low-velocity Doppler shift signals from myocardium and valves [17].

Doppler equation

If a transmitted frequency is changed by the Doppler effect, the resulting frequency change is dependent on the flow direction, flow velocity and flow characteristics. This is expressed in the Doppler equation:

$$f_d = 2 \times f_0 \times V \times \cos \alpha / c \qquad (2.9)$$

where

f_d = Doppler shift (Hz)
f_0 = transmitted sound frequency (Hz)
V = blood flow velocity (m/s)
$\cos \alpha$ = cosine of the angle between blood flow direction and ultrasound beam
c = velocity of sound (1540 m/s)

From the Doppler equation, we can see that the Doppler shift is directly proportional to:

- transmitted sound frequency
- velocity of blood
- intercept angle

For practical application in Doppler echocardiography, the emitted frequency is known and the velocity of sound is constant at 1540 m/s. Therefore, the velocity causing the Doppler shift can be calculated by:

$$V = f_d \times c/2 \times f_0 \times \cos \alpha \qquad (2.10)$$

Intercept angle and Doppler shift

When the ultrasound equipment calculates the velocity using the above-mentioned Doppler equation, it assumes that optimal measurement conditions have been achieved and that the intercept angle α was 0, for which the cos α is 1. If this is not the case, the measured velocity will always be underestimated, as cos α decreases below 1 and will be 0 at an angle α of 90° (Table 2.4). Therefore, the intercept angle between blood flow and ultrasound beam should be as parallel as possible. It is important to remember that we see a 2D image, but are measuring a 3D flow. Because of this, the angle correction feature available with some equipment can only be recommended for vascular ultrasound, not if blood flow in the heart is to be measured. An intercept angle up to 20° may be tolerated, as the cos α of 20° is 0.94 and the resulting error will not be more than 6% of the actual velocity.

Analysis and display of Doppler signals

The received primary signal is a complex mixture of the transmitted frequency and multiple overlying Doppler shifts. It is broken down into individual frequencies by fast Fourier transformation. Frequencies of Doppler shifts in the heart are below 20 kHz and are therefore audible. The Doppler signal comprises a spectrum of frequencies with varying intensities. The graphic display of the spectral analysis shows velocities recorded against time. The signal intensity

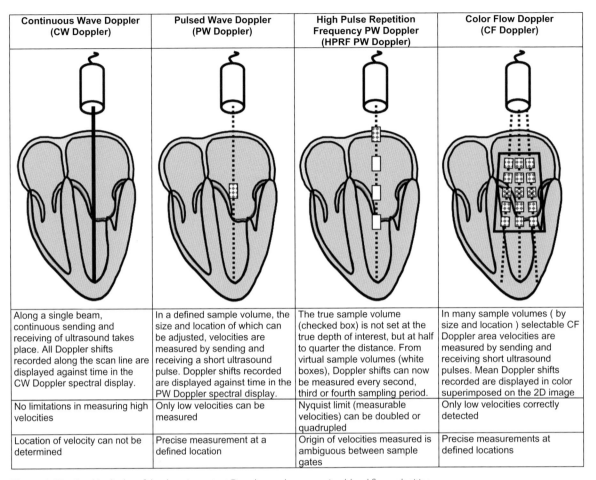

Continuous Wave Doppler (CW Doppler)	Pulsed Wave Doppler (PW Doppler)	High Pulse Repetition Frequency PW Doppler (HPRF PW Doppler)	Color Flow Doppler (CF Doppler)
Along a single beam, continuous sending and receiving of ultrasound takes place. All Doppler shifts recorded along the scan line are displayed against time in the CW Doppler spectral display.	In a defined sample volume, the size and location of which can be adjusted, velocities are measured by sending and receiving a short ultrasound pulse. Doppler shifts recorded are displayed against time in the PW Doppler spectral display.	The true sample volume (checked box) is not set at the true depth of interest, but at half to quarter the distance. From virtual sample volumes (white boxes), Doppler shifts can now be measured every second, third or fourth sampling period.	In many sample volumes (by size and location) selectable CF Doppler area velocities are measured by sending and receiving short ultrasound pulses. Mean Doppler shifts recorded are displayed in color superimposed on the 2D image
No limitations in measuring high velocities	Only low velocities can be measured	Nyquist limit (measurable velocities) can be doubled or quadrupled	Only low velocities correctly detected
Location of velocity can not be determined	Precise measurement at a defined location	Origin of velocities measured is ambiguous between sample gates	Precise measurements at defined locations

Figure 2.15. Graphic display of the three important Doppler modes measuring blood flow velocities.

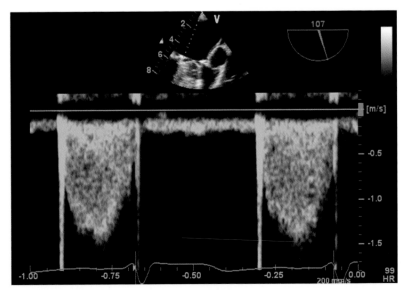

Figure 2.16. Continuous-wave Doppler recording of blood flow across a mechanical mitral valve prosthesis. The characteristic CWD spectrum consists of filled-in diastolic flow curves, as many different velocities are recorded along the scan line at each moment in time. This is because blood flow is accelerating from the left atrium towards the valve orifice and decelerating after it reaches the left ventricle. The maximal velocity is achieved at the narrowest section, which is assumed to be the orifice of the prosthetic mitral valve.

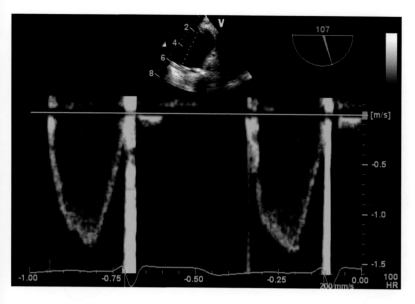

Figure 2.17. Pulsed-wave Doppler recording of blood flow across a mechanical mitral valve prosthesis (similar to Fig. 2.16). The characteristic PWD spectrum consists of clearly framed diastolic flow curves, since with a homogenous flow profile only very similar velocities are recorded in the sample volume at each moment in time.

is coded through the brightness of the spectral display. In the acoustic display, the sound frequency codes velocity, and the volume codes signal intensity.

Continuous-wave Doppler (CWD)

Two separate crystals in one transducer are used to transmit and receive ultrasound continuously and independently along a single ultrasound beam (Fig. 2.15). All velocities causing Doppler shifts along this scan line are measured, with the result being displayed as a characteristic filled-in spectrum (Fig. 2.16), as many different velocities are measured along the scan line at one time. The origin of an individual velocity cannot be located. This is called range ambiguity.

- Advantage: very high velocities (Doppler shifts) can be measured accurately.
- Disadvantage: the origin of the velocity along the scan line cannot be located, as no time delay is measured.

Pulsed-wave Doppler (PWD)

One crystal in a transducer sends a short ultrasound burst and acts intermittently as transmitter and receiver. Only Doppler shifts caused by velocities within a defined sample volume are measured. The result is a characteristic framed spectrum if laminar flow is measured, as all velocities are within a narrow range at a given time (Fig. 2.17). This allows precise location and timing of blood flow with a low velocity. The length of one measuring cycle depends on the distance

of the sample volume from the transducer, as the equipment needs to wait for the returning reflected signal. This will limit the pulse repetition frequency with increasing depth of interest [18].

- Advantage: velocity can be measured at a precise location (depth of interest, sample volume of choice).
- Disadvantage: the maximal measurable velocity (V_{max}) is limited by the pulse repetition frequency (Nyquist limit, at 10 cm depth the correct measurable V_{max} is approximately 1.5 m/s).

In order to partially overcome the limitation of a low pulse repetition frequency with PWD, high pulse repetition frequency PWD (HPRF-PWD) can be used. Instead of setting the sample volume at the depth of interest, it is set at half, third, or quarter of this distance. Doppler-shift signals from the actual depth of interest will now reach the transducer every second, third, or fourth listening period, thereby doubling, tripling, or quadrupling the Nyquist limit. As this method induces range ambiguity into PWD, it can only be used if the investigator can be certain that no significant Doppler shifts are caused by velocities in the position of the real or other virtual sample volumes except the one of interest.

Color-flow Doppler (CFD)

The working principle of the PWD is used, but now with many sample volumes next to each other in a sector freely adjustable by size and position. Increased

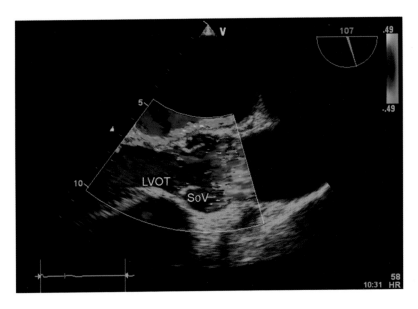

Figure 2.18. Color-flow Doppler recording of blood flow across the left ventricular outflow tract (LVOT) and an insufficient mitral valve in systole using the mid-esophageal long-axis view. The LVOT is covered with homogeneous red color indicating laminar flow towards the transducer. A bright green jet starts at the level of the closed mitral valve and reaches into the left atrium, indicating turbulent and fast flow towards the transducer caused by blood accelerated by the pressure difference between left ventricle and left atrium causing turbulent flow in the left atrium. Note that a little turbulence is indicated by some color changes in the sinus of Valsalva (SoV) area.

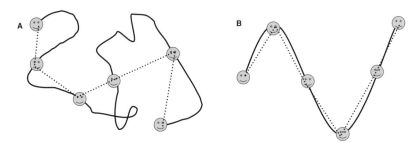

Figure 2.19. (A) If a fast and irregularly moving object (such as a flying butterfly) is imaged at a few time points (smiling faces), the path actually taken (solid line) cannot be determined. From the registered waypoints the dotted line seems to be the traveled path, which in reality, besides the waypoints, has nothing in common with the actual path. The periodic observation of an irregular motion gives no realistic impression of the motion itself. (B) If a slow periodic motion is imaged at certain time points, the path actually taken (solid line) and the assumed path connecting the waypoints (dotted line) are very similar. The frequent periodic observation of a periodic motion allows a realistic impression of the motion itself.

distance of the furthest sample volume from the transducer, as well as a wide color-flow sector will result in prolonging the time needed to collect and calculate all data in the sample volume. Therefore the frame rate is low and extremely dependent on the size and position of the color sector selected, which should always be chosen as small as possible. To display the velocities in each sample volume simultaneously and continuously, the spectral display used for the PWD is not practical. Instead, flow direction and velocity is now displayed using a color scale, with the velocity indicated being the mean velocity measured in the sample volume. Red is used if flow towards the transducer is measured, with dark shades of red showing low velocities, bright shades of red showing high velocities. Blue

indicates flow away from the transducer, and again dark shades show low velocities, while bright shades indicate high velocities. A homogeneous color spectrum is seen with laminar flow. If flow velocities in neighboring sample volumes differ significantly, yellow or green colors are added to the red or blue color spectrum. This is usually an indicator for non-laminar, turbulent flow. As flow direction changes rapidly with turbulence, this will lead to markedly different intercept angles between blood flow direction and ultrasound beam for neighboring sample volumes. Therefore, markedly different Doppler shifts will be measured, resulting in markedly different mean velocities calculated. The CFD sector is displayed overlying the 2D echocardiographic image on the screen, thereby allowing the attribution of the measured flow velocity to the respective anatomic area in the heart (Fig. 2.18).

- Advantage: flow velocity and flow direction is displayed in relation to the anatomy on the 2D display.
- Disadvantage: low image update frequency (low frame rate).

Aliasing phenomenon

In order to describe a movement precisely, we would normally watch the moving object continuously. In echocardiography, objects are imaged by sending out short ultrasound pulses and registering their reflection. This is comparable to watching a moving structure in complete darkness with a stroboscope light. With each flash of light, we would see the object at a different position, and from the change in position, we would infer the underlying movement. If the underlying movement and speed is irregular, we would not be able to describe the actual path taken, but only describe waypoints during this movement. If the underlying movement is periodic and the speed is constant, we would be able to describe the movement correctly despite the fact that we only see the object assuming different positions at different times, as long as we have enough flashes of light showing multiple positions of the object during one cycle (Fig. 2.19). For our echocardiographic imaging system, the number of flashes in unit time translates into the pulse repetition frequency.

For PWD and CFD, the pulse repetition frequency is limited and is dependent on the depth of the sample volume in PWD as well as on the number of sample lines selected. Figure 2.20 illustrates what happens if the pulse repetition frequency is reduced. A slight reduction (Fig. 2.20A,B) will show fewer positions during the cycle, but will still describe the movement correctly. If the pulse repetition frequency is reduced to twice the frequency of the cycling motion, the frequency of the cycle is still correctly described, but we lose the knowledge about the direction of the movement (Fig. 2.20C). The maximal frequency which can be described correctly with a given pulse repetition frequency is called the Nyquist limit, which can be calculated as:

Nyquist Limit = Pulse Repetition Frequency / 2 (2.11)

Lowering the pulse repetition frequency further suddenly gives the impression that the cyclic movement is running backwards at a much lower frequency (Fig. 2.20D). This is called signal aliasing. In Doppler echocardiography, aliasing occurs if the frequency of the Doppler shift is higher than half of the pulse repetition frequency. In PWD, aliasing will be depicted as cutoff PWD envelopes which are continued upside-down on the opposite side of the base line. For CFD, aliasing signals are shown with an inverted color coding [19].

Imaging artifacts and pitfalls

Imaging artifacts occur with all imaging modalities (2D, M, Doppler). The most frequent causes of artifacts are:

- ultrasound physics (and insufficient consideration of its laws)
- inappropriate instrument settings
- inappropriate alignment of the ultrasound beam with regard to the structure being investigated
- inappropriate equipment (sector defects of transducers, transducers of wrong frequency)

2D-echo imaging artifacts

Echo imaging artifacts can be grouped into three major categories:

- failure to visualize structures that are present
- extraneous ultrasound signals mimicking structures that are not actually present, at least not in the imaged plane
- image of a structure that differs in size and/or shape from its actual appearance

Suboptimal image quality

The main reason for suboptimal image quality is an insufficient echocardiographic window. This may be caused simply by transducer malposition, but may also be due to individual biological circumstances such as interposition of adipose tissue, lung, bone, or gastric contents between transducer and cardiac structures, or insufficient filling of cardiac chambers. Technical reasons include inadequate penetration due to the use of high ultrasound frequencies, incorrect gain settings (either time or lateral gain controls), and maladjusted settings of imaging modes, contrast, and post-processing modes.

Motions across the imaging plane

The heart shows a twisting motion in the pericardium during the cardiac cycle. In addition, with respiration

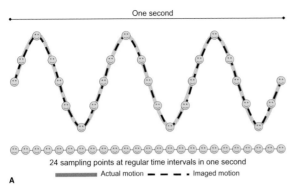

One second

24 sampling points at regular time intervals in one second

━━━ Actual motion ━ ━ ━ Imaged motion

A

Figure 2.20. (A). A ball bouncing up and down at a constant speed is imaged at 24 time points in one second. The position is recorded against time on the *x*-axis in the graph. The solid gray line shows the actual path, the yellow dots the position of the ball at the time of imaging. The dotted line shows the impression of the movement the viewer gets from the individual positions watched over time. If the sampling frequency is much higher (24/s) than the cycling frequency (3/s), the movement is correctly recognized.

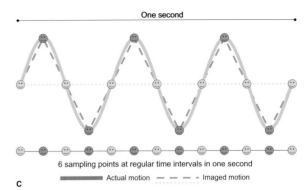

One second

6 sampling points at regular time intervals in one second

━━━ Actual motion ━ ━ ━ Imaged motion

C

Figure 2.20. (C). Now only six time points in one second are available to image the ball, which means that the imaging frequency is exactly twice the cycle frequency. If the yellow time points are used to look at the ball, it is always seen in the same position, and no motion is recognized. At the green time points, it is seen either at the upper or at the lower turn-around point. The actual movement can only be approximated. This marks the point where the motion frequency equals the Nyquist limit of the sampling rate (Nyquist limit = sampling rate / 2).

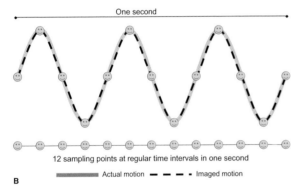

One second

12 sampling points at regular time intervals in one second

━━━ Actual motion ━ ━ ━ Imaged motion

B

Figure 2.20. (B). the bouncing ball is now imaged at 12 time points in one second. Although the sampling frequency is reduced, the movement is still correctly recognized.

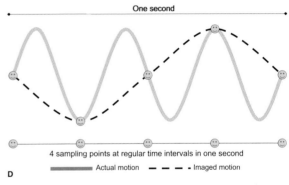

One second

4 sampling points at regular time intervals in one second

━━━ Actual motion ━ ━ ━ Imaged motion

D

Figure 2.20. (D). With the imaging frequency dropped to four per second, it seems that the ball is now bouncing again, but with a much slower frequency (1cycle per second) and in the inverse direction, as it bounces down first and then up. The motion frequency (3 per second) is higher than the Nyquist limit (sampling rate/2 = 2/s).

the heart is dislocated laterally. Both effects cause the heart to move across or in and out of the imaging plane during the cardiac cycle. The echocardiographer needs to minimize or eliminate this effect by optimal selection of the imaging plane, or at least to recognize it.

Acoustic shadowing

At tissue boundaries or structures with significant differences in acoustic impedance, total reflection of the ultrasound beam may occur. This may be due, for example, to bone or tissue calcification, air, prosthetic valves, cannulas, or tubes. Ultrasound may not travel through and hence beyond these structures, and this causes a fan-shaped shadow devoid of reflected signals following the direction of the scan line. Structures close to the transducer will cast large shadows, peripheral structures small shadows.

Reverberations

Reverberations are linear high-amplitude echo signals originating from two strong specular (mirror) reflectors, extending in the far field along the scan lines. Ultrasound is reflected back and forth between reflectors before it travels back to the transducer. The resulting increased time delay mimics structures distal to the reflectors extending into the far field. Prominent reverberations can obliterate information from structures in the far field. This is also called "comet tail" artifact.

Beam-width artifact

As the ultrasound beam widens with increasing imaging depth, lateral resolution decreases with depth. Point targets distant to the transducer appear as lines, and two close neighboring points appear as one line. In addition, the 3D volume of the ultrasound beam is displayed in a single tomographic plane. While the "slice" thickness is small near the transducer, it increases in the far field with penetration depth. Structures in different spatial planes are superimposed in one imaging plane.

Side-lobe artifact

Strong specular (mirror) reflectors such as calcifications or prosthetic material produce echo signals if they are hit by the side lobes of neighboring ultrasound beams. Side-lobe echoes are depicted lateral to the object at the same distance from the transducer, resulting in arched lines extending laterally beyond the object in equidistance to the transducer.

Refraction artifact

The ultrasound beam is deviated from its straight path (the scan line) by refraction in tissue between transducer and object. The equipment assumes that the reflected beam has originated from the transmitted scan line, and the object is displayed on the image in the wrong location, often as a double image next to the correctly displayed object.

Range-ambiguity artifact: mirror-image artifact

In good imaging conditions, with a good window and little interposition of other tissue, minimal attenuation of the ultrasound signal takes place. Therefore, a strong, specular reflector in the near field sends large amounts of reflected ultrasound energy back to the transducer, a part of which is reflected at the transducer or at a second specular reflector close to the transducer. With a depth setting at least twice that distance (resulting in a long listening period), ultrasound travels twice to this reflector, but the equipment assumes reflection has originated from twice as far. The result is a mirror image at double distance from the transducer [20].

Range-ambiguity artifact: doubled-image artifact

With a low depth setting and little attenuation, a part of the ultrasound energy travels beyond the depth setting (beyond the extend of the listening period). If deeper structures act as strong reflectors, ultrasound reflections from an earlier impulse will reach the transducer during the next sampling (listening) cycle. The equipment assumes that the signal has originated from a reflector closer to the transducer within depth range, and the image from the deeper structure is displayed overlying other structures close to the transducer.

Doppler imaging artifacts

Similar to 2D imaging artifacts, Doppler imaging artifacts can be grouped into three major categories:

- failure to visualize flow velocity and flow direction that is present
- extraneous ultrasound signals that mimic flow velocities and directions that are not present, at least not in the imaged plane
- measurements of flow velocities and directions that differ from their absolute values

Intercept-angle artifact

A non-parallel angle between blood flow and ultrasound beam leads to underestimation of the flow velocity. Applying the formula $V = f_d \times c/2 \times f_0 \times \cos \alpha$, the equipment assumes that $\cos \alpha$ is 1 (Table 2.4).

Signal-aliasing artifact

If the actual velocity exceeds the adjusted Nyquist limit (maximal measurable velocity) in PWD or CFD, the signal is displayed with inverted +/– signs:

- with PWD the spectral display is upside down or wrapped around
- with CFD the colors are inverted or show multiple changes

Practical points to prevent aliasing artifacts are to attain maximum pulse repetition frequency by decreasing the measuring depth with PWD, paying attention to the sector area of CFD, and to use the baseline shift to double the maximal Nyquist limit.

Range-ambiguity artifact

If the PWD sample volume is close to the transducer, and little attenuation takes place, for example in a blood-filled cavity, strong signals from double or triple the distance may be recorded in the next receiver phase and misinterpreted as originating from the sample volume depth. This is constructively used in

HPRF-PWD and always present in CWD. Another form of range-ambiguity artifact arises from flow signals from two adjacent structures that are superimposed in one Doppler signal due to the 3D volume of the ultrasound beam. Examples are LV outflow and inflow signals in one recording, or situations where the flow signal from an adjacent structure is projected into another structure without flow. This artifact is more pronounced with increased sample volume depth and also appears as a side-lobe artifact.

Mirror-image artifact

This may appear with spectral Doppler if strong signals are recorded from a low sample volume depth. A symmetric signal of somewhat less intensity is recorded in the opposite direction of the actual flow signal (i.e. an upside-down mirror image). This artifact can be reduced or eliminated by using less gain or power output at the instrument.

Shadowing artifact

Structures that are strong reflectors may cause total ultrasound reflection, with no signals penetrating to and reflecting from beyond these structures. No velocities and flow directions can be measured in the area of the ultrasound shadow.

Ghosting artifact

Brief large color patterns overlying anatomic structures with no underlying flow patterns, appearing inconsistent from beat to beat and mostly monochromatic (blue or red), caused by strong moving reflectors.

Gain-settings artifact

This is very important with the use of color-flow Doppler. Excessively high gain settings cause random background noise, whereas gain settings that are too low result in smaller flow areas than are actually present being displayed.

Electronic interference artifact

These artifacts in the 2D and Doppler modes result from other electric instruments with inadequate shielding, for example electric cauterizing and continuous cardiac output devices.

References

1. Ludwig GD. The velocity of sound through tissues and the acoustic impedance of tissues. *J Acoust Soc Am* 1950; **22**: 862–6.

2. Goldman DE, Hueter TF. Tabular data of the velocity and absorption of high-frequency sound in mammalian tissues. *J Acoust Soc Am* 1956; **28**: 35–40.

3. Goss SA, Johnston RL, Dunn F. Comprehensive compilation of empirical ultrasonic properties of mammalian tissues. *J Acoust Soc Am* 1978; **64**: 423–57.

4. Gregg EC, Palagallo GL. Acoustic impedance of tissue. *Invest Radiol* 1969; **4**: 357–63.

5. Duck FA. Nonlinear acoustics in diagnostic ultrasound. *Ultrasound Med Biol* 2002; **28**: 1–18.

6. Fry WJ. Mechanism of the acoustic absorption in tissue. *J Acoust Soc Am* 1952; **24**: 412–15.

7. Goss SA, Frizzell LA, Dunn F. Ultrasonic absorption and attenuation in mammalian tissues. *Ultrasound Med Biol* 1979; **5**: 181–6.

8. Roelandt J, van Dorp WG, Bom N, Laird JD, Hugenholtz PG. Resolution problems in echocardiography: a source of interpretation errors. *Am J Cardiol* 1976; **37**: 256–62.

9. Shung KK. The principle of multidimensional arrays. *Eur J Echocardiogr* 2002; **3**: 149–53.

10. Vogel L, Bom N, Ridder J, Lancée C. Transducer design considerations in dynamic focusing. *Ultrasound Med Biol* 1979; **5**: 187–93.

11. Hertz CH. Ultrasonic engineering in heart diagnosis. *Am J Cardiol* 1967; **19**: 6–16.

12. Griffith JM, Henry WL. A sector scanner for real time two-dimensional echocardiography. *Circulation* 1974; **49**: 1147–52.

13. Tranquart F, Grenier N, Eder V, Pourcelot L. Clinical use of ultrasound tissue harmonic imaging. *Ultrasound Med Biol* 1999; **25**: 889–94.

14. Wang XF, Deng YB, Nanda NC, *et al*. Live three-dimensional echocardiography: imaging principles and clinical application. *Echocardiography* 2003; **20**: 593–604.

15. Sugeng L, Weinert L, Thiele K, Lang RO. Real-time three-dimensional echocardiography using a novel matrix array transducer. *Echocardiography* 2003; **20**: 623–35.

16. Hung J, Lang R, Flachskampf F, *et al*. 3D echocardiography: a review of the current status and future directions. *J Am Soc Echocardiogr* 2007; **20**: 213–33.

17. Burns PN. The physical principles of Doppler and spectral analysis. *J Clin Ultrasound* 1987; **15**: 567–90.

18. Baker DA, Rubenstein SA, Lorch GS. Pulsed Doppler echocardiography: principles and applications. *Am J Med* 1977; **63**: 69–80.

19. Bom K, de Boo J, Rijsterborgh H. On the aliasing problem in pulsed Doppler cardiac studies. *J Clin Ultrasound* 1984; **12**: 559–67.

20. Yeh EL. Reverberations in echocardiograms. *J Clin Ultrasound* 1977; **5**: 84–6.

Further reading

Feigenbaum H, Armstrong WF, Ryan T. *Feigenbaum's Echocardiography*, 6th edn. Philadelphia, PA: Lippincott Williams and Wilkins, 2004.

Hedrick WR, Hykes DL, Starchman DE. *Ultrasound Physics and Instrumentation*, 4th edn. St. Louis, MO: Elsevier Mosby, 2005.

Otto CM. *Textbook of Clinical Echocardiography*, 3rd edn. Philadelphia, PA: Saunders, 2004.

3

Safety and complications; probe maintenance

Robert Feneck

Introduction

The development of transesophageal echocardiography (TEE) has been of great importance to the care of the cardiac patient. In the non-surgical setting, TEE has made a substantial contribution to the diagnostic modalities available to cardiologists. In the cardiac surgery patient, the impact has been such that the widespread uptake of intraoperative TEE has been one of the most important developments in cardiac anesthesia in the last 20 years [1]. In the USA, TEE has a very high rate of routine use amongst cardiac anesthesiologists in academic institutions [2,3]. Although similar data for Europe are less authoritative, the use of intraoperative TEE is widespread amongst academic institutions throughout Europe.

This suggests that TEE is both effective and safe. Whilst that assumption may be correct, we should recognize that TEE does in fact have a complication rate measurable in terms of both morbidity and mortality [4]. Identifying those at greatest risk of adverse outcomes and complications from TEE will help us to reduce the risk still further.

Serious complications related to TEE are rare, with a reported rate of up to 0.5% [5]. In an analysis of intraoperative complications associated with TEE, Kallmeyer *et al.* found an overall complication rate of 0.2% [6]. In more difficult circumstances, such as in an emergency department, the complication rate may increase, up to 12% [7] (Table 3.1). Early studies have concluded that in terms of morbidity and mortality the procedure is similar to upper gastrointestinal endoscopy [4].

Safety of TEE: sedation or general anesthesia

In current practice, TEE may be undertaken in a variety of clinical locations, including the echo laboratory, the operating room, the post-anesthetic recovery area,

the intensive care and high dependency units, and the accident and emergency department.

In a surgery-related setting, TEE will usually be undertaken under general anesthesia or deep sedation. In both situations, the airway will need to be secured, usually with an endotracheal tube, and anesthesia (e.g. during surgery) or deep sedation (e.g. in the intensive care unit) will in any case be required for purposes other than TEE. There may be safety issues related to the passage of the probe in anesthetized patients. Trauma to the lips, teeth, and soft tissues of the oropharynx may occur. Care should always be taken to minimize this risk. It is preferable if the probe can be passed under controlled conditions before surgery, rather than after the patient has been "prepped and draped," when access is substantially limited. This subject is dealt with in greater detail below.

In the diagnostic cardiology setting, TEE will be performed under mild sedation, although increasingly clinicians have reported carrying out the procedure

Table 3.1. TEE-associated complications

A. Intraoperative complications [6]	Incidence
Odynophagia	0.1%
Dental injury	0.03%
Endotracheal tube malpositioning	0.03%
Upper gastrointestinal hemorrhage	0.03%
Esophageal perforation	0.01%
B. Complications in emergency department [7]	**Rate**
Respiratory failure	4.9%
Emesis	2.8%
Hypotension	2.1%
Agitation	1.4%
Cardiac dysrhythmias	0.7%
Death	0.7%

Core Topics in Transesophageal Echocardiography, ed. Robert Feneck, John Kneeshaw, and Marco Ranucci.
Published by Cambridge University Press. © Cambridge University press 2010.

with no sedation at all [4,8]. In either situation, it should be recognized that the patient may experience some discomfort, and the duration of the procedure may need to be limited [9]. Thus a TEE study may be goal-directed towards only those questions that cannot be adequately answered by a transthoracic (TTE) study. In particular, it is wise to address the key issues first [10]. In this clinical setting, it is therefore recommended that a TEE should always be accompanied by a TTE: not only are the two examinations best considered as complementary, but also images and data acquired during a TTE study will reduce the time required for the TEE study, resulting in less discomfort for the patient [11].

The requirements for an echo laboratory undertaking TEE have recently been described in detail, and are shown in Table 3.2.

TEE is frequently undertaken outside the operating room. Some patients find the procedure too uncomfortable without any sedation at all, and it has been usual to undertake TEE in the conscious patient under some form of sedation. In judging the needs of the procedure, and with regard to untoward effects and outcomes, a TEE can be compared to an upper gastrointestinal endoscopy [4]. The overall stimulus of the two procedures is comparable, and hence the sedative requirements of the patient will be similar also. The usual sedation offered includes topical anesthesia to the mouth and oropharynx, and one or more intravenous sedatives. It is important to recognize, however, that there are safety issues concerning the use of sedative drugs [8]. These are considered below.

Topical anesthesia

Antisialogogue premedication may be useful to reduce secretions, which if excessive may provoke aspiration and coughing. They will also reduce tone in the gastroesophageal sphincter, which could theoretically ease the passage of the TEE probe. However, in practice antisialogogue drugs are frequently omitted. Atropine, hyoscine, and glycopyrollate are available. Atropine and hyoscine may be given orally; both cross the blood–brain barrier and may produce central

Table 3.2. Summary of criteria for rating transesophageal laboratories [11]

Standard	Advanced
Staff	
Designated head of TEE	Head of TEE performs/supervises >50 studies each year
Designated head should be performing or supervising at least 50 TEE annually	Head of TEE has EAE/national accreditation
Designated person, usually a nurse, to manage airway and recover the patient	
Organization/equipment	
Established protocols	Recovery area
Written informed consent	Minimum standards for studies established
Resuscitation equipment	List of indications for TEE agreed internally
Multiplane probe	Quality control of results, e.g. against surgery, pathology, other imaging
Routine use of:	
• Suction, oxygen, and pulse oximeter	Room at least 20 m² in area
• BP monitor	Regular audits
Patient preparation including letter and pre-procedure checklist	Written standard operating procedures
Provision for continuing education	History of success in training students
Provision for quality control	Digital storage and retrieval
Sedation used according to published guidelines	Provision of intraoperative services
Lockable drug cupboard	
Facilities for cleaning/sterilizing the probe	

anticholinergic effects which may be undesirable, particularly in the elderly. Glycopyrollate does not cross the blood–brain barrier but it is not absorbed from the gastrointestinal tract and must be given parenterally. If an antisialogogue is required, glycopyrollate is probably the agent of choice [9]. However, an anticholinergic should always be drawn up and available for intravenous administration in case either the passage of the probe or the use of other drugs provokes a vagal bradycardia during the procedure.

Topical anesthesia to the pharynx reduces the gag reflex, preventing retching and laryngospasm, but may facilitate pulmonary aspiration in susceptible individuals. Topical anesthesia may be administered in a number of ways, for example as 2% viscous lidocaine, or as a 10% lidocaine spray. Its efficacy may be improved by anticholinergic premedication, which will prevent dilution of the anesthetic with saliva. In contrast to awake fiberoptic endotracheal intubation, which requires anesthesia to the airway below the vocal cords, topical anesthesia for TEE need be no more extensive than the oropharynx, and this can usually be easily achieved well within the recommended dosing of local anesthetic, thus avoiding the risk of toxicity.

Intravenous sedation

Propofol has been widely used for intravenous sedation, particularly by the anesthesia community, where it is also used as an intravenous induction agent and for maintenance of surgical anesthesia, usually in conjunction with other agents. For intravenous sedation it is given by continuous infusion using an electronic syringe pump, with the dose adjusted as necessary. As with all intravenous techniques, there will be a delay between a dose adjustment and effect, and a common error is to fail to allow sufficient time for the drug to take effect.

Propofol is useful and effective, and is noted for its good quality of recovery. The main caveats to its use are in judging the dose, in particular in recognizing that excessive dosage may lead to inducing an anesthetic state with loss of airway protection and control, and cardiorespiratory depression. In common with most anesthetics, there is no "antidote" to propofol and the anesthetized patient must be supported until the effects of the drug wear off. Propofol has vasodilator effects on the peripheral circulation, and may depress cardiac contractility. These features should be borne in mind if the TEE study is being undertaken for evaluation of a cardiac condition that may be significantly affected by these hemodynamic changes.

Opioid drugs may also be useful. Apart from their analgesic effect, patients may benefit from the euphoric effect that usually accompanies their use. Although fentanyl has previously been recommended, remifentanil is a drug that has been introduced relatively recently, and has been shown to be particularly useful in intravenous sedation, due to its ultra-short duration of action. Remifentanil shares the same mechanism for the termination of its action as the β-blocker esmolol, although there is no evidence that the two drugs effectively compete for that mechanism, and thus they can be used together if desired.

Remifentanil is also given by continuous infusion using an electronic syringe pump. It has the classic effects of a μ-opioid receptor agonist, and thus the side effects will include respiratory depression, hypercapnia and unconsciousness. It is therefore imperative to monitor the patient closely during remifentanil administration. That said, the duration of effect is ultra-short once administration is terminated, and so overdosage may be managed simply by discontinuing the infusion, usually without requiring a specific opioid antagonist such as naloxone.

Intravenous benzodiazepines have been the mainstay of intravenous sedative techniques over the years, particularly for non-anesthetists, and they are still frequently used. Intravenous midazolam may be easily titrated to effect, although enough time should be allowed for the full onset of action. Intravenous benzodiazepines are best administered by a small intravenous bolus dose in this situation, repeated as necessary. Apart from sedative effects, they also have a useful anterograde amnesic effect, and may combine usefully with an opioid such as remifentanil.

Benzodiazepines are relatively long-acting drugs, and their potency and duration of action may be much less predictable in the frail and elderly. Overdosage will eventually lead to unconsciousness and cardiorespiratory depression. It is certainly possible to administer an inadvertent general anesthetic with benzodiazepines, with all the consequences that will entail. However, one safety feature is that there is a specific benzodiazepine antagonist – flumazenil – which may be useful in antagonizing the effects of an inadvertent overdose.

Monitoring and prophylaxis

Although practitioners will have different levels of competence and experience with performing TEE in

Table 3.3. Specimen technique for TEE under conscious sedation

Equipment

- Oxygen, suction, and resuscitation equipment
- Trolley with negative Trendelenberg facility
- Clean and intact TEE probe
- TEE probe sheath if appropriate
- Bite guard

Patient management

- Nil by mouth for 4 hours
- Intravenous access
- Glycopyrrollate 200 μg slowly intravenously (allow 3–5 minutes for antisialogogue effect)
- Topical lidocaine 10% spray or 2–4% viscous lidocaine ("swish and swallow")
- Midazolam 1–3 mg intravenously and/or
- Remifentanil infusion @ 0.05–1 μg/kg/min and/or
- Propofol infusion TCI (target controlled infusion) @ 1–2 μg/mL
- Flumazenil for midazolam reversal

the awake patient, safety is enhanced by ensuring a minimum level of non-invasive monitoring even in the patient in whom the procedure is planned as a procedure without sedation at all. Minimum monitoring should include ECG, non-invasive blood pressure measurement, and pulse oximetry. Although the necessity for pulse oximetry in patients receiving mild sedation has been questioned, it has also been noted that relative hypoxia may occur even in those patients undergoing TEE without any sedation at all [12].

The use of antibiotic prophylaxis in patients undergoing TEE remains the subject of debate. However, at the present time the European Society of Cardiology [9], the British Society of Echocardiography [13,14], and the American Heart Association [15] all recommend that routine prophylaxis is not given for any patient group, but may be given on individual grounds.

A specimen technique for conducting TEE in the awake patient is shown in Table 3.3.

Complications and contraindications

TEE may be associated with both minor and severe complications. Gastrointestinal injury and perforation are rare but serious complications, and may be associated with direct and indirect trauma [5,16–18]. Direct trauma may be more common following blind insertion of the probe, and it is always prudent to insert the probe at the beginning of the surgical procedure and under controlled conditions. Spahn et al. [19] described a case of esophageal perforation in a surgical patient in whom the probe was inserted after separation from cardiopulmonary bypass, with the TEE probe visible in the anterior mediastinum (Fig. 3.1). Poor matching of the probe size to the patient (i.e. the use of a large probe in a small patient),

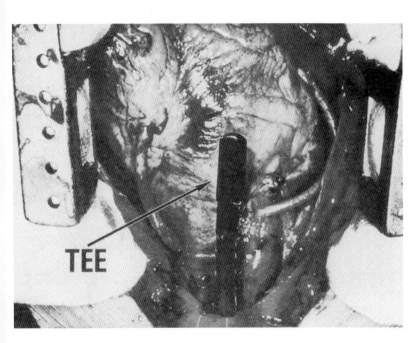

Figure 3.1. TEE probe following perforation of the left side of the hypopharynx, with the probe in the upper anterior mediastinum. The patient was a female aged 75 years undergoing emergency CABG surgery. The probe was passed during surgery after difficulty in weaning from cardiopulmonary bypass. The perforation was identified and repaired, and the patient discharged from hospital. Reproduced with permission from Spahn et al., Anesthesiology 1995; **82**: 581–3 [19].

37

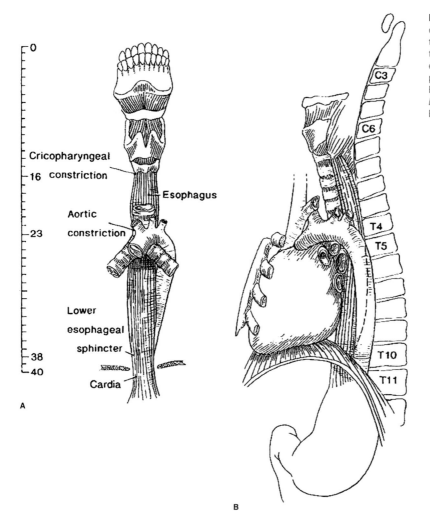

Figure 3.2. Anterior (A) and lateral (B) diagrams showing the esophagus and the levels of the cricopharyngeal constriction, the aortic constriction, and the lower esophageal sphincter. Reproduced with permission from Freeman WK, Seward JB, Khandeheria BK, Tajik AJ. *Transesophageal Echocardiography*. New York, NY: Little, Brown, 1994.

excessive flexion of the probe tip, and pre-existing esophageal pathology have also been implicated in causing esophageal trauma and perforation.

The main anatomical areas of risk are at the cricopharyngeal constriction (approximately 15 cm from the teeth – level of C6), at the level of the aortic arch (23 cm from teeth – level of T4/5), and at the lower esophageal sphincter (38 cm from teeth – level of T10/11) (Fig. 3.2).

Trauma and perforation are the major risks at the cricopharyngeal constriction and at the lower esophageal sphincter, whereas there is a risk of vascular damage to the aortic arch in the case of an aneurysm.

Safe practice should include checking the probe tip for any damage before insertion, good lubrication, and the use of a protective sheath. At all times forcefully advancing the probe *must* be avoided – firm but

gentle is the necessary technique. Manipulating the probe once it is in a flexed position should also be avoided.

The risk factors for TEE-associated gastroesophageal injury are shown in Table 3.4. There are over 15 cases of esophageal perforation reported in the literature, almost all occurring in patients undergoing cardiac surgery. Pharyngeal or esophageal perforation carries a 10–25% mortality, and late onset of symptoms (> 24 hours) may be more common than early onset (< 24 hours). Pre-existing gastrointestinal pathology may be contributive, but it should be noted that difficulty in advancing the probe and poor image quality are not invariable findings in patients with esophageal perforation [5].

Hemorrhage is another serious complication. Most lacerations associated with TEE are Mallory–Weiss

Table 3.4. Risk factors for TEE-associated gastroesophageal injury

- Gastroesophageal pathology
- Difficulty with TEE probe insertion
- Advanced age
- Small body size
- Child
- Chronic steroid therapy
- Previous thoracic radiotherapy
- Chronic vasculopathy
- Cervical arthritis
- Hypertrophy of cricopharyngeal sphincter
- Prolonged surgery/TEE insertion

tears near the gastroesophageal junction or in the gastric cardia [20,21]. It may present as "coffee grounds" or bright red blood. Splenic and parapharyngeal injuries have also been reported [22]. However, one should beware of attributing all GI hemorrhage in cardiac surgery patients to TEE, since the risk of GI hemorrhage in cardiac surgery patients is approximately 2% independent of the use of TEE [23].

Dysphagia (difficulty) and odynophagia (pain) are less serious complications, and the incidence in cardiac surgery patients undergoing TEE is more difficult to predict. In a study of 1245 cardiac surgery patients, Messina *et al.* found no difference between TEE and non-TEE patients [24]. By contrast, Rousou *et al.* and Hogue *et al.* found a significant increase in symptoms in patients who had undergone intraoperative TEE [25,26].

Airway obstruction is a potentially dangerous complication. It is more common in children, owing to the relative size of the probe and the airways, and to anatomical variants, and airway pressure increases and evidence of gas trapping may be indicative. Airway obstruction has been noted in adult non-surgical patients, particularly in the elderly and in those who are poorly sedated, and anticoagulation may predispose to hematoma formation if there is trauma to the submucosa.

Indirect trauma has been associated with prolonged mucosal pressure and thermal injury.

Finally, a number of miscellaneous serious complications have been described including thromboembolism [27,28], aortic dissection [29], and vascular compression [30,31].

One complication that must be considered is failure to pass the probe at all [5]. This may occur in both awake and anesthetized patients. In the latter group it is more common in children than in adults. Whilst failure to pass the probe may seriously complicate intraoperative management, including surgical decision making, it is wise to reflect that this is a better situation than generating a serious introperative complication such as a gastrointestinal perforation through the use of undue force in trying to advance the probe.

Suggested absolute contraindications to TEE include esophageal disease (stricture, diverticula, tumor, esophagitis, Mallory–Weiss tear, esophageal varices), external vascular compression by a thoracic aortic aneurysm, and recent esophageal surgery. Suggested relative contraindications include gastroesophageal reflux and hiatus hernia, and severe dysphagia/odynophagia. However, the issue of contraindication to TEE probe insertion should be seen as a risk–benefit ratio, and in some specific circumstances, for example liver transplantation, TEE may be used even in the presence of esophageal varices, since the benefits of the procedure may outweigh the risks [32].

Thus far, it seems that insertion of a TEE probe in a patient under general anesthesia and mechanical ventilation is accompanied by a very low complication rate. A sedated, conscious patient may experience a similar or higher rate of complications, but this is increased when TEE is performed under emergency conditions.

Probe care and cleaning

TEE has been described as a semi-invasive procedure, presumably to identify it as less invasive than intravascular monitoring and diagnostic procedures. In fact, an upper GI endoscopy carries risks to the patient, as summarized above, and we must take care not to compound these with a cross-infection risk. Furthermore, TEE equipment is expensive and delicate, and probe care should be a natural part of our routine work.

Probe care

During a TEE exam in the echo laboratory, the probe is in place for a relatively short period – rarely more than 10 minutes, often much less. By contrast, during cardiac surgery, if the probe is placed at the beginning of the procedure and kept *in situ* until the end, the probe may be in place for 3–5 hours or more. If an institution does not have one probe per machine, the probe may be disconnected from the machine, exposing the

39

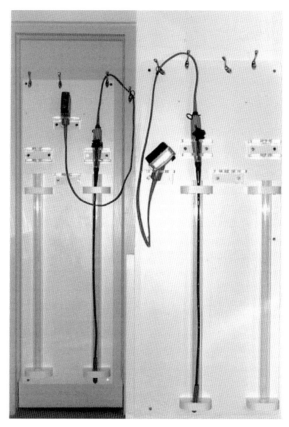

Figure 3.3. Storage devices for TEE probes, maintaining the probe straight, not flexed.

electronics to damage and contamination. Operating rooms are crowded areas, and accidental damage is a real risk. The risks to the probe may be minimized by using a protective box to protect the probe connector in the operating room when it is disconnected from the machine, and by stabilizing the probe in a non-flexed position when it is in the patient for long periods. After use, the probes should be stored in a protective environment, and the case used for transportation is not the best device for this. When it is not in use it is better to store the probe hung straight – that is, with no flexion of the probe shaft – in a dedicated holder (Fig. 3.3). This may be used for storing soiled probes before cleaning, and for storing clean probes thereafter.

Cleaning

A TEE probe should never be used without proper cleaning. This process should involve the following steps:

1. Clean the probe and probe tip with warm soapy water to perform a gross decontamination and remove all obvious protein material.

2. Use an enzymatic cleaner to assist in removing protein residuals. A common enzymatic cleaner is one with a pH of 6.0–8.0 and contains diluted concentrations of surfactants, alcohols, salts, and acids. These cleaners are further diluted during use, and any specific instructions from the manufacturers should be followed.
3. Rinse the distal tip and shaft thoroughly, taking care not to immerse the control housing, cable or connector.
4. Disinfect the probe tip and shaft using a glutaraldehyde-based disinfectant. Commonly, 2.4% glutaraldehyde is used.

Glutaraldehyde is a potentially toxic chemical, and whilst adequate concentrations and exposure are required for appropriate disinfection, healthcare workers should be protected from glutaraldehyde vapor. Conventional probe cleaners usually are vented such that waste vapor is removed. The probes themselves are exposed to glutaraldehyde for a limited amount of time recommended by the disinfectant manufacturer, and then washed extensively, usually with three wash cycles to remove any residual glutaraldehyde.

It is recommended that a disposable protective sheath is used for each TEE exam. Both latex and latex-free sheaths are available.

More recently, a simpler method of cleaning has been developed [33], involving the use of sachets of chlorine dioxide-based disinfectant that are claimed to be sporicidal, mycobactericidal, bactericidal, virucidal, and fungicidal within a 30-second contact time. The only significant drawback to this technique is that, since it is carried out by a person and not a machine, there is no objective record of it having being completed conscientiously. However, as with cabinet-based techniques, accurate records of the date, time, name of the patient, and name of the individual carrying out the cleaning should be maintained.

Conclusion

TEE is a relatively safe procedure that can be undertaken on a wide range of patients and with minimal complications. These complications can be minimized by paying close attention to the details outlined in this chapter. Close attention to probe care, maintenance, and disinfection also plays an important role in maintaining the effectiveness of each study and of the TEE service, whether in the echo lab or in the operating room.

References

1. Feneck RO. Cardiac anaesthesia: the last 10 years. *Anaesthesia* 2003; **58**: 1171–7.

2. Thys DM. Updated indications for intraoperative TEE. In: Savage RM, Aronson S, eds., *Comprehensive Textbook of Intraoperative Transesophageal Echocardiography*. Philadelphia, PA: Lippincott Williams & Wilkins, 2005: 95–102.

3. Poterack KA. Who uses transesophageal echocardiography in the operating room? *Anesth Analg* 1995; **80**: 454–8.

4. Daniel WG, Erbel R, Kasper W, *et al.* Safety of transesophageal echocardiography: a multicenter survey of 10,419 examinations. *Circulation* 1991; **83**: 817–21.

5. Shernan SK. Safety of intraoperative transoesophageal echocardiography. In: Konstadt SN, Shernan S, Oka Y, eds., *Clinical Transesophageal Echocardiography: a Problem-Oriented Approach*, 2nd edn. Philadelphia, PA: Lippincott Williams & Wilkins, 2003: 25–36.

6. Kallmeyer IJ, Collard CD, Fox JA, *et al.* The safety of intraoperative transesophageal echocardiography: a case series of 7200 cardiac surgical patients. *Anesth Analg* 2001; **92**: 1126–30.

7. Gendreau MA, Triner WR, Bartfield J. Complications of transesophageal echocardiography in the ED. *Am J Emerg Med* 1999; **17**: 248–51.

8. Blondheim DS, Levi D, Marmor AT. Mild sedation before transesophageal echo induces significant hemodynamic respiratory depression. *Echocardiography* 2004; **21**: 241–5.

9. Flachskampf FA, Decoodt P, Fraser AG, *et al.* Working Group on Echocardiography of the European Society of Cardiology. Guidelines from the Working Group. Recommendations for performing transesophageal echocardiography. *Eur J Echocardiogr* 2001; **2**: 8–21.

10. Stewart WJ. Willie Sutton and the completeness and priorities of the Ideal Transoesophageal Echo Study in the year 2001. *Eur J Echocardiogr* 2001; **2**: 6–7.

11. Nihoyannopoulos P, Fox K, Fraser A, Pinto F. EAE laboratory standards and accreditation. *Eur J Echocardiogr* 2007; **8**: 80–7.

12. Kassimatis A, Tsoukas A, Ikonomidis I, Joshi J, Nihoyannopoulos P. Routine arterial oxygen saturation monitoring is not necessary during transesophageal echocardiography. *Clin Cardiol* 1997: **20**: 547–52.

13. Chambers JB, Klein JL, Bennett SR, Monaghan MJ, Roxburgh JC. Is antibiotic prophylaxis ever necessary before transesophageal echocardiography? *Heart* 2006; **92**: 435–6.

14. Statement on antibiotic prophylaxis before transoesophageal echocardiography. Approved by the Councils of British Society of Echocardiography, Association of Cardiothoracic Anaesthetists and the Society of Cardiothoracic Surgeons. www.bsecho.org (accessed September 2009).

15. Dajani AS, Bisno AL, Chung KJ, *et al.* Prevention of bacterial endocarditis: recommendations by the American Heart Association. *JAMA* 1990; **264**: 2919–22.

16. Badaoui R, Choufane S, Riboulot M, Bachelet Y, Ossart M. [Esophageal perforation after transesophageal echocardiography.] *Ann Fr Anesth Reanim* 1994; **13**: 850–2.

17. Jougon J, Gallon P, Dubrez J, Velly JF. [Esophageal perforation during transesophageal echocardiography.] *Arch Mal Coeur Vaiss* 2000; **93**: 1235–7.

18. Massey SR, Pitsis A, Mehta D, Callaway M. Oesophageal perforation following perioperative transesophageal echocardiography. *Br J Anaesth* 2000; **84**: 643–6.

19. Spahn DR, Schmid S, Carrel T, Pasch T, Schmid ER. Hypopharynx perforation by a transesophageal echocardiography probe. *Anesthesiology* 1995; **82**: 581–3.

20. St-Pierre J, Fortier LP, Couture P, Hébert Y. Massive gastrointestinal hemorrhage after transoesophageal echocardiography probe insertion. *Can J Anaesth* 1998; **54**: 1196–9.

21. Kihara S, Mizutani T, Shimizu T, Toyooka H. Bleeding from a tear in the gastric mucosa caused by transoesophageal echocardiography during cardiac surgery: effective haemostasis by endoscopic argon plasma coagulation. *Br J Anaesth* 1999; **82**: 948–50.

22. Olenchock SA, Lukaszczyk JJ, Reed J, Theman TE. Splenic injury after intraoperative transesophageal echocardiography. *Ann Thorac Surg* 2001; **72**: 2141–3.

23. Hulyalkar AR, Ayd JD. Low risk of gastrointestinal injury associated with transesophageal echocardiography during cardiac surgery. *J Cardiothorac Vasc Anesth* 1993; **7**: 175–7.

24. Messina AG, Paranicas M, Fiamengo S, *et al.* Risk of dysphagia after transesophageal echocardiography. *Am J Cardiol* 1991; **67**: 313–14.

25. Rousou JA, Tighe DA, Garb JL, *et al.* Risk of dysphagia after transesophageal echocardiography during cardiac operations. *Ann Thorac Surg* 2000; **69**: 486–9.

26. Hogue CW, Lappas GD, Creswell LL, *et al.* Swallowing dysfunction after cardiac operations. Associated adverse outcomes and risk factors including intraoperative transesophageal

echocardiography. *J Thorac Cardiovasc Surg* 1995; **110**: 517–22.

27. Kwak KD, Mosher SF, Willis CL, Kimura BJ. Witnessed embolization of a right atrial mass during transesophageal echocardiography: implications regarding the safety of esophageal intubation. *Chest* 1999; **115**: 1462–4.

28. Cavero MA, Cristóbal C, González M, *et al.* Fatal pulmonary embolism of a right atrial mass during transesophageal echocardiography. *J Am Soc Echocardiogr* 1998; **11**: 397–8.

29. Silvey SV, Stoughton TL, Pearl W, Collazo WA, Belbel RJ. Rupture of the outer partition of aortic dissection during transesophageal echocardiography. *Am J Cardiol* 1991; **68**: 286–7.

30. Janelle GM, Lobato EB, Tang Y. An unusual complication of transesophageal echocardiography. *J Cardiothorac Vasc Anesth* 1999; **13**: 233–4.

31. Bensky A, O'Brien W, Hammon J. Transesophageal echo probe compression of an aberrant right subclavian artery. *J Am Soc Echocardiogr* 1995; **8**: 964–6.

32. Wax DB, Torres A, Scher C, Leibowitz AB. Transesophageal echocardiography utilization in high-volume liver transplantation centers in the United States. *J Cardiothorac Vasc Anesth.* 2008; **22**: 811–13.

33. Hernández A, Carrasco M, Ausina V. Mycobactericidal activity of chlorine dioxide wipes in a modified prEN 14563 test. *J Hosp Infect* 2008; **69**: 384–8.

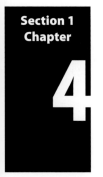

The transesophageal echo examination

Robert Feneck, Luca Lorini

Introduction

A transesophageal echo (TEE) examination may serve as an adjunct to a transthoracic study, or it may serve as a stand-alone examination. The patient's clinical circumstances will determine the nature of the examination. A patient who has just undergone a diagnostic transthoracic echo (TTE) in the laboratory may require an abbreviated TEE study which is directed primarily towards the pathology in question, with the aim of answering a specific question. Such a study may be conducted with minimal or even no sedation [1].

By contrast, an intraoperative examination should not only focus on the relevant pathology in question, but should also be seen as an opportunity to check the preoperative findings, and perform a more complete echocardiographic evaluation of the heart. Intraoperative TEE is increasingly being used to assess ventricular function in patients about to undergo coronary revascularization, and it should always be used to assess the result of surgery and cardiac function both following bypass and/or at the time of chest closure.

Preliminary factors

Despite a good safety record, TEE may be associated with an incidence of both minor and serious complications. The latter are fortunately rare, and have been dealt with in Chapter 3. However, it is essential to keep the risks of TEE to a minimum, and to that end all patients should be assessed to identify any relevant factors. The medical history should be reviewed and any relevant tests noted. Previous esophageal surgery and a history of dysphagia or hematemesis are especially important. Where there is any doubt about a relevant pre-existing pathology, this may be further investigated in an elective case. In an urgent or emergency situation, a careful balance must be struck between the value of the investigation and the potential for any damage to the patient. It may be that modifying the procedure – for example, limiting the exam

to the upper and mid-esophagus – may be useful in patients with lower esophageal or gastric pathology. The presence of an increased risk should always be noted and discussed with the patient, and the patient's consent obtained.

Manipulating the probe

The modern omniplane TEE probe is a highly versatile instrument for acquiring images. The electronics of the probe are described in Chapter 2. The probe itself is easily manipulated in the patient, and it is important that a uniform terminology is used for clarification (Fig. 4.1).

The following terms have been agreed for describing manipulations of the probe. It is assumed that the

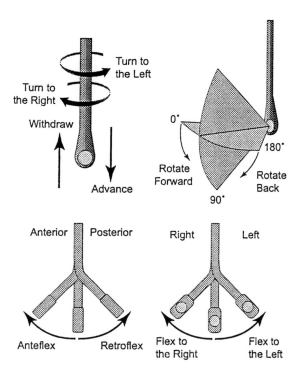

Figure 4.1. Conventional terminology used to describe manipulation of the TEE probe and transducer.

Core Topics in Transesophageal Echocardiography, ed. Robert Feneck, John Kneeshaw, and Marco Ranucci.
Published by Cambridge University Press. © Cambridge University Press 2010.

patient is in the supine position and that the imaging plane is directed anteriorly from the esophagus.

- advancing the probe – pushing the probe further into the patient
- withdrawing the probe – pulling the probe out of the patient
- turning the probe to the right/left – clockwise/counterclockwise turning the probe
- rotation of the transducer (transducer angle) – increasing/decreasing the omniplane angle of the transducer
- anteflexion – flexing the tip of the probe by clockwise turning of the large wheel
- retroflexion – flexing the tip of the probe by counterclockwise turning of the large wheel
- flexing to left and right – flexing the tip of the probe using the small wheel

These terms will be used to describe acquiring the views in the following section.

The 20 standard views

In 1997, the American Society of Echocardiography Council for Intraoperative Echocardiography set about creating a set of guidelines for performing a comprehensive intraoperative multiplane TEE examination. These guidelines were formally published in 1999, and include a set of 20 cross-sectional views of the heart and great vessels [2]. The guidelines have since formed the basis of teaching and learning TEE. There are limitations to their value, most notably that they are based on patients with relatively normal anatomy, so that the recommendations for acquiring the views may not be accurate in the presence of severe structural heart disease. In complex cases, and particularly in congenital heart disease, a series of non-standard views may be necessary in order to visualize the required structures. Even in relatively normal patients, some minor adjustments to the probe depth and positioning, and the transducer angulation, are frequently necessary. Despite these limitations, the standard views will be sufficient for a comprehensive examination in the majority of adult patients, and they form the basis of any modified views that may be necessary in complex cases.

An overview of the 20 standard views described by Shanewise *et al.* [2] is shown in Figure 4.2.

The title of each view, and its echo-anatomical correlation, is part of a standard nomenclature. Figure 4.3 (a–t) shows a drawing of each view and a link to the relevant echo image on video. The optimal or usual transducer position for acquiring each view is described.

Examining structures

The echocardiographer can perform a comprehensive examination in the majority of patients using the standard views described above. In certain circumstances, some modification of the view, or additional non-standard views, may be required. A detailed examination of the relevant cardiac anatomy and pathology may be found in each of the relevant chapters in this book. However, the following is intended as a simple guide to using the standard views to obtain a comprehensive evaluation of the majority of patients.

Left ventricle

Echocardiographic examination of left ventricular function is a valuable technique that can reveal useful information when the heart is at rest or under stress with a pharmacological agent such as dobutamine.

In order to evaluate each part accurately, the left ventricle has been divided into a number of segments. Recently, the convention for naming the walls and segments of the left ventricle has changed [3]. This change has come about in order to standardize the description of the segments of the myocardium throughout the different imaging modalities, including nuclear and magnetic resonance techniques. The main changes between the new and old descriptive terminology is that the new classification defines 17 myocardial segments, not 16, and the starting point (i.e. segment 1) in the new classification is the basal anterior segment, in contrast to the old system which defined segment 1 as the basal anteroseptal segment.

Furthermore, a number of descriptive changes have occurred, as shown in Table 4.1.

Although the older convention is still commonly used [4], the European Association of Echocardiography recognizes the new convention for accreditation purposes.

The six walls of the left ventricle and 17 segments are shown in Figure 4.4. These segments can be seen in the long axis using the standard views shown in Figures 4.3a, 4.3b, and 4.3c. Since these are all mid-esophageal views, they can be developed by placing the transducer at a mid-esophageal depth of 30–40 cm, and then rotating the multiplane transducer from the start position of 0–20°, through to approximately

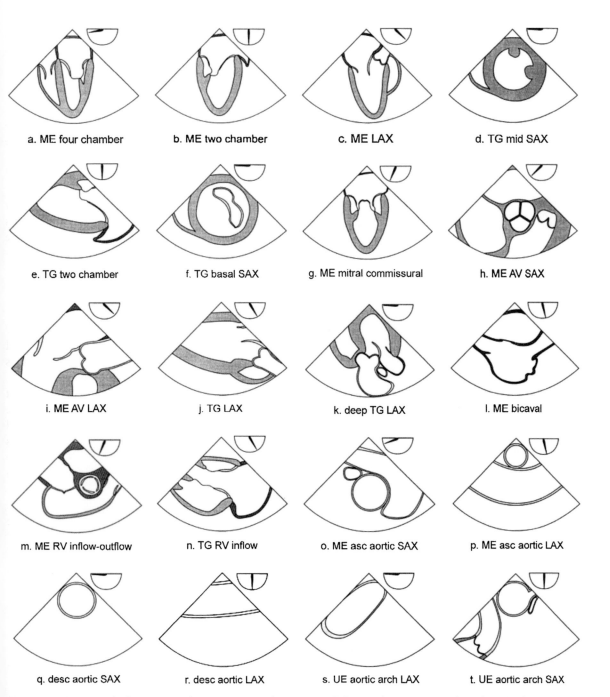

a. ME four chamber

b. ME two chamber

c. ME LAX

d. TG mid SAX

e. TG two chamber

f. TG basal SAX

g. ME mitral commissural

h. ME AV SAX

i. ME AV LAX

j. TG LAX

k. deep TG LAX

l. ME bicaval

m. ME RV inflow-outflow

n. TG RV inflow

o. ME asc aortic SAX

p. ME asc aortic LAX

q. desc aortic SAX

r. desc aortic LAX

s. UE aortic arch LAX

t. UE aortic arch SAX

Figure 4.2. The 20 standard cross-sectional views comprising the recommended comprehensive transesophageal examination.

120°. The depth of the transducer will not need to be altered, although some retroflexion of the tip may be required to visualize the true apex and prevent a fore-shortened image (Video 4.21).

The human heart has a branching network of coronary arteries with a good collateral supply. Nonethe-less, it is possible to predict which coronary artery supplies which area of the myocardium at the mid-cavity (mid-papillary) level, as shown in Figure 4.5. The short axis of the left ventricle may be assessed by developing the standard short-axis transgastric mid-cavity and basal views (Figs. 4.3d and 4.3f respectively).

45

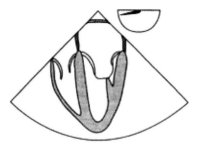

a. ME four chamber

Figure 4.3 (a). Mid-esophageal four-chamber view.
Usual probe tip depth: 30–40 cm.
Transducer angle: 0–20°.
Transducer tip: some retroflexion may be needed to visualize the true LV apex. For the left and right pulmonary vein, the probe may need to be withdrawn a few centimetres and turned to left and right respectively. For the coronary sinus view, the probe should be advanced and turned to right.
Anatomy imaged: left ventricle, left atrium, mitral valve leaflets, interatrial septum, interventricular septum, lateral wall of the left ventricle, free wall of the right ventricle, tricuspid valve leaflets, left and right pulmonary veins, coronary sinus.
Video 4.1.

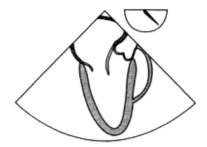

c. ME LAX

Figure 4.3 (c). Mid-esophageal long-axis view.
Usual probe tip depth: 30–40 cm.
Transducer angle: 120–160°.
Transducer tip: some retroflexion may be needed to visualize the true LV apex.
Anatomy imaged: left atrium, mitral valve leaflets, anteroseptal and inferolateral (posterior) walls of the left ventricle, left ventricular outflow tract, aortic valve, part or all of the aortic root, ascending aorta.
Video 4.3.

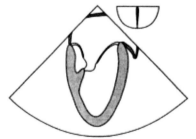

b. ME two chamber

Figure 4.3 (b). Mid-esophageal two-chamber view.
Usual probe tip depth: 30–40 cm.
Transducer angle: 80–100°.
Transducer tip: some retroflexion may be needed to visualize the true LV apex. The probe should be turned to the right to visualize the left pulmonary veins.
Anatomy imaged: left atrium, anterior and posterior mitral valve leaflets, left atrial appendage, anterior and inferior walls of the left ventricle.
Video 4.2.

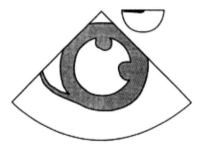

d. TG mid SAX

Figure 4.3 (d). Transgastric mid short-axis view.
Usual probe tip depth: 40–50 cm.
Transducer angle: 0–20°.
Transducer tip: probe anteflexion usually required.
Anatomy imaged: left and right ventricle at the level of the papillary muscles, anterolateral and posteromedial papillary muscles.
Video 4.4.

From the mid-cavity position (40–50 cm, transducer angle 0–20°, marked anteflexion) the probe is withdrawn gently and slowly until the basal view is developed and the mitral annulus becomes visible. The probe does not usually have to be rotated or turned.

Although the apical segments of the left ventricle are often difficult to visualize, this may be attempted by gently advancing the probe, without rotation of transducer, 2–4 cm from the mid-cavity position.

However, frequently the view is either poor or the deep transgastric view (Fig 4.3k) becomes apparent. The apical segments are therefore often best seen using the long-axis mid-esophageal views.

Global left ventricular function can be assessed by measuring the size of the chamber and observing left ventricular motion in the relevant views. Global ventricular wall motion may be assessed by measuring fractional shortening, fractional area change, or

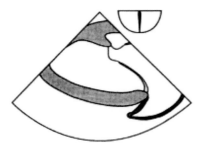

e. TG two chamber

Figure 4.3 (e). Transgastric two-chamber view.
Usual probe tip depth: 40–50 cm.
Transducer angle: 80–110°.
Transducer tip: anteflexion of the tip may be required.
Anatomy imaged: left ventricle (inferior and anterior walls), mitral valve including chordae and papillary muscles, left atrium.
Video 4.5.

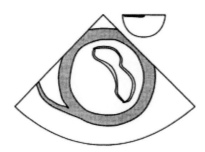

f. TG basal SAX

Figure 4.3 (f). Transgastric basal short-axis view.
Usual probe tip depth: 40–50 cm.
Transducer angle: 0–20°.
Transducer tip: anteflexion of the probe tip usually required.
Anatomy imaged: left and right ventricle, mitral valve, tricuspid valve.
Video 4.6.

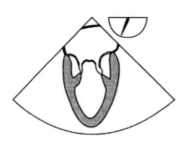

g. ME mitral commissural

Figure 4.3 (g). Mid-esophageal mitral commissural view.
Usual probe tip depth: 30–40 cm.
Transducer angle: 60–70°.
Transducer tip: retroflexion may be required to view the true left ventricular apex. Neutral tip position for viewing the mitral valve.
Anatomy imaged: left ventricle, left atrium, mitral valve.
Video 4.7.

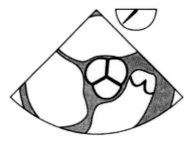

h. ME AV SAX

Figure 4.3 (h). Mid-esophageal aortic valve short-axis view.
Usual probe tip depth: 25–35 cm; usually needs to be 5–10 cm withdrawn from optimal ME four-chamber view.
Transducer angle: 30–60°.
Transducer tip: usually neutral position.
Anatomy imaged: aortic valve, coronary ostia and coronary arteries, interatrial septum, right ventricular outflow tract and pulmonary valve.
Video 4.8.

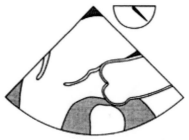

i. ME AV LAX

Figure 4.3 (i). Mid-esophageal aortic valve long-axis view.
Usual probe tip depth: 25–35 cm; at same level as aortic valve short-axis view.
Transducer angle: 120–160°.
Transducer tip: usually neutral position.
Anatomy imaged: aortic valve, aortic root and proximal ascending aorta. Left ventricular outflow tract, mitral valve, pulmonary artery.
Video 4.9.

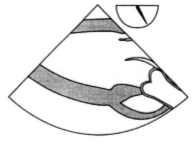

j. TG LAX

Figure 4.3 (j). Transgastric long-axis view.
Usual probe tip depth: 40–50 cm; at same level as transgastric short-axis view.
Transducer angle: 90–120°.
Transducer tip: neutral position or mild anteflexion.
Anatomy imaged: Left ventricle and left ventricular outflow tract, aortic valve, aortic root, mitral valve.
Video 4.10.

47

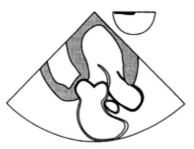

k. deep TG LAX

Figure 4.3 (k). Deep transgastric long-axis view.
Usual probe tip depth: 45–55 cm.
Transducer angle: 0–20°.
Transducer tip: pronounced anteflexion.
Anatomy imaged: left atrium, mitral valve, interventricular septum, left ventricle and left ventricular outflow tract, right ventricle, aortic valve and aortic root.
Video 4.11.

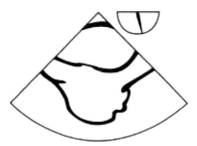

l. ME bicaval

Figure 4.3 (l). Mid-esophageal bicaval view.
Usual probe tip depth: 25–35 cm; at same level as aortic long-axis view.
Transducer angle: 80–110°.
Transducer tip: turn probe to the right; neutral probe tip position.
Anatomy imaged: superior vena cava, inferior vena cava, right atrium, crista terminalis, tricuspid valve, Eustachian valve, interatrial septum, left atrium.
Video 4.12.

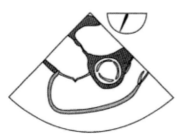

m. ME RV inflow-outflow

Figure 4.3 (m). Mid-esophageal right ventricular inflow–outflow view.
Usual probe tip depth: 30–40 cm; slightly advanced from aortic short-axis view.
Transducer angle: 60–90°.
Transducer tip: usually neutral probe tip position.
Anatomy imaged: right atrium, tricuspid valve, right ventricle, right ventricular outflow tract, pulmonary valve, main pulmonary artery.
Video 4.13.

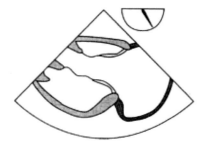

n. TG RV inflow

Figure 4.3 (n). Transgastric right ventricular inflow view.
Usual probe tip depth: 40–45 cm.
Transducer angle: 100–120°.
Transducer tip: from the transgastric short-axis view, the probe is turned to the right to place the right ventricle in the center of the display. The transducer is rotated as described above; anteflexion of the tip may be required.
Anatomy imaged: right atrium, tricuspid valve including chordae and papillary muscles, right ventricle.
Video 4.14.

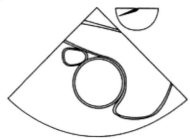

o. ME asc aortic SAX

Figure 4.3 (o). Mid-esophageal ascending aortic short-axis view.
Usual probe tip depth: 25–35 cm; usually approximately 5 cm less than mid-esophageal aortic valve short-axis view.
Transducer angle: 0–60°.
Transducer tip: turned to left to view left pulmonary artery.
Anatomy imaged: ascending aorta, pulmonary valve, main pulmonary artery, right pulmonary artery, left pulmonary artery.
Video 4.15.

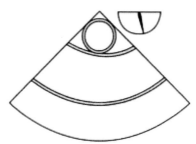

p. ME asc aortic LAX

Figure 4.3 (p). Mid-esophageal ascending aortic long-axis view.
Usual probe tip depth: 25–35 cm; usually at same level as mid-esophageal ascending aortic short-axis view.
Transducer angle: 100–150°.
Transducer tip: neutral position.
Anatomy imaged: ascending aorta, pulmonary artery.
Video 4.16.

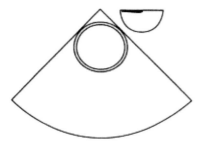

q. desc aortic SAX

Figure 4.3 (q). Descending aortic short-axis view.
Usual probe tip depth: 30–40 cm.
Transducer angle: 0°.
Transducer tip: neutral position. Probe rotated approximately 180° from mid-esophageal four-chamber view.
Anatomy imaged: descending thoracic aorta.
Video 4.17.

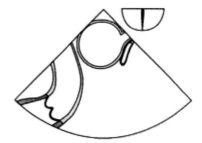

t. UE aortic arch SAX

Figure 4.3 (t). Upper esophageal aortic arch short-axis view.
Usual probe tip depth: 20–25 cm; at same level as upper esophageal aortic arch long-axis view.
Transducer angle: 90°.
Transducer tip: usually neutral position.
Anatomy imaged: main pulmonary artery and pulmonary valve, aortic arch, left subclavian and carotid arteries.
Video 4.20.

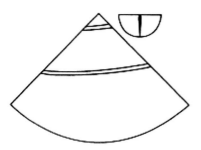

r. desc aortic LAX

Figure 4.3 (r). Descending aortic long-axis view.
Usual probe tip depth: 30–40 cm.
Transducer angle: 90–110°.
Transducer tip: neutral position; probe rotated approximately 180° from mid-esophageal four-chamber view.
Anatomy imaged: descending thoracic aorta.
Video 4.18.

Table 4.1. Myocardial segments as defined by the new [3] and old [4] classifications

New	Old
Anterior	Anterior
Anteroseptal	Anteroseptal
Inferoseptal	Septal
Inferior	Inferior
Inferolateral	Posterior
Anterolateral	Lateral

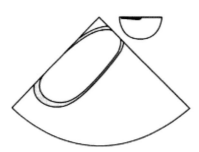

s. UE aortic arch LAX

Figure 4.3 (s). Upper esophageal aortic arch long-axis view.
Usual probe tip depth: 20–25 cm.
Transducer angle: 0°.
Transducer tip: neutral position.
Anatomy imaged: aortic arch, left subclavian and carotid arteries.
Video 4.19.

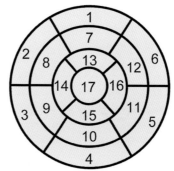

1. basal anterior
2. basal anteroseptal
3. basal inferoseptal
4. basal inferior
5. basal inferolateral
6. basal anterolateral
7. mid anterior
8. mid anteroseptal
9. mid inferoseptal
10. mid inferior
11. mid inferolateral
12. mid anterolateral
13. apical anterior
14. apical septal
15. apical inferior
16. apical lateral
17. apex

Figure 4.4. New convention of myocardial segmentation. Reproduced with permission from Cerqueira *et al., Circulation* 2002; **105**: 539–42 [3]. See Video 4.19 (ME long-axis views, rotating from 0° to 130°; all six left ventricular walls are shown in the long axis).

Coronary Artery Territories

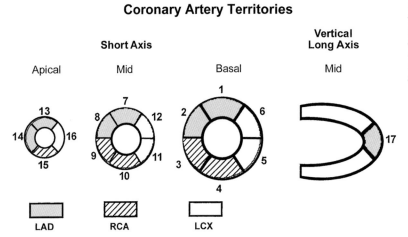

Figure 4.5. Distribution of coronary blood flow according to the 17 left ventricular segment convention. LAD, left anterior descending coronary artery; RCA, right coronary artery; LCX, left circumflex artery. Reproduced with permission from Cerqueira *et al.*, *Circulation* 2002; **105**: 539–42 [3].

ejection fraction. In fact, many of these techniques have been found to be no more accurate than the visual assessment of an experienced echocardiographer [5].

The function of each left ventricular segment can be assessed using a semi-quantitative technique. This assesses segmental motion, radial shortening, and wall thickening, and is described in detail in Chapter 9. In perioperative practice, wall motion abnormalities are not uncommon and may be related to preload [6], but a significant change may be an indication for considering either further coronary revascularization, or improving coronary blood flow with an intra-aortic balloon pump or relevant pharmacologic therapy.

The function of the right ventricle is generally more difficult to assess. The right ventricular free wall and the interventricular septum can be visualized in the mid-esophageal four-chamber view. Semi-quantitative assessment is possible, but in fact it is rarely undertaken formally. Right ventricular dilation is almost invariably a feature of severe ventricular dysfunction, and this can be easily seen and assessed. Prolonged right ventricular dilation may lead to dilation of the tricuspid annulus and tricuspid regurgitation, seen both on color-flow and continuous-wave Doppler.

Mitral valve

TEE is particularly useful for examining the mitral valve. The mid-esophageal long-axis views (Figs. 4.3a, 4.3b, 4.3c) enable the mitral valve to be examined in great detail. The mid-esophageal four-chamber view allows the mitral valve to be positioned in the center of the display, at which point the anterior leaflet is

seen on the left of the screen and the posterior leaflet on the right. As the transducer angle is increased, a transition point is reached, usually at about 60–80°, after which the anterior leaflet is seen on the right and the posterior on the left.

Also, the mid-esophageal four-chamber view can reveal valuable information about the mitral valve in the monoplane view; that is, without rotating the transducer [7]. By advancing and withdrawing the probe by approximately 3 cm, one can develop a view which focuses more predictably on the anatomical cross-section of the mitral valve. Thus withdrawing the probe, to the point where the non-standard five-chamber view (which includes the aortic valve and part of the aortic root) becomes visible, allows us to view the lateral scallop (P1) of the posterior leaflet and the lateral segment (A1) of the anterior leaflet (Video 4.22). Advancing the probe by 1–2 cm allows us to view the middle scallop (P2) of the posterior leaflet and the middle third (A2) of the anterior leaflet (Video 4.23). If we advance the probe further, the view will become disrupted as the probe enters the lower esophagus and stomach, but if we then gently withdraw the probe the four-chamber view reappears and the medial scallop (P3) of the posterior leaflet and the medial third (A3) of the anterior leaflet are seen (Fig. 4.6, Video 4.24).

The mid-esophageal views are particularly valuable for Doppler studies, since it is usually simple to align the Doppler beam directly parallel to the direction of blood flow through the mitral valve. The severity of mitral valve disease and the impact it may have on left atrial pressure can also be evaluated by studying

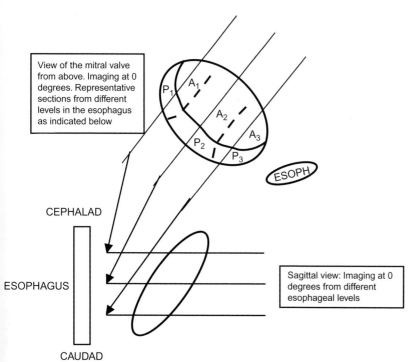

View of the mitral valve from above. Imaging at 0 degrees. Representative sections from different levels in the esophagus as indicated below

ESOPH

CEPHALAD

ESOPHAGUS

Sagittal view: Imaging at 0 degrees from different esophageal levels

CAUDAD

Figure 4.6. Advancing the TEE probe from the non-standard five-chamber view reveals the anterior leaflet segments and posterior leaflet scallops of the mitral valve. See also Chapter 7. See Video 4.23 (TG LAX), Video 4.24 (ME four-chamber rotated to right to focus on the tricuspid valve).

the Doppler waveform of blood flow through the superior pulmonary vein. This can usually be imaged from the mid-esophageal four-chamber view, although the probe may need to be turned slightly to the left.

The transgastric basal short-axis view (Fig. 4.3f) may be useful for viewing the full circumference of the mitral annulus, thus revealing any calcification or disruption of the annulus, in addition to abnormalities of the leaflets. Although it is possible to measure the annular circumference and the mitral valve area by planimetry, the nature of the mitral valve is such that this is rarely an accurate method, and it is not recommended.

The transgastric long-axis view (Fig. 4.3j) will position the mitral valve at approximately 90° to the direction of blood flow, but it will allow visualization of the papillary muscles and the chordae tendineae (Video 4.25). Although the deep transgastric view (Fig. 4.3k) will also allow visualization of the mitral leaflets, this view rarely adds to the evaluation of the mitral valve.

For more detail on TEE evaluation of the mitral valve the reader is referred to Chapters 7 and 16.

Aortic valve and aortic root

Imaging the aortic valve with TEE is not as comprehensive as imaging the mitral valve, but nonetheless a large amount of valuable information may be obtained and the study is usually successful. The aortic valve may be seen in the short axis using the mid-esophageal short-axis view shown in Figure 4.3h. This view may be acquired from the mid-esophageal four-chamber view simply by withdrawing the probe 2–5 cm and then rotating the transducer by up to 30° to bring the cross-sectional image in full view. In the patient with a normal valve, the three leaflets of the aortic valve should be easily seen to open and close.

In the long axis, the valve may be seen by rotating the transducer by 80–100°, thereby developing the mid-esophageal aortic valve long-axis view (Fig. 4.3i). Changing the probe depth is not usually necessary. However, withdrawing the probe slightly may be valuable in revealing the aortic root and the proximal part of the ascending aorta.

The mid-esophageal long-axis view (Fig. 4.3c) will also show the aortic valve leaflets, but this view is usually less useful than the mid-esophageal aortic valve long-axis view.

The aortic valve may also be visualized using the transgastric views. Figure 4.3j shows the transgastric long-axis view, and Figure 4.3k shows the deep transgastric view. The former is acquired by obtaining the transgastric mid-chamber short-axis view (Fig. 4.3d) and then rotating the transducer from zero to approximately

120°; minor alterations in probe depth may be necessary. The latter view is acquired by advancing the probe to a depth of 45–55 cm and then anteflexing the probe tip. This view may appear similar to the apical four-chamber view on transthoracic echo.

Mid-esophageal views do not allow for an alignment of the Doppler beam parallel to the direction of blood flow through the aortic valve. This is necessary for accurate calculations based on blood flow velocity in the left ventricular outflow tract and aorta. The transgastric views are valuable for a TEE assessment of the aortic valve. Either the transgastric long-axis or the deep transgastric view could be selected, but in practice it may be necessary to choose whichever gives the best signal and alignment.

The right heart

Starting with the mid-esophageal four-chamber view, the probe may be turned to the right to bring the tricuspid valve into the center of the display (Video 4.26). Thus the apical portion of the right ventricular free wall is on the right of the display and the basal section is on the left. The septal leaflet of the tricuspid valve is seen on the right. The leaflet on the left is either the anterior or the posterior leaflet, depending on the image orientation. Gently advancing or withdrawing the probe a few centimetres may be necessary to visualize all the leaflets adequately.

The mid-esophageal right ventricular inflow–outflow view (Fig. 4.3m) allows further examination of the tricuspid valve, the pulmonary valve, and the right ventricular free wall. It is often easily acquired from the mid-esophageal aortic valve short-axis view (Fig. 4.3h) simply by further rotating the probe by 20–30°, although it may be necessary to gently withdraw the probe by a few centimetres. The anterior leaflet of the tricuspid valve is visible on the right of the display and the posterior leaflet on the left. Thus the mid-esophageal four-chamber view (Fig. 4.3a) and the mid-esophageal RV inflow–outflow view (Fig. 4.3m) should allow visualization of all three leaflets of the tricuspid valve.

The pulmonary valve is also imaged using the mid-esophageal RV inflow–outflow view, where the valve is visible on the right-hand side of the display. The valve is seen in the long axis. The pulmonary valve is a semilunar trileaflet structure similar to the aortic valve, although less clearly visible on TEE.

The right atrium may be visualized using the mid-esophageal four-chamber view (Fig. 4.3a), which allows direct comparison of the size of the right and left atria. The right atrium may also be seen in part in the mid-esophageal AV short-axis view (Fig. 4.3h) and the mid-esophageal RV inflow–outflow view (Fig. 4.3m), which may be useful views for checking the integrity of the atrial septum. However, this may be better seen by developing the mid-esophageal bicaval view (Fig. 4.3l), which can simply be acquired from the mid-esophageal long-axis view (Fig. 4.3c) by turning the probe to the right (rotating the probe clockwise).

Finally, the transgastric right ventricular inflow view (Fig. 4.3n) may give usueful information about the inferior right ventricular free wall, the tricuspid valve, and the tricuspid chordae tendineae. It is acquired by obtaining the transgastric short-axis mid-papillary view (Fig. 4.3d) and turning the probe to the right to center the right ventricle in the image display (Videos 4.27, 4.28). The transducer is then rotated to between 100 and 120° until the apex of the right ventricle appears in the left-hand side of the display (cf. left ventricle in Fig. 4.3j).

Thoracic aorta

At the level of the diaphragm (i.e. just as the mid-esophageal four-chamber image is lost by advancing the probe) the probe is turned to the left, maintaining the angle of the transducer at 0°. The descending aorta is seen in cross-section as the decending aorta short-axis view is acquired (Fig. 4.3q). It may be useful to alter the image focus and depth to more clearly examine the aortic wall. The probe may be withdrawn and re-advanced, thus examining the descending aorta in cross-section. The transducer may then be rotated through 90° to acquire the long-axis view (Fig. 4.3r). Again, the probe may be withdrawn and advanced to examine the length of the descending aorta. The lack of anatomical landmarks in close proximity may make it difficult to accurately locate an abnormality. This may be facilitated either by noting the depth of the probe from the incisors, or by rotating the probe to orientate oneself to a cardiac landmark at a similar depth.

The ascending aorta may be viewed in the short and long axis. The mid-esophageal ascending aorta short-axis view (Fig. 4.3o) may be acquired from the mid-esophageal aortic valve short-axis view (Fig. 4.3h) by withdrawing the probe 3–5 cm and rotating the transducer, usually reducing the angle of rotation by 20–30°. Gently advancing and withdrawing the probe will bring the aortic root and ascending aorta into view in the center of the display. Rotating the transducer tip through a further 90–100° will develop the mid-esophageal ascending aorta long-axis view (Fig. 4.3p).

If the probe is withdrawn to a depth of 20–25 cm, with the transducer at 0° rotation, the upper esophageal aortic arch long-axis view may be acquired (Fig. 4.3s). With the probe turned to the right, the distal arch is seen on the right of the display and the proximal arch to the left. Rotating the probe through 90° allows the upper esophageal short-axis view (Fig. 4.3t) to be developed. Turning the probe to the right allows the proximal aortic arch to be viewed, and turning to the left views the distal arch. Turning the probe and retroflexing may bring the pulmonary artery and pulmonary valve into view on the left of the display.

TEE examination: sequence of view acquisition

For a comprehensive TEE exam it is not necessary, and many may deem it unusual, to acquire all the views in the sequence from Figures 4.3a–t as described above. Although there are a number of options when considering the sequence of views, it should be recognized that the goal of an echo study is to provide a comprehensive examination of the anatomy and physiology of the heart and great vessels. This may be achieved solely by one echo imaging modality, or by a combination of TTE and TEE.

Regarding the optimal TEE sequence, there is no universally agreed protocol, although many experts have recommended a logical sequence which may in certain circumstance be abbreviated. The following alternatives are worthy of consideration:

1. **Limited and goal-directed examination concentrating on the pathology in question**. This should only be considered when a recent and thorough TTE has already been performed and the relevant anatomical structures identified. A limited TEE examination may then be directed towards specific pathology. This is more common in the cardiological setting than during an intraoperative study.
2. **Structuring the acquisition sequence such that each anatomical structure is examined fully before moving on to the next structure** (e.g. mitral valve, aortic valve, left ventricle, etc.). This has the advantage of allowing the

sonographer to concentrate on each structure in turn, thus facilitating a full assessment. The disadvantage is that it may take longer, as the same view may be required repeatedly for an analysis of different structures, and numerous positional changes of the probe from the mid-esophagus to the stomach may affect image quality and be less well tolerated in a non-anesthetized patient. This can be miminized by recording a comprehensive examination and doing the analysis offline.

3. **Structuring the acquisition sequence based on the probe depth**, so that all the upper esophageal views, all the mid-esophageal views, and all the transgastric views are acquired without the need to continually advance and withdraw the probe. A comprehensive examination is undertaken at each of the three levels, although it probably does not matter if the study commences with the probe in the upper or mid-esophagus, or in the stomach.

In practice, cardiologists may carry out a combined study such as outlined in (1) above, and perioperative echocardiographers will perform a study based on an approach that combines both (2) and (3) above. This is practically convenient, allows for all the views to be obtained with least probe movement and manipulation, and yet allows the sonographer to concentrate on the relevant pathology. It thus reconciles two approaches which otherwise might appear contradictory

Normal values

A comprehensive echo examination will identify the relevant anatomy. However, cardiac disease will cause echocardiographic abnormalities, many of which can be measured and thus numerical values applied. These may be very useful, since they may help to identify and quantify chamber enlargement and hypertrophy, valve abnormalities, and abnormal patterns of flow on Doppler investigation.

Normal values of commonly measured and important parameters are shown in Appendix 4.1.

The abbreviated TEE exam in the operating room

The operating room is not an echo-friendly environment. Pressure for space is at a premium, particularly

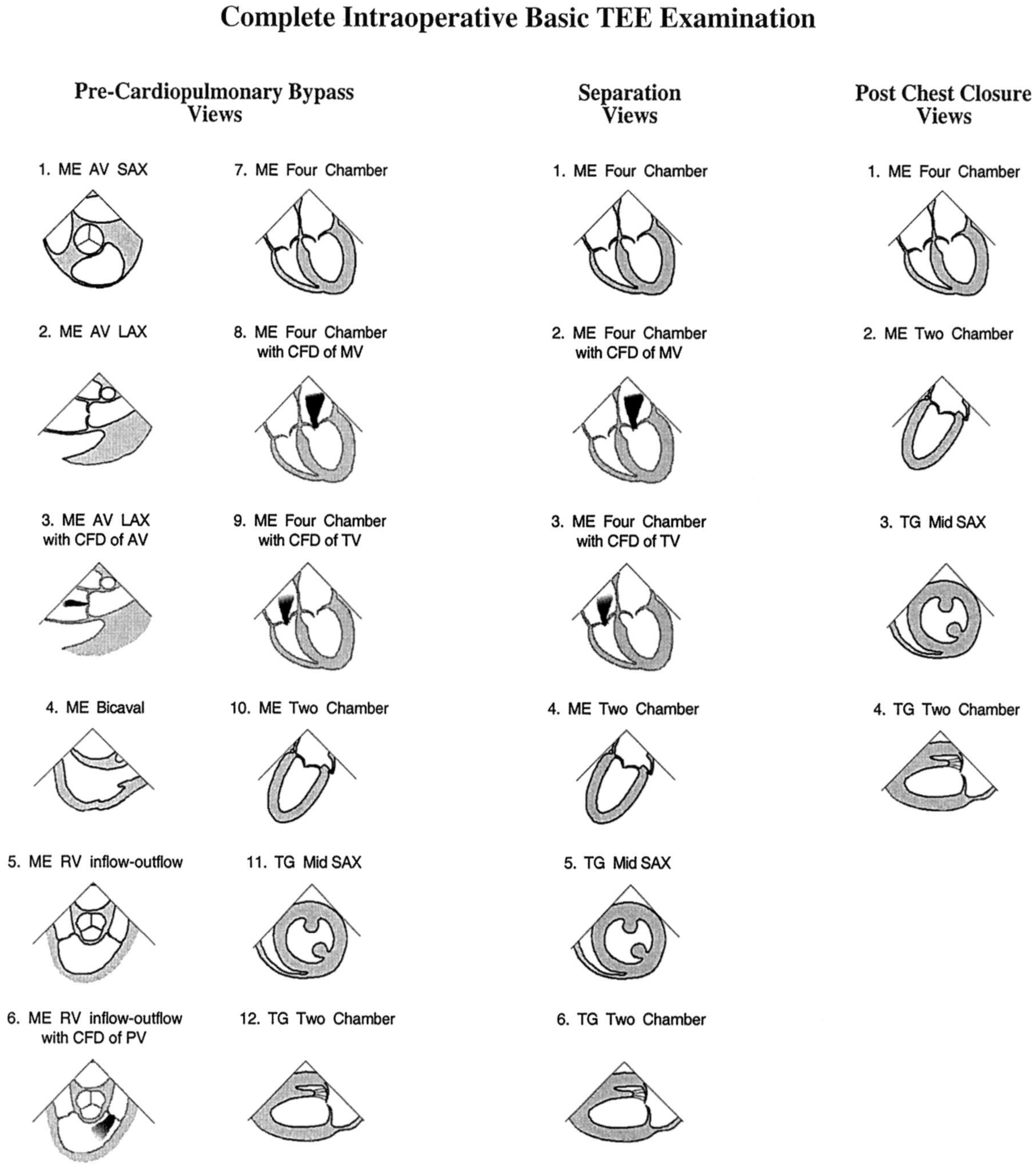

Complete Intraoperative Basic TEE Examination

Pre-Cardiopulmonary Bypass Views		Separation Views	Post Chest Closure Views
1. ME AV SAX	7. ME Four Chamber	1. ME Four Chamber	1. ME Four Chamber
2. ME AV LAX	8. ME Four Chamber with CFD of MV	2. ME Four Chamber with CFD of MV	2. ME Two Chamber
3. ME AV LAX with CFD of AV	9. ME Four Chamber with CFD of TV	3. ME Four Chamber with CFD of TV	3. TG Mid SAX
4. ME Bicaval	10. ME Two Chamber	4. ME Two Chamber	4. TG Two Chamber
5. ME RV inflow-outflow	11. TG Mid SAX	5. TG Mid SAX	
6. ME RV inflow-outflow with CFD of PV	12. TG Two Chamber	6. TG Two Chamber	

Figure 4.7. Suggested protocol for an abbreviated study in the cardiac surgery patient. Reproduced with permission from Miller *et al.*, *Anesth Analg* 2001; **92**: 1103–10 [9].

at the head of the patient, and necessary access to the patient during surgery may limit the possibility of conducting a painstaking and complete transesophageal exam utilizing all 20 standard views. However, recent guidelines on continuous quality improvement have recommended that a full TEE exam be under-

taken whenever possible, not least to establish a baseline and to allow for later remote consultation if necessary [8]. Nonetheless, an abbreviated study may be both indicated and useful, and such a study should yield the maximum of information in the least possible time. One example is shown in Figure 4.7 [9].

Table 4.2. Abbreviated transesophageal echo study for patients undergoing cardiac surgery

View	Modality	Structures	Timing
1. ME four-chamber	2D	LV inferoseptal and lateral walls; LV, LA, RV, RA dimensions; atrial septum; MV, TV	Pre & post surgery
	CFD	MV, TV	Pre & post surgery
	PWD	MV and TV blood flow	Pre surgery
2. ME two-chamber	2D	LV inferior and anterior walls, MV, LA appendage	Pre & post surgery
3. ME LAX	2D	LV anteroseptal and inferolateral walls, MV esp. prolapse, AV	Pre & post surgery
4. Bicaval view	2D	Superior and inferior venae cavae, RA, TV, atrial septum	Pre surgery
	CWD	TV	Pre surgery
5. ME AV SAX	2D	AV, coronary arteries, LA, RA	Pre surgery
6. ME RV inflow–outflow	2D	TV, RA, RV, PV, PA	Pre surgery
	CFD	TV, PV	Pre surgery
7. ME AV LAX	2D	AV, aortic root, LVOT	Pre surgery
	M-mode	LVOT dimension (where possible)	Pre surgery
	CFD	AV	Pre surgery
8. Descending aorta SAX/LAX	2D	Descending aorta	Pre surgery
9. Transgastric mid-cavity SAX	2D	LV wall segments (mid-cavity anterior, anteroseptal, inferoseptal, inferior, inferolateral, lateral)	Pre & post surgery
	M-mode	LV mid-cavity dimension, wall thickness	Pre surgery
10. Transgastric LAX (deep transgastric for CWD)	2D	LV anterior and inferior walls, MV papillary muscles and chordae	Pre & post surgery
	CWD	AV blood flow	Pre surgery
	PWD	LVOT blood flow	Pre surgery

2D, two-dimensional; AV, aortic valve; CFD, color-flow Doppler; CWD, continuous-wave Doppler; LA, left atrium; LAX, long-axis; LV, left ventricle; LVOT, left ventricular outflow tract; ME, mid-esophageal; MV, mitral valve; PA, pulmonary artery; PV, pulmonary valve; PWD, pulsed-wave Doppler; RA, right atrium; RV, right ventricle; SAX, short-axis; TV, tricuspid valve.

Such an approach is useful, although a patient-centered approach will be necessary to ensure that each study is appropriate to the individual patient.

The concept of an abbreviated study has spawned many others. Valuable additions to the approach described by Miller *et al.* [9] include transgastric long-axis views to enable accurate calculation of left ventricular stroke output and aortic valve area, and views of the descending aorta. These alternatives are included in Table 4.2, which represents a routine examination which we frequently use in the absence of any further pathology.

It should be noted that the sequence described is by no means mandatory. The choice of starting with the transgastric views may be considered, particularly if the probe is positioned under direct vision and advanced to 50 cm before the patient is "prepped and draped" for surgery. However, others may prefer to start with the mid-esophageal views.

Every study should be recorded and archived. Modern echo machines may record echo clips digitally, and these clips may be used to make measurements and calculations offline once the study is completed. This is very useful, since the echocardiographer can initially devote him- or herself to acquiring the best images without the need to hurry through the calculations.

One disadvantage of digital echo clip storage is that it is usually only possible to record and store specific and chosen clips rather than the whole study.

Where video tape is available, it may be useful to tape the whole study (Table 4.2).

Intraoperative echocardiographers should consider an echo examination and recording of the relevant clips following surgery as mandatory. However, the nature of the examination and the clips to be recorded will vary markedly depending on the nature of the surgery. Routine examination and recording of views 1–3 and 9 in Table 4.2 following surgery will give a good evaluation of left ventricular and mitral valve function. Other views may be examined and recorded as necessary.

The protocol described above utilizes 10 of the 20 standard views, but this could be further reduced if necessary. The recommended number of echo clips recorded as described above is 19. Some of these may be deleted offline if they simply duplicate normal anatomy.

The abbreviated study described above has not concentrated on any single pathology or anatomical structure, but it clearly is able to fulfill the criteria of a basic study – that is, to detect markedly abnormal ventricular filling or function, to identify extensive myocardial ischemia or infarction, to detect severe valve dysfunction, to identify cardiac masses or thrombi, to detect large air embolism, large pericardial effusions, and major abnormalities of the great vessels [2]. Interpatient variability will always be a factor in acquiring the necessary views speedily, and in both cardiology [10] and cardiac anesthesiology [2] experts have underlined the need for concentrating on the most pressing problem first. But we usually find it possible to examine and record the images as described before the onset of surgical diathermy damages the image quality.

Conclusion

The development of standard echocardiographic views, coupled with agreed terminology for describing manipulation of the TEE probe, has been essential for the development of TEE into an effective imaging modality. The 20 standard views described in 1999 form the basis of the TEE study. However, we should remember that in individual patients some modification of these views may be necessary to demonstrate the relevant pathology.

References

1. Daniel WG, Erbel R, Kasper W, et al. Safety of transesophageal echocardiography: a multicenter survey of 10,419 examinations. Circulation 1991; **83**: 817–21.

2. Shanewise JS, Cheung AT, Aronson S, et al. ASE/SCA guidelines for performing a comprehensive intraoperative multiplane transesophageal echocardiography examination: recommendations of the ASE Council for intraoperative echocardiography and the SCA Task Force for certification in perioperative transesophageal echocardiography. Anesth Analg 1999; **89**: 870–84.

3. Cerqueira MD, Weissman NJ, Dilsizian V, et al. Standardized myocardial segmentation and nomenclature for tomographic imaging of the heart: a statement for healthcare professionals from the Cardiac Imaging Committee of the Council on Clinical Cardiology of the American Heart Association. Circulation 2002; **105**: 539–42

4. Schiller NB, Shah PM, Crawford M, et al. Recommendations for quantitation of the left ventricle by two-dimensional echocardiography. American Society of Echocardiography Committee on Standards, Subcommittee on Quantitation of Two-Dimensional Echocardiograms. J Am Soc Echocardiogr 1989; **2**: 358–67.

5. London MJ. Ventricular function. In: Konstadt SN, Shernan S, Oka Y, eds., Clinical Transesophageal Echocardiography: a Problem-Oriented Approach, 2nd edn. Philadelphia, PA: Lippincott Williams & Wilkins, 2003: 63–78.

6. Seeberger MD, Cahalan MK, Rouine-Rapp K, et al. Acute hypovolemia may cause segmental wall motion abnormalities in the absence of myocardial ischemia. Anesth Analg 1997; **85**: 1252–7.

7. Maslow AD, Schwartz C, Bert A. Pro: single-plane echocardiography provides an accurate and adequate examination of the native mitral valve. J Cardiothoracic Vasc Anesth 2002; **16**: 508–14.

8. Mathew JP, Glas K, Troianos CA, et al. American Society of Echocardiography/Society of Cardiovascular Anesthesiologists recommendations and guidelines for continuous quality improvement in perioperative echocardiography. J Am Soc Echocardiogr 2006; **19**: 1303–13.

9. Miller JP, Lambert AS, Shapiro WA, et al. The adequacy of basic intraoperative transesophageal echocardiography performed by experienced anesthesiologists. Anesth Analg 2001; **92**: 1103–10.

10. Stewart WJ. Willie Sutton and the completeness and priorities of the Ideal Transoesophageal Echo Study in the year 2001. Eur J Echocardiogr 2001; **2**: 6–7.

Appendix 4.1: Reference values

Many of the normal dimensions have been derived from TTE data and are not validated for TEE.

Left ventricle

Normal

	Diastole	Systole
Short axis transgastric (cm)	2.4–5.4	1.8–4.2
Long axis (cm)	6.5–10.0	4.6–8.4
Wall thickness	0.6–1.1 (end diastolic)	

Mitral valve

Stenosis

	Normal	Mild	Moderate	Severe
Valve area (cm^2)	4–6	1.5–2.5	1–1.5	< 1
Mean pressure gradient (mmHg)	< 3	3–6	6–12	> 12
Pressure half-time (ms)	< 89	90–149	150–219	> 220

Regurgitation

	Mild	Moderate	Severe
CW jet density	Faint	Variable density parabolic shape	Dense
PW mitral inflow	A > D		Dominant E (V_{max} > 1.2 m/s)
Pulmonary vein flow	S > D	Blunted S	Reversed S
Jet area (cm^2)	< 4	4–8	> 8
Jet area/LA area	< 20	20–40	> 40 (or wall hugging to back wall)
Pressure half-time (ms)	90–149	150–219	> 220
VC (cm)	< 0.3	0.3–0.7	> 0.7
Regurg vol (mL)	< 35	35–59	> 60
Regurgitant fraction (%)	< 30	30–49	> 50
EROA (cm^2)	< 0.2	0.20–0.39	> 0.4

Aortic valve

Normal

Annulus (cm)	1.4–2.6
Sinus diameter (cm)	2.1–3.5
Sinotubular junction	1.7–3.4
Valve area (cm²)	2 – 4
V_{max} (m/s)	1.0–1.7
LVOT diameter (cm)	1.8–2.2
LVOT velocity (m/s)	0.7–1.1

Stenosis

	Mild	Moderate	Severe
Aortic valve area (cm²)	1.2–1.5	0.7–1.2	< 0.7
V_{max} (m/s)	2.5–3.0	3.0–4.0	> 4.0
Peak instantaneous pressure gradient (mmHg)	25–35	35–60	> 60
Mean pressure gradient (mmHg)	15–20	20–35	> 35
Velocity ratio LVOT/AV	0.35–0.4	0.25–0.35	< 0.25

Regurgitation

	Mild	Moderate	Severe
Jet deceleration pressure half-time (ms)	> 500 slow	500–250	< 200 very steep
VC width (cm)	< 0.3	0.3–0.6	> 0.6 (LAX)
Jet width/LVOT width (%)	< 25	25–65	> 65
Regurgitant volume (mL)	< 30	30–60	> 60
Regurgitant fraction (%)	< 30	30–50	> 50
EROA (cm²)	< 0.1	0.1–0.3	> 0.3

Tricuspid valve

Regurgitation

	Mild	Moderate	Severe
Jet area (cm²)	< 5	5–10	> 10
VC width (cm)		< 0.7	> 0.7
Hepatic vein flow	Systolic dominant	Systolic blunting	Systolic reversal

5

Normal valves

Dominique Bettex, Pierre-Guy Chassot

Introduction

Transesophageal echocardiography (TEE) is a well-known and accepted technique to assess valvular anatomy, function, and pathology. A detailed and comprehensive assessment of the different valves of the heart should be part of routine TEE examination. The American Society of Echocardiography Council for Intraoperative Echocardiography created guidelines for performing a comprehensive examination, consisting of a set of anatomically directed cross-sectional views [1]. This document is the collective result of an effort that represents the consensus views of both anesthesiologists and cardiologists who have extensive experience in perioperative echocardiography. We will be using mostly their standardized approach to assess the four valves of the heart.

Mitral valve

Anatomy

The mitral valve (MV) is a complex entity constituted of six different parts: two leaflets, 120 chordae tendineae, two papillary muscles, the annulus, the fibrous skeleton of the heart, and the left ventricular walls. During diastole, the MV allows rapid filling of the left ventricle under conditions of low pressure with minimal gradient (< 4 mmHg). The degree of opening of the leaflets reaches about 70° and the MV opening surface is 4–6 cm². During systole, the MV has to act as a resistance to oppose high left ventricular pressures (up to 200 mmHg). The intraventricular pressure forces the leaflets against each other on the coaptation surface, called the zona rugosa. The coaptation surface results from an active balance between closing and tethering forces (Fig. 5.1). Dilation of the annulus will lead to a diminution of this coaptation surface and to an imbalance of these forces; mitral regurgitation (MR) will ensue.

Normal MV function depends upon the complex interactions of all the different components of the valve.

The anterior leaflet covers two-thirds of the valve orifice but occupies one-third of the annulus circumference. The posterior leaflet occupies approximately two-thirds of the annulus circumference but covers only one-third of the valve orifice. The base of the anterior leaflet lies in close proximity to the left and non-coronary cusps of the aortic valve. The combined surface area of the mitral leaflets is twice that of the mitral orifice, permitting large areas of coaptation. The two leaflets are joined at the anterolateral and posteromedial commissures, each of which is associated with a corresponding papillary muscle. Following the Carpentier nomenclature (Fig. 5.2), the posterior leaflet consists of three scallops: lateral (P1), middle (P2), and medial (P3). For descriptive purposes, the anterior leaflet is also divided into three parts: lateral third (A1), middle third (A2), and medial third (A3).

The annulus is composed of fibroelastic tissue and completely encircles the orifice in a cone-like shape. During systole, the annulus is a saddle-shaped ellipse, whereas it is almost round at end-diastole. This saddle shape is particularly relevant for the diagnosis of mitral valve prolapse, since the level of the annulus will appear deeper in the ventricular cavity in the transverse view (0°) than in the longitudinal view (120°) (Fig. 5.3) [2]. To avoid false positives, the diagnosis of mitral valve prolapse should be made exclusively in the longitudinal view.

The mean mitral valve annular diameter for normal individuals is between 20 and 38 mm at early diastole. Because of its elliptical or D-shape, it also varies depending on the plane of visualization (Fig. 5.4). The annulus fibrosus of the mitral annulus becomes thinner and poorly defined as it extends posteriorly from the left and right trigones. This portion of the annulus is poorly supported and is prone to dilation. The posterior leaflet of the mitral valve is attached to this portion of the annulus. Dilation of the

59

Core Topics in Transesophageal Echocardiography, ed. Robert Feneck, John Kneeshaw, and Marco Ranucci.
Published by Cambridge University Press. © Cambridge University Press 2010.

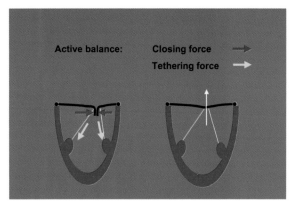

Figure 5.1. Mitral leaflets coaptation.

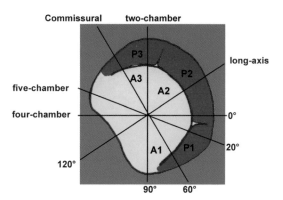

Figure 5.2. Carpentier nomenclature: mitral valve viewed from the left ventricle as in a basal transgastric view, showing the positions of the different examination planes of a multiplane transesophageal probe.

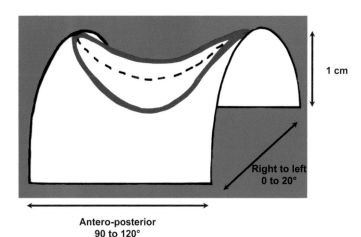

Figure 5.3. Saddle shape of the mitral annulus.

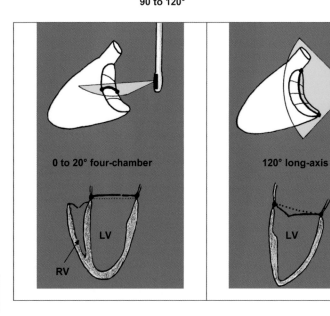

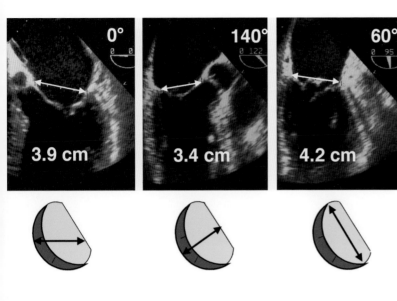

Figure 5.4. Diameter of the mitral valve annulus: the diameter of the valve varies as a function of the plane of the view, due to the D-shape of the valve.

annular attachment of the posterior leaflet creates an increase in tension on the middle scallop (P2) of the posterior leaflet, thus explaining why 60% of chordal tears occur at the P2 scallop.

The chordae tendineae are strong fibrous cords extending from the margins of the leaflets to the papillary muscles. They are divided as follows:

- first-order chordae – insert into the free edge of the leaflets
- second-order chordae – insert into the ventricular side of the leaflets
- third-order chordae – insert into the base of the leaflets

Chordae from both papillary muscles insert into both leaflets.

The papillary muscles are large trabeculae carneae. Each papillary muscle has a consistent relationship with its respective commissural area (anterolateral and posteromedial). The anterolateral papillary muscle is more commonly supplied by two separate arteries, the left anterior descending and circumflex coronary arteries, while the posterior descending coronary artery, arising usually from the right coronary artery, alone supplies the posterior papillary muscle. This explains the greater incidence of posterior papillary muscle dysfunction or rupture due to ischemia.

The subvalvular apparatus pulls the annulus and base of the heart toward the ventricular apex during systole, thereby shortening the longitudinal axis of the left ventricle (LV). It provides support for the leaflets, facilitating coaptation and preventing prolapse.

Two-dimensional imaging

Lambert *et al.* developed a systematic MV examination to improve intraoperative identification of mitral segments, identify the precise localization of the pathology, and determine the mechanism of MR [3]. TEE correctly identified 96% of mitral segments as being normal or abnormal in the prospective group. In the retrospective study (non-systematic assessment), only 70% of segments were correctly identified. They concluded that a systematic approach improves both the identification of mitral segments and the precise localization of pathologies, and may improve the diagnosis of the mechanism of MR.

The MV is examined through four mid-esophageal and two transgastric views. The mid-esophageal views are all developed by first positioning the transducer posterior to the mid level of the left atrium (LA), approximately 30–35 cm distal to the incisors, and directing the imaging plane through the mitral annulus parallel to the transmitral flow. Retroflexion of the probe is often necessary. The multiplane angle is then rotated forward to develop the mid-esophageal four-chamber view (Fig. 5.5). The posterior leaflet P1 is to the right of the image display, and the anterior mitral leaflet A3 is to the left. The multiplane angle is further rotated to 60°; a transition in the image occurs, beyond which the posterior leaflet is to the left of the display and the anterior to the right (Fig. 5.6). At this transition angle, the imaging plane is parallel to the line that intersects the two commissures of the MV and forms the mid-esophageal mitral commissural

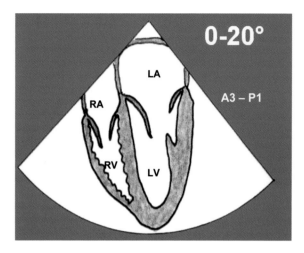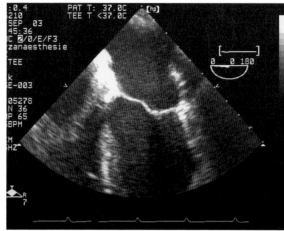

Figure 5.5. Four-chamber view (0–20°). LA, left atrium; LV, left ventricle; RA, right atrium; RV, right ventricle. Video 5.1.

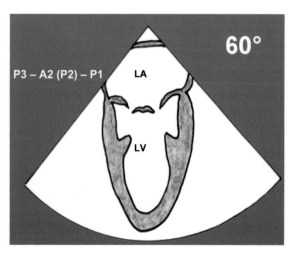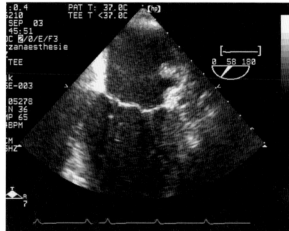

Figure 5.6. Commissural view (60°). LA, left atrium; LV, left ventricle. Video 5.1.

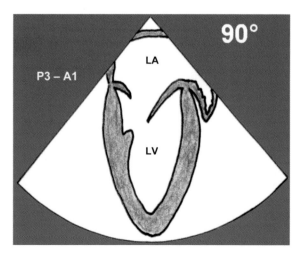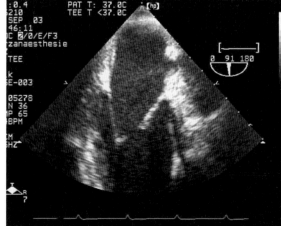

Figure 5.7. Two-chamber view (90°). LA, left atrium; LV, left ventricle. Video 5.1.

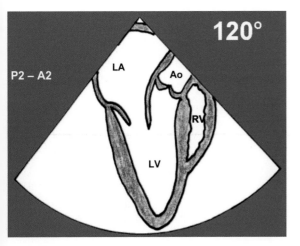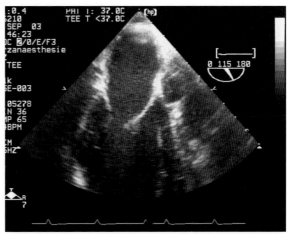

Figure 5.8. Longitudinal view (120°). LA, left atrium; LV, left ventricle; RV, right ventricle; Ao, aorta. Video 5.1.

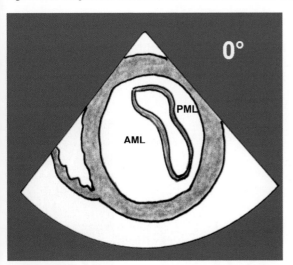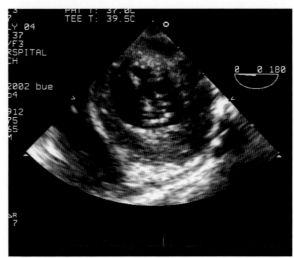

Figure 5.9. Transgastric short-axis view (0°). AML, anterior mitral leaflet; PML, posterior mitral leaflet. Video 5.2.

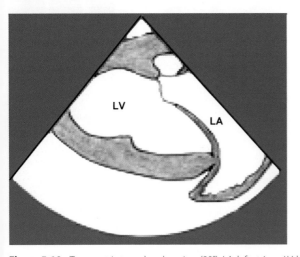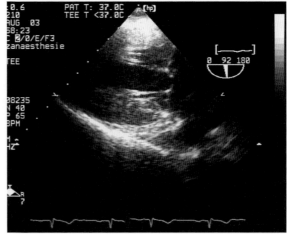

Figure 5.10. Transgastric two-chamber view (90°). LA, left atrium; LV, left ventricle. Video 5.2.

view. P1 is to the right of the display, P3 is to the left, and A2 or P2 is in the middle of the display, depending on the level of the cross-section.

Further rotating the angle of the probe will gradually show a different part of the MV with the mid-esophageal two-chamber view (Fig. 5.7) and the mid-esophageal longitudinal view (Fig. 5.8). In the two-chamber view, P3 is to the left of the display and A1 is to the right; the longitudinal view shows P2 on the left of the display and A2 on the right.

Transgastric views of the MV are developed by advancing the probe until the transducer is level with the base of the LV, approximately 35–40 cm distal to the incisors (Fig. 5.9). Anteflexion of the tip of the probe and a slight withdrawing of the probe will usually be required to obtain an orthogonal short-axis view of the MV; the posteromedial commissure is in the upper left of the display, the anterolateral commissure is to the lower right of the display, the posterior leaflet is to the right, and the anterior leaflet to the left. A true orthogonal view of the MV is often difficult to obtain. In this case, the probe is withdrawn to visualize the posteromedial commissure, then further advanced in the stomach to obtain the anterolateral commissure.

Rotating the multiplane angle forward to 90° will show the transgastric two-chamber view (Fig. 5.10). This view is useful for assessing the chordae tendineae (posterior chordae on the top of the screen, anterior on the bottom) and the papillary muscles.

Doppler imaging

Color Doppler should be used in every cross-section to detect, localize, and semi-quantify MV flow abnormalities.

The transmitral Doppler spectral flow depends upon the instantaneous relationship between the left atrial and the left ventricular pressures (Fig. 5.11). It will vary according to both pre- and afterload, aging, and heart rate. To assess the maximal velocity of transmitral flow accurately, the sampling point of the pulsed-wave Doppler (PWD) should be placed at the tip of the mitral leaflets (if measuring stroke volume at this site, the sample should be placed at the level of the annulus) and kept to a minimal size (around 3–5 mm; Fig. 5.12). The Doppler beam should be aligned such that the angle between the beam and the direction of flow is as close to zero as possible. Flow across the mitral valve should be assessed in four different periods: the isovolumic relaxation time (IVRT), the rapid filling phase or E wave, diastasis, and the

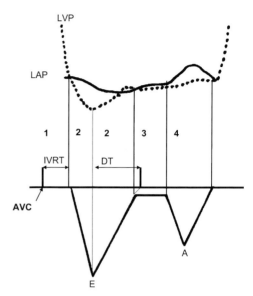

Figure 5.11. Normal transmitral flow and transvalvular pressure gradient: (1) isovolumic relaxation time (IVRT) from the aortic valve closure (AVC) to the mitral valve opening; (2) rapid filling phase (E wave); (3) diastasis; (4) atrial contraction (A wave). DT, deceleration time.

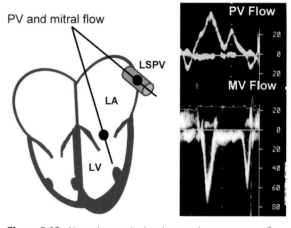

Figure 5.12. Normal transmitral and transpulmonary venous flow. LA, left atrium; LV, left ventricle; PV, pulmonary vein; LSPV, left superior pulmonary vein; MV, mitral valve.

active filling phase or atrial contraction or A wave (Figs. 5.11, 5.12; Table 5.1).

To complete a functional assessment of the mitral valve, pulmonary venous flow should be interrogated (Fig. 5.12; Table 5.1). The sampling point of the PWD should be placed 1–2 cm into preferably the upper left pulmonary vein. The pulmonary venous flow consists of four different waves: the systolic wave, divided into S1 (depending upon atrial relaxation)

Table 5.1 Normal Doppler values in adults

Localization		Velocity and times
Mitral valve flow	E	0.6–1.3 m/s
	A	0.4–0.8 m/s
	E/A	1.2–1.4
	DT	180–210 ms
	IVRT	75–90 ms
Pulmonary venous flow	S	0.5 m/s
	D	0.4–0.5 m/s
	A	– 0.15 m/s
LVOT flow		0.8–1.3 m/s
Aortic valve flow		1–1.7 m/s
Tricuspid valve flow	E	0.3–0.7 m/s
	A	0.3 m/s
Pulmonary artery flow		0.6–0.9 m/s

DT, deceleration time; IVRT, isovolumic relaxation time.

and S2 (depending upon LV function), the diastolic passive wave or D, and the diastolic retrograde wave during atrial systole or rA. The diastolic part of the pulmonary flow varies in accordance with transmitral flow.

Aortic valve

Anatomy

The aortic valve is a semilunar valve with three cusps of similar size. Each cusp is attached to the aortic root at its lower edge along a U-shaped line with its upper free edge protruding into the lumen of the aorta. Behind each cusp is a pocket-like dilation of the aortic root called the sinus of Valsalva. The three cusps are named according to their relationship with the coronary arteries: the left, right, and non-coronary cusps. The adjacent portions of the left and non-coronary cusps are in continuity with the base of the anterior leaflet of the mitral valve. The anterior halves of the right and left cusps are in contact with the muscular interventricular septum. The region where the aortic valve joins the cylindrical portion of the ascending aorta is called the sinotubular junction. The left ventricular outflow tract (LVOT) is situated just inferior to the aortic valve. The whole aortic root is generally considered during assessment of the aortic valve. It includes the aortic valve annulus, the cusps, the sinuses of Valsalva, the right and left coronary ostia, the sinotubular junction, and the proximal ascending aorta.

Two-dimensional and Doppler imaging

The aortic root is usually easy to visualize with TEE and needs three cross-sections for a complete evaluation. The mid-esophageal five-chamber view (0°) should initially be obtained, approximately 30–35 cm distal to the incisors. With the aorta brought into the middle of the display, the multiplane angle is rotated forward between 30° and 60° to develop the mid-esophageal short-axis view of the valve (Fig. 5.13). The left coronary cusp is then at the top of the screen (posterior), the right coronary cusp is at the bottom (anterior), and the non-coronary cusp is situated on the left of the display, facing the interatrial septum. Planimetry

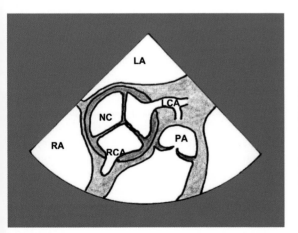
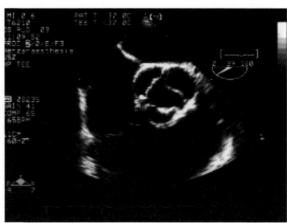

Figure 5.13. Short-axis view of the aortic valve and coronary arteries. RA, right atrium; LA, left atrium; PA, pulmonary artery; LCA, left coronary artery; RCA, right coronary artery; NC, non-coronary cusp. Video 5.3.

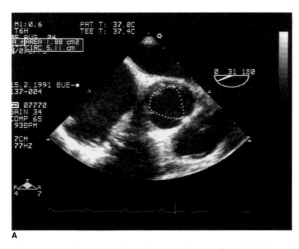
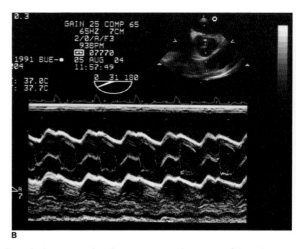

Figure 5.14. (A) Aortic valve planimetry (1.88 cm²) and (B) M-mode through the aortic valve showing a normal opening of the valve in a 14-year-old patient.

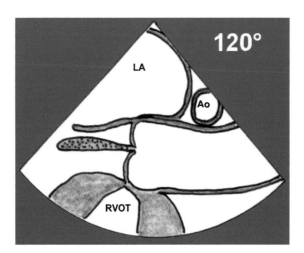
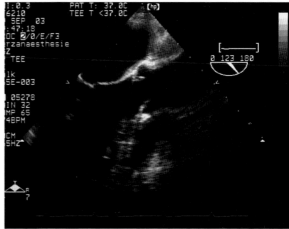

Figure 5.15. Long-axis view of the aortic root. LA, left atrium; Ao, aorta; RVOT, right ventricular outflow tract. Video 5.3.

of the opening surface of the valve may be traced in this view (Fig. 5.14A). The correct opening and closure of the aortic valve, as well as the exclusion of a LVOT obstruction, may also be assessed in this view, using M-mode perpendicularly to the valve (Fig. 5.14B). Color-flow Doppler is applied in this cross-section to assess the presence of aortic regurgitation and to estimate the size and location of the regurgitation orifice.

The probe is withdrawn or anteflexed slightly to move the imaging plane superiorly through the sinuses of Valsalva to show the right and left coronary ostia and arteries. The probe is then advanced through and then inferiorly to the valve to produce a short-axis view of the LVOT.

As the multiplane angle is further rotated to 120–160°, the long axis of the aortic valve will be obtained with a good view of the LVOT, the sinotubular junction, and the proximal ascending aorta (Fig. 5.15). The LVOT is on the left of the display and the ascending aorta on the right. The cusp on the bottom of the screen (anterior) is the right coronary cusp. The cusp situated superiorly is usually the non-coronary cusp, but may be the left coronary cusp, depending upon the location of the imaging plane. In this view we can measure the dimensions of the aortic annulus, sinotubular junction, and proximal ascending aorta. The aortic annulus is measured during systole at the point of attachment of the aortic valve cusps to the LVOT (Fig. 5.16). The normal aortic annulus dimension in

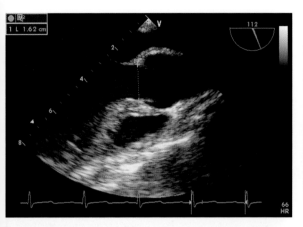

Figure 5.16. Aortic valve annulus diameter: the diameter is 1.62 cm.

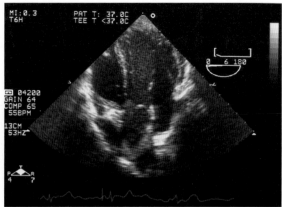

Figure 5.18. Deep transgastric long-axis 0° view. Video 5.5.

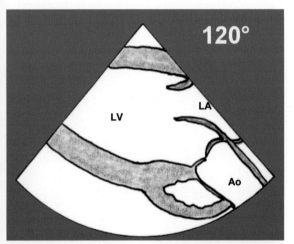

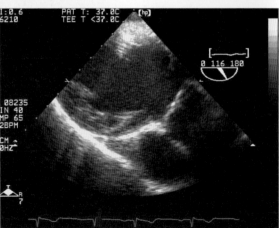

Figure 5.17. Transgastric long-axis 120° view. LA, left atrium; LV, left ventricle; Ao, aorta. Video 5.4.

systole is usually between 1.8 and 2.5 cm. Color-flow Doppler applied in this view will allow the detection and semi-quantification of aortic regurgitation.

The transgastric long-axis view is obtained by advancing the probe in the stomach, approximately 35–40 cm distal to the incisors, to obtain the classical short-axis basal view of the LV. The multiplane angle is then rotated forward to 90–120° to visualize the aortic valve on the bottom right of the display (Fig. 5.17). The LV outflow is directed away from the transducer in this view. Finally, a deep transgastric view may be obtained by advancing the probe deep into the stomach and positioning the probe adjacent to the LV apex at 0°. The probe is then maximally anteflexed and slightly rotated to obtain the aortic valve in long-axis centered at the bottom of the display (Fig. 5.18). The aortic valve is located in the far field at the bottom of the display with the LV outflow directed away from the transducer. These last two views offer the best alignment with the aortic flow for Doppler assessment. Detailed assessment of the anatomy of the valve is difficult in these views, however, because the LVOT and the aortic valve are located too far from the transducer.

Peak outflow velocity at the aortic valve is obtained most easily with continuous-wave Doppler, assuming there is no obstruction to outflow proximal to the valve such as a subaortic membrane or hypertrophic obstructive cardiomyopathy. Blood flow velocity in the LVOT is measured using PWD, positioning the sample point in the middle of the LVOT, just inferior to the aortic cusps. Normal LVOT and aortic outflow velocities are less than 1.5 m/s (Fig. 5.19; Table 5.1).

Tricuspid valve

Anatomy

The tricuspid valve consists of three leaflets (anterior, posterior, and septal), attached via multiple chordae

67

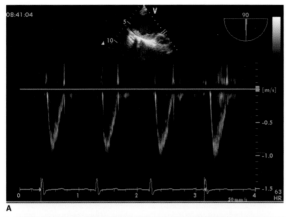

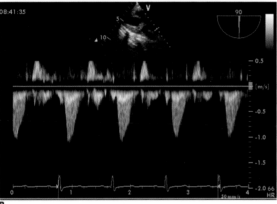

Figure 5.19. (A) Pulsed-wave Doppler through the LVOT; (B) continuous-wave Doppler through the aortic valve.

tendineae to three small papillary muscles, a supporting annular ring, and a portion of the myocardium of the right ventricular (RV) free wall. The septal insertion of the tricuspid valve is normally slightly (1–2 cm) more apical than the insertion of the anterior mitral leaflet (Fig. 5.5). Exceptions to this rule are the atrioventricular canal, in which case both valves are inserted at the same level, and the Ebstein anomaly, where parts of the tricuspid valve are inserted much lower in the ventricular cavity. The tricuspid valve has chordae tendineae inserted on three papillary muscles, one of which is on the interventricular septum: another way to differentiate it from the mitral valve.

Two-dimensional imaging

The tricuspid valve can be visualized with TEE from three main views. The probe should be positioned in the mid or lower esophagus to obtain a four-chamber view (Fig. 5.20). The septal and posterior leaflets will be visualized. The probe should be advanced and withdrawn as appropriate to map the entire tricuspid annulus from its inferior to superior extent.

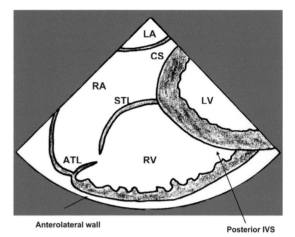

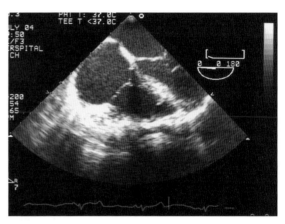

Figure 5.20. Low-esophageal view (0°). LA, left atrium; LV, left ventricle; RA, right atrium; RV, right ventricle; STL, septal tricuspid leaflet, ATL, anterior tricuspid leaflet; CS, coronary sinus; IVS, interventricular septum. Video 5.6.

The multiplane angle is then rotated forward to 60° to obtain the RV inflow–outflow view, with the anterior (close to the aorta) and posterior (on the free wall of the RV) leaflets of the tricuspid valve on the left of the screen as well as the pulmonary valve on the right of the screen (Fig. 5.21). The use of color Doppler will allow the detection of tricuspid flow abnormalities.

The probe should then be further advanced in the transgastric position and rotated to 30° to obtain a short-axis view of the valve, with the anterior and posterior leaflets seen at the top of the screen and the septal leaflet at the bottom of the screen (Fig. 5.22). Further rotating the multiplane angle to 110° will show the RV inflow long-axis view, with the posterior wall at the top of the screen, the anterior wall with the papillary muscles at the bottom of the screen, and the posterior and anterior leaflet of the tricuspid valve (Fig. 5.23).

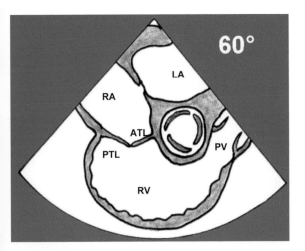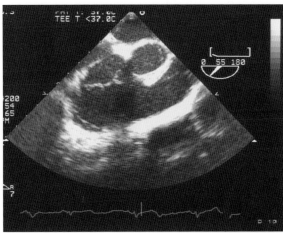

Figure 5.21. RV inflow–outflow view (60°). LA, left atrium; RA, right atrium; RV, right ventricle; PTL, posterior tricuspid leaflet; ATL, anterior tricuspid leaflet; PV, pulmonary valve. Video 5.6.

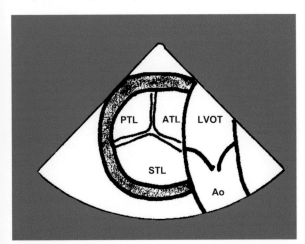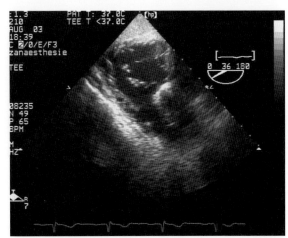

Figure 5.22. Transgastric short-axis view of tricuspid valve. Ao, aorta; LVOT, left ventricular outflow tract; PTL, posterior tricuspid leaflet; ATL, anterior tricuspid leaflet; STL, septal tricuspid leaflet. Video 5.7.

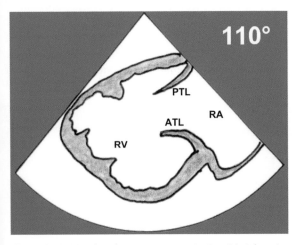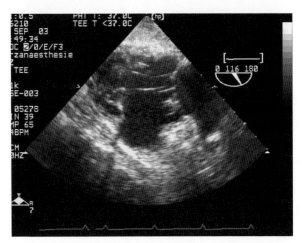

Figure 5.23. RV inflow, long-axis transgastric view. RA, right atrium; RV, right ventricle, ATL, anterior tricuspid leaflet; PTL, posterior tricuspid leaflet. Video 5.8.

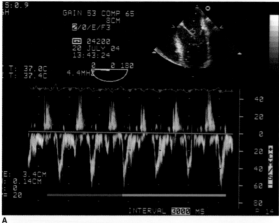

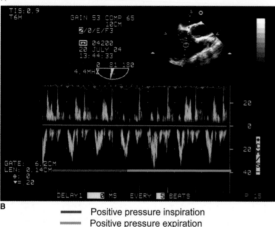

▬ Positive pressure inspiration
▬ Positive pressure expiration

Figure 5.24. (A) Mitral and (B) tricuspid Doppler flow variations during respiration.

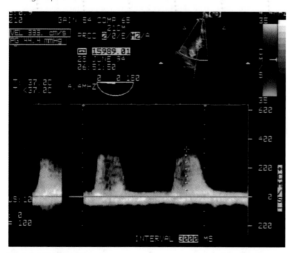

Figure 5.25. Pulmonary pressure assessment with continuous Doppler through the tricuspid regurgitation. The maximal velocity of the tricuspid regurgitation is 3.33 m/s, giving a pressure gradient of 44 mmHg between the right ventricle and the right atrium. Assuming a central venous pressure of 10 mmHg, the systolic pulmonary pressure in this case would be around 54 mmHg.

Doppler imaging

The transtricuspid Doppler flow will be optimally obtained in the mid-esophageal view between 0° and 60°, using PWD. Normal tricuspid blood flow is M-shaped, similar to that of transmitral blood flow, with the two characteristic waves, E and A, occurring in early diastole and during atrial systole (Table 5.1). Tricuspid blood flow velocities are usually lower than transmitral blood flow velocities and show a greater variation during ventilation, particularly during positive pressure ventilation. During mechanical ventilation, the E/A peak velocity ratio exhibits cyclic changes within the respiratory cycle so that an accurate analysis is difficult. During positive pressure inspiration, transmitral blood flow peak velocities will increase while tricuspid blood flow peak velocities will decrease. The reverse is true during expiration (Fig. 5.24).

Color Doppler at the tricuspid level allows rapid detection of tricuspid regurgitation, which is a frequent and often normal finding, particularly in mechanically ventilated patients. Using continuous Doppler recording parallel to the regurgitant flow allows the determination of the maximal velocity of the backward flow (V_{max}). Applying the Bernoulli equation, the gradient between RV and atrium may be assessed:

$$\Delta P = 4V_{max}^2 \tag{5.1}$$

In the absence of a VSD, adding the central venous pressure value to this gradient will give a good estimation of the RV systolic pressure. In the absence of any pathology of the RV outflow tract or of the pulmonary valve, the systolic ventricular pressure will be the same as the systolic pulmonary pressure (Fig. 5.25). When the quality of the tricuspid regurgitant flow envelope is not good enough for an accurate measurement, it may be enhanced by saline or contrast-medium injection through a peripheral or central venous line.

Pulmonary valve

Anatomy

The pulmonary valve is a semilunar valve consisting of three cusps and an annulus. The RV infundibulum and the pulmonary valve are part of the right ventricular outflow tract (RVOT) that extends from the crista supraventricularis to the bifurcation of the main pulmonary artery.

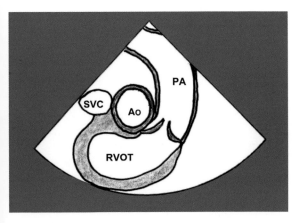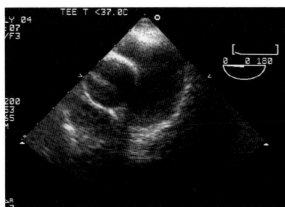

Figure 5.26. Basal view of the pulmonary valve. PA, pulmonary artery; RVOT, right ventricular outflow tract; Ao, aorta; SVC, superior vena cava. Video 5.9.

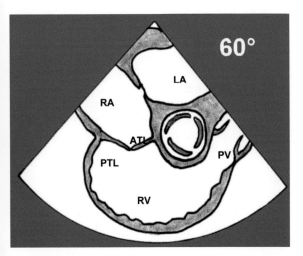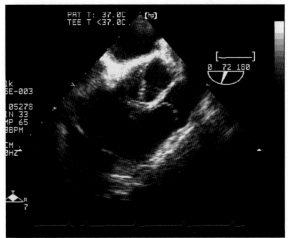

Figure 5.27. Mid-esophageal inflow–outflow view (60°). LA, left atrium; RA, right atrium; RV, right ventricle; PTL, posterior tricuspid leaflet; ATL, anterior tricuspid leaflet, PV, pulmonary valve. Video 5.10.

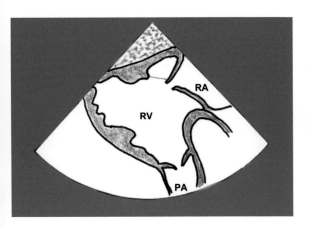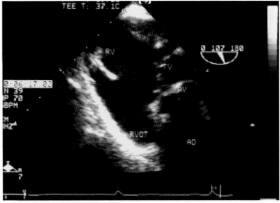

Figure 5.28. Transgastric view of the RVOT and pulmonary valve (120°). RA, right atrium; RV, right ventricle; PA, pulmonary artery; RVOT, right ventricular outflow tract; TV, tricuspid valve; AO, aorta; AV, aortic valve. Video 5.11.

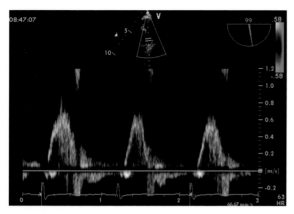

Figure 5.29. Transpulmonary pulsed-wave Doppler flow (basal view 0°).

Two-dimensional and Doppler imaging

The pulmonary valve and the main pulmonary artery can be assessed with TEE in the basal view (Fig. 5.26). The probe is placed in the upper-esophagus 0° to 30–40° plane, approximately 28–30 cm distal to the incisors. Pulmonary artery flow velocity can be assessed in this view, using pulsed Doppler. Other views to assess the pulmonary valve are the mid-esophageal inflow–outflow 60° view previously described (Fig. 5.27), as well as the deep transgastric 120° view (Fig. 5.28). This last view offers the best alignment for Doppler interrogation of the pulmonary valve. Transpulmonary flow is similar to transaortic flow with lower velocity (Table 5.1). Normally, RV ejection velocity increases more gradually, exhibits a peak occurring close to mid-ejection, and decreases more slowly than LV ejection velocity (Fig. 5.29). Pulmonary insufficiency or stenosis should be excluded applying color Doppler in each of these views.

Conclusion

A systematic approach should be applied to a TEE assessment of the cardiac valves, as it should for every TEE examination. The standardized approach outlined in this chapter provides a useful framework for such an assessment.

References

1. Shanewise JS, Cheung AT, Aronson S, *et al.* ASE/SCA guidelines for performing a comprehensive intraoperative multiplane transesophageal echocardiography examination: recommendations of the ASE Council for intraoperative echocardiography and the SCA Task Force for certification in perioperative transesophageal echocardiography. *Anesth Analg* 1999; **89**: 870–84.

2. Levine RA, Triulzi MO, Harrigan P, Weyman AE. The relationship of mitral annular shape to the diagnosis of mitral valve prolapse. *Circulation* 1987; **75**: 756–67.

3. Lambert AS, Miller JP, Merrick SH, *et al.* Improved evaluation of the location and mechanism of mitral valve regurgitation with a systematic TEE examination. *Anesth Analg* 1999; **88**: 1205–12.

Further reading

1. Savage RM, Aronson S, eds. *Comprehensive Textbook of Intraoperative Transesophageal Echocardiography.* Philadelphia, PA: Lippincott Williams & Wilkins, 2005: 65–93.

2. Zoghbi WA, Enriquez-Sarano M, Foster E, *et al.* Recommendations for evaluation of the severity of native valvular regurgitation with two-dimensional and Doppler echocardiography. *J Am Soc Echocardiogr* 2003; **16**: 777–802.

6

Aortic valve disease

Justiaan Swanevelder

Introduction

Every complete transesophageal echocardiographic (TEE) examination should include a careful assessment of the aortic valve. TEE can define the severity and mechanisms of aortic stenosis (AS) and aortic regurgitation (AR). Although in general cardiology TEE is rarely needed for evaluating the aortic valve, it may be appropriate when transthoracic image quality is poor and to evaluate other structures more fully, including the mitral valve [1].

In perioperative practice, many surgeons appreciate the ability of TEE to define the abnormality preoperatively, confirm their intraoperative impression, and assess the postoperative results, even in routine valve replacement procedures.

Aortic valve anatomy

The aortic valve (AV) forms part of the aortic root, together with the three sinuses of Valsalva, two coronary ostia, and sinotubular junction (Fig. 6.1).

It consists of a crown-shaped aortic annulus (annulus fibrosa) and three similar semilunar cusps – the right coronary cusp (RCC), left coronary cusp (LCC), and non-coronary cusp (NCC). The leaflets are composed of a dense collagen layer, covered by a thin avascular collagen layer, and endothelium. The RCC and right sinus of Valsalva are positioned anteriorly and give rise to the right coronary artery (RCA). The left coronary artery (LCA) originates from the LCC and left sinus of Valsalva. The posterior of the three cusps, the NCC, lies adjacent to the interatrial septum. The fibrous thickenings seen at the central portion of the free edges of the normal leaflets are called the nodules of Arantius. After years of function the leaflets may develop this thickening of the edges, as well as filamentous strands on them. These small filamentous strands, called Lambl's excrescences, up to 5 mm in length, are connected to the aortic valve and may appear in the left ventricular outflow tract during diastole, or on the aortic side during systole. They may be mistaken for vegetations, and are usually an incidental finding in elderly patients who are otherwise well [2].

The sinotubular junction (STJ) connects the root to the proximal ascending aorta. It is circular and thicker than the adjacent sinuses, defining the start of the ascending aorta. The STJ plays an important role in suspending the semilunar aortic valve leaflets. The upper limit of the normal aortic valve annulus diameter is 2.6 cm, and the STJ is 3.4 cm. Together with the sinuses of Valsalva and ascending aorta diameters, these are important measurements for surgical decision making. The plane of the AV is oblique, with the right posterior side more inferior than the left anterior side. Therefore the origin of the LCA is superior to that of the RCA.

The normal AV area (AVA) is 2.5–3.5 cm^2 with a normal echo pressure gradient across the valve of 2–4 mmHg assuming a flow velocity of 60–100 cm/s. The opening and closing of the leaflets inside a normal

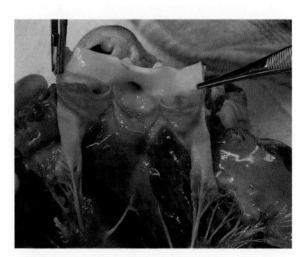

Figure 6.1. Pathology specimen demonstrating the aortic root with the crown-shaped annulus fibrosa, three semilunar cusps (LCC, RCC, and NCC), three sinuses of Valsalva, and the sinotubular junction.

73

Core Topics in Transesophageal Echocardiography, ed. Robert Feneck, John Kneeshaw, and Marco Ranucci.
Published by Cambridge University Press. © Cambridge University Press 2010.

aortic root is smooth and symmetrical. During systole in a compliant aorta, root dilation precedes and aids in the opening of the leaflets. This root dilation pulls the closed leaflets apart and reduces the frictional forces at the commissures [3]. A minimal pressure gradient of around 2 mmHg is therefore enough to open the aortic valve. At maximum displacement of the leaflets during early systole, the aortic valve opening is nearly circular, which is followed by a triangular shape in later systole. The echocardiography appearance of the normal valve orifice may therefore be circular or triangular, depending on whether it was observed earlier or later in systole (Fig. 6.2).

There is a gap between the body of the leaflets and the aortic wall (sinuses of Valsalva). If the pressure gradient is increased in a compliant root from 2 to 8 mmHg, the valve area increases strikingly by about 25%. This effect is absent in a stiff, non-compliant

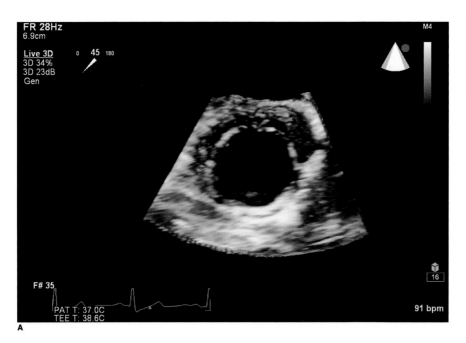

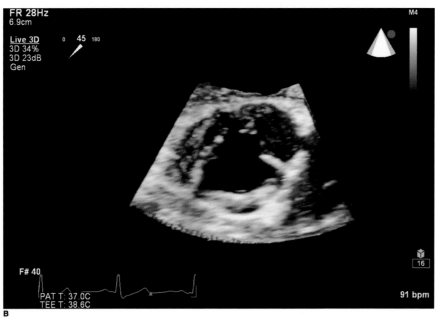

Figure 6.2. The short axis of the aortic valve demonstrating (A) an almost circular opening during early systole and (B) a triangular opening later in systole.

root. When the cardiac output is increased under certain physiological conditions (e.g. exercise), the normal aortic valve therefore copes by increased dilation of the root, and increased pushing and bending of the leaflets towards the aortic wall.

In a stiff, non-compliant aortic root the valve opening tends to be asymmetric and delayed, with considerable wrinkling of the leaflets [4]. The systolic aortic root dilation with the active "pull-release" open-

ing mechanism of the leaflets is absent. The leaflets show a lot of inertia and therefore open much later after the development of a gradient between the left ventricle (LV) and the aorta. The valve opening remains circular and does not become triangular, as seen in a compliant root. There has been speculation that the leaflet wrinkling inside a non-compliant root may increase leaflet stresses and may be responsible for earlier calcification. A stiff root seems to function

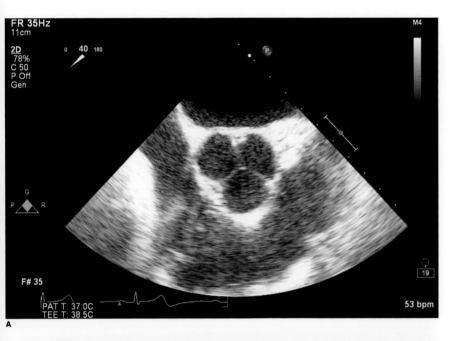

Figure 6.3. Mid-esophageal short-axis (ME AV SAX) views of the aortic valve in (A) diastole and (B) systole.

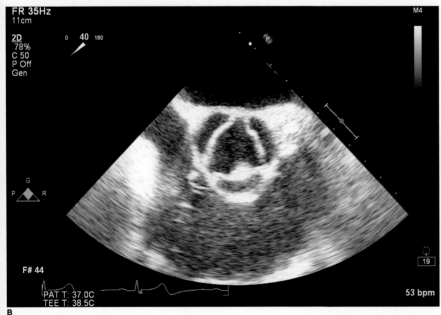

at maximum level of efficiency and is not able to increase the valve area during a period of increased cardiac output. The compliance of the aorta and root also has a very important role in directing coronary blood flow to the myocardium [5].

The AV is continuous with the anterior leaflet of the mitral valve (MV). It connects the aortic root to the left ventricular outflow tract (LVOT). The left atrium is immediately posterior to the AV while the pulmonary valve (PV) is anterior. Abnormalities of any of the components of the AV or the adjacent structures can affect the function of the valve.

TEE examination of the AV

Evaluation of the AV should include two-dimensional (2D) images from several views and angles together with color-flow Doppler (CFD) and spectral Doppler

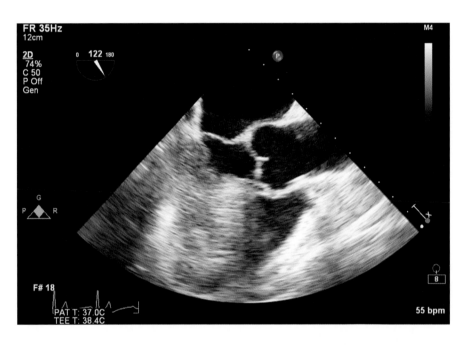

Figure 6.4. Mid-esophageal long-axis (ME AV LAX) view of the aortic valve, demonstrating its continuity with anterior leaflet of the mitral valve.

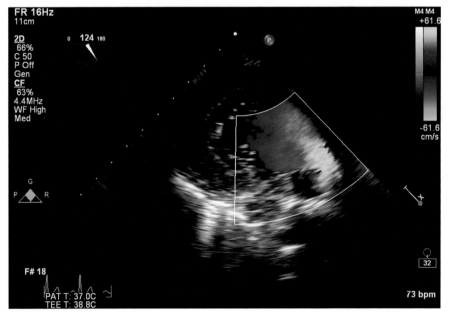

Figure 6.5. Transgastric long-axis (TG LAX) view of the aortic valve.

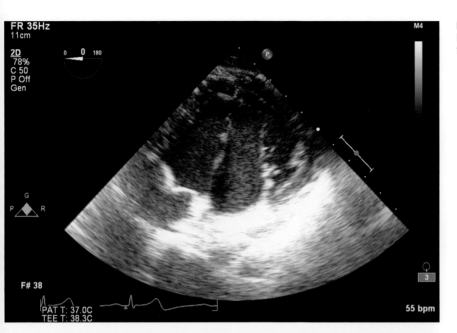

Figure 6.6. Deep transgastric long-axis (deep TG LAX) view of the aortic valve.

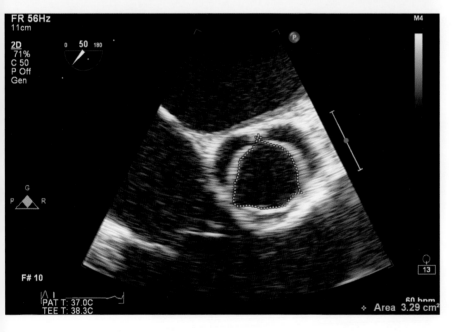

Figure 6.7. Planimetry of the aortic valve area in the mid-esophageal short-axis view.

displays. By assessing the AV in the short-axis and long-axis views all the different components of the valve and root can be examined.

The aortic valve can be imaged using the following standard views [6]:

1. mid-esophageal short-axis view (ME AV SAX; Fig. 6.3)
2. mid-esophageal long-axis view (ME AV LAX; Fig. 6.4)
3. transgastric long-axis view (TG LAX; Fig. 6.5)
4. deep transgastric long-axis view (deep TG LAX; Fig. 6.6)

The ME AV SAX view is used to assess the structure and function of each of the three individual cusps and to perform planimetry (Fig. 6.7).

The typical "Mercedes Benz" sign during diastole is an easy image to obtain at approximately 40° by advancing and withdrawing the transducer slowly

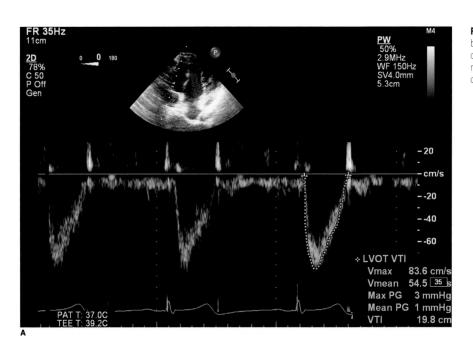

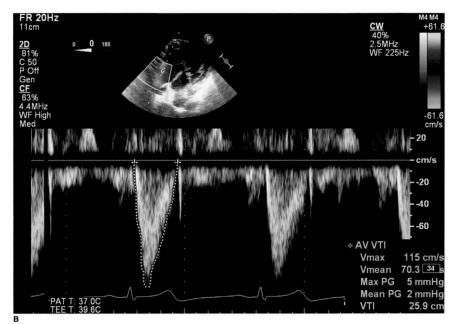

Figure 6.8. Spectral Doppler image of blood flow velocity across the aortic valve, demonstrating a pressure drop within normal limits. (A) Pulsed-wave Doppler; (B) continuous-wave Doppler.

until all three commissures of the valve and the leaflet bodies are visible. The RCC is viewed in the anterior position at the bottom of the display, with the LCC on the right side of the image and the NCC on the left side of the image adjacent to the interatrial septum.

From the ME AV SAX view it is easy to demonstrate the ME AV LAX view by keeping the probe in the same position and rotating the angle to around 120–140°. The LVOT is visible together with the long-axis view of the valve, the whole aortic root, and the ascending aorta. The RCC is anterior at the bottom of the screen with the NCC seen above it. The ME AV LAX view clearly demonstrates the function of the NCC and RCC. If the transducer is slightly rolled to the patient's left side, the LCC will be visible instead of the NCC. In the ME AV LAX view it is easy to measure the diameter of the annulus, sinuses of Valsalva, STJ, and ascending aorta. The mid-esophageal short-axis,

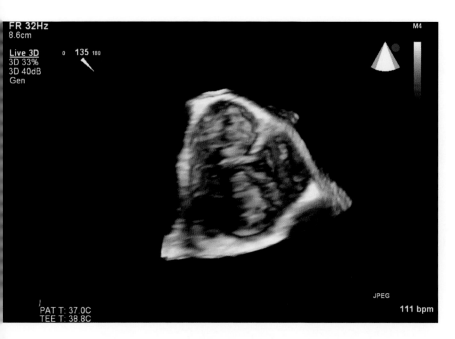

Figure 6.9. A 3D dataset cropped to demonstrate the aortic valve in 3D.

long-axis and five-chamber views cannot be used for Doppler measurements of flow velocity, because the ultrasound wave is perpendicular to the blood flow.

By advancing the transducer into the stomach and flexing slightly, the transgastric mid-papillary short-axis view can be seen. If the operator then rotates the transducer to approximately 110° the TG LAX view is found, with the LVOT and AV towards the bottom right of the image. The deep TG LAX view is more difficult to obtain. At 0° the transducer is advanced until the echo image disappears, and it is then fully flexed. By gentle withdrawal the transducer will make contact with the superior wall of the stomach, and the deep TG LAX view should appear. The LVOT and AV will be seen in the bottom left part of the conventional image. It is important to find this view very gently in order to avoid damage to the stomach, gastroesophageal junction, or esophagus. In the two transgastric views the Doppler signal can be aligned almost parallel to blood flow through the AV and flow velocity can usually be measured using one or both of the views to calculate the pressure gradient via the Bernoulli equation (Fig. 6.8). It is important for the echocardiographer to be familiar with both transgastric approaches, because they require considerable practice and expertise and are often difficult to obtain.

When evaluating the aortic valve for stenosis or regurgitation, it is always essential to assess the geometry and contractility of the LV in all the views. The recent introduction of real-time 3D (RT3D) trans-esophageal echocardiography will certainly advance our knowledge of both normal AV physiology and pathology (Fig. 6.9).

Aortic stenosis

Aortic valve disease is very common in Western populations. About 25% of people over 65 years of age have aortic sclerosis, and 3% of those over 75 years have severe stenosis [7]. Aortic sclerosis is diagnosed when there is an ejection systolic murmur present in the aortic valve region due to calcification in the ascending aorta, with associated turbulent flow. In this condition there is minor disruption of the aortic valve and minimal obstruction to flow. There may be thickening or calcification of one or more leaflets of a tricuspid AV, but in contrast to aortic stenosis, leaflet opening is not markedly restricted and the velocity through the valve is less than 2.5 m/s (Fig. 6.10; Videos 6.1–6.3). Aortic sclerosis is not innocent because it is an antecedent to clinically significant aortic valve stenosis and it acts as a marker of increased risk of cardiovascular events [8]. Aortic stenosis (AS) is differentiated from sclerosis when significant restriction of cusp movement and a raised transaortic peak velocity is seen on echocardiography [9].

Mechanisms of aortic stenosis

Calcific "degeneration" is the most common cause of AS in the elderly Western adult population (70–90 years

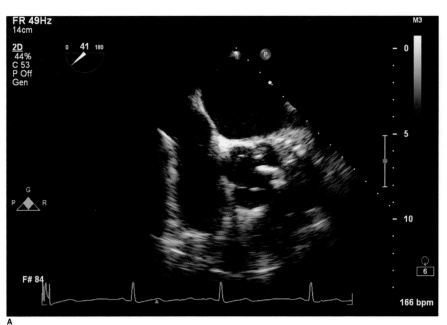

A

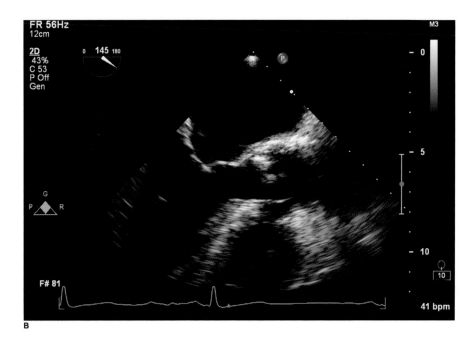

B

Figure 6.10. (A) Mid-esophageal short-axis (ME AV SAX) view of a patient with aortic sclerosis diagnosed by an ejection systolic murmur on examination, with subsequent confirmation on TEE, i.e. calcified immobile LCC with AVA around 2.8 cm² on planimetry. (B) ME AV LAX view of the same patient. (C) ME AV LAX view with added color-flow Doppler.

old). It begins with annular and leaflet thickening, which gradually becomes calcified (Fig. 6.11).

Although it seems that most patients with AS start off with aortic sclerosis, the rate of progression is not very clear [10]. The RCC is affected most commonly and often undergoes calcific fusion together with the NCC. These calcified leaflets have decreased mobility and are very echogenic. AS was once viewed as a "degenerative" disease but is now seen as an active inflammatory process which resembles atherosclerosis, and many of the risk factors are the same for both processes. Inflammation, lipid infiltration, dystrophic calcification, ossification, platelet deposition, and endothelial dysfunction have been observed in both diseases. Hypercholesterolemia, lipoprotein Lp(a), smoking, hypertension, and diabetes have been

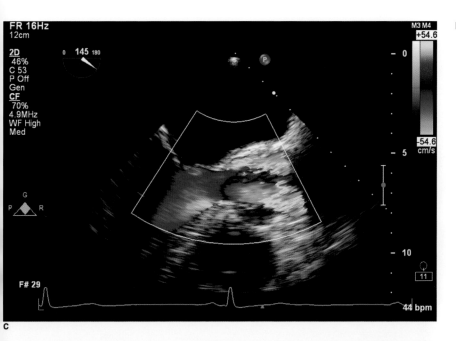

Figure 6.10 (*Cont.*)

C

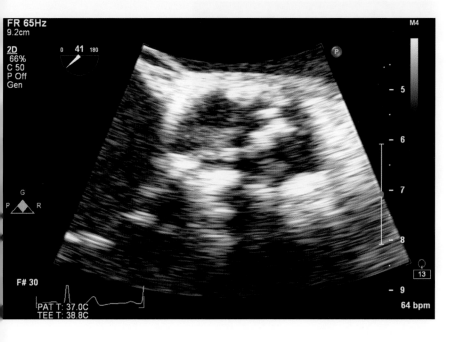

Figure 6.11. Mid-esophageal short-axis view of calcific degenerative aortic stenosis in systole, showing calcified, echogenic leaflets.

reported to be common risk factors for both of them [11]. Aortic valve disease is also a marker for coronary artery disease. Although controversial, it seems that higher doses of lipid-lowering statins may slow down the process of this disease, similar to their effect on coronary artery pathology [12]. There is some evidence that this effect occurs without a consistent relationship to cholesterol levels, suggesting that the beneficial result of statins may be caused by their anti-inflammatory effects rather than simply by lowering cholesterol [13,14]. Angiotensin converting enzyme (ACE) has also been shown to be involved not only in an unfavorable LV remodeling response in AS patients, but also in the progression of valve degeneration itself. A potential benefit has therefore been suggested for ACE inhibitors [15].

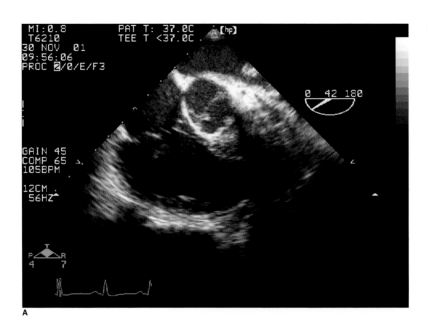

Figure 6.12. Bicuspid aortic valve: (A) mid-esophageal short-axis view, in systole; note raphe and secondary calcification; (B) mid-esophageal long-axis view, in systole.

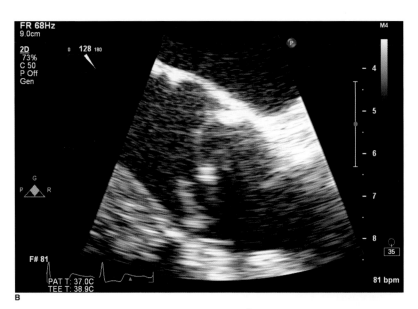

The congenital bicuspid AV has a 1–2% incidence, making it the most common cardiovascular malformation in humans [16]. These patients are usually male, and the high heritability of bicuspid aortic valve suggests that its determination is almost entirely genetic [17–20]. Patients may present with stenosis as a child or may undergo accelerated calcification of the abnormal AV and present in adulthood (50–60 years old). The two leaflets typically show either fusion of right and non-coronary cusps (19%) or fusion of right and left coronary cusps (80%), with a variation in coronary arrangement. Fusion of the left and non-coronary cusps is rare (Fig. 6.12; Videos 6.4–6.6) [21].

Patients with the most severely malformed bicuspid valves may require intervention during childhood. The bicuspid aortic valve is also associated with other congenital abnormalities including coarctation of the aorta (50–80%), interruption of the aortic arch (36%), and isolated ventricular septal defect (20%) [19,20,22]. Although a non-stenotic bicuspid aortic valve is often considered a benign lesion earlier in life,

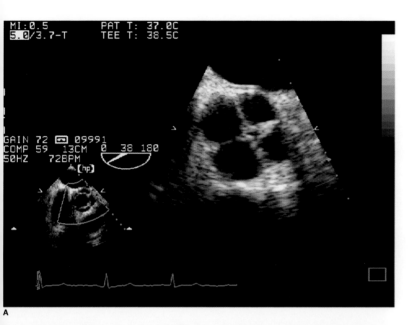

Figure 6.13. Quadricuspid aortic valve: (A) mid-esophageal short-axis view, in diastole; (B) mid-esophageal short-axis view, in diastole, with CFD.

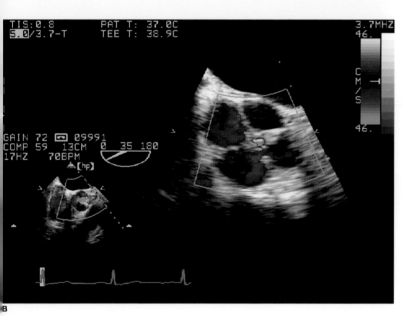

it has potential complications including aortic regurgitation, infective endocarditis, aortic dilation and dissection, resulting in considerable morbidity and mortality later in life. Unicuspid valves are very rare and may be a cause of stenosis. Quadrileaflet valves are also rare and are most frequently associated with mixed aortic valve disease (Fig. 6.13; Videos 6.7, 6.8) [23].

Although rheumatic heart disease may affect the AV, with leaflet thickening and decreased movement, it preferentially involves the mitral valve. Rheumatic

degeneration of the AV therefore rarely occurs in isolation. Commissural fusion occurs together with thickening and fibrosis of the leaflet edges, while the leaflet bodies are less affected in the earlier stage (Fig. 6.14; Video 6.9).

It is very clear that symptoms alone are not an adequate guide for the management of valve heart disease, and lack of symptoms does not predict an uncomplicated course. For example, patients with severe AS may remain completely asymptomatic but

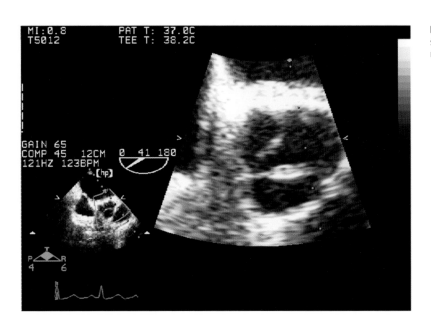

Figure 6.14. Rheumatic aortic valve stenosis, mid-esophageal short-axis view; note commissural fusion.

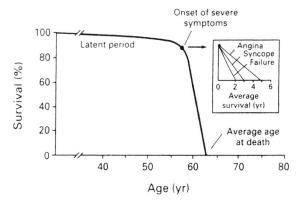

Figure 6.15. At the onset of symptoms survival is greatly reduced in the AS patient (see text for details).

are at risk of sudden death. Once angina, syncope, or heart failure develops, survival is greatly reduced (Fig. 6.15) [24].

About 75% of patients with symptomatic AS will be dead three years after the onset of symptoms, unless the AV is replaced [25]. When the peak flow velocity is more than 4.0 m/s, the likelihood of an asymptomatic AS patient being alive without a valve replacement in two years' time is only 21% (± 18%) [26]. In the era of modern echocardiography it is no longer appropriate to wait for a change in symptoms to guide management [1,27]. Even in the elderly, the prognosis for a patient with AS who receives valve replacement surgery is excellent. Age should therefore not be a contraindication in these patients, in the absence of

comorbid conditions [28,29]. The same principle applies to patients with poor LV function due to AS. Although patients with more severe stenosis, worse LV function, and more severe symptoms experience the greatest benefit from surgical relief of the obstruction, they also have a higher operative mortality [30].

TEE evaluation of aortic stenosis

TEE evaluation of AS starts with a 2D examination of the ME SAX and LAX views of the valve [31]. The leaflets may be thickened and calcified with a bright echogenic appearance and reduced mobility (Fig. 6.11). It may be difficult to recognize the leaflet edges, and planimetry of the open calcified AV is often very inaccurate, but it should be performed whenever feasible [32]. The calcification often creates acoustic shadows obscuring certain areas of the valve. Calcification of the annulus is an important finding, particularly in the intraoperative study. Doming of the leaflets during systole is another important sign of AS. Post-stenotic dilation of the aortic root and ascending aorta is common. It is important to look for LV hypertrophy or dilation, and for LA dilation as a result of the pressure overload. All findings must be communicated to the surgeon, because they will affect surgical options.

RT3D echocardiography is an exciting new development and will in future most likely become part of a complete AV examination dataset. The LVOT, root, origin of the coronary arteries, and STJ can be visualized well. However, the normal AV leaflets are thin and

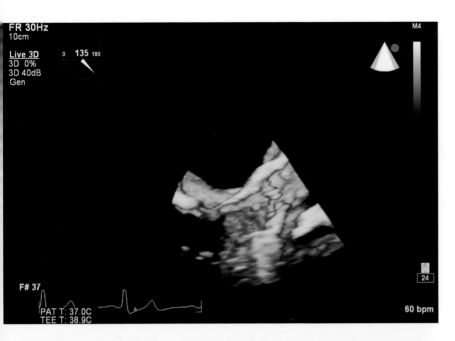

Figure 6.16. 3D ME LAX view of the aortic valve.

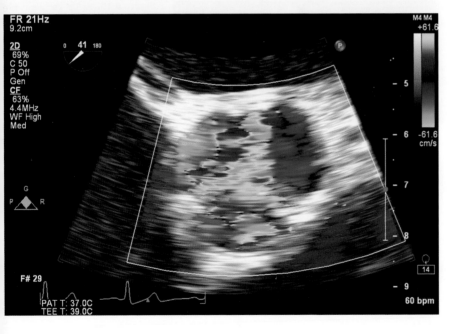

Figure 6.17. Calcific degenerative aortic stenosis. The mid-esophageal short-axis view in systole, with color-flow Doppler.

are at the lower limit of current 3D spatial and temporal resolution (see Chapter 22). This means that the leaflets cannot always be clearly investigated without artifact. RT3D echo has also not yet been validated to quantify severity of AS (Fig. 6.16) [33].

Color-flow Doppler usually demonstrates turbulence across the valve but does not quantify its severity (Figs. 6.17, 6.18). With the 2D image in the ME LAX AV view, the M-mode cursor can be aligned through the aortic valve and used to assess leaflet separation directly and as a percentage of aortic root diameter.

Quantification of severity of aortic stenosis

Continuous-wave Doppler (CWD) is applied to measure flow velocity across the valve and then calculate a pressure gradient using the Bernoulli equation (pressure gradient = $4V^2$) (see Chapter 13). The color Doppler

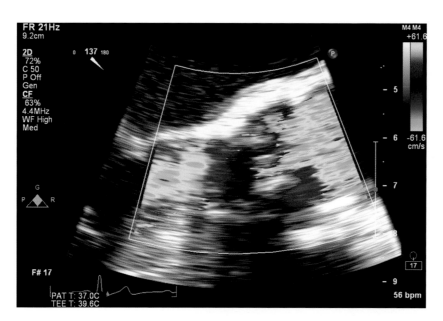

Figure 6.18. Calcific degenerative aortic stenosis. The mid-esophageal long-axis view in systole, with color-flow Doppler.

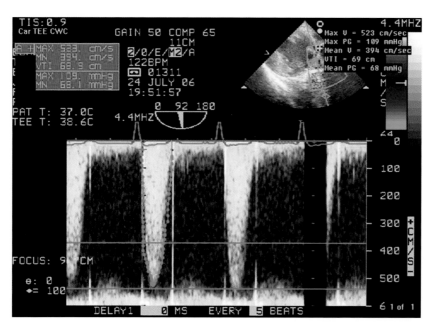

Figure 6.19. In this deep TG view, continuous-wave Doppler across a severely stenotic aortic valve measures an increased flow velocity and demonstrates a high pressure drop calculated with the Bernoulli equation. Note that the angle of the Doppler beam must be as parallel as possible to ensure an accurate measurement.

sector is useful to guide the echocardiographer towards the outflow tract and AV. To make an accurate measurement it is very important that the CWD wave is parallel to the direction of blood flow. Although it is more difficult to align the ultrasound beam correctly with TEE than with transthoracic echocardiography (TTE), this angle can usually be obtained in the TG LAX and deep TG views (Fig. 6.19).

A meticulous search for the maximal aortic flow velocity signal is essential. The high flow velocity jet of severe AS will have a typical audible sound. The flow pattern is helpful, because in severe AS the peak will occur during mid-systole, while in more moderate AS it will occur during early systole. The mean pressure gradient is obtained by accurately tracing the outline of the flow velocity signal. Severe AS is defined as a flow velocity more than 4.0 m/s, a mean pressure gradient more than 40 mmHg, and a peak pressure gradient more than 80 mmHg [34]. There is excellent anatomical and physiological correlation between

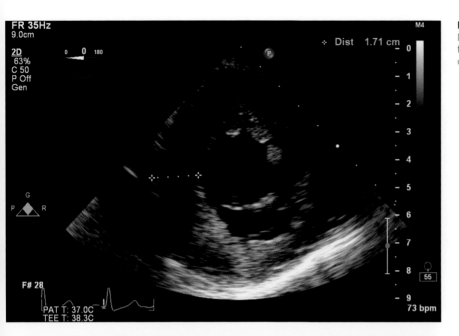

Figure 6.20. Severe concentric LV hypertrophy compensating for the pressure overload conditions of severe aortic stenosis.

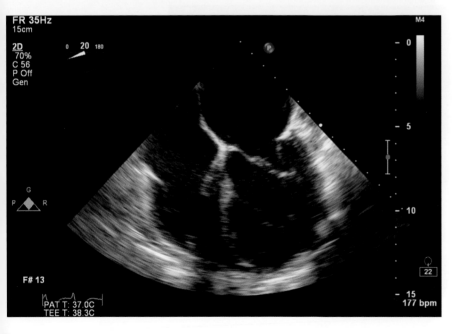

Figure 6.21. End-stage LV systolic dilation and failure due to longstanding severe aortic stenosis. In this situation the transvalvular pressure gradient may be decreasing due to a decreased stroke volume and flow velocity.

echocardiography and cardiac catheterization findings [35]. The "peak-to-peak," "peak," and "mean" gradients can be reported from catheterization data. It is important to distinguish between maximum instantaneous peak gradient obtained with echocardiography and peak-to-peak gradient obtained in the catheter laboratory. The peak-to-peak gradient is obtained by measuring the difference between peak LV pressure and peak aortic pressure with a pressure transducer, at different times in the cardiac cycle. The maximum instantaneous echo pressure gradient is higher than the peak-to-peak gradient. It has been shown that the best correlation is between mean Doppler gradient and mean cardiac catheter gradient measured simultaneously [36]. Technical quality of the echocardiography examination, however, has an important influence on the reliability of the information and subsequent surgical decision making. Maximum Doppler

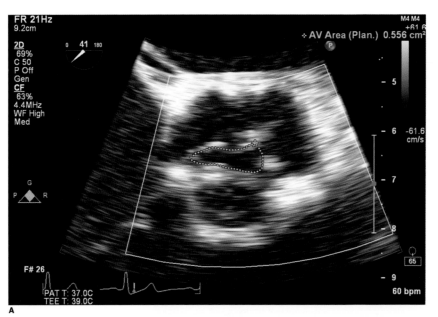

A

Figure 6.22. Calculation of aortic valve area (AVA) by continuity equation. In (A) this patient with aortic stenosis, (B) the LVOT diameter (leftmost dotted line) is measured, together with flow velocities across the LVOT and aortic valve. These are used in the continuity equation (Chaper 13). The dimensionless severity index (DSI) can be calculated by using the ratio of (C) velocity time integral (VTI) through the LVOT (measured with PWD) to (D) VTI through the aortic valve (measured with CWD). Aortic stenosis is considered severe when the ratio is less than 0.25.

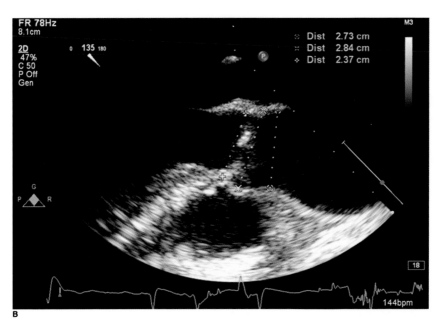

B

velocity through the AV will be underestimated if the ultrasound beam is not parallel to aortic blood flow [37].

On the other hand, the pressure recovery phenomenon may lead to overestimation of Doppler pressure gradient measurements [38–40]. Pressure will be lowest where velocity is highest. This is at the vena contracta, which corresponds to the minimal cross-sectional valve area. Distal to the stenosis, as velocity decreases, pressure will increase. The total amount of

pressure recovery is related to viscous and turbulence energy losses across the stenotic valve. Doppler gradients that are measured at the vena contracta will be significantly higher than catheter measurements taken downstream in the ascending aorta after pressure has completely recovered [41]. The Doppler pressure drop will depend on where flow velocity is sampled. When quantifying AS using CWD, the highest velocity at the vena contracta may therefore overestimate pressure gradient (PG) across the valve. In mild to moderate

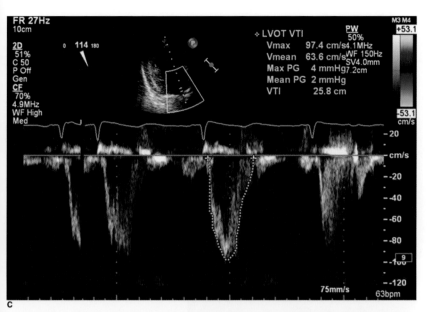

Figure 6.22 (Cont.)

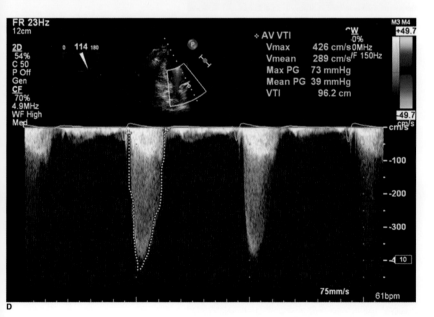

aortic stenosis the three cusps of the valve form a funnel rather than a diaphragm, as would be found in severe stenosis. This leads to greater pressure recovery. The pressure recovery phenomenon is more significant in prosthetic aortic valves than in native valves [42].

Due to pressure overload, the LV responds to AS with myocardial fibrosis, concentric hypertrophy, and impaired diastolic relaxation. This will be followed by systolic LV dilation, and failure later in the disease (Figs. 6.20, 6.21; Videos 6.10–6.12).

The transvalvular PG or pressure drop is only a reliable indicator of severity in the presence of good ventricular function. The PG will decrease if the LV function deteriorates in end-stage disease.

The differential diagnosis of a high PG will include LVOT obstruction (subaortic membrane or muscular subaortic stenosis), hypertrophic obstructive cardiomyopathy (HOCM), and any form of supravalvular stenosis in the root or aorta.

The effective valve area is far less flow-dependent than the pressure gradient, and should therefore be

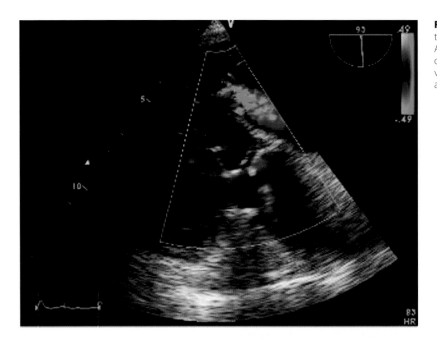

Figure 6.23. When measuring the systolic flow velocity with CWD across the AV in the transgastric long-axis view of the LVOT, the presence of a high-velocity mitral regurgitant jet may lead to a wrong diagnosis.

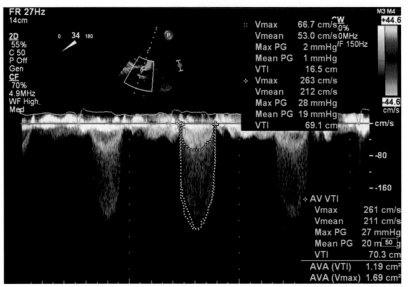

Figure 6.24. The "double-envelope" continuity equation technique to measure flow velocities across the AV and LVOT on a single Doppler signal.

the index of choice for quantifying AS in the presence of abnormal flow rate or elevated blood pressure [34]. Planimetry is relatively reliable in the valve with healthy leaflets, but more inaccurate in the calcified valve. A perfect short-axis view should be obtained, and the three-dimensional anatomy of the crown-shaped AV should be kept in mind when using this technique. The AVA remains fairly constant whatever the flow across the valve.

The continuity equation is most commonly used to calculate AVA. This is based on the conservation of mass and is detailed in Chapter 13. AS is severe when the AVA is less than 1.0 cm^2 (Fig. 6.22) [34].

It may be difficult to measure the LVOT diameter accurately because of heavy calcification. This measurement can then easily be underestimated. Another pitfall of the continuity equation occurs when the ultrasound beam is not parallel to blood flow and

Doppler measurements are therefore inaccurate. One of the most common causes of misinterpretation of echocardiography findings in this condition is the presence of a jet of mitral regurgitation (MR). When attempting examination of the aortic valve in the transgastric views, the CWD beam may accidentally cross the mitral valve flows. The orientation and high velocity of a mitral regurgitant jet will be similar to that of an aortic stenosis jet (Fig. 6.23).

If a patient is not in sinus rhythm the AV and LVOT flow velocities will vary with each cardiac cycle. Multiple measurements should then be made and the average obtained. Small errors in measurement may result in large errors in calculated values, because of the squaring of linear dimensions. These may lead to wrong diagnosis with severe implications, particularly in small elderly patients.

The Doppler velocity index (DVI), dimensionless severity index (DSI), and double-envelope technique are all similar in principle and use the continuity equation to find the ratio between LVOT and AV flow velocities [31]. The aim is to simplify the continuity equation measurement and avoid the influence of flow on the measurement.

The DVI is the ratio of peak velocity in the LVOT to peak velocity across the AV, being proportional to the cross-sectional area of both of these structures [43]. AS is considered to be severe when the ratio is less than 0.25.

The DSI (Fig. 6.22) is similar in that it uses the ratio of velocity–time integral (VTI) through the LVOT (measured with pulsed-wave Doppler, PWD) to VTI through the aortic valve (measured with CWD):

$$DSI = VTI_{LVOT}/VTI_{AT} \qquad (6.1)$$

Again, a ratio of less than 0.25 indicates severe AS [43].

The double-envelope continuity equation technique has been described for use in prosthetic valves [44]. Using this technique, the high-velocity VTI_{AV} is obtained from the outside edge of the CWD signal. Instead of using PWD to obtain the LVOT velocity, the denser low-velocity signal in the same envelope is used to represent the VTI_{LVOT} (Fig. 6.24).

This technique has the advantage of simplicity and minimizing error due to beat-to-beat variability in blood flow. It may also be useful in the stenotic AV.

Other novel methods of quantifying AS severity including aortic valve resistance [45], percentage stroke work loss [46], and energy loss coefficient [47] have been described. However, these are mainly research-based and theoretical, and are not necessary for routine use in clinical practice [31].

Many patients with aortic stenosis also have aortic regurgitation (AR). This leads to increased transaortic blood flow during systole with a higher gradient for a given aortic valve orifice. The AR, however, does not affect the continuity equation calculations because the increase in systolic flow is measured both in the LVOT and across the AV. On the other hand, coexisting mitral stenosis will cause a low aortic valve gradient because the fixed cardiac output will lead to a decrease in transvalvular blood flow [48]. AS is a disease continuum and there is no one specific value which defines severity. Recent ACC/AHA guidelines have used aortic jet velocity, mean pressure gradient, and AVA to grade AS into mild, moderate, and severe [34]. Severe AS is defined as a flow velocity greater than 4.0 m/s, a mean pressure gradient more than 40 mmHg, and an AVA of less than 1.0 cm² (Table 6.1).

It is both important and difficult to distinguish the patient with truly severe low-flow AS responsible for low ejection fraction (EF) from "pseudo-severe AS," where an LV damaged by another process such as coronary artery disease or cardiomyopathy is unable to open a mildly stenotic AV [49]. The patient with true low-gradient, low-EF AS is defined where there is afterload mismatch with a mean gradient < 30 mmHg, an AVA < 1 cm², and an EF < 35% [50]. Common current practice to distinguish between this scenario and pseudo-severe AS is to increase the cardiac output pharmacologically and assess ventricular reserve during dobutamine stress echocardiography. An increase of stroke volume (SV) > 20% with dobutamine indicates contractile reserve. Any patient with severe AS and LV contractile reserve should benefit from afterload reduction obtained through

Table 6.1. ACC/AHA classification of severity of aortic stenosis in adults. Adapted from Bonow et al., Circulation 2008; **118**: e523–661 [34]

Index	Mild	Moderate	Severe
Jet velocity (m/s)	< 3.0	3.0–4.0	> 4.0
Mean gradient (mmHg)	< 25	25–40	> 40
Valve area (cm²)	> 1.5	1.0–1.5	< 1.0
Valve area index (cm²/m²)			< 0.6
Dimensionless severity index (VTI_{LVOT}/VTI_{AV})		0.25–0.5	< 0.25

aortic valve replacement (AVR) surgery. AVR may not always be beneficial in patients with pseudo-severe AS. However, AS patients without contractile reserve should be carefully discussed and not automatically turned down for surgery [51–53]. In the near future, percutaneous AVR could be a valuable alternative for surgical high-risk patients with low-gradient, low-EF AS (see Chapter 17) [54].

Systemic hypertension can modify the physical examination findings in the AS patient [55]. It may also affect the echo findings by inducing a significant reduction in transvalvular flow rate, an increase in effective valve area, and consequently a reduction in pressure gradient [56–58]. This can be misleading when quantifying the severity of stenosis.

The assessment of AV pathology is very much affected by intraoperative changes in hemodynamic conditions, including the level of anesthesia, ventricular filling, inotropic support, and cardiopulmonary bypass.

Aortic regurgitation

Mechanisms of aortic regurgitation

Aortic regurgitation (AR) results from a primary valve lesion, an abnormal aortic root and/or ascending aorta, or a combination of both. The etiology of primary valve lesions includes calcific or rheumatic AV disease, or infective endocarditis. Stenotic AV leaflets often do not completely coapt during diastole, leading to regurgitation. The most common cause of aortic regurgitation in developing countries is rheumatic disease, with clinical presentation in the second or third decade of life [59]. In Western countries it is most frequently due to degenerative (Fig. 6.25) or congenital (bicuspid valve) causes, with patients presenting in the fourth to sixth decades. The prevalence of aortic regurgitation increases with age. Infective endocarditis of the AV typically presents with mobile vegetations connected to a damaged cusp. This is best visible on the ventricular side of the valve when it prolapses into the LVOT during diastole (Fig. 6.26; Videos 6.13, 6.14). The diagnosis of aortic valve prolapse is made when any part of a leaflet appears in the LVOT below the level of the aortic annulus (Fig. 6.27). As the endocarditis progresses the cusps are damaged, resulting in an increasing severity of AR. Destruction of the AV may occur, caused either by a mycotic aneurysm of the aortic root or by a perivalvular abscess infiltrating the transverse sinus (Fig. 6.28; Video 6.15).

In patients with pure aortic regurgitation secondary to rheumatic disease, the essential lesion is retraction and thickening of the edges of the cusps with preservation of the hinge mechanism [60]. The hemodynamic lesion may result in progressive dilation of the aortic annulus, with worsening of the regurgitation over time.

A dilated or abnormal aorta and aortic root may occur due to hypertension, Marfan syndrome, a con-

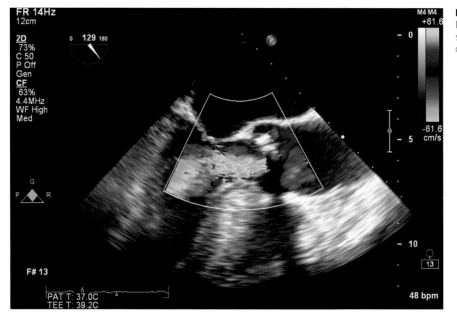

Figure 6.25. A mid-esophageal long-axis view with CFD of a severely regurgitant AV due to degenerative valve disease.

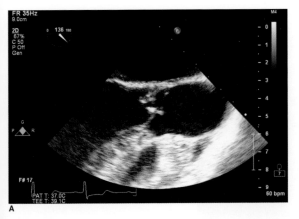

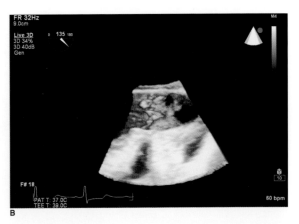

Figure 6.26. (A) A 2D image and (B) a 3D image of a patient with severe AR due to destruction of the AV by endocarditis. Note the vegetation on the LVOT side of the AV during diastole.

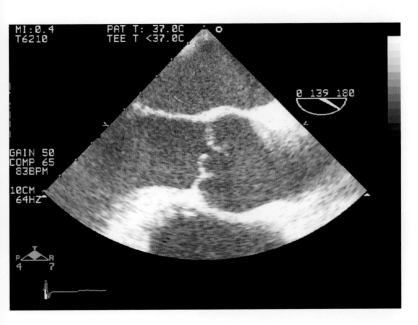

Figure 6.27. A mid-esophageal long-axis view demonstrating severe prolapse of RCC below the level of the aortic annulus.

genital bicuspid AV, or trauma. Aneurysmal dilation of the ascending aorta can cause AR without annular dilation, through a tethering effect on the cusps (Fig. 6.29). Four potential mechanisms of AR in a patient with acute type A aortic dissection have been described (Table 6.2) [61]. Some patients can have more than one mechanism of AR. In aortic dissection the intimal flap prolapsing through the valve may keep the leaflets in the open position, causing severe AR. However, sometimes the flap acts as a valve during diastole with remarkably little AR although the leaflets are open. The risk of aortic dissection or rupture is increased in

patients with a dilated aorta with diameter more than 5.5 cm [62]. The diameter of the ascending aorta should therefore be routinely assessed and any dilation should be carefully followed. In the patient with a bicuspid AV (congenital) or Marfan syndrome (connective tissue disease) there is an integral weakness of the ascending aorta, and risk of dissection will be much higher. Recent ESC guidelines [1] have recommended surgery in a patient with *any* degree of AR and ascending aorta disease in the following situations:

- maximum ascending aorta or root diameter > 4.5 cm in a Marfan patient

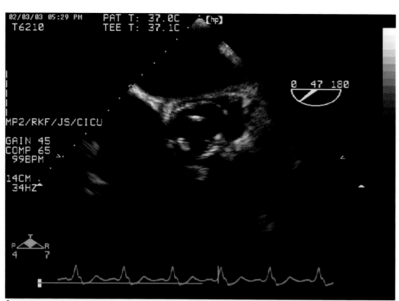

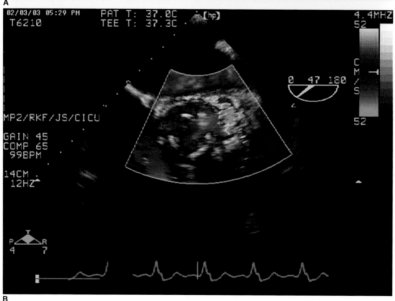

Figure 6.28. (A) A mid-esophageal short-axis view (and (B) with added CFD) of an infected AV demonstrating thickening into the transverse sinus and a potential abscess cavity.

- maximum ascending aorta or root diameter > 5.0 in a patient with a bicuspid valve
- maximum ascending aorta or root diameter > 5.5 in any other patient (Figs. 6.30, 6.31)

Although the congenital bicuspid valve usually undergoes premature heavy calcification, a proportion of these patients present with severe regurgitation and pliable cusps, which may be treated by valve repair. The bicuspid aortic valve also predisposes to infective endocarditis, which can lead to its destruction with subsequent AR. In another form of congenital AR, the AV is in close relationship to a perimembranous sub-arterial ventricular septal defect (VSD). In this situation there is usually a degree of prolapse, more commonly of the right coronary cusp due to inadequate fibrous support and in some cases due to the Venturi effect of the VSD. On current evidence it is very important not only to repair the VSD, but also to resuspend the prolapsing cusp, to prevent rapid progression of aortic insufficiency [63]. Quadricuspid aortic valves are rare, but significant aortic insufficiency is common with this lesion because of the uneven

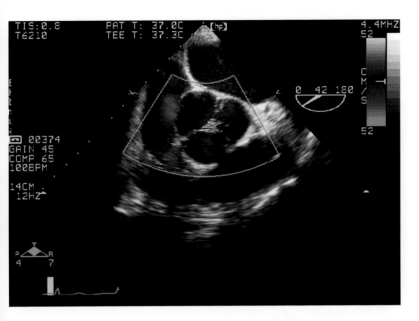

Figure 6.29. A mid-esophageal short-axis view of a severely regurgitant AV due to a dilated aortic root with tethering of the cusps.

Table 6.2. Mechanisms of functional aortic regurgitation in type A aortic dissection. From Movsowitz *et al., J Am Coll Cardiol* 2000; **36**: 884–90 [61].

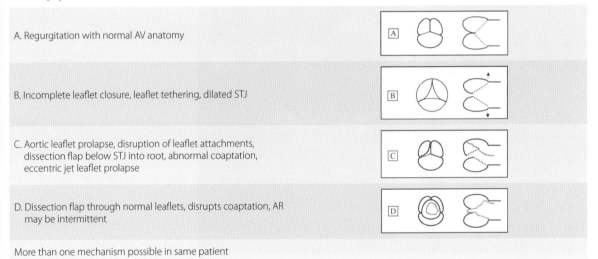

A. Regurgitation with normal AV anatomy	
B. Incomplete leaflet closure, leaflet tethering, dilated STJ	
C. Aortic leaflet prolapse, disruption of leaflet attachments, dissection flap below STJ into root, abnormal coaptation, eccentric jet leaflet prolapse	
D. Dissection flap through normal leaflets, disrupts coaptation, AR may be intermittent	

More than one mechanism possible in same patient

distribution of mechanical stress leading to incomplete cusp coaptation [23] (Fig. 6.13).

On clinical examination the patient with aortic regurgitation will have a characteristic decrescendo diastolic murmur over the left sternal border. In some patients a mid- to late-diastolic apical rumble (Austin–Flint murmur) is heard, possibly due to vibration of the anterior mitral leaflet as it is struck by an eccentric directed AR jet [59,64]. A third heart sound is due to regurgitant flow throughout diastole with subsequent rapid filling of the LV. Because of the increased left ventricular end-diastolic volume, there is also an increase in the systolic flow across the valve. This leads to a wide pulse pressure with a collapsing pulse and often an ejection systolic murmur [65].

TEE evaluation of aortic regurgitation

The mainstay of aortic regurgitation assessment is based on the integration of the information obtained by 2D echocardiography, CFD, PWD, and CWD.

95

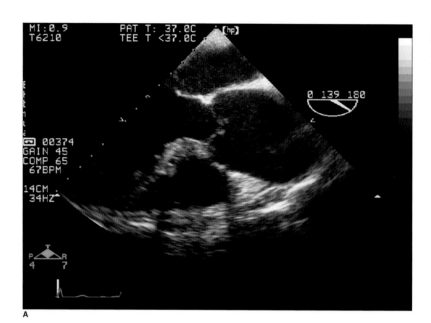

Figure 6.30. (A) A mid-esophageal long-axis view (and (B) with added CFD) of a severely regurgitant AV due to a dilated aortic root. Note the poor coaptation of the leaflets.

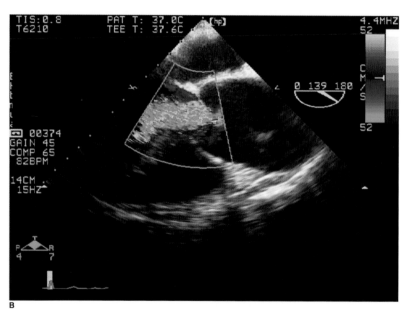

Qualitative diagnosis of AR with TEE is relatively easy, but quantitative evaluation is much more difficult and time-consuming, and is used more selectively. There is no one specific technique to accurately quantify AR severity and it is therefore important to examine multiple imaging planes and use several parameters. In future RT3D echo may be a useful additional tool to confirm the mechanism of regurgitation and simplify grading of severity.

Assessment of AR starts with an accurate 2D examination in the ME SAX and LAX views of the

AV. This includes an evaluation of the cusps, LVOT, aortic root, and ascending aorta. Poor coaptation, vegetations, cusp prolapse or perforations, and annular dilation should be noted. The regurgitant jet causes a rapid rise in left ventricular end-diastolic pressure (LVEDP) and may impair opening of the anterior mitral valve leaflet ("reverse doming") by direct restriction leading to "functional" mitral stenosis [66]. Early closure of the MV is sometimes seen before the onset of systole, which can in severe cases even lead to diastolic mitral regurgitation,

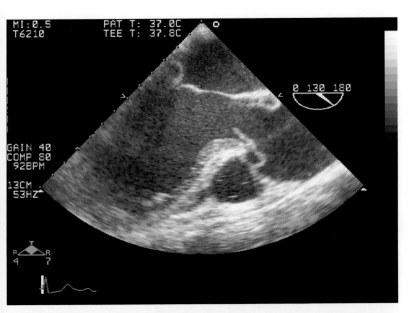

Figure 6.31. A mid-esophageal long-axis view demonstrating a dilated ST junction and ascending aorta together with dilation of the aortic root and annulus. This aorta has dissected, with the intimal flap prolapsing through the AV during diastole, causing severe regurgitation.

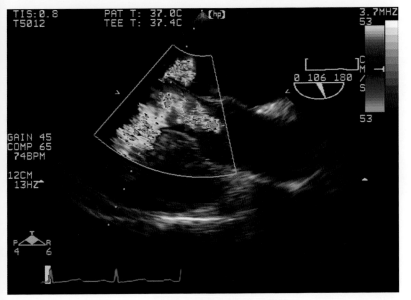

Figure 6.32. A mid-esophageal long-axis view with CFD demonstrating a severe eccentric AR jet onto the anterior leaflet of the mitral valve causing "reverse doming" and end-diastolic mitral regurgitation.

demonstrated with CFD [67]. On M-mode a high frequency fluttering of the anterior MV leaflet may be seen during diastole as a result of this jet. Left atrial dilation would indicate severe AR, except in acute AR in which the chambers have not had time to dilate. The LV should be carefully assessed for function and any dilation resulting from chronic volume overload, which provides valuable clues to the acute or chronic nature of the AR. The 2D examination is now repeated with CFD. The color-flow jet is imaged in multiple planes to assess its direction, length, and height/width. A central jet usually implies aortic root dilation while an eccentric jet is caused by leaflet pathology (Figs. 6.32, 6.33; Videos 6.16, 6.17). Measurement of its penetration into the LV cavity or jet area alone is not reliable in quantifying AR. The severity of an eccentric jet is easily underestimated [68], so when assessing a regurgitant jet there are three components to consider: the flow convergence in the aorta, the vena contracta through the regurgitant orifice, and the jet direction and size in the LV.

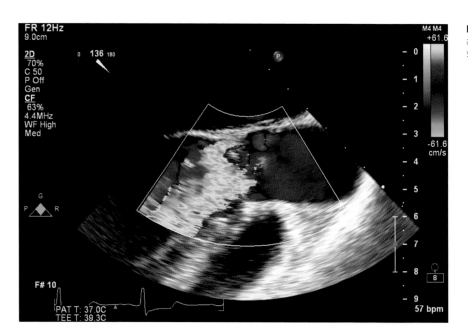

Figure 6.33. A mid-esophageal long-axis view with CFD demonstrating a severe central AR jet.

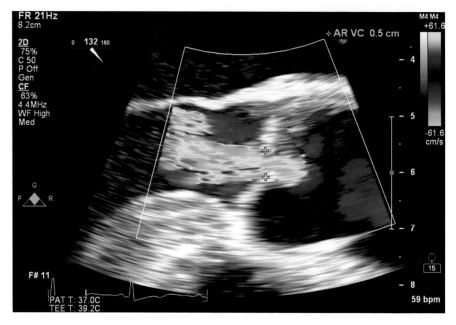

Figure 6.34. The vena contracta is the narrowest component of the jet, positioned at or just distal to the effective orifice.

Quantification of severity of aortic regurgitation

The vena contracta is the narrowest central flow region of the jet, located at or just distal to the valve orifice, immediately below the flow convergence area (Fig. 6.34) [69]. It is independent of flow rate and driving pressure for a fixed orifice, and should therefore be less influenced by loading conditions than traditional indices of AR severity, such as regurgitant volume and fraction. The vena contracta is also not affected much by the Nyquist limit. To assess the vena contracta appropriately all three components of the jet (flow convergence, vena contracta, and jet body) need to be visualized, usually seen best in the mid-esophageal long-axis view of the AV and LVOT (140°). A vena contracta diameter of more than 0.5 cm is highly sensitive, while a diameter of more than 0.7 cm

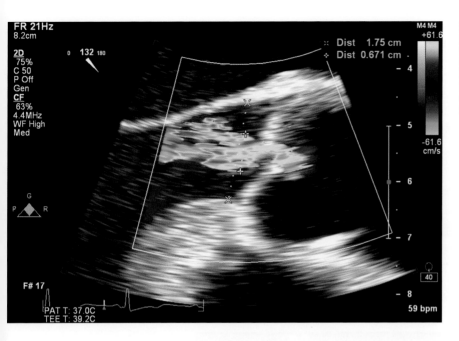

FR 21Hz
8.2cm

2D
75%
C 50
P Off
Gen
CF
63%
4.4MHz
WF High
Med

0   132 180

G

P ◄ R

F# 17

PAT T: 37.0C
TEE T: 39.2C

Dist 1.75 cm
Dist 0.671 cm

M4 M4
+61.6

-4

-5

-6

-7

-8

-61.6
cm/s

40

59 bpm

Figure 6.35. AR index. If the jet width takes up more than 65% of the LVOT the regurgitation is severe; if the ratio is less than 25% it is mild. This image shows moderate AR, with the jet width occupying around 40% of the LVOT.

has high specificity as a measure of severe AR [70]. It may not be accurate in the presence of multiple regurgitant jets, eccentric jets, or jets with irregular shapes [68]. Its cross-sectional area is equivalent to the effective regurgitant orifice area. If planimetry of the jet performed in the AV SAX view is more than 0.3 cm², AR is severe [71]. The vena contracta has also been shown to correlate well with direct measurements of the regurgitant volume and fraction by aortic flow probe [72].

The height of the AR jet as a ratio of the LVOT diameter has a good correlation with severity [73]. This is different from the vena contracta, which is measured at the valve orifice. The jet width in the LVOT is bigger than the vena contracta because the jet expands after passing through the regurgitant orifice. Although this is a semi-quantitative index, it became the clinical standard for echocardiographic grading of AR. When the jet width takes up more than 65% of the LVOT diameter it is severe (Fig. 6.35; Videos 6.18–6.20). The jet width is superior to jet length or jet area and is more accurate in the setting of eccentric jets [74]. Limitations of the jet width/LVOT ratio method are that the regurgitant jet orifice may not be in the same imaging plane as the true LVOT diameter, or the regurgitant orifice may be asymmetric in shape. The jet may therefore be wider in one plane than another, leading to an inaccurate estimate. Both the vena contracta and jet width should preferably be evaluated with the Nyquist limit set at 50–60 cm/s. Color M-mode can be used to deter-

mine the jet width/LVOT ratio, and it is also useful to determine the duration of the AR jet during diastole (Fig. 6.36; Video 6.21).

CWD is used to assess the AR jet from TG LAX or deep TG views because the beam can be aligned relatively parallel to blood flow. CFD is useful to demonstrate the location and direction of the AR jet. The deceleration time (slope) of the diastolic regurgitant jet should now be measured. The rate of decrease of the velocity profile is influenced by severity of AR, decreasing more rapidly with more severe AR because the larger regurgitant orifice allows a more rapid equilibration of pressures leading to a collapsing pulse. A slope of greater than 3 m/s demonstrates severe AR, and a pressure half-time (PHT) of less than 200 ms acts as confirmation (Figs. 6.37, 6.38). LV compliance and systemic vascular resistance will affect these measurements.

The continuity equation can be used to calculate regurgitant volume (RV) and regurgitant fraction (RF). The RV is the difference between systolic stroke volumes across the aortic and mitral valves. The stroke volume through each valve is obtained by multiplying valve area by velocity–time integral across each valve. In the absence of mitral regurgitation and intracardiac shunts, flow across the mitral valve equals cardiac output. AR is severe if the RV is more than 60 mL/beat across the AV.

$$RV = AV\ stroke\ volume - MV\ stroke\ volume \quad (6.2)$$

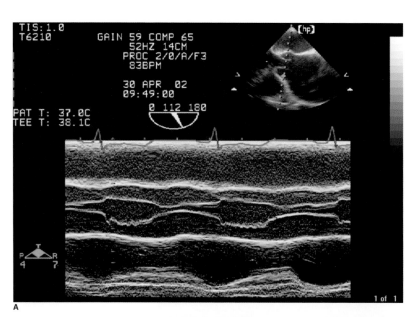

A

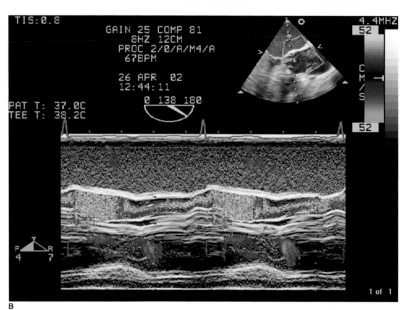

B

Figure 6.36. (A) M-mode, and (B) with CFD added, across the AV leaflets, demonstrating the jet width/LVOT ratio and also the duration of the jet throughout diastole.

The RF is the ratio of RV to stroke volume across the AV. If RF is more than 50%, AR is considered severe.

$$RF = RV \, / \, AV \text{ stroke volume} \qquad (6.3)$$

Holodiastolic flow reversal demonstrated with PWD in the descending aorta is a sensitive confirmation of severe AR [75]. The long-axis view of the descending aorta is used and the PWD cursor is placed as parallel as possible so that flow can be demonstrated.

The more distal the holodiastolic flow in the aorta, the more significant is the finding (Fig. 6.39).

The proximal flow convergence area or proximal isovelocity surface area (PISA) can be used to calculate effective regurgitant orifice area and regurgitant volume. This method is derived from the principle that, as blood approaches an orifice, its velocity increases, forming concentric, roughly hemispheric shells of increasing velocity and decreasing surface area [76]. The PISA technique has been validated to

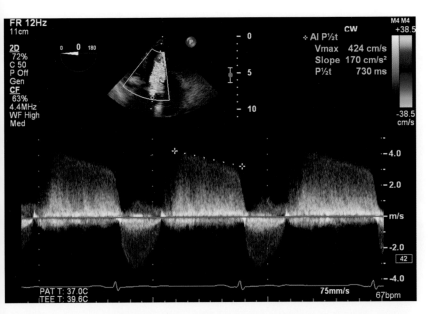

Figure 6.37. A CWD signal across the LVOT and AV in the TG LAX view, demonstrating mild–moderate AR as measured with the pressure half-time (PHT) and deceleration slope techniques. The slope is flat and the PHT is long.

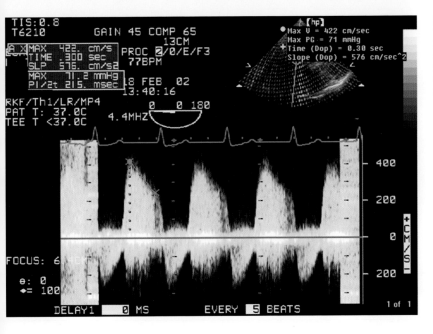

Figure 6.38. A CWD signal across the LVOT and AV in the TG LAX view, demonstrating severe AR as measured with the pressure half-time (PHT) and deceleration slope techniques. The slope is steep and the PHT is short.

provide a reasonably accurate quantification of the AR [76]. It is, however, less easy to identify a clear proximal flow convergence in AR than in MR (Figs. 6.40, 6.41; Table 6.3).

The threshold of severe AR is an effective regurgitant orifice area (EROA) more than 0.3 cm² and RV more than 60 mL. Because of the small values measured, the slightest measurement error may lead to a large percentage calculation error and therefore misclassification of AR severity. It is less accurate for eccentric than for central jets, and a circular orifice with perfect flow convergence hemisphere is assumed. PISA also depends very much on the Nyquist limit. Another limitation is that in the presence of an ascending aorta aneurysm the PISA measurement appears to overestimate the RV.

The evaluation of severity of AR using quantitative indices such as RV, RF, and EROA with the PISA

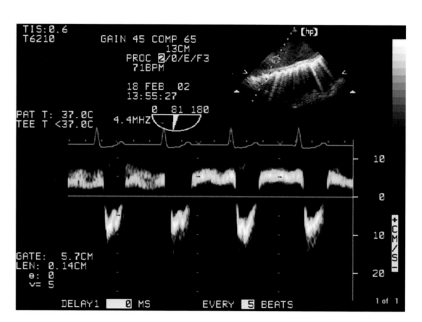

Figure 6.39. Holodiastolic flow reversal demonstrated in the descending thoracic aorta with PWD. Aortic flow is from right to left on the 2D image and appears below the spectral Doppler baseline as flow away from the transducer.

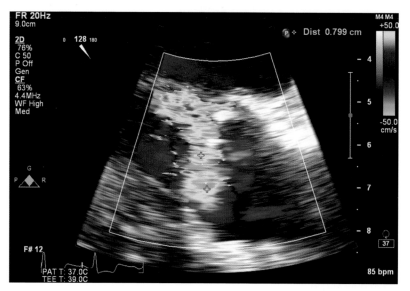

Figure 6.40. ME LAX AV (128°) (zoom on AV) demonstrating proximal flow convergence with CFD. Nyquist velocity shifted in direction of jet producing PISA area as large as possible. Measure radius (r) from alias line to regurgitant orifice. Calculate PISA surface area with $2\pi r^2$. Calculate regurgitant flow (RF) by multiplying this value by aliasing velocity obtained from color scale.

technique is much less established than in MR, and should therefore be integrated with supporting qualitative data [1,68] (Table 6.4). The 2D PISA technique does appear to underestimate the volume of regurgitant flow when compared to 3D volumes. Due to often difficult measurement conditions and acute changes in loading conditions under anesthesia, PISA has never been very popular for intraoperative quantification of AR. The technique is simple in theory, but complicated in practice. With technology rapidly

improving, 3D color Doppler assessment of EROA and RV will probably replace the 2D PISA technique in the near future.

Patients with severe left-sided regurgitant lesions can remain relatively asymptomatic while the left ventricle dilates and develops irreversible functional impairment. In AR the LV experiences an increased afterload. There is both volume and pressure overload and therefore an increase not only in chamber size but also in wall thickness [78]. In chronic aortic

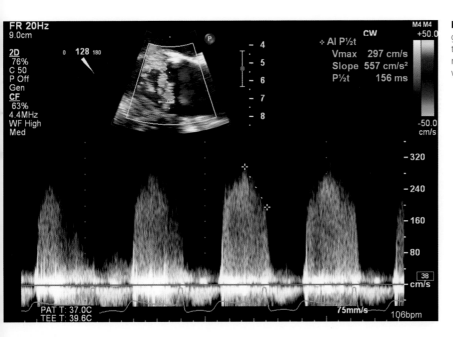

Figure 6.41. Effective regurgitant orifice area (EROA) is equal to peak RF divided by peak regurgitant velocity, measured with CWD in TG LAX view.

Table 6.3. Calculation of regurgitant flow and effective regurgitant orifice area using PISA method. Derived from Bargiggia GS et al., Circulation 1991; **84**: 1481–9 [77]

Step 1. Zoom in on AV in ME LAX AV (140°) and find clear proximal flow convergence

Step 2. Shift Nyquist velocity in the direction of the jet to produce PISA area as large as possible

Step 3. Calculate PISA surface area = $2\pi r^2$ assuming a perfect hemisphere (r is radius from alias line to regurgitant orifice)

Step 4. Calculate regurgitant flow (RF) = $2\pi r^2 \times$ aliasing velocity obtained from color scale

Step 5. Effective regurgitant orifice area (EROA) = peak RF divided by peak regurgitant velocity measured with CWD (TG LAX or deep TG views)

Table 6.4. Grading of severity of aortic regurgitation in adults. Modified from Zoghbi et al., J Am Soc Echocardiogr 2003; **16**: 777–802 [68]

Index	Mild	Moderate	Severe
CFD ratio jet width/LVOT (Perry index)	< 25%	25–65%	> 65%
CFD vena contracta (cm)	< 0.3	0.3–0.6	> 0.6
PWD holodiastolic flow reversal in descending aorta	No	No	Yes
CWD AR jet pressure half-time			< 200 ms
LV enlargement (cm)			LVIDs >5.0, LVIDd >7.0
RV (mL/beat)	< 30		> 60
RF (%)	< 30		> 50
EROA (cm²)	< 0.1		> 0.3

regurgitation the LV will be more dilated and spherical in shape but not necessarily in the acute case. If the LV end-systolic diameter is less than 5.0 cm, the patient has a better long-term prognosis. Marked left ventricular enlargement with an end-diastolic diameter of 7 cm or more is generally accompanied by overt dysfunction and associated with increased risk of sudden death [34,79]. In symptomatic AR urgent AVR surgery should be performed. In asymptomatic patients surgery is recommended when the end-systolic diameter reaches 5.0 cm or more, the end-diastolic diameter reaches 7.0 cm, and/or when the ejection fraction decreases below 50% [1,34]. Left ventricular dysfunction continues to predict a very

poor outcome in spite of technically successful valve surgery. However, despite the higher risk in patients with severe AR and reduced LV ejection fraction, many will enjoy several years of event-free survival after AV replacement and should not be denied its benefits [80,81].

Conclusion

In conclusion, TEE is valuable in revealing important aspects of aortic valve disease. Whilst TEE may not be appropriate as the primary technique for aortic valve evaluation in the echo laboratory, it is indicated if TTE windows are poor. TEE evaluation of the aortic valve has now become invaluable in the perioperative setting. It provides definite information on the mechanisms of pathology, aids planning in aortic valve surgery, and is used by the surgical team to screen patients undergoing other cardiac procedures. However, quantitative assessment by Doppler techniques may be difficult in the perioperative setting using TEE, and measurements should be made with meticulous care if errors are to be avoided. RT3D imaging will certainly change our approach to evaluating the AV in the foreseeable future.

References

1. Vahanian A, Baumgartner H, Bax J, *et al.* Guidelines on the management of valvular heart disease: the Task Force on the Management of Valvular Heart Disease of the European Society of Cardiology. *Eur Heart J* 2007; **28**: 230–68.

2. Bollen B, Duran C, Savage RM. Surgical anatomy of the heart: correlation with echocardiographic imaging planes In: Savage RM, Aronson S, eds., *Comprehensive Textbook of Intraoperative Transesophageal Echocardiography.* Philadelphia, PA: Lippincott Williams & Wilkins, 2005: 65–79.

3. Robicsek F, Thubrikar MJ. Role of sinus wall compliance in aortic leaflet function. *Am J Cardiol* 1999; **84**: 944–6.

4. Sripathi VC, Kumar RK, Balakrishnan KR. Further insights into normal aortic valve function: role of a compliant aortic root on leaflet opening and valve orifice area. *Ann Thorac Surg* 2004; **77**: 844–51.

5. Davies JE, Parker KH, Francis DP, Hughes AD, Mayet J. What is the role of the aorta in directing coronary blood flow? *Heart* 2008; **94**: 1545–7.

6. Shanewise JS, Cheung AT, Aronson S, *et al.* ASE/SCA guidelines for performing a comprehensive intraoperative multiplane transesophageal echocardiography examination: recommendations of the ASE Council for intraoperative echocardiography and the SCA Task Force for certification in perioperative transesophageal echocardiography. *Anesth Analg* 1999; **89**: 870–84.

7. Lindroos M, Kupari M, Heikkila J, Tilvis R. Prevalence of aortic abnormalities in the elderly: an echocardiographic study of a random population sample. *J Am Coll Cardiol* 1993; **21**: 1220–5.

8. Nightingale AK, Horowitz JD. Aortic sclerosis: not an innocent murmur but a marker of increased cardiovascular risk. *Heart* 2005; **91**: 1389–93.

9. Chambers J. Aortic stenosis. *BMJ* 2005; **330**: 801–2.

10. Cosmi JE, Kort S, Tunick PA, *et al.* The risk of development of aortic stenosis in patients with "benign" aortic valve thickening. *Arch Intern Med* 2002; **162**: 2345–7.

11. Mohler ER. Mechanisms of aortic valve calcification. *Am J Cardiol* 2004; **94**: 1396–402.

12. Novaro GM, Tiong IY, Pearce GL, *et al.* Effect of hydroxymethylglutaryl coenzyme A reductase inhibitors on the progression of calcific aortic stenosis. *Circulation* 2001; **104**: 2205–9.

13. Rosenhek R, Rader F, Loho N, *et al.* Statins but not angiotensin-converting enzyme inhibitors delay progression of aortic stenosis. *Circulation* 2004; **110**: 1291–5.

14. Rajamannan NM, Otto CM. Targeted therapy to prevent progression of calcific aortic stenosis. *Circulation* 2004; **110**: 1180–2.

15. Caulfield MT, Budoff MJ, Takasu J, *et al.* Angiotensin converting enzyme inhibitor use is associated with a decreased rate of aortic valve calcium accumulation. *Circulation* 2002; **106** (suppl II): 640 (abstract).

16. Roberts WC. The congenitally bicuspid aortic valve: a study of 85 autopsy cases. *Am J Cardiol* 1970; **26**: 72–83.

17. Cripe L, Andelfinger G, Martin LJ, Shooner K, Benson DW. Bicuspid aortic valve is heritable. *J Am Coll Cardiol* 2004; **44**: 138–43.

18. Clementi M, Notari L, Borghi A, Tenconi R. Familial congenital bicuspid aortic valve: a disorder of uncertain inheritance. *Am J Med Genet* 1996; **62**: 336–8.

19. Huntington K, Hunter AG, Chan KL. A prospective study to assess the frequency of familial clustering of congenital bicuspid aortic valve. *J Am Coll Cardiol* 1997; **30**: 1809–12.

20. Duran AC, Frescura C, Sans-Coma V, *et al.* Bicuspid aortic valves in hearts with other congenital heart disease. *J Heart Valve Dis* 1995; **4**: 581–90.

21. Schaefer BM, Lewin MB, Stout KK, *et al.* The bicuspid aortic valve: an integrated phenotypic classification of leaflet morphology and aortic root shape. *Heart* 2008; **94**: 1634–8.

22. Warnes CA. Bicuspid aortic valve and coarctation: two villains part of a diffuse problem. *Heart* 2003; **89**: 965–6.

23. Tutarel O. The quadricuspid aortic valve: a comprehensive review. *J Heart Valve Dis* 2004; **13**: 534–7.

24. Ross J, Braunwald E. Aortic stenosis. *Circulation* 1968; **38** (Suppl 5): 61–7.

25. O'Keefe JH, Vlietstra RE, Bailey KR, Holmes DR. Natural history of candidates for balloon valvuloplasty. *Mayo Clin Proc* 1987; **62**: 986–91.

26. Otto CM, Burwash IG, Legget ME, *et al.* Prospective study of asymptomatic valvular aortic stenosis: clinical, echocardiographic, and exercise predictors of outcome. *Circulation* 1997; **95**: 2262–70.

27. Wilkins GT. Valvular heart disease: putting guidelines into practice. *BMJ* 1997; **314**: 1428–9.

28. Carabello BA, Crawford FA. Valvular heart disease. *N Engl J Med* 1997; **337**: 32–41.

29. Carabello BA. Evaluation and management of patients with aortic stenosis. *Circulation* 2002; **105**: 1746–50.

30. Pereira JJ, Lauer MS, Bashir M, *et al.* Survival after aortic valve replacement for severe aortic stenosis with low transvalvular gradients and severe left ventricular dysfunction. *J Am Coll Cardiol* 2002; **39**: 1356–63.

31. Baumgartner H, Hung J, Bermejo J, *et al.* Echocardiographic assessment of valve stenosis: EAE/ASE recommendations for clinical practice. *Eur J Echocardiogr* 2009; **10**: 1–25.

32. Hoffmann R, Flachskampf FA, Hanrath P. Planimetry of orifice area in aortic stenosis using multiplane transesophageal echocardiography. *J Am Coll Cardiol* 1993; **22**: 529–34.

33. Sugeng L, Shernan SK, Salgo IS, *et al.* Live three-dimensional transesophageal echocardiography: initial experience using the fully-sampled matrix array probe. *J Am Coll Cardiol* 2008; **52**: 446–49.

34. Bonow RO, Carabello BA, Chatterjee K, *et al.* Focused update incorporated into the ACC/AHA 2006 guidelines for the management of patients with valvular heart disease. A Report of the ACC/AHA Task Force on Practice Guidelines. *Circulation* 2008; **118**: e523–661.

35. Roger VL, Tajik AJ, Reeder GS, *et al.* Effect of Doppler echocardiography on utilization of hemodynamic cardiac catheterization in the preoperative evaluation of aortic stenosis. *Mayo Clin Proc* 1996; **71**: 141–9.

36. Currie PJ, Seward JB, Reeder GS, *et al.* Continuous-wave Doppler echocardiographic assessment of severity of calcific aortic stenosis: a simultaneous Doppler-catheter correlative study in 100 adult patients. *Circulation* 1985; **71**: 1162–9.

37. Hatle L, Angelsen BA, Tromsdal A. Non-invasive assessment of aortic stenosis by Doppler ultrasound. *Br Heart J* 1980; **43**: 284–92.

38. Niederberger J, Schima H, Maurer G, Baumgartner H. Importance of pressure recovery for the assessment of aortic stenosis by doppler ultrasound: role of aortic size, aortic valve area, and direction of the stenotic jet in vitro. *Circulation* 1996; **94**: 1934–40.

39. Gjertsson P, Caidahl K, Svensson G, Wallentin I, Bech-Hanssen O. Important pressure recovery in patients with aortic stenosis and high Doppler gradients. *Am J Cardiol* 2001; **88**: 139–44.

40. Baumgartner H, Stefenelli T, Niederberger J, Schima H, Maurer G. "Overestimation" of catheter gradients by Doppler ultrasound in patients with aortic stenosis: a predictable manifestation of pressure recovery. *J Am Coll Cardiol* 1999; **33**: 1655–61.

41. Popescu WM, Prokop E, Elefteriades JA, Kett K, Barash PG. Phantom aortic valve pressure gradient: discrepancies between cardiac catheterization and Doppler echocardiography. *Anesth Analg* 2005; **100**: 1259–62.

42. Chambers J. Is pressure recovery an important cause of "Doppler aortic stenosis" with no gradient at catheterisation? *Heart* 1996; **76**: 381–3.

43. Oh JK, Taliercio CP, Holmes DR, *et al.* Prediction of the severity of aortic stenosis by Doppler aortic valve area determination: prospective Doppler–catheterization correlation in 100 patients. *J Am Coll Cardiol* 1988; **11**: 1227–34.

44. Maslow AD, Haering JM, Heindel S, *et al.* An evaluation of prosthetic aortic valves using transesophageal echocardiography: the double-envelope technique. *Anesth Analg* 2000; **91**: 509–16.

45. Antonini-Canterin F, Faggiano P, Zanuttini D, Ribichini F. Is aortic valve resistance more clinically meaningful than valve area in aortic stenosis? *Heart* 1999; **82**: 9–10.

46. Tobin JR, Rahimtoola SH, Blundell PE, Swan HJ. Percentage of left ventricular stroke work loss: a simple haemodynamic concept for estimation of severity in valvular aortic stenosis. *Circulation* 1967; **35**: 868–79.

47. Garcia D, Pibarot P, Dumesnil JG, Sakr F, Durand LG. Assessment of aortic valve stenosis severity: a new index based on the energy loss concept. *Circulation* 2000; **101**: 765–71.

48. Troianos CA. Assessment of the aortic valve. In: Savage RM, Aronson S, eds., *Comprehensive Textbook of Intraoperative Transesophageal Echocardiography.* Philadelphia, PA: Lippincott Williams & Wilkins, 2005: 205–18.

49. Carabello BA. Is it ever too late to operate on the patient with valvular heart disease? *J Am Coll Cardiol* 2004; **44**: 376–83.

50. Tribouilloy C, Levy F. Assessment and management of low-gradient, low ejection fraction aortic stenosis. *Heart* 2008; **94**: 1526–7.

51. Monin JL, Quéré JP, Monchi M, *et al.* Low-gradient aortic stenosis: operative risk stratification and predictors for long-term outcome: a multicenter study using dobutamine stress hemodynamics. *Circulation* 2003; **108**: 319–24.

52. Levy F, Laurent M, Monin JL, *et al.* Aortic valve replacement for low-flow/low-gradient aortic stenosis

105

operative risk stratification and long-term outcome: a European multicenter study. *J Am Coll Cardiol* 2008; **51**: 466–72.

53. Burwash IG, Lortie M, Pibarot P, *et al.* Myocardial blood flow in patients with low-flow, low-gradient aortic stenosis: differences between true and pseudo-severe aortic stenosis. Results from the multicentre TOPAS (Truly or Pseudo-severe Aortic Stenosis) study. *Heart* 2008; **94**: 1627–33.

54. Rosengart TK, Feldman T, Borger MA, *et al.* Percutaneous and minimally invasive valve procedures: a scientific statement from the American Heart Association Council on Cardiovascular Surgery and Anesthesia, Council on Clinical Cardiology, Functional Genomics and Translational Biology Interdisciplinary Working Group, and Quality of Care and Outcomes Research Interdisciplinary Working Group. *Circulation* 2008; **117**: 1750–67.

55. Chambers J. Can high blood pressure mask severe aortic stenosis? *J Heart Valve Dis* 1998; **7**: 277–8.

56. Bermejo J. The effects of hypertension on aortic valve stenosis. *Heart* 2005; **91**: 280–2.

57. Little SH, Chan KL, Burwash IG. Impact of blood pressure on the Doppler echocardiographic assessment of severity of aortic stenosis. *Heart* 2007; **93**: 848–55.

58. Pibarot P, Dumesnil JG. Assessment of aortic valve severity: check the valve but don't forget the arteries! *Heart* 2007; **93**: 780–2.

59. Enriquez-Sarano M, Tajik AJ. Aortic regurgitation. *N Engl J Med* 2004; **351**: 1539–46.

60. Yacoub MH, Cohn LH. Novel approaches to cardiac valve repair: from structure to function: part II. *Circulation* 2004; **109**: 1064–72.

61. Movsowitz HD, Levine RA, Hilgenberg AD, Isselbacher EM. Transesophageal echocardiographic description of the mechanisms of aortic regurgitation in acute type A aortic dissection: implications for aortic valve repair. *J Am Coll Cardiol* 2000; **36**: 884–90.

62. Davies RR, Goldstein LJ, Coady MA, *et al.* Yearly rupture or dissection rates for thoracic aortic aneurysms: simple prediction based on size. *Ann Thorac Surg* 2002; **73**: 17–28.

63. Cheung YF, Chiu CS, Yung TC, Chau AK. Impact of preoperative aortic cusp prolapse on long-term outcome after closure of subarterial ventricular septal defect. *Ann Thorac Surg* 2002; **73**: 622–7.

64. Rahko PS. Doppler and echocardiogaphic characteristics of patients having an Austin Flint murmur. *Circulation* 1991; **83**: 1940–50.

65. Bekeredjian R, Grayburn PA. Valvular heart disease: aortic regurgitation. *Circulation* 2005; **112**: 125–34.

66. Riedel BJ, Dixon S, Lovell AT. Echocardiographic evidence for valvular abnormalities. *J Cardiothorac Vasc Anesth* 2003; **17**: 549–51.

67. Emi S, Fukuda N, Oki T, *et al.* Genesis of the Austin–Flint murmur: relation to mitral inflow and aortic regurgitant flow dynamics. *J Am Coll Cardiol* 1993; **21**: 1399–405.

68. Zoghbi WA, Enriquez-Sarano M, Foster E, *et al.* Recommendations for evaluation of the severity of native valvular regurgitation with two-dimensional and Doppler echocardiography. *J Am Soc Echocardiogr* 2003; **16**: 777–802.

69. Baumgarten H, Schima H, Kuhn P. Value and limitations of proximal jet dimensions for the quantitation of valvular regurgitation: an in vitro study using Doppler flow imaging. *J Am Soc Echocardiogr* 1991; **4**: 57–66.

70. Tribouilloy CM, Enriquez-Sarano M, Bailey KR, Seward JB, Tajik AJ. Assessment of severity of aortic regurgitation using the width of the vena contracta: a clinical Doppler imaging study. *Circulation* 2000; **102**: 558–64.

71. Enriquez-Sarano M, Seward JB, Bailey KR, Tajik AJ. Effective regurgitant orifice area: a noninvasive Doppler development of an old hemodynamic concept. *J Am Coll Cardiol* 1994; **23**: 443–51.

72. Willett DL, Hall SA, Jessen ME, Wait MA, Grayburn PA. Assessment of aortic regurgitation by transesophageal color doppler imaging of the vena contracta: validation against an intraoperative aortic flow probe. *J Am Coll Cardiol* 2001; **37**: 1450–5.

73. Perry GJ, Helmcke F, Nanda NC, Byard C, Soto B. Evaluation of aortic insufficiency by Doppler color flow mapping. *J Am Coll Cardiol* 1987; **9**: 952–9.

74. Ishii M, Jones M, Shiota T, *et al.* Quantifying aortic regurgitation by using the color Doppler-imaged vena contracta: a chronic animal model study. *Circulation* 1997; **96**: 2009–15.

75. Sutton DC, Kluger R, Ahmed SU, Reimold SC, Mark JB. Flow reversal in the descending aorta: a guide to intraoperative assessment of aortic regurgitation with transesophageal echocardiography. *J Thorac Cardiovasc Surg* 1994; **108**: 576–82.

76. Tribouilloy CM, Enriquez-Sarano M, Fett SL, *et al.* Application of the proximal flow convergence method to calculate the effective orifice area in aortic regurgitation. *J Am Coll Cardiol* 1998; **32**: 1032–9.

77. Bargiggia GS, Tronconi L, Sahn DJ, *et al.* A new method for quantitation of mitral regurgitation based on color flow Doppler imaging of flow convergence proximal to regurgitant orifice. *Circulation* 1991; **84**: 1481–9.

78. Bonow RO, Lakatos E, Maron BJ, Epstein SE. Serial long-term assessment of the natural history of

asymptomatic patients with chronic aortic regurgitation and normal left ventricle systolic function. *Circulation* 1991; **84**: 1625–35.

79. Klodas E, Enriquez-Sarano M, Tajik AJ, *et al.* Aortic regurgitation complicated by extreme left ventricular dilation: long-term outcome after surgical correction. *J Am Coll Cardiol* 1996; **27**: 670–7.

80. Chaliki HP, Mohty D, Avierinos JF, *et al.* Outcomes after aortic valve replacement in patients with severe aortic regurgitation and markedly reduced left ventricular function. *Circulation* 2002; **106**: 2687–93.

81. Bonow RO, Carabello BA, Kanu C, *et al.* ACC/AHA 2006 guidelines for the management of patients with valvular heart disease: a report of the American College of Cardiology/American Heart Association task force on practice guidelines. *Circulation* 2006; **114**: e84–231.

Mitral valve disease

John Kneeshaw

Introduction

Blood in the left atrium forms an ideal acoustic window onto the mitral valve for a transesophageal echocardiographic (TEE) probe. This, and the short distance between the TEE transducer and the mitral valve apparatus, allows the use of high frequencies to produce excellent spatial resolution [1]. Since the ultrasound beam is perpendicular to the mitral valve leaflets in systole, and parallel to diastolic transmitral blood flow (and regurgitant flow), it is almost always possible to obtain high-quality images and accurate spectral Doppler data [2]. The anatomy of the mitral apparatus and a systematic sequence for acquiring images is described in Chapter 5.

Mitral valve leaflet nomenclature

There are two systems of nomenclature available to describe the architecture of the mitral valve leaflets, Carpentier and Duran (Fig. 7.1).

The Duran classification is an anatomically based system of nomenclature [3]. The anterolateral commissure is named C1 and the posteromedial commissure C2, and accordingly the anterolateral papillary muscle (ALPM) is described as M1 and the posteromedial papillary muscle (PMPM) is M2. Consequently segments of the anterior leaflet (AL) and posterior leaflet (PL), which receive chordae that arise from M1, are annotated A1 and P1, respectively. The same principle applies to M2, so the parts of leaflets where its chordae insert onto the AL and PL are A2 and P2. The middle scallop of the PL receives chordae from both papillary muscles, and hence is divided into PM1 and PM2 segments.

The older Carpentier classification is considered by many to be easier to understand; it is certainly in wider use [4]. Each of the mitral valve leaflets is divided into three segments. The three scallops of the PL are named P1, P2, and P3, where P1 is the most anterior and P3 the most posterior. The AL is arbitrarily divided into three portions, A1, A2, and A3, to indicate those portions of the AL which coapt with the three scallops of the PL. Note that, unlike the PL, there are no morphological divisions in the AL.

The Carpentier system of nomenclature is favored by the European Association of Echocardiography and the American Society of Echocardiography, and is the system used in this chapter.

Imaging considerations in mitral valve disease

The basic views required for examination of the mitral valve are described in Chapter 5. This section describes the additional views and maneuvers that may help to further delineate the mitral valve without lengthening the image acquisition time. A complete TEE interrogation of the mitral valve also involves an examination of left atrial pulmonary venous inflow, especially in the case of mitral regurgitation. Although the examination of the mitral valve is usually described in terms of specific standard views, the aim in mitral disease is to scan the whole of the valve apparatus at several multiplane angles.

For accurate interpretation of perioperative abnormalities, it is important that preload, afterload, and especially blood pressure are as close to the patient's pre-anesthetized level as possible.

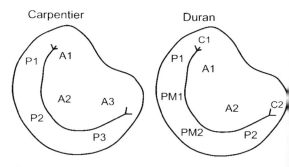

Figure 7.1. The Carpentier and Duran classifications [3,4]. See text for details.

Core Topics in Transesophageal Echocardiography, ed. Robert Feneck, John Kneeshaw, and Marco Ranucci.
Published by Cambridge University Press. © Cambridge University Press 2010.

Mid-esophageal five-chamber view (0°)

This view, although not a standard view, is easily obtained and a useful starting point (Fig. 7.2). The probe is advanced 30–35 cm into the esophagus, with the sector scan at 0° and the transducer very lightly anteflexed. The five chambers seen are the LVOT, LA, LV, RA, and RV. The aortic valve is seen in oblique cross-section. Since the AV and LVOT are anterior cardiac structures, the scan plane usually passes through the anterior segments of the mitral valve, i.e. A1 and P1, with A1 (near the aortic valve) on the left and P1 on the right of the image.

In many patients, imaging from different levels in the esophagus at 0° may be valuable in demonstrating the coaptation point. Thus, with the probe withdrawn to a level that develops the five-chamber view, the visible coaptation point of the anterior and posterior leaflets is at A1 and P1. As the probe is advanced, A2 and P2 come into view, and further advancing the probe until the ME view is nearly lost reveals A3 and P3 [5] (Fig. 7.3).

Mid-esophageal four-chamber view (0–15°)

From the above position, and with the sector scan still at 0°, advance the probe 3–5 cm and retroflex the

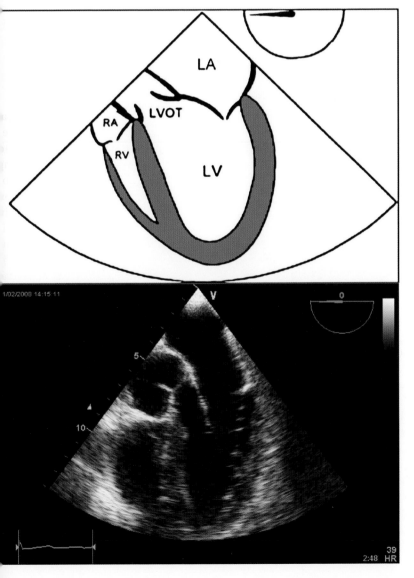

Figure 7.2. The (non-standard) mid-esophageal five-chamber view. RA, right atrium; RV, right ventricle; LA, left atrium; LV, left ventricle; LVOT, left ventricular outflow tract.

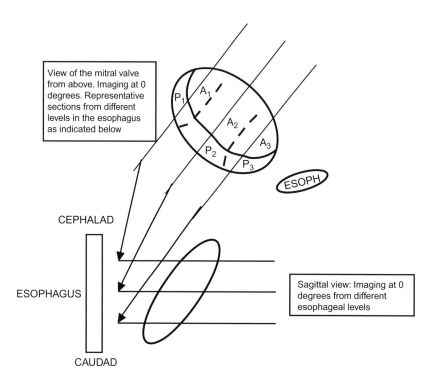

Figure 7.3. Schematic representation of the mitral valve as seen using single plane (0°) imaging from three different locations in the esophagus. A1, A2, and A3 refer to the three scallops of the anterior leaflet; P1, P2, and P3 refer to the scallops of the posterior leaflet. The three-dimensional structure of the mitral valve shows that it does not lie in one plane. The valve is shown in the sagittal plane, and it extends from a cephalad position to a caudad one. Three different echocardiographic beams are depicted at three different levels within the esophagus.

Within the figure:
- View of the mitral valve from above. Imaging at 0 degrees. Representative sections from different levels in the esophagus as indicated below
- CEPHALAD
- ESOPHAGUS
- CAUDAD
- ESOPH
- Sagittal view: Imaging at 0 degrees from different esophageal levels

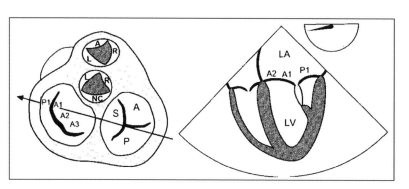

Figure 7.4. Mid-esophageal four-chamber long-axis view (0–15°) and corresponding short-axis cross-sectional view.

probe, until the AV and LVOT disappear (Fig. 7.4). Since the apex of the LV is located inferior to the base of the heart in many patients, retroflexion of the probe will prevent foreshortening of the LV, and the resultant image plane should be parallel to transmitral flow. At 0° the scan plane should intersect the coaptation line perpendicularly at A2 and P2. However, this may not always be the case in this view. By advancing the multiplane angle to 15°, the scan line now cuts the coaptation line obliquely through the A2, A1, and P1 segments. The anterolateral papillary muscle should also come into view at 15°. The LV lateral wall is on the right and the septal wall on the left of the display.

Mid-esophageal commissural view (60°) (trapdoor view)

As the multiplane angle is rotated from 15° to 60°, a transition in the image occurs where the PL appears on the left of the display and the AL on the right (Fig. 7.5). At this transition angle (often around 60°), the scan plane is parallel to the line that intersects the two commissures of the mitral valve. Hence the scan plane intersects the coaptation line twice, at A1/P1 and A3/P3. The A2 segment of the AL is seen flicking in and out of the LV inflow, with P1 on the right and P3 on the left of the display. Both papillary muscles should be visible, and the RV disappears from the image. From this neutral position, by

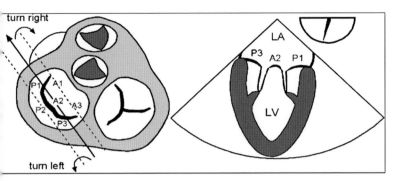

Figure 7.5. Mid-esophageal commissural view (60°) and corresponding short-axis cross-section.

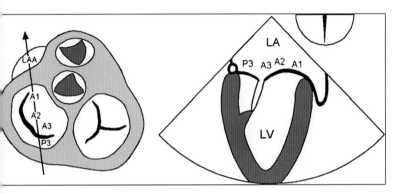

Figure 7.6. Mid-esophageal two-chamber view (90°) and corresponding short-axis cross-section.

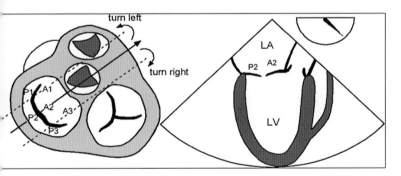

Figure 7.7. Mid-esophageal long-axis view (120–150°) and corresponding short-axis cross-section.

urning the probe clockwise, the scan plane passes through he body of the posterior leaflet (P1, P2, P3). Going back to he neutral position and then turning the probe counter-clockwise, the scan plane now passes through the body of he anterior leaflet (A3, A2, A1), and the left atrium should lso come into view.

Mid-esophageal two-chamber view (90°)

Next, the multiplane angle is rotated forward to 90° rom the above position to develop this view (Fig. 7.6). This image is characterized by the appearance of the

posteromedial papillary muscle and coronary sinus on the left, and the left atrial appendage on the right. The anterior wall of the left ventricle is on the right and the inferior wall on the left. The scan plane intersects the coaptation line at P3/A3, and cuts through the remaining body of the anterior leaflet. Therefore P3 is on the left and A3, A2, A1 on the right.

Mid-esophageal long-axis view (120–150°)

From the two-chamber position, the multiplane angle is rotated forward until the mitral valve, aortic valve,

111

and LVOT are visualized (Fig. 7.7). No papillary muscles should be seen, and the inferolateral (posterior) and anteroseptal LV walls are seen respectively on the left and right of the display. The sector scan intersects the mitral valve coaptation line perpendicularly at P2 (on the left) and A2 (on the right). As with the mid-esophageal commissural view, rotation of the probe clockwise from this neutral position will cause the scan plane to pass through the P3/A3 coaptation point. Rotation of the probe counterclockwise from the neutral position will cause the scan plane to pass through the P1/A1 coaptation point, and also through the left atrial appendage. The mid-esophageal long-axis view is the recommended view for measuring the mitral end-systolic annular diameter, the width of the vena contracta, and the length of the mitral valve leaflets, and for assessing whether the leaflets are prolapsing. An end-systolic mitral annular diameter greater than 37 mm is by definition annular dilation.

At each of these mid-esophageal views of the mitral valve, color-flow Doppler (CFD) should be deployed. It is necessary to ensure that the color sector includes a large portion of the LA in order to detect mitral regurgitant jets and the flow convergence of mitral stenosis. Figure 7.8 summarizes the mid-esophageal mitral views, and shows the relevant structural details.

Transgastric basal short-axis view (0°)

The multiplane angle should now be returned to 0° and the probe advanced into the stomach (Fig. 7.9). The probe may then be anteflexed in order to maintain contact with the gastric mucosa and hence the base of the heart. Better basal short-axis cross-sectional views are often obtained if the transducer is pushed slightly deeper into the stomach and the probe anteflexed more in order to orientate the scanning plane parallel to the mitral annulus. This view produces the typical "fishmouth" appearance of the mitral valve orifice. It is the only TEE view in which all six leaflet segments can be seen at the same time, with the posteromedial commissure (P3/A3) at the top left of the display, and the anterolateral commissure (P1/A1) at the bottom right of the display. The posterior and anterior leaflets occupy the right and left of the display respectively. Basal LV segments are also seen, and regional wall motion abnormalities may be noted. The fishmouth view with added CFD is useful for identifying the source of a regurgitant jet (Fig. 7.10; Video 7.1).

Advancing the probe slightly, or decreasing the amount of anteflexion, or a combination of both, produces the transgastric mid short-axis view. This view is important for detecting regional wall motion abnormalities adjacent to the papillary muscles, or hypermobility indicating rupture of a papillary muscle or its components. From this view the LV mid-papillary diameter can be ascertained.

Transgastric two-chamber view (90°)

From the basal short-axis view, the multiplane angle is rotated forward to 90° (Fig. 7.11). This view is especially useful for interrogating the subvalvular apparatus, as the scan plane is perpendicular to the papillary

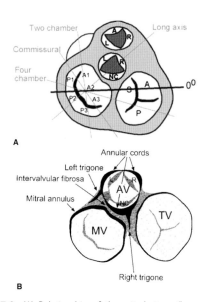

Figure 7.8. (A) Relationship of the mitral views (long-axis, two-chamber, four-chamber, and commissural) as viewed in the short axis. (B) Important structural details relevant to (A). The fibrous skeleton provides the structural framework for the heart valves. It consists of the left, right, and non-coronary cords that form the aortic annulus. The left trigone extends from the left annular cord, and the right trigone from the non-coronary annular cord.

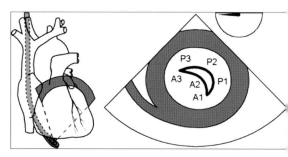

Figure 7.9. Transgastric basal short-axis view (0°).

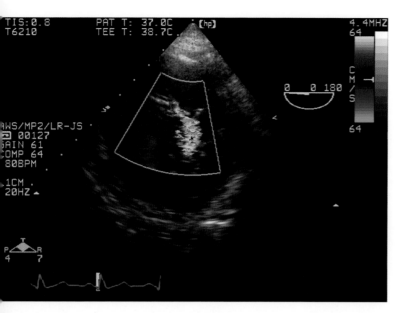

Figure 7.10. Transgastric basal view with color-flow Doppler showing all six segments of the mitral leaflets. See Video 7.1.

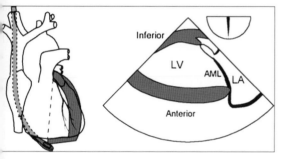

Figure 7.11. Transgastric two-chamber view (90°).

muscles and chordae tendineae. Basal and mid segments of the anterior LV wall (bottom of display), and inferior LV wall (top of display) are also visualized. The posteromedial papillary muscle is usually clearly seen.

From the 2D images described above, the mitral valve can be critically assessed. Morphological characteristics of interest are leaflet mobility, leaflet thickening, subvalvular thickening, and calcification. Scoring systems have been developed with these characteristics in mind (Table 7.1) [6]. These may play a role in the management of mitral valve disease, especially mitral stenosis, where they can predict procedure-related morbidity and mortality.

Mitral stenosis

Mitral stenosis is obstruction of left ventricular inflow at the level of the mitral valve, as a result of structural abnormalities of the mitral valve apparatus that limit proper opening during diastole. The etiology of mitral stenosis is shown in Table 7.2.

Pathophysiology

Narrowing of the valve area to less than 2.5 cm^2 usually occurs before symptoms develop [7]. As the valve area is reduced, blood flow from the left atrium (LA) to the left ventricle (LV) can only occur if it is propelled by an increased pressure gradient. This diastolic transmitral pressure gradient is the key to the pathophysiology of mitral stenosis, and reflects an increased LA pressure [8]. The LA dilates to accommodate this increased pressure. This pressure increase is reflected back into the pulmonary venous circulation. The hydrostatic pressure in the pulmonary veins and capillaries increases, causing pulmonary venous hypertension and pulmonary edema. The increase in pulmonary venous pressure results in an increase in pulmonary artery pressure, which is initially *passive*, i.e. there is a normal transpulmonary pressure gradient (pulmonary artery to LA pressure) as pulmonary artery and LA pressures increase by an equal amount. In this situation, although the pulmonary artery pressure is increased, pulmonary vascular resistance is normal, and the pulmonary artery pressure will fall if the stenosis is relieved [8].

When the pulmonary venous hypertension becomes long-standing, the pulmonary arterioles react with vasoconstriction, intimal hyperplasia, and medial hypertrophy, which leads to *active* pulmonary

113

Table 7.1. Scoring system to assess mitral valve morphology and mobility. From Wilkins *et al., Br Heart J* 1988; **60**: 299–308 [6]

Grade	Mobility of leaflets
0	Normal
1	Highly mobile valve with only leaflet tips restricted
2	Leaflet middle and base portions have normal mobility
3	Valve continues to move forward in diastole, mainly from the base
4	No or minimal forward movement of the leaflets in diastole

Grade	Thickening of leaflets
0	Normal
1	Leaflets near normal in thickness (4–5mm)
2	Midleaflets normal, marked thickening of margins (5–8mm)
3	Thickening extending through the entire leaflet (5–8mm)
4	Marked thickening of all leaflet tissue (8–10mm)

Grade	Subvalvular thickening
0	Normal
1	Minimal thickening just below the mitral leaflets
2	Thickening of chordal structures extending up to one third of the chordal length
3	Thickening extending to the distal third of the chordal length
4	Extensive thickening and shortening of all chordal structures extending to papillary muscles

Grade	Calcification of leaflets
0	Normal
1	A single area of increased echo brightness
2	Scattered areas of brightness confined to leaflet margins
3	Brightness extending into the mid-portion of the leaflets
4	Extensive brightness throughout much of the leaflet tissue

Total score is obtained by adding the scores for each of the four features.

Table 7.2. Etiology of mitral stenosis

1. Congenital
a. Congenital mitral stenosis
2. Acquired
b. Rheumatic carditis*
c. Degenerative/calcific mitral stenosis*
c. SLE
d. Malignant sarcoid
e. Mucopolysaccharidosis
f. Gout

* commonest causes.

is a spectrum of mitral annular calcification, which in its most trivial form appears as an isolated area of calcification at the base of the posterior mitral annulus. In its most severe form, the calcification involves the entire posterior mitral annulus. The anterior mitral annulus is often spared. The calcification may extend to involve the base of the posterior mitral leaflet, resulting in functional mitral stenosis. Mitral regurgitation may also be present, due to the inflexibility of the posterior mitral annulus secondary to calcification. Unlike rheumatic mitral stenosis, the leaflet tips remain thin and mobile with no commissural fusion (Fig. 7.12; Video 7.2).

Rheumatic mitral stenosis

Rheumatic carditis is the commonest cause of mitral stenosis in both developed and developing countries. However, the disease profile in developed countries tends to be milder, with a delayed onset of symptoms. The mitral valve is affected in isolation in 40% of cases of rheumatic carditis [8], and there is a 2 : 1 female preponderance. Once symptoms develop, usually in the fifth or sixth decade, there is a period of approximately a further decade before these symptoms become disabling. Overall, the 10-year survival for untreated mitral stenosis is 50–60%.

TEE features of rheumatic mitral stenosis

Valvular and subvalvular features

Two-dimensional leaflet morphology abnormalities include loss of leaflet mobility due to fusion of the anterior and posterior leaflet tips along the medial and lateral commissures, i.e. commissural fusion. Hence the base and mid-section of the leaflets are free to move towards the ventricular apex in diastole. This create

artery hypertension, which persists despite relief of the stenosis. Consequent upon persistent pulmonary artery hypertension, the right ventricle hypertrophies and enlarges, resulting in tricuspid annular dilation and eventually tricuspid regurgitation.

Mitral annular calcification/calcific mitral stenosis

Mitral annular calcification is a degenerative process, and is a common incidental finding in the elderly. There

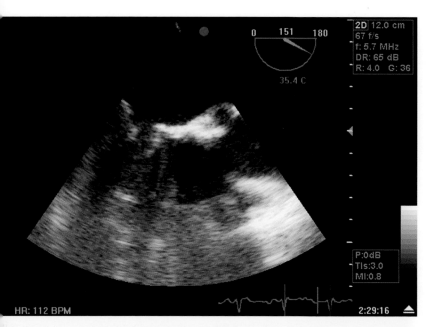

Figure 7.12. Long-axis view showing calcific mitral stenosis. Only the leaflet tips remain mobile. See Video 7.2.

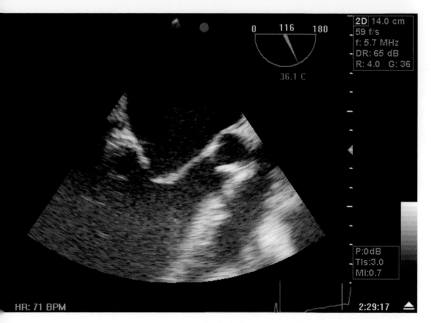

Figure 7.13. Long-axis view in a patient with rheumatic mitral stenosis, showing the "hockey stick" deformity of the anterior leaflet. The disease has also affected the aortic valve. See Video 7.3.

The appearance of diastolic doming of the body of the leaflets, especially in the AL, as it is longer than the PL. Reverse doming occurs in systole as the valve moves in the opposite direction. With the restricted movement of its tip and the associated thickening, the anterior leaflet often resembles a "hockey stick" in diastole. Although thickening of the leaflet tips due to valvitis occurs frequently, the remainder of the leaflet can show variable degrees of thickening and/or calcification. The subvalvular region is also frequently involved, with fusion, shortening, fibrosis, and calcification of the chordae. The combination of valvular and subvalvular abnormalities results in a funnel-shaped deformity of the mitral apparatus. These features are best appreciated in the mid-esophageal and transgastric views. Rheumatic carditis may affect other heart valves. The aortic valve is the next most frequently involved, followed by the tricuspid valve (Fig. 7.13, Video 7.3).

115

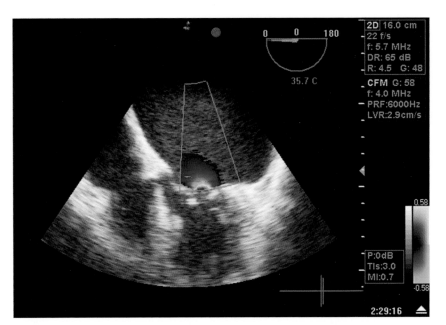

Figure 7.14. Mid-esophageal four chamber view with color-flow Doppler showing flow acceleration and PISA formation in mitral stenosis. See Video 7.4.

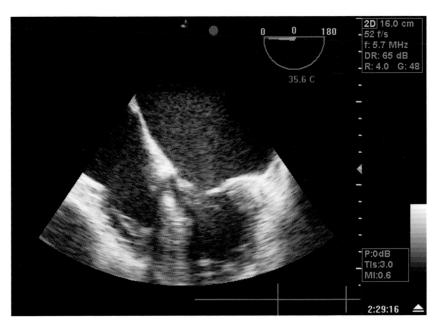

Figure 7.15. Mid-esophageal four chamber view of the classic appearances of mitral stenosis. There is a large left atrium with spontaneous echo contrast thickening and reduced leaflet motion, and a small left ventricle. See Video 7.5.

Using **color-flow Doppler**, flow acceleration marked by color aliasing and PISA formation may be seen on the left atrial side of the stenotic mitral valve. There may also be concomitant mitral regurgitation, which is often trivial to mild (Fig. 7.14; Video 7.4).

Non-valvular features

With increased LA pressure, **LA dilation** occurs, with pronounced left-to-right bowing of the interatrial septum. Spontaneous echo contrast (SEC), sometime described as "smoke," may be seen within the left atrium. SEC is caused by slow-moving blood, and may result in thrombus formation, which commonly occurs in the left atrial appendage (LAA) but can occur anywhere in the LA chamber, including the free atrial wall or interatrial septum. LAA thrombus may protrude into the LA chamber, whereas thrombus in other parts of the LA has a laminated appearance. Atrial fibrillation in patients with mitral stenosis is highly thrombogenic, but thrombus formation can also occur in patients in sinus rhythm. TEE has a high sensitivity (> 99%), and a high specificity (> 99%), for the detection of LAA thrombus [7] (Fig. 7.15; Video 7.5).

Chronic exposure of the right ventricle (RV) to pulmonary artery hypertension results in **RV hypertrophy** and **enlargement**. Increased RV pressure produces paradoxical septal motion. RV chamber enlargement culminates in tricuspid annular dilation, with consequent tricuspid regurgitation. Continuous-wave Doppler (CWD) analysis of this regurgitant jet and application of the modified Bernoulli equation allows the systolic pressure gradient to be calculated across the tricuspid valve. If the pulmonary valve is normal, the systolic pressure gradient across the tricuspid valve plus right atrial (RA) pressure approximates to systolic pulmonary artery pressure.

The **LV** is frequently **small** and **underfilled**, with normal wall thickening and apparently normal systolic function. If the LV is dilated, other valvular abnormalities including mitral and/or aortic regurgitation, or a primary myocardial problem such as cardiomyopathy or ischemia, should be considered [2].

Quantification of the severity of mitral stenosis

Most of the techniques for assessing the severity of mitral stenosis have their origins in transthoracic echo, and have been transferred to TEE (Box 7.1).

Transmitral pressure gradient

Using an appropriate mid-esophageal view, the mean diastolic transmitral velocity can be estimated using pulsed or continuous-wave Doppler, provided the Doppler flow signal is parallel to transmitral blood flow. The mean velocity is obtained by tracing the area under the transmitral Doppler spectrum. Since spectral Doppler often underestimates velocity, several measurements should be taken and the mean transmitral diastolic pressure gradient calculated using the modified Bernoulli equation (Fig. 7.16).

Accurate pressure gradients depend on accurate velocity measurements, which are dependent on a near-parallel intercept angle between the spectral Doppler beam and blood flow.

All calculated pressure gradients are highly dependent on volume, flow rate, and valve area. Therefore

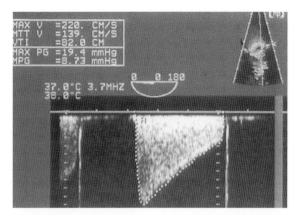

Figure 7.16. The use of spectral Doppler to estimate the mean mitral gradient in mitral stenosis.

conditions which increase transmitral flow rate (e.g. an increase in cardiac output and heart rate, mitral regurgitation [MR], and restrictive diastolic filling defects) will increase the transmitral pressure gradient. Conversely, factors which decrease flow rate will reduce the transmitral pressure gradient.

Mitral valve orifice area

The MV orifice is normally between 4 and 6 cm² in area. Below are four methods to estimate valve area.

Planimetry

In the transgastric basal short-axis view the largest mitral orifice area can be identified, and then measured using the 2D area trace modality. Although well validated for transthoracic echo, this method cannot be recommended for routine TEE assessment of the mitral valve orifice area. As the mitral valve becomes progressively more stenotic, it assumes a funnel shape, with the narrowest orifice at the tips of the valve leaflets. The transgastric basal short-axis view is more often than not an oblique cut through the mitral valve, and thus planimetry overestimates the valve orifice area.

Pressure half-time (PHT) and deceleration time (DT)

These methods are based on the concept that the rate of decline of a pressure gradient across an orifice is determined in part by the cross-sectional area of the orifice. The smaller the orifice, the slower the rate of decline of the pressure gradient. This decline in pressure is also influenced by the compliance of the left atrium and ventricle. It may be obtained from the

Box 7.1. Quantification of mitral stenosis

(a) Calculation of mean diastolic transmitral pressure gradient

$$P = \frac{4\left(V_1^2 + V_2^2 + V_3^2 + V_n^2\right)}{n} \tag{7.1}$$

(see also Fig. 7.16)

(b) Derivation of pressure half-time (PHT)

PHT is the time taken for the velocity (V_{max}) to fall to $\frac{1}{\sqrt{2}} V_{max}$.($\frac{1}{\sqrt{2}} = 0.7$).

A PHT of 220 ms corresponds well to a valve area of 1 cm², leading to the derivation of Hartle's formula:

$$\text{Mitral valve orifice area (MVOA)} = 220/\,PHT \tag{7.2}$$

Deceleration time is the interval from the maximum transmitral diastolic pressure gradient to zero pressure gradient (see Fig. 7.17).

$$PHT = \text{deceleration time} \times 0.29 \tag{7.3}$$

Substituting this for PHT in Equation 7.2 yields:

$$MVOA = 220/0.29 \times DT \implies MVOA = 759/DT \tag{7.4}$$

Implying that if DT = 759 ms, MVOA= 1 cm².

(c) Calculation of mitral valve area using the continuity equation

Since flow (Q) through an orifice (cm³/s) = calculated orificial area (COA) (cm²) × velocity (V) (cm/s):

$$Q_{mean} = COA \times V_{mean} \tag{7.5}$$

$$Q_{max} = COA \times V_{max} \tag{7.6}$$

Dividing each side of the equation by time (s) reveals:

$$\text{Stroke Volume (SV) (cm}^3) = (COA) \text{ (cm}^2) \times VTI \text{ (cm)} \tag{7.7}$$

Mitral valve velocity–time integral (VTI_{mv}):
  • is a measure of distance (in cm)
  • is obtained by integrating the area under the transmitral diastolic velocity–time curve
  • is a function of mean velocity of flow ($V_{mean} \times$ time).
SV is a derivative of mean velocity.
Rearranging equation 7.6 yields:

$$MVOA \text{ (cm}^2) = SV/\,VTI_{mv} \tag{7.8}$$

But SV through the mitral valve in diastole should be equal to SV through the LVOT (in systole) and pulmonary artery (in systole)
Since

$$SV_{LVOT} = COA_{LVOT} \times VTI_{LVOT} \tag{7.9}$$

Therefore, combining Equations 7.8 and 7.9:

$$MVOA = COA_{LVOT} \times VTI_{LVOT}/VTI_{mv} \tag{7.10}$$

(d) Proximal isovelocity surface area (PISA)

Fluid converging towards the orifice accelerates, reaching a peak velocity at the orifice.
Consider a series of hemispheres centered on the orifice. The velocity of flow at the surface of each of these hemispheres will be constant.
These surfaces are called a proximal isovelocity surface area (PISA).

Box 7.1. (*cont.*)

Since the surface area of a sphere is $4\pi r^2$:

$$\text{Calculated surface area of PISA (hemisphere) } (CSA_{PISA}) = 2\pi r^2 \text{ (cm}^2\text{)} \qquad (7.11)$$

where r = radius of the hemisphere, i.e. distance from the center of the orifice to the outer shell of the outermost hemisphere.
Therefore:

$$\text{Flow rate at PISA } (Q_{PISA}) = CSA_{PISA} \times NL \qquad (7.12)$$

where NL = aliasing velocity = Nyqvist limit
By application of the continuity principle, volume flow rate through the mitral valve orifice (Q_{MVO}) must equal volume flow rate at PISA (Q_{PISA}).
Therefore:

$$MVOA = CSA_{PISA} \times NL / V_{max-mv} \qquad (7.13)$$

where V_{max-mv} is maximum transmitral diastolic velocity, measured by CWD
  • If the mitral valve leaflets have restricted mobility, they may open incompletely.
  • The resultant PISA has a cone-shaped base formed by the mitral valve leaflets.
  • This decreases the CSA_{PISA}, which needs to be amended accordingly [9]:

$$CSA_{PISA} = 2\pi r^2 \times a / 180 \qquad (7.14)$$

where a = the angle formed by the mitral valve leaflets in diastole.

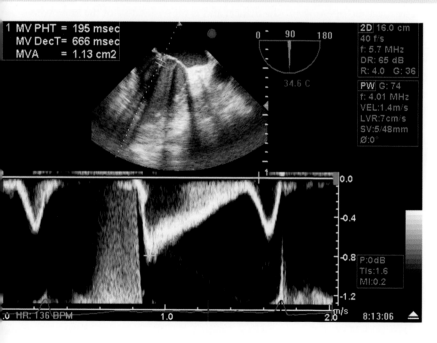

Figure 7.17. Estimation of valve area by pressure half-time (PHT) using pulsed-wave Doppler in mitral stenosis.

spectral Doppler transmitral diastolic velocity–time curve.

• **PHT** is the time in milliseconds for the transmitral diastolic pressure gradient to fall from any particular value to half that value. The maximum early diastolic transmitral pressure

gradient is commonly used for convenience, but any point along the velocity–time curve can be used (see also Chapter 13).
• **DT** is the interval in milliseconds from the maximum transmitral diastolic pressure gradient to zero pressure gradient. DT is more flow-dependent than PHT (Fig. 7.17).

Table 7.3. Quantitative assessment of severity of mitral stenosis

	Mean transvalvular gradient (mmHg)	Mitral valve area (cm²)	Pressure half-time (ms)
Mild	< 6	1.5–4	100–150
Moderate	6–12	1.0–1.5	150–200
Severe	> 12	< 1.0	> 200

The PHT method may be misleading or inaccurate in certain clinical situations. Any condition which increases left ventricular end-diastolic pressure (LVEDP), for example coexisting aortic or mitral regurgitation, will decrease the pressure gradient across the mitral valve and therefore *increase* the rate of decay of the transmitral diastolic pressure gradient, leading to a decreased PHT and hence an overestimation of the mitral valve area. PHT may also be decreased by an increase in cardiac output or heart rate and by restrictive diastolic filling defects. If there is severe coexisting aortic regurgitation, the regurgitant jet will paradoxically impede diastolic opening of the anterior mitral leaflet, causing functional mitral stenosis to be superimposed on anatomical mitral stenosis. This will result in prolongation of the PHT and therefore underestimate the mitral valve orifice area. Other technical considerations that may hamper PHT interpretation include arrhythmias, especially fast atrial fibrillation, and a non-linear transmitral velocity–time curve, in which case the mid-diastolic part of the curve should be used for measurements.

The relationships between mitral valve area, transmitral pressure gradient, PHT, and severity of mitral stenosis are shown in Table 7.3.

Continuity method

This is based on the **law of conservation of mass**. When applied to blood flow in the context of echocardiography it can be expressed as: *In the absence of shunts, or valvular regurgitation, and under conditions of cardiovascular stability, net forward stroke volume (SV) (or maximum instantaneous flow or mean flow) at any point in the circulation must equal net forward SV (or maximum instantaneous flow or mean flow) at any other point in the circulation, provided blood is neither added to nor removed from the system.*

The flow through the mitral valve in diastole is the same as the flow through the LVOT in systole, assuming no flow is lost through an anatomical shunt or returned via a regurgitant valve.

The continuity method is unreliable with coexistent mitral and aortic regurgitation, and is highly dependent on accurate diameter measurements, since these values have to be squared to calculate areas.

Proximal isovelocity surface area (PISA)

This refers to the organized area of flow acceleration proximal to an orifice [9]. If we consider a column of fluid approaching a point orifice on a flat surface, as the fluid flow converges towards the orifice, it accelerates along a series of multidirectional streamlines, reaching a peak velocity at the orifice itself. At any distance (r), in any direction, proximal to the orifice, the velocity of flow will be constant. Hence a series of arcs or hemispheres centered on the orifice will have constant flow velocity at the surface of each hemisphere. These surfaces are called proximal isovelocity surface areas (PISA).

If color Doppler is used to image this flow convergence zone, an abrupt area of color change, signifying aliasing, will be seen a certain distance (r), from the center of the orifice. This outermost area of aliasing will assume the shape of an arc, or hemisphere, centered on the orifice, and is representative of the zone where the flow velocity exceeds the Nyquist limit (Fig. 7.14). As flow continues to accelerate towards the orifice, further hemispheres of progressively smaller radii will appear each time the flow velocity exceeds a multiple of the Nyquist limit. It is possible to adjust the echo machine Nyquist limit to better define the PISA and, using the freeze and scroll function of the TEE machine, to measure the radius (r) of the PISA (Fig. 7.18). In the case of mitral stenosis, as the mitral valve leaflets have restricted mobility they open incompletely in diastole. Hence the resultant PISA, centered across the stenotic mitral valve orifice, has a cone-shaped base formed by the mitral valve leaflets. This decreases the surface area of the PISA, which needs to be amended accordingly (Box 7.1; Fig. 7.19; Video 7.6). Valve orifice area calculations based on PISA methods are unaffected by coexistent regurgitant lesions.

Mitral regurgitation

Mitral regurgitation is the most commonly encountered valvular lesion in modern clinical practice. Dysfunction or altered anatomy of any one of the components of the mitral valve may result in valvular incompetence. Mitral regurgitation may be **organic** if there is intrinsic valve disease causing regurgitation, or **functional** if the valve is structurally normal and regurgitation is due to an extra-valvular abnormality [10]. The etiology of mitral regurgitation is shown in Table 7.4.

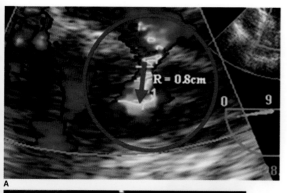

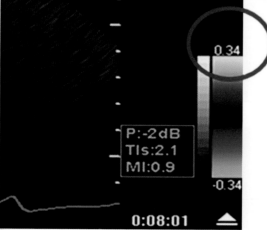

Figure 7.18. Measurement of PISA: (A) *r* = radius to first PISA; (B) Nyquist limit (velocity at first PISA).

Table 7.4. Etiology of mitral regurgitation

1. Organic/valvular

  a. Congenital (*is the MV in AVSD really a mitral valve? It is usually referred to as a left AV valve*)

    i. Cleft or fenestrated mitral leaflet

    ii. Double mitral valve orifice

    iii. Parachute mitral valve (endocardial cushion defects/endocardial fibroelastosis)

  b. Acquired

    i. Rheumatic heart disease

    ii. Mitral valve prolapse syndrome/myxomatous degeneration

    iii. Marfan syndrome

    iv. Erler–Danlos syndrome

    v. Endocarditis

    vi. Collagen vascular disease (SLE, rheumatoid arthritis)

2. Functional

  a. Annulus

    i. Mitral annular calcification

    ii. Mitral annular dilation (DCM)

  b. Papillary muscles

    i. Rupture secondary to myocardial infarction

  c. Left ventricle

    i. Myocardial ischemia or infarction

    ii. Primary myocardial dysfunction (DCM, HOCM)

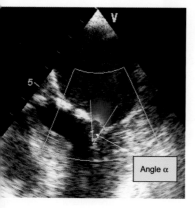

Figure 7.19. Color-flow Doppler showing PISA formation in mitral stenosis. The PISA is not an exact hemispherical shell, and an angulation adjustment will be required. See Video 7.6.

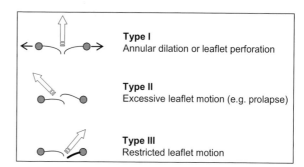

Type I
Annular dilation or leaflet perforation

Type II
Excessive leaflet motion (e.g. prolapse)

Type III
Restricted leaflet motion

Figure 7.20. The mechanisms of mitral regurgitation and consequent jet direction.

Some of the disease processes shown may affect more than one component of the mitral apparatus concomitantly.

Mechanisms of mitral regurgitation

Based on their experience of mitral valve repair, Carpentier *et al.* devised a system detailing the anatomical changes in the mitral apparatus [4,11]. This system is based entirely upon the motion of the mitral valve leaflets. Three mechanisms of MR are described (Fig. 7.20):

Type I describes **normal leaflet motion**, with annular dilation or leaflet perforation. Annular dilation is likely to result in a central regurgitant

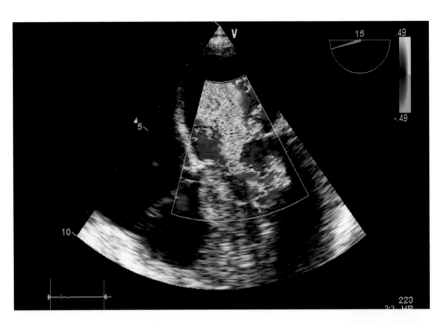

Figure 7.21. Annular dilation causing central mitral regurgitation. See Video 7.7.

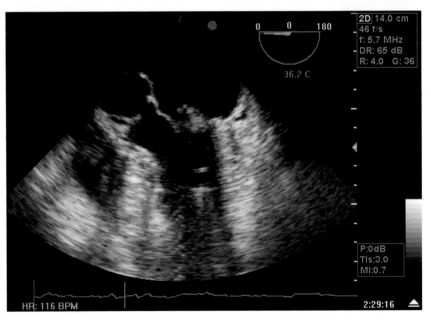

Figure 7.22. Excess leaflet motion. A long-axis view showing myxomatous degeneration with flail of the P2 (or possibly P1) segment. See Video 7.8.

jet, whereas leaflet perforation may result in an eccentric jet (Fig. 7.21; Video 7.7).

Type II describes **excessive motion**, flail, or prolapsing leaflets (most commonly P2). The excessive motion may result from leaflet degeneration, elongated chordae, ruptured chordae, or papillary muscle rupture. Suboptimal leaflet coaptation leads to an eccentric regurgitant jet, directed away from the affected leaflet (Fig. 7.22; Video 7.8).

Type III refers to **restricted leaflet motion**, where the coaptation point is typically apically displaced below the mitral annular plane. The leaflets appear tethered or tented in systole. The regurgitant jet is directed towards the side of the restricted leaflet, or it may be central if both leaflets are equally tethered (Fig. 7.23; Video 7.9). **Type IIIb** is also described, in which the restriction of leaflet motion occurs as a result of an abnormality of LV geometry that causes

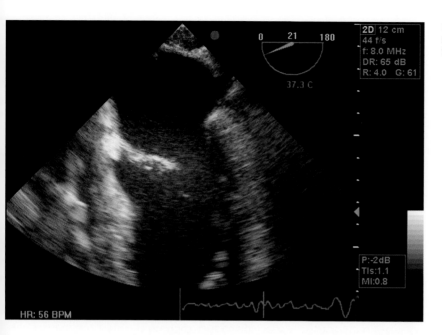

Figure 7.23. Four-chamber view showing restriction of motion of the posterior leaflet. See Video 7.9.

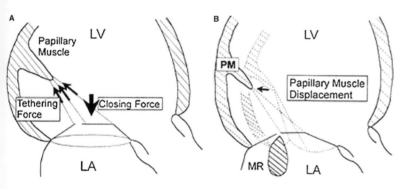

Figure 7.24. Restriction of leaflet motion occurs as a result of an abnormality of LV geometry that causes displacement of the papillary muscles. The result is tethering of the cords and mitral regurgitation.

displacement of the papillary muscles and hence chordal tethering (Fig. 7.24).

Descriptive criteria for excessive leaflet motion

The diagnostic criteria for mitral valve prolapse have long been controversial [12]. Recently, greater understanding of the 3D shape and size of the mitral annulus has allowed these definitions to be refined. The saddle shape of the mitral annulus means that two axes can be described: a high basal axis which is visualized in the mid-esophageal long-axis view, and a low apical axis which is seen in the mid-esophageal commissural view. The diagnostic criteria for prolapse are made with reference to the high axis. If any other view is used, prolapse may be overdiagnosed.

Prolapse (Fig. 7.25) is defined as maximum superior displacement of the body of one or both of the mitral valve leaflets, of greater than or equal to 2 mm, relative to a line connecting the annular hinge points of the mitral annular plane at end systole. The leaflet tips are directed towards the LV, and a coaptation defect may or may not be visible. **Flail** is characterized by a visible 2D coaptation defect, with the leaflet tip directed towards the LA in systole. It is frequently associated with severe MR. Systolic **leaflet billowing** refers to hooding of the body of the mitral valve leaflet, less than 2 mm, above the mitral annular plane. It may represent a pre-prolapse state.

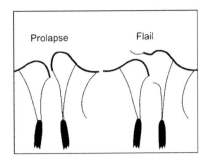

Figure 7.25. Schematic differentiation between prolapse and flail leaflets.

Mitral valve pathology

Organic mitral regurgitation

Rheumatic heart disease

This has the characteristic 2D features of restricted leaflet mobility, thickened and calcified leaflet tips, and commissural fusion, usually with some degree of MR. The restricted leaflet and chordal shortening may result in an eccentric MR jet directed towards the side of the restricted leaflet. If both leaflets are affected equally, there may be a central MR jet. In rheumatic carditis, if prolapse does occur, it is more likely to affect the anterior leaflet.

Primary mitral valve prolapse syndrome (MVPS) / myxomatous degeneration

MVPS refers to a disease spectrum with frank myxomatous degeneration at one extreme. It is characterized by systolic prolapse of one or both mitral leaflets into the LA, with or without MR. Myxomatous degeneration should be a histological diagnosis, not an echocardiographic one, but there are some characteristic 2D echo features, which are grouped under the heading of primary MVPS. MVPS is the most common form of valvular heart disease, accounting for 2–6% of the population. Whilst it often produces little or no MR, it is also the commonest cause of significant MR.

The basic microscopic feature of primary MVPS is marked proliferation of the spongiosa. This is the delicate myxomatous connective tissue between the atrialis and the fibrosa or ventricularis. The atrialis is a thick layer of collagen and elastic tissue forming the atrial aspect of the leaflet, and the ventricularis is the dense layer of collagen that forms the basic support of the leaflet [13]. Myxomatous proliferation of the acid mucopolysaccharide-containing spongiosa causes focal interruption of the fibrosa. Hence the leaflet, most commonly P2, and chordae become thickened and redundant, but with reduced tensile strength, so that they are prone to progressive elongation or rupture. With time, leaflet or chordal tissue rupture will result in a flail coaptation defect and severe MR. A large proportion of these patients will require mitral valve surgery. The gradual progression of MR in patients with primary MVPS results in progressive dilation of the left atrium and ventricle. Atrial dilation may result in atrial fibrillation, and ventricular dilation may progress to dysfunction and congestive cardiac failure if untreated. The myxomatous process in primary MVPS may also involve the tricuspid, pulmonary, and aortic valves in 40%, 10%, and 2% of cases respectively

Valvular endocarditis

MR occurs as a consequence of leaflet destruction, deformity, or perforation [2]. Vegetations typically develop on the low-pressure atrial side of the mitral valve. The papillary muscles and chordae may also be affected and may rupture. The most common mechanism of MR in endocarditis is a flail leaflet. Leaflet perforation is a little more difficult to diagnose, but CFD may help to detect regurgitant jets, which arise from perforations of the body of the leaflet rather than from the coaptation point. This, together with one or more proximal flow convergence phenomena centered along the body of the leaflet and not at the closure line, should alert the echocardiographer to the possibility of leaflet perforation. The endocarditic process may frequently involve other valves, which should be examined carefully.

Marfan syndrome

MR occurs secondary to a long redundant anterior leaflet, which is displaced into the left atrium in systole.

Functional mitral regurgitation

Unlike structural mitral valve disease, functional MR is characterized by normal leaflets that remain apically displaced within the ventricle. MR, ranging in severity, occurs in 20–25% of such patients. Several mechanisms have been proposed for this apical displacement or tenting of the leaflets below the mitral annular plane, termed **incomplete mitral leaflet closure** [14].

The mitral valve leaflets are acted upon by a series of opposing forces, and when these forces are balanced, valvular competence is achieved. In diastole, the predominant force is the LA-to-LV pressure gradient, which opens the valve leaflets. In systole, however, there are two opposing forces: firstly the force generated by increased LV chamber pressure secondary to LV contraction, which acts to close the leaflets, and secondly the restrictive force exerted by the subvalvular apparatus to prevent excessive excursion of the leaflets.

The potential mechanisms for functional MR include:

- global LV dysfunction, which decreases LV systolic pressure and hence the force acting to close the leaflets
- forces restricting leaflet closure, including geometric changes in mitral leaflet attachments due to abnormal wall motion and distortion of the region of the LV from which the papillary muscles (PMs) arise

A change in the ventricular geometric shape that makes it more spherical, rather than simple dilation, is associated with non-organic MR. Furthermore, MR is considered a potent stimulus for adverse spherical LV remodeling, which results in even more MR. Increased sphericity causes a splaying of the interpapillary angle; that is, the PMs are displaced apically and laterally. This results in the valve leaflets, which are restricted by the chordae, being displaced apically

Although the primary and predominant problem is that of leaflet tethering secondary to geometric changes in LV shape, it is recognized that the problem is compounded by LV dysfunction, which decreases the force available to close the leaflets.

Ischemic mitral regurgitation (IMR)

This has a 50% five-year survival if left untreated. IMR is a complication of ischemic systolic LV dysfunction [12]. However, the severity of IMR is not related to the severity of the LV dysfunction. Local remodeling leads to apical and posterior displacement of the PMs, which results in excess valvular tethering or tenting, independent of global LV remodeling. A dilated annulus in IMR is a non-specific finding. PM dysfunction is inapplicable in the context of IMR, because with acute ischemia the PM actually elongates in response to the forces exerted by the chordae, balancing out wall displacement and hence paradoxically reducing MR. It may be characterized by a dynamic regurgitation, in that in patients with IMR the degree of MR may increase during exercise, since the resulting ischemia may produce a decrease in regional or global LV function.

Mitral annular calcification

This causes increased rigidity of the posterior mitral annulus, which impairs systolic descent and the consequent decrease in mitral annular circumference, culminating in valvular incompetence [15]. It is characterized by increased echogenicity of the ventricular surface of the posterior mitral annulus, immediately adjacent to the insertion of the posterior leaflet. It is commonly seen as an incidental finding in the elderly, but renal failure and hypertension may accelerate the calcification process.

Mitral annular dilation

This may occur secondary to any cause of left atrial or ventricular distension. As coaptation is incomplete, a central regurgitation jet is usually seen.

Dilated cardiomyopathy (DCM)

Left ventricular dilation secondary to an intrinsic myocardial muscle dysfunction results in geometric changes that result in valvular tethering. In conjunction with poor systolic function and mitral annular dilation, this further increases the tendency to regurgitation.

Hypertrophic obstructive cardiomyopathy (HOCM)

Functional MR may occur due to systolic anterior motion (SAM) of the anterior leaflet. In this situation, the leaflet partially obstructs the LVOT. This is characteristically worse in mid-systole.

Circulatory pathophysiology of mitral regurgitation

In **acute severe MR**, a sudden volume overload is imposed on the LA. The total LV stroke volume (SV), which is the sum of LA regurgitant volume and the forward SV through the LVOT, is actually very slightly increased. This small increase is mainly due to LA regurgitant volume, as the LA has a lower resistance to flow than the LVOT. The forward SV and cardiac output (CO) are reduced because compensatory eccentric hypertrophy, i.e. an increase in LV wall thickness in proportion to the increase in chamber size, has not had time to develop. Simultaneously the LA cannot acutely accommodate the increased regurgitant volume, because it has not had time to dilate. This results in a significant increase in atrial pressure. This pressure is transmitted into the pulmonary venous circulation and may result in pulmonary edema.

The left ventricle on 2D echo may appear hyperdynamic as it empties into the low-resistance left atrium. The acute hemodynamic overload imposed on the LV is often poorly tolerated, necessitating urgent valve surgery.

In **chronic severe MR**, the insidious onset of the condition allows time for the development of eccentric hypertrophy. This compensatory increase in LV end-diastolic volume (LVEDV) allows for an increase in total LV stroke volume, with restoration of forward SV and CO. At the same time, LA dilation accommodates the regurgitant volume at a lower or normal LA pressure, preventing the development of symptoms of pulmonary edema. LV function may also appear vigorous and hyperdynamic. However, this may be a partial compensatory mechanism, and LV function with apparently normal contractility may in fact be impaired. The duration of this compensatory phase, when even vigorous exercise may fail to elicit symptoms, is varied but may last for many years. Eventually the prolonged burden of volume overload results in LV dysfunction and an increase in LV end-systolic volume (LVESV). Forward SV decreases and pulmonary congestion ensues. MR should be treated before this decompensation occurs.

Irrespective of the duration of onset of severe MR, the increase in **pulmonary artery pressure** is initially passive, but if the lesion is not corrected, secondary changes may occur to the pulmonary vasculature. This may result in persistent pulmonary artery hypertension, even after the lesion is corrected. The increased pulmonary artery pressure will result in changes to the RV and eventual **tricuspid regurgitation**.

Assessment of the severity of mitral regurgitation

The TEE variables used in the assessment of MR severity can be classified as **semi-quantitative** or **quantitative**. In common with mitral stenosis, most of these methods have their origins in transthoracic echo. Most, if not all, of these parameters have their limitations, especially with TEE. For this reason, no single method should be used in isolation to estimate the severity of MR.

For the rapid assessment of MR severity, semi-quantitative methods are often used, as they are less time-consuming. These methods are also prone to inter-observer variability. It is therefore best to keep any grading system simple (i.e. mild, moderate, or severe), with clear institutional guidelines for each grade of severity [12].

Semi-quantitative methods

2D features

This involves assessment of the mitral valves leaflets and the four cardiac chambers [2,15]. These 2D features, coupled with spectral Doppler, can also help to establish whether the MR is acute or chronic.

A visible 2D **leaflet** coaptation defect, due to leaflet segment flail, is indicative of severe MR. A 2D

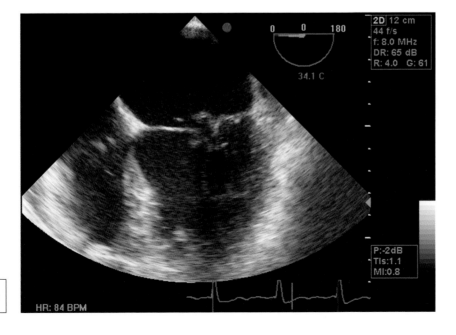

Figure 7.26. Four-chamber view showing myxomatous degeneration and annular dilation. There is a large coaptation defect which will result in severe regurgitation. See Video 7.10.

coaptation defect in the setting of prolapse or tethering may not always be representative of severe MR (Fig. 7.26; Video 7.10).

In the patient with acute severe MR, **LV systolic function** should be hyperdynamic, except where there is clear concurrent coronary artery disease, primary myocardial disease, or aortic valve lesions. With chronic severe MR, LV systolic function may initially be hyperdynamic, but with sustained volume overload systolic function will normalize and eventually become depressed. Preoperative LV systolic function is a powerful predictor of postoperative outcome in patients with chronic severe MR [16]. A left ventricular ejection fraction (LVEF) $\geq$ 60% equates to a 10-year postoperative survival rate of 72 $\pm$ 4%, whereas LVEF < 50% equates to a 10-year postoperative survival rate of 32 $\pm$ 12%. Hence consensus opinion is that LVEF <55% represents impaired LV systolic function

With chronic severe MR, the **LV dilates** and becomes spherical. The LV is considered dilated when the end-systolic short-axis diameter is > 4.5 cm. In this situation, LV end-systolic chamber size is a more sensitive marker of impending LV dysfunction than end-diastolic dimensions. The American Heart Association and American College of Cardiology recommend valve surgery in those patients with severe MR and LV end-systolic diameter $\geq$ 4.5 cm, even if the patient is asymptomatic [8].

As the LV dilates in chronic severe MR, annular dilation and/or leaflet tethering may occur, resulting in further MR.

In chronic severe MR, the **LA diameter** is increased to accommodate the regurgitant volume, with a normalized or reduced LA pressure. LA size may be a predictor of postoperative morbidity and mortality [17]. If the LA diameter is > 5.5 cm, it is unlikely to normalize after surgery and the patient is at risk of atrial fibrillation, if not already present.

Irreversible **pulmonary hypertension** is more likely to occur in the setting of chronic severe MR.

Secondary to pulmonary artery hypertension, the **RV and RA** undergo morphological changes, culminating in RV enlargement, dilation, and then tricuspid regurgitation with RA dilation.

Color Doppler imaging of regurgitant jet dimensions

Color-flow Doppler (CFD) imaging can detect the direction and extent of regurgitant jets into the left atrium [18]. Jet dimensions (length and area) have been proposed as semi-quantitative indices of mitral regurgitation severity. A regurgitant jet, however, is a complex 3D entity the dimensions of which will vary depending on the TEE interrogating plane. CFD imaging provides an instantaneous velocity map of the regurgitant jet rather than an absolute instantaneous regurgitant volume. Despite this, several studies have

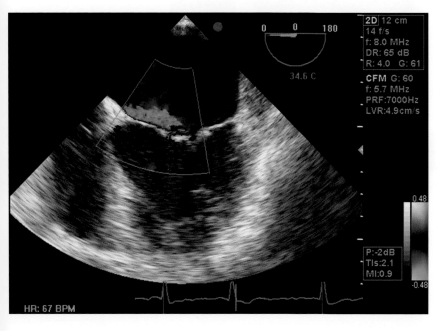

Figure 7.27. A constrained anteriorly directed regurgitant jet. See Video 7.11.

demonstrated a relationship between color jet dimensions and regurgitation severity. This relationship is most accurate under conditions of unconstrained or free jet flow. **Free jets** refer to flow into the center of a chamber, for example in functional MR. In this setting the cross-sectional area is large compared to that of the jet [2]. Consequently the jet is able to expand freely in the center of the LA. **Constrained jets** are also described as eccentric jets, for example due to mitral valve prolapse, flail or tethering (Fig. 7.27; Video 7.11) [2]. These are projected against the wall of the receiving chamber, and are unable to expand freely. Hence a so called "wall-hugging" jet of a given regurgitant volume will have a smaller area by color Doppler imaging than the equivalent free jet. The phenomenon of jet direction being changed by a solid surface (the atrial wall) is known as the Coanda effect.

Jet area, when averaged over several interrogating planes, appears to correlate reasonably well with angiographic grades of the severity of mitral regurgitation, and seems to be more robust than jet length alone.

Accurate assessment of MR severity can be further improved by indexing the jet area to the LA area.

Accepted signs of severe MR include a wall-hugging jet whose length encircles the LA, or which is seen to enter a pulmonary vein.

In addition to flow constraint, the dimensions of the color Doppler jet may also be affected by physiological, technical, and instrumentation factors. Since the regurgitant jet velocity is dependent on the transmitral pressure gradient, physiological factors which may directly or indirectly influence MR severity assessment include LA pressure, LA compliance, LV systolic function, and LV pressure (Fig. 7.28; Video 7.12). Instrumentation and technical factors that may affect the assessment of MR by Doppler color jets include the color gain setting, wall filter, transducer frequency, pulse repetition frequency, and the alignment of the transducer with jet flow. Therefore, assessment of the jet size and extent in a number of views, plus an appreciation of physiological and technical factors, is important for accurate assessment of lesion severity (Table 7.5).

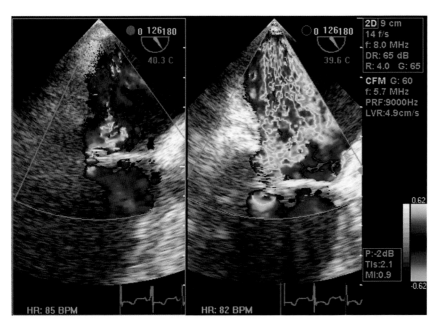

Figure 7.28. The effect of blood pressure on regurgitant jet size. The left panel was recorded when the patient's mean systemic blood pressure was 75 mmHg. The right panel was recorded with identical settings, except that the mean blood pressure had been pharmacologically elevated to 95 mmHg. See Video 7.12.

Table 7.5. Quantitative assessment of severity of mitral regurgitation

Grade of MR	Jet area (cm²)	Jet area % of left atrial area	Regurgitant volume (mL)	PISA radius (mm)	EROA (cm²)	Width of vena contracta (mm)
Mild	< 3	< 20	< 44	< 6	< 0.2	2–4
Moderate	3–7	20–40	45–59	7–9	0.2–0.39	4–5.9
Severe	> 7	> 40	≥ 60	≥ 10	≥ 0.4	≥ 6

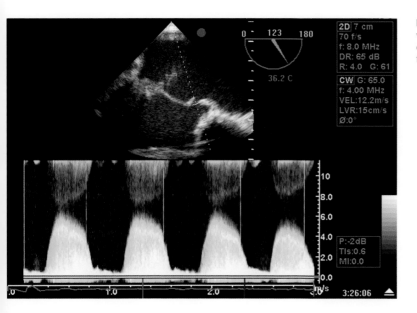

Figure 7.29. A densely filled continuous-wave Doppler signal indicating a severe degree of regurgitation through a perforated anterior leaflet

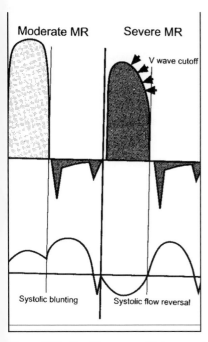

Figure 7.30. The "V-wave cutoff" sign, seen in acute severe MR, signifying a marked decrease in MR jet velocity in mid- to late systole.

Continuous-wave spectral Doppler

Analysis of the **intensity and the shape** of the continuous-wave Doppler (CWD) envelope of transmitral flow in both systole and diastole can be used for a semi-quantitative/qualitative assessment of the severity of MR [2,12]. The intensity or brightness of a Doppler signal is proportional to the number of scatterers, in this case the number of red blood cells, encountered in a unit volume of blood. Thus a large volume of blood will produce a brighter Doppler signal. Doppler gain settings and beam alignment will also influence the brightness of the CWD envelope of transmitral flow. By comparing the intensity of the CWD envelope produced by MR to that of transmitral diastolic inflow in any given patient, an assessment of the lesion severity can be made, which is independent of spectral Doppler gain settings (Fig. 7.29).

A regurgitant CWD envelope that is complete and of equal intensity to the transmitral diastolic inflow CWD envelope may be considered to be consistent with severe MR. An MR Doppler envelope that is complete, but of less intensity than the transmitral diastolic Doppler envelope, may be consistent with moderate MR. If the MR Doppler envelope is incomplete and faint, this may be consistent with mild MR.

The **shape** of the CWD envelope may also provide a clue to the presence of acute severe MR. The mitral regurgitation jet velocity is determined by the transmitral pressure gradient (LVP/LAP). This gradient is normally maintained throughout systole, resulting in a smoothly rounded contour of the CWD envelope consistent with mild to moderate MR. With acute severe MR, a larger regurgitant volume is expelled into a non-dilated LA in systole. This results in a precipitous decrease in the mid- to late- systolic transmitral pressure gradient, due to the sudden increase in LA pressure. Consequently MR jet velocity decreases markedly in mid- to late systole, producing an asymmetric shape to the MR CWD tracing. This is the so-called "V-wave cutoff" sign, and it is most obvious in acute severe MR, as the LA is poorly compliant and has not had time to dilate to accommodate the increased regurgitant volume. The V-wave cutoff sign is uncommon in chronic severe MR (Fig. 7.30).

Diastolic **transmitral E wave** (E_{max}) velocity is increased in cases of MR, due to the regurgitant volume loading the LA in systole. Accordingly, the LA-to-LV pressure gradient is maximum during early diastolic filling, hence the increased transmitral E_{max} velocity. An E_{max} > 1.2 m/s is indicative of severe MR, with a sensitivity and specificity of 86%, a positive predictive value of 75% and a negative predictive value of 92% [19]. However, to further reduce the possibility of false positives, an E_{max} value of 1.4 m/s is used instead to denote severe MR. This sign is unreliable, however, in the setting of a hyperdynamic circulation or even minor degrees of mitral stenosis.

Pulmonary vein flow velocity profile

TEE is the imaging modality of choice for measuring pulmonary flow velocities [20]. The S wave represents venous inflow into the LA in systole, and the D wave represents the venous inflow pattern in diastole. Using pulsed-wave spectral Doppler (PWD), variation in the **S- and D-wave patterns** can be used to assess the severity of MR.

1. **Trivial or mild MR**. This is associated with a normal pulmonary vein inflow pattern; that is, S-wave velocity > D-wave velocity.

2. **Moderate MR**. As MR worsens, the LA pressure increases, decreasing the gradient for venous inflow into the LA from the pulmonary veins in systole; hence the S-wave velocity is blunted in moderate MR. Thus S-wave velocity < D-wave velocity. This finding is also seen in patients with reduced LA compliance, secondary to LV diastolic dysfunction, and should be treated with caution.

3. **Severe MR**. Flow reversal may be seen in the pulmonary veins in systole as MR jets reflux into pulmonary veins, producing a reversal of the S wave. Which pulmonary veins are affected by S-wave reversal will depend on the direction of the MR jets. Conversely, pulmonary vein flow reversal may be absent in almost 41% of patients with severe MR. Therefore, although a useful sign of severe MR when present, it has a relatively low sensitivity (Fig. 7.31).

Quantitative methods

These are more time-consuming and have a greater inherent propensity for errors because of the calculations and measurements involved. However, they may be necessary for a formal quantitative assessment.

The three parameters which lend themselves to quantitative measurement are:

1. regurgitant volume and fraction
2. effective regurgitant orifice area (EROA)
3. vena contracta

Data relating these variables to the severity of mitral regurgitation are shown in Table 7.5.

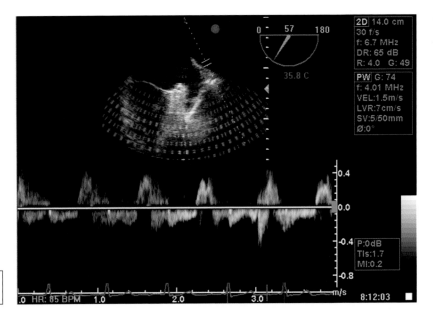

Figure 7.31. Pulsed-wave Doppler spectrum from the upper left pulmonary vein demonstrating systolic wave reversal in severe mitral regurgitation.

Regurgitant volume/regurgitant fraction

This is a measurement of the volume of blood regurgitating through the mitral valve into the LA in one systole [10,12,15]. **Regurgitant fraction** represents this volume as a percentage of total mitral inflow in diastole. Regurgitant fraction is probably a more reliable guide to the severity of the lesion than simple regurgitant volume, which depends on hemodynamic status and chamber dimensions.

In order to calculate regurgitant volume and regurgitant fraction, the transmitral SV or total LV stroke volume, and systemic SV at another cardiac site, need to be measured. Commonly the systemic SV is measured at the LVOT, but theoretically the pulmonary artery or tricuspid valve may also be used. PWD should be deployed in the optimal TEE view which allows for parallel alignment of the beam with the flow in question (see Chapter 13).

Several measurements of each parameter should be made and these averaged. This will tend to minimize errors. This methodology is of doubtful value in the presence of severe aortic regurgitation.

Effective regurgitant orifice area (EROA)

This can be calculated by two methods, **quantitative Doppler** and PISA (**flow convergence**).

The quantitative Doppler method [10] yields the effective area available for regurgitant flow, and is the mean EROA value over one cardiac cycle. Again, several measurements of each individual parameter should be taken and then averaged. The calculation is shown in Box 7.2.

In contrast to the quantitative Doppler method of EROA calculation, the flow convergence or PISA method [21,22] measures **instantaneous** EROA. The mitral regurgitation orifice area is dynamic and changes size and shape significantly from early to late systole, as does the peak regurgitant jet velocity. This methodology is based on the law of **conservation of mass**.

Flow convergence refers to the organized area of flow just proximal to an orifice, in this case a regurgitating mitral orifice. Three-dimensional flow approaching an orifice does so in a series of arcs or hemispheres centered on the orifice. The outer surface of these hemispheres can be visualized in 2D by CFD as abrupt changes in color, due to aliasing. The hemisphere has a radius (r), in any direction proximal to the orifice. In the case of MR, these hemispheres will be on the LV side of the mitral valve, in contrast to MS (Fig. 7.32).

The outermost flow convergence zone most closely resembles a hemisphere, compared to successive smaller zones, and therefore the radius of this outermost zone should be used for flow calculations. Also, the outermost zone is assumed to correspond to the peak regurgitant jet velocity (V_{max-mv}) through the mitral orifice. In this way it can be assumed that flow convergence and orifice flow rates correspond to the

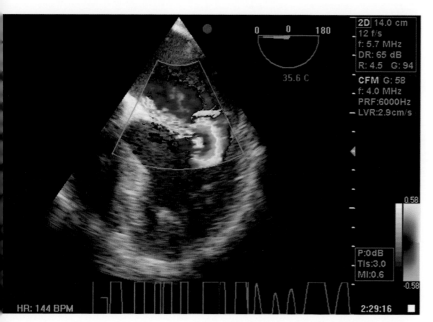

Figure 7.32. PISA formation proximal to the regurgitant orifice in mitral regurgitation.

Box 7.2. Quantitative methods for assessing the severity of mitral regurgitation

(1) Calculation of mitral regurgitant volume and regurgitant fraction

(a) Regurgitant volume (mL) = Total LV SV − Systemic SV

$$= (CSA_{mitral\ annulus} \times VTI_{mitral\ annulus}) - (CSA_{LVOT} \times VTI_{LVOT})$$

The mitral annulus is assumed to have a circular geometry.

Hence calculated surface area (CSA) of mitral annulus = $\pi(D/2)^2 = \pi D^2/4$.

(b) Regurgitant fraction = (Regurgitant volume / Total LV SV) × 100.

(2) Effective regurgitant orifice area (EROA)

(a) Quantative Doppler

Given that:

$$SV = CSA \times VTI$$

Rearranging this equation:

$$CSA = SV/VTI$$

Solving this equation for regurgitant volume:

$$CSA = EROA$$

Therefore:

$$EROA = SV / VTI$$

where SV = Regurgitant volume (calculated as shown above); VTI = the VTI of mitral regurgitant jet (measured by CW Doppler, mid-esophageal long-axis view)

Therefore:

$$EROA = \text{Regurgitant volume} / VTI_{mitral\ regurgitant\ jet}$$

(b) Proximal isovelocity surface area (PISA)

By application of the continuity principle:

(i) PISA flow rate (Q_{PISA}) = Orifice flow rate $(Q_{orifice})$

$$2\pi r^2 \times Va = EROA \times V_{max\text{-}mv}$$
$$EROA = (2\pi r^2 \times Va)/V_{max\text{-}mv}$$

where:

Va is the aliasing velocity or Nyqvist limit if the first/outermost aliasing hemisphere is used

r is the radius of the outermost flow convergence hemisphere

$V_{max\text{-}mv}$ refers to the peak mitral regurgitant jet velocity, measured with CW spectral Doppler in the MOLA view

(ii) Regurgitant volume = $EROA \times VTI_{regurgitant\ jet}$

(iii) Simplified flow convergence calculation

Assume normal LV function, i.e. LV–LA pressure gradient of 100 mmHg

Peak MR jet velocity is therefore 5 m/s ($V_{max\text{-}mv} = 500$ cm/s)

Aliasing velocity (NL) is set at 40 cm/s

$$EROA = EROA = (2\pi r^2 \times Va)/V_{max\text{-}mv}$$
$$= 2 \times 40 \times \pi r^2/500 = \frac{80 \times 3.146 \times r^2}{500}$$
$$= \frac{r^2}{2}$$

same point in time, hence generating an instantaneous EROA.

The flow convergence method is comparable in accuracy to the quantitative Doppler technique.

The regurgitant volume can also be derived from PISA, once the EROA is calculated. In addition, the flow convergence method can also be simplified as shown in Box 7.2, without any loss of accuracy.

Vena contracta

The vena contracta (VC) refers to the narrowest portion or neck of the regurgitant jet, which occurs at or just beyond the regurgitant orifice. Although flow in this region is of high velocity, the flow pattern is organized into a series of parallel flow lines. Distal to the VC, flow becomes progressively more turbulent and disorganized as blood in the receiving chamber (LA), is entrained by the expanding jet [23] (Fig 7.33).

The vena contracta has been shown to increase directly in accordance with the size of the EROA. This relationship is relatively independent of the driving pressure and flow rates in the normal clinical range, and hence VC is probably superior to jet dimension measurement for assessing the severity of the lesion [24]. The relationship between VC and EROA appears to hold true even with eccentric jets.

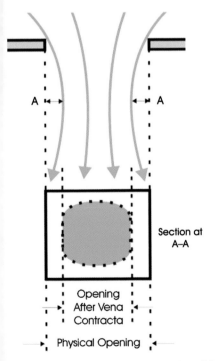

Figure 7.33. Diagrammatic representation of the vena contracta phenomenon.

Measurement of the VC should be undertaken in the mid-esophageal long-axis view, in order to avoid cutting the coaptation plane obliquely and in so doing overestimating the width of the VC. A VC width ≥ 6 mm has a sensitivity of 95% and specificity of 98% for severe MR [21].

Limitations to this technique include the fact that localizing the VC may be difficult, requiring off-axis views. The VC in absolute dimensions is very small, and measurement may be prone to errors due to issues regarding axial or lateral resolution, depending on the interrogating angle. The vena contracta method is not recommended with multiple jets of MR.

References

1. Peterson GE, Brickner ME, Reimold SC. Transesophageal echocardiography: clinical indications and applications. *Circulation* 2003; **107**: 2398–402.

2. Sidebotham D, Merry A, Legget M. Mitral valve. In: *Practical Perioperative Transoesophageal Echocardiography*. Edinburgh: Butterworth Heinemann, 2003: 131–70.

3. Kumar N, Kumar M, Duran C. A revised terminology for describing surgical findings of the mitral valve. *J Heart Valve Dis* 1995; **4**: 70–5.

4. Carpentier A. Cardiac valve surgery: the 'French Correction'. *J Thorac Cardiovasc Surg* 1983; **86**: 323–37.

5. Maslow AD, Schwartz C, Bert A. Pro: single-plane echocardiography provides an accurate and adequate examination of the native mitral valve. *J Cardiothorac Vasc Anesth* 2002; **16**: 508–14.

6. Wilkins GT, Weyman AE, Abascal VM, Block PC, Palacios IF. Percutaneous balloon dilatation of the mitral valve: an analysis of echocardiographic variables related to outcome and the mechanism of dilatation. *Br Heart J* 1988; **60**: 299–308.

7. Otto CM. Valvular stenosis: diagnosis, quantitation and clinical approach. In: *Textbook of Clinical Echocardiography*. Philadelphia: Saunders, 2000; 249–59.

8. Bonow RO, Carabello BA, Chatterjee K, *et al.* ACC/AHA guidelines for the management of patients with valvular heart disease. *J Am Coll Cardiol* 2006; **48**: e1–148.

9. Oku K, Utsunomiya T, Mori H, Yamachika S, Yano K. Calculation of mitral valve area in mitral stenosis using the proximal isovelocity surface area method: comparison with two-dimensional planimetry and Doppler pressure half time method. *Jpn Heart J* 1997; **38**: 811–19.

10. Thomson H, Enriquez-Sarano M. Echocardiographic assessment of mitral regurgitation. *Cardiol Rev* 2001; **9**: 210–16.

11. Carpentier A, Deloche A, Dauptain J, *et al*. A new reconstructive operation for correction of mitral and tricuspid insufficiency. *J Thorac Cardiovasc Surg* 1971; **61**: 1–13.

12. Irvine T, Li X, Sahn D, Kenny A. Assessment of mitral regurgitation. *Heart* 2002; **88**(Suppl iv): 11–19.

13. Tamura K, Fukuda Y, Ishizaki M, *et al*. Abnormalities in elastic fibers and other connective-tissue components of floppy mitral valve. *Am Heart J* 1995; **129**: 1149–58.

14. Levine RA, Hung J, Otsuji Y, *et al*. Mechanistic insights into functional mitral regurgitation. *Curr Cardiol Rep* 2002; **4**: 125–9.

15. Otto CM. Valvular regurgitation: diagnosis, quantitation, and clinical approach. In: *Textbook of Clinical Echocardiography*. Philadelphia, PA: Saunders, 2000: 265–93.

16. Enriquez-Sarano M, Tajik AJ, Schaff HV, *et al*. Echocardiographic prediction of survival after surgical correction of organic mitral regurgitation. *Circulation* 1994; **90**: 830–7.

17. Chua YL, Schaff HV, Orszulak TA, Morris JJ. Outcome of mitral valve repair in patients with preoperative atrial fibrillation: should the maze procedure be combined with mitral valvuloplasty? *J Thorac Cardiovasc Surg* 1994; **107**: 408–15.

18. Baumgartner H, Schima H, Kuhn P. Value and limitations of proximal jet dimensions for the quantitation of valvular regurgitation: an in vitro study using Doppler flow imaging. *J Am Soc Echocardiogr* 1991; **4**: 57–66.

19. Thomas L, Foster E, Schiller N. Peak mitral inflow velocity predicts mitral regurgitation severity. *J Am Coll Cardiol* 1998; **31**: 174–9.

20. Enriquez-Sarano M, Dujardin KS, Tribouilloy C, *et al*. Determinants of pulmonary venous flow reversal in mitral regurgitation and its usefulness in determining the severity of regurgitation. *Am J Cardiol*. 1999; **83**: 535–41.

21. Recusani F, Bargiggia GS, Yoganathan A, *et al*. A new method for quantification of regurgitant flow rate using color flow Doppler imaging of the flow convergence region proximal to a discrete orifice: an in vitro study. *Circulation* 1991; **83**: 594–604.

22. Pu M, Vandervoort PM, Griffin BP, *et al*. Quantification of mitral regurgitation by the proximal convergence method using transesophageal echocardiography: clinical validation of a geometric correction for proximal flow constraint. *Circulation* 1995; **92**: 2169–77.

23. Grayburn PA, Fehske W, Omran H, Brickner ME, Lüderitz B. Multiplane transesophageal echocardiographic assessment of mitral regurgitation by Doppler color flow mapping of the vena contracta. *Am J Cardiol* 1994; **74**: 912–17.

24. Zhou X, Jones M, Shiota T, *et al*. Vena contracta imaged by Doppler color flow mapping predicts the severity of eccentric mitral regurgitation better than color jet area: a chronic animal study. *J Am Coll Cardiol* 1997; **30**: 1393–8.

The tricuspid valve, pulmonary valve, and pulmonary artery

Alfredo Pazzaglia, Patrick Wouters

Introduction

The tricuspid and pulmonary valves are the most difficult valves to image with transesophageal echocardiography (TEE). Although there are fewer specific indications for obtaining a TEE of these valves than of the mitral or aortic valves, it is important to inspect them as a routine part of each examination.

The tricuspid valve

The tricuspid valve (TV) apparatus consists of three leaflets: a large anterior leaflet, a septal leaflet, and a smaller posterior leaflet. These three leaflets are attached to their papillary muscles through their associated chordae tendineae. The anterior papillary muscle is large and gives rise to the moderator band. The posterior papillary muscle is frequently small and may be absent.

The tricuspid annulus lies more apically than the mitral valve, with its inferior margin in proximity to the coronary sinus and the inferior vena cava (Fig. 8.1).

Because the two-dimensional sector may initially miss the major axis of the TV, it is important to scan the valve from different windows, using small changes in transducer angle, probe rotation, and probe position to obtain the maximum diameter.

Images of the tricuspid valve can be obtained with the TEE probe in the lower esophageal position or from a number of additional transgastric windows obtained by rotating the transducer from 0° to 145° in order to improve assessment of the TV annulus and function. The imaging windows are shown in Table 8.1.

In the mid-esophageal four-chamber view, the septal leaflet is seen on the right and either the anterior or posterior leaflet on the left of the display, depending on the degree of probe retroflexion. It may be necessary to advance the probe slightly to prevent the tricuspid valve from being shaded by the aortic valve. Color-flow Doppler may be deployed to test for tricuspid regurgitation (Videos 8.1, 8.2).

Rotating the transducer to acquire the right ventricular (RV) inflow–outflow view, the posterior leaflet then appears from the left side of the annulus and the anterior leaflet from the right. The tricuspid valve may be viewed via the mid-esophageal bicaval view, particularly if the probe is slightly rotated counterclockwise. This view may be appropriately aligned, thus allowing accurate spectral Doppler measurements.

The transgastric RV inflow view may be developed from the transgastric short-axis view as desribed in Chapter 4. This view shows the right ventricle on the left of the display and the right atrium on the right, and is an excellent view for showing the chordae tendineae and papillary muscle. A non-standard TV

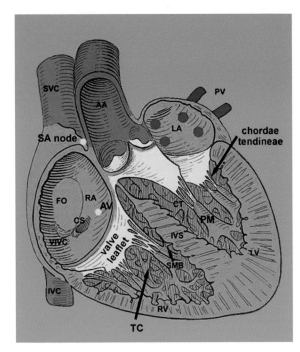

Figure 8.1. The tricuspid valve leaflet is shown, in relation to the inferior vena cava (IVC) coronary sinus (CS), and fossa ovalis (FO). See text for further details.

135

Core Topics in Transesophageal Echocardiography, ed. Robert Feneck, John Kneeshaw, and Marco Ranucci.
Published by Cambridge University Press. © Cambridge University Press 2010.

Table 8.1. TEE imaging of the tricuspid valve

View	Image	Transducer position (degrees)	Structures imaged
Mid-esophageal four-chamber	a. ME four chamber	0–10	RA, RV, TV, IAS, IVS, LA, LV
Mid-esophageal RV inflow–outflow	m. ME RV inflow-outflow	60–90	TV, RV, RVOT, PV, AV
Mid-esophageal bicaval view	l. ME bicaval	100–120	RA, LA, IAS, SVC, IVC
Transgastric long-axis RV inflow	n. TG RV inflow	110–130	RV, TV, RA
Transgastric short-axis tricuspid (non-standard)		0–20	TV (anterior, posterior, septal leaflets)
Mid-esophageal RV inflow (non-standard)		100–120	RV, TV, RA, chordae, papillary muscles
Transgastric hepatic veins (non-standard)		100–120	Hepatic veins

AV, aortic valve; IAS, interatrial septum; IVC, inferior vena cava; IVS, interventricular septum; LA, left atrium; LV, left ventricle; PV, pulmonary valve; RA, right atrium; RV, right ventricule; RVOT, right ventricular outflow tract; SVC, superior vena cava; TV, tricuspid valve.

short-axis view may be acquired by withdrawing the probe, which should reveal the three leaflets of the tricuspid valve seen in the short axis (Videos 8.3–8.7).

Using these windows, it is important to remember that it may be necessary to manipulate and rotate the transducer to obtain the clearest images of the TV and its insertion into the annulus

Tricuspid valve disease

Tricuspid valve disease can be caused by the following:

- Infection, i.e. rheumatic fever or infective endocarditis.
- Right ventricular dilation, causing the annulus (a ring of tough fibrous tissue which is attached to and supports the leaflets of the valve) to enlarge.
- Increased pressure through the tricuspid valve; this is commonly seen with pulmonary hypertension.
- Less common causes include congenital defects, trauma, carcinoid heart disease, tumor, tricuspid valve prolapse, Ebstein's anomaly, systemic lupus, and trauma.

Rheumatic tricuspid valve disease is often combined with mitral and/or aortic valve disease.

Tricuspid stenosis

Tricuspid stenosis (TS) is a relatively uncommon valvular lesion in North America and Western Europe. It is more common in tropical and subtropical climates, especially in southern Asia and in Latin America. It is generally rheumatic in origin, and it is more common in females than in males.

Rheumatic heart disease causes tricuspid stenosis in up to 8% of affected patients. Two-dimensional (2D) echocardiography can detect doming of the leaflets in diastole, thickened tricuspid valve leaflets, and a reduced tricuspid valve orifice diameter. Continuous-wave Doppler (CWD) allows estimation of the tricuspid transvalvular pressure gradient, and increased peak inflow velocities, with an E wave velocity of > 1.5 m/s [1]. The pressure gradient across the stenotic valve is determined according to the modified Bernoulli equation (see also Chapter 13):

$$\Delta P = 4 \times V^2 \qquad (8.1)$$

A mean diastolic pressure gradient of 4 mmHg is usually sufficient to elevate the mean right atrial (RA) pressure to levels that result in systemic venous congestion.

Nevertheless, in contrast to its use in the evaluation of mitral stenosis, short-axis 2D imaging of the TV orifice is often unsatisfactory, as it is not possible to visualize all three TV leaflets simultaneously. However, real-time three-dimensional echocardiography can demonstrate each separate TV leaflet, and thus they can be assessed with regard to thickness, mobility, calcification, and the relationship to other tricuspid valve leaflets (Videos 8.8, 8.9).

Tricuspid regurgitation

Unlike tricuspid stenosis, tricuspid regurgitation (TR) is common and can be primary or secondary to annular dilation. However, TR is a frequent echocardiographic finding in normal individuals [2], particularly in the elderly, where TR may be seen in more than 90% of patients over 70 years of age [3]. Primary causes of TR include rheumatic disease, endocarditis, carcinoid heart disease, Ebstein's anomaly, and traumatic injury.

Tricuspid valve dysfunction is not usually accompanied by leaflet malformation. Functional tricuspid regurgitation (FTR) in the absence of leaflet pathology commonly occurs with pulmonary hypertension, which may be primary or secondary to left-sided valve disease and/or left ventricular (LV) dysfunction. Dilation of the right ventricle then follows, resulting in dilation of the tricuspid annulus [4,5]. Surgical management of functional TR at the time of correction of left-sided heart disease is recommended because, if

significant TR remains, postoperative morbidity and mortality rise considerably (Videos 8.10–8.12).

TR severity is associated with worse survival in men regardless of the left ventricular ejection fraction (LVEF) or pulmonary artery pressure. However, assessing the severity of TR may be difficult. Normal (physiological) TR jet velocity is 2.0–2.5 m/s. Higher velocities may suggest pulmonary hypertension, whereas lower values may be seen with more severe degrees of regurgitation. Severe TR is associated with a poor prognosis, independent of age, biventricular systolic function, RV size, and dilation of the inferior vena cava [6]. Moderate and severe TR should be repaired surgically, since it has been widely demonstrated that in these patients tricuspid annuloplasty provides better symptomatic results and may improve survival [7,8].

Although TV tethering is an important determinant of recurrent or residual TR, LV and RV function and pressures may have an impact on the durability of the repair. These factors may identify patients at risk for recurrent TR after annuloplasty [9]. After significant pulmonary artery pressure reduction by pulmonary thromboendarterectomy, severe functional TR with a dilated annulus may improve without annuloplasty despite dilated tricuspid annulus diameters [10].

Carcinoid syndrome

Carcinoid syndrome originates from carcinoid tumors located in the gastrointestinal system, pancreas, biliary vessels, bronchi, ovaries, and testes. The condition is characterized by flushing, telangiectasia, diarrhoea, bronchoconstriction, and cardiac involvement. Cardiac lesions may occur in 50% of patients. Right-sided valvular heart disease occurs frequently in patients with carcinoid syndrome, but left-sided involvement, pericardial effusion, and myocardial metastases may also occur [11,12]. The development of right-sided valve stenosis may be rapid, leading to right heart failure, but death usually occurs from progressive systemic disease and rarely from pulmonary stenosis. Surgery is the most effective treatment, and balloon valvulotomy is only palliative. However, therapy of the systemic condition is predominantly the treatment of choice [13].

The main predictor of clinical outcome in patients with carcinoid syndrome is the extent and severity of the cardiac involvement. The TV leaflets and subvalvular structures are often thickened, shortened, and retracted, leading to incomplete coaptation and usually moderate or severe TR. The pulmonary valve may also be thickened and retracted. Interestingly, calcification of the affected valves is rare and may be considered a notable negative echocardiographic feature of carcinoid heart disease (Video 8.13).

Endocarditis

The majority of cases of endocarditis involving intravenous drug users occur on the right side of the heart. In contrast, only 5–10% of all endocarditis cases occur on the left. *Streptococcus* viridans is the most common cause overall, while *Staphylococcus aureus* is the most common cause in intravenous drug users. It is possible that these patients exhibit a greater expression of matrix molecules that bind to microbial surface components, recognizing adhesive matrix molecules on the right-sided valvular surface and predisposing these valves to increased adherence. The chordae tendineae appear thickened and fused, and friable prolapsing vegetations may be present. There is evidence of significant tissue destruction. Because of extensive leaflet destruction, TV replacement may be the procedure of choice in most surgical centers. This subject is dealt with more fully in Chapter 18.

Ebstein's anomaly

Ebstein's anomaly was first described by Wilhelm Ebstein in 1866. It is a rare congenital heart disorder occurring in 1 in 200 000 live births, and consists of a malformation of the tricuspid valve and right ventricle characterized by the following:

- adherence of the septal and posterior leaflets to the underlying myocardium (failure of delamination, namely splitting of the tissue by detachment of the inner layer during embryologic development)
- downward (apical) displacement of the functional annulus
- dilation of the "atrialized" portion of the right ventricle, with variable degree of hypertrophy and thinning of the wall
- redundancy, fenestrations, and tethering of the anterior leaflet
- dilation of the right atrioventricular junction (true tricuspid annulus).

Echocardiography allows accurate evaluation of the TV leaflets. In normal human hearts, the downward displacement of the septal and posterior leaflets in relation to the anterior mitral valve leaflet is < 8 mm/m^2

body surface area. The principal feature of Ebstein's anomaly is apical displacement of the septal leaflet of the tricuspid valve from the insertion of the anterior leaflet of the mitral valve by at least 8 mm/m^2 body surface area. Marked enlargement of the RA and atrialized RV is present. The site and degree of regurgitation of the TV, and the feasibility of valve repair, may also be assessed with echocardiography. The outcome for patients with Ebstein's malformation depends mainly on the severity of the TV malformation.

Precise description of the tricuspid anatomy may be difficult from only the 2D planes, and once again greater definition may be achieved by 3D echocardiography (Video 8.14).

Traumatic tricuspid valve regurgitation

Traumatic TV regurgitation (TTR) is a rare complication of non-penetrating chest trauma, and has been associated with high-speed automobile accidents. Transthoracic echocardiography (TTE) is often difficult in the patient with blunt chest trauma because of coexisting chest injuries. However, TEE allows better visualization of much of the cardiac anatomy involved.

The etiology of tricuspid injury is straightforward. The right ventricle is immediately posterior to the sternum, and thus may be inured by blunt chest trauma. Acute elevation of the right intraventricular pressure results in injury to the TV apparatus. The most frequently reported mechanism of injury is chordal rupture, followed by rupture of the anterior papillary muscle and leaflet tear, primarily of the anterior leaflet.

Other causes

Although cardiac valve disease is frequent in the antiphospholipid syndrome, isolated TV pathology is uncommon. TV stenosis and insufficiency with concomitant vegetations in association with primary antiphospholipid syndrome has been reported [14] (Video 8.15).

Grading tricuspid regurgitation

Color Doppler echocardiography is a sensitive technique for detecting valvular regurgitation, and provides a semi-quantitative method for estimating the severity of regurgitation (Table 8.2).

Tricuspid regurgitation may be graded as follows:

- **mild** – regurgitant jet area/right atrial area $\leq 19\%$
- **moderate** – regurgitant jet area/right atrial area 20–40%
- **severe** – regurgitant jet area/right atrial area $\geq 41\%$.

Table 8.2. Grading the severity of tricuspid regurgitation

Parameter	Mild	Moderate	Severe
Tricuspid valve	Usually normal	Normal or abnormal	Abnormal / flail leaflet / poor coaptation
RV/RA/IVC size	Normal	Normal or dilated	Usually dilated
Jet area: central jets (cm^2) (not eccentric jets)	< 5	5–10	> 10
VC width (cm) (Nyquist limit c. 50–60 cm/s)	Not defined	Not defined, but < 0.65	> 0.65
PISA radius (cm) (Nyquist limit 28 cm/s)	≤ 0.5	0.6–0.9	> 0.9
Jet density and contour: CWD peaking	Soft and parabolic	Dense, variable contour	Dense, triangular with early peaking
Hepatic vein flow (may be affected by atrial fibrillation or elevated RA pressure)	Systolic dominance	Systolic blunting	Systolic reversal

CWD, Continuous-wave Doppler; IVC, inferior vena cava; RA, right atrium; RV, right ventricle; VC, vena contracta width.

The color Doppler jet size is widely used for assessment of the degree of TR, but it has important limitations [15]. The regurgitant jet area, even when corrected for the receiving chamber size, is strongly influenced by its dependence on hemodynamic conditions, by jet interaction with the receiving chamber, and by the settings, including gain, on the echo machine.

Enlargement of the RV may be an important feature of tricuspid regurgitation, and may be graded as follows:

- **mild** – the RV area is greater than two-thirds of the LV but less than the LV area
- **moderate** – the RV area is equal to the LV area
- **severe** – the RV area is greater than the LV area

Systolic flow reversal in the vena cava and hepatic veins is a useful sign of severe TR but is not quantitative and does not provide a full description of the entire spectrum of TR.

Color Doppler imaging has also been used to quantify the size of the vena contracta, which has been used to quantify valve regurgitation. The vena contracta is the narrowest neck of the regurgitant flow just distal to the flow convergence region and corresponds hydrodynamically with the effective regurgitant orifice area (EROA). The narrowest sector angle of imaging should be selected in order to optimize the imaging frame rate, and the position of the transducer modified to optimize visualization of the flow convergence region and the regurgitant flow proximal and distal to the TV. Measurement of the vena contracta is then made in mid-systole.

Data suggest that the vena contracta width correlates well with the EROA by the flow convergence method, even when restricted to patients with eccentric jets. The vena contracta width also showed significant correlations with hepatic venous flow and right atrial area. A vena contracta width ≥ 6.5 mm identified severe TR with 88.5% sensitivity and 93.3% specificity. In comparison with jet area or jet/RA area ratio, the vena contracta width showed better correlations with EROA [16].

Determination of right ventricular systolic pressure

During the examination, it is also important to measure the TR velocity with CWD, to provide an estimation of RV systolic pressure.

Patients with clinical signs of elevated right-sided pressures have jets of tricuspid regurgitation clearly recorded by CWD ultrasound. By use of the maximum velocity (V) of the regurgitant jet, the systolic pressure gradient between RV and RA is calculated by the modified Bernoulli equation. Adding the transtricuspid gradient to the mean RA pressure allows us to determine RV systolic pressure, which is equal to pulmonary artery systolic pressure in the absence of pulmonary stenosis. The technique is dependent on close alignment between the Doppler beam and the direction of blood flow. The most commonly used views for this purpose may be the mid-esophageal four-chamber view, the mid-esophageal short-axis RV inflow–outflow view, and the mid-esophageal bicaval view. In each case, the TEE view may need to be modified in order to achieve the best alignment (Fig. 8.1).

Doppler techniques have been used in a variety of clinical settings, including those where the diagnosis of pulmonary hypertension is critical [17–19].

The pulmonary valve and pulmonary artery

Anatomy

The pulmonary valve (PV) is a trileaflet semilunar valve with an anterior, a left, and a right leaflet, and is similar to the aortic valve in basic structure and function. It is positioned anterosuperiorly and to the left of the aortic valve and oriented perpendicularly to it. In comparison to the aortic valve, the PV is thinner and has a slightly larger valve orifice area. While the other three cardiac valves are in fibrous continuity with each other, the pulmonary valve stands alone, separated by the infundibulum.

The pulmonary artery (PA) trunk is approximately 4–5 cm long and 2–3 cm wide in normal adults. It arises anteriorly to the aortic valve and runs posterior to and underneath the aortic arch, where it divides into a T-shape, giving right and left branches. The right PA forms a 90-degree angle with the pulmonary trunk whereas the left PA projects as an extension of the trunk. The ductus arteriosus leaves the superior portion of the PA bifurcation on the left side and joins the junction of the distal aortic arch and descending aorta.

2D echocardiographic assessment of the PV and PA

Since the pulmonary valve is located in the far field of TEE, it is sometimes difficult to accurately visualize the thin leaflets. This is best achieved using the mid-esophageal RV inflow–outflow view, and the mid-esophageal AV short-axis view (Fig. 8.2), and by slight adjustments of the probe's position and the multiplane angle. Withdrawal of the probe to the mid-esophageal ascending aorta short-axis view (at 0°) shows the pulmonary trunk and the PA bifurcation in a T-shape on the right side of the aortic arch and superior vena cava. The upper esophageal aortic arch short-axis view may be useful and can be achieved by further withdrawal of the probe and rotation of the multiplane probe to 90°. This shows the pulmonary artery in long axis on the left side of the screen (behind

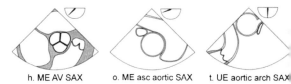

h. ME AV SAX   o. ME asc aortic SAX   t. UE aortic arch SAX

Figure 8.2. Standard TEE views for assessing the pulmonary valve mid-esophageal AV short-axis view, mid-esophageal ascending aorta short-axis view, upper esophageal aortic arch short-axis view.

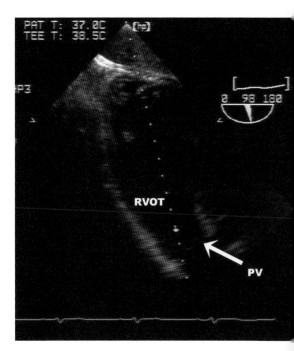

Figure 8.3. Modified deep transgastric right ventricular infundibular view. Note the parallel alignment of the Doppler beam to blood flow in the right ventricular outflow tract and across the pulmonary valve.

the aortic arch). The modified deep transgastric RV infundibular view is very useful to study flow characteristics in the RV outflow tract (RVOT) and PA, as it is the best window to align the Doppler beam with the PV flow (Fig. 8.3).

Doppler study of the PV and PA

Pulmonary insufficiency is seen with color Doppler as a diastolic regurgitant flow through the PV into the RVOT in the mid-esophageal inflow–outflow view and a modified deep transgastric RV infundibular view. A minor degree of pulmonary insufficiency can be seen in 40–78% of normal subjects as a small central jet that extends less than 1 cm into the RV (Fig. 8.4) [20]. Exclusion of significant pulmonary regurgitation may be important, for example prior to a Ross procedure, where the pulmonary valve is used as an autograft into the systemic circulation to replace a diseased aortic valve.

The assessment of the PA flow profile and flow velocities with pulsed-wave Doppler may be difficult due to malalignment. It can be performed using the mid-esophageal ascending aorta short-axis (at 0–40°) and the upper esophageal aortic arch short-axis views with the sample placed centrally in the pulmonary artery 1–2 cm distal to the pulmonary valve (Fig. 8.5) [21]. The normal blood flow profile in the RVOT is laminar, with velocities between 0.6 and 0.9 m/s. The time from the start of the signal to peak velocity is termed the acceleration time (AcT) and is normally approximately 134 ± 24 ms. RV ejection time (RVET) is normally 304 ± 38 ms and the ratio of AcT to RVET is 0.45 ± 0.05 (Fig. 8.6). Subtle changes in the PA flow profile may indicate the presence of increased pulmonary vascular impedance. However, correct positioning of the sample is crucial, as the flow profile of the PA is significantly skewed. When the sample is placed closer to the wall, time to peak velocity decreases, and this may be misinterpreted as a sign of elevated pulmonary artery pressures.

From the PA flow velocity signal, stroke volume and cardiac output can be calculated from the velocity–time integral (VTI) and the PA diameter. Due to the irregular shape of the flow profile, this method is subject to significant error [22].

Finally, CWD can be used to measure the pressure gradient across a stenosed pulmonary valve using the modified Bernouilli equation, and to measure the deceleration rate of the PV regurgitant jet. This can be performed using the mid-esophageal aortic arch short-axis, or preferably the modified deep transgastric infundibular view.

Pulmonary valve disease

Severe pulmonary regurgitation (PR) is usually caused by dilation of the PA and PV annulus, for example as a result of acute or chronic pulmonary hypertension. However, it may also result from endocarditis, rheumatic disease, carcinoid syndrome, trauma, or congenital heart disease. Estimation of the severity of PR is made semi-quantitatively by measuring the size and depth of penetration of the PR jet (> 10 mm = moderate) or the jet width relative to the RVOT diameter. With severe PR, the pulmonary systolic VTI is significantly greater than the aortic systolic VTI, the jet is dense with a steep deceleration, and there is also RV dilation [23].

Repair of the tetralogy of Fallot using a transannular patch results in a variable degree of PR, and a

Figure 8.4. Mild (normal) degree of pulmonary regurgitation.

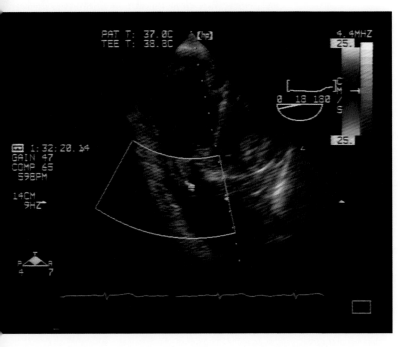

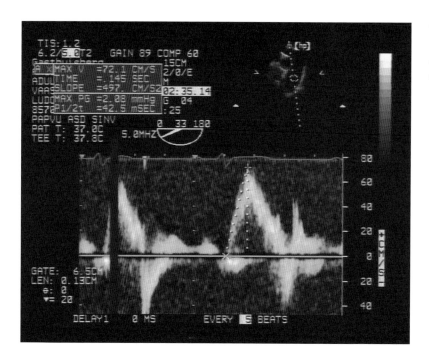

Figure 8.5. Doppler assessment of pulmonary artery blood flow using the upper esophageal aortic arch short-axis view. The Doppler beam/blood flow angle is at the upper acceptable limit.

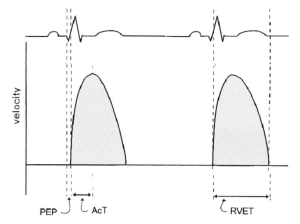

Figure 8.6. Pre-ejection phase (PEP), acceleration time (AcT), and RV ejection time (RVET) are shown timed to the ECG.

and/or supravalvular level. A substantial number of patients with tetralogy of Fallot need further surgery of the RVOT due to homograft stenosis in adulthood. Pulmonary stenosis is diagnosed with color-flow Doppler showing flow turbulence distal to the obstruction. The pulmonary valve area may be measured by the vena contracta method, assuming a circular stenotic PV orifice, but can be quantified with CWD measurement of the transvalvular gradient [24]. Severity of pulmonary stenosis is classified according to transvalvular pressure gradients as follows:

- peak systolic gradients ≤ 29 mmHg = mild stenosis
- peak systolic gradients 30–64 mmHg = moderate stenosis
- peak systolic gradients ≥ 65 mmHg = severe stenosis

Examples of disease of the pulmonary valve can be seen in Videos 8.16–8.18.

Conclusion

Although in surgical practice right-sided valve disease is less common than diseases of the mitral and aortic valves, the importance of imaging particularly the tricuspid valve is evident in patients with endocarditis and immunosupression from any cause. Imaging of the tricuspid and pulmonary valves, and of the pulmonary artery, may be difficult with TEE, and standard views are frequently unable to reveal sufficient

substantial number of these patients develop chronic volume overload. At a later age, this often requires further surgical intervention, with placement of a PA homograft.

The incidence of acquired pulmonary stenosis is low compared to the incidence of acquired stenosis of other valves. Rheumatic disease, infective endocarditis, and carcinoid syndrome may all produce pulmonary stenosis. In congenital heart disease RV obstruction can occur at the subvalvular, valvular, nformation. However, simple modifications of the standard views may be valuable, particularly in achieving parallel alignment for Doppler studies in cases where this is required.

References

1. Schroeder RA, Grichnik KP, Mark JB. Assessment of the tricuspid and pulmonic valves. In: Konstadt SN, Shernan S, Oka Y, eds., *Clinical Transesophageal Echocardiography: a Problem-Oriented Approach*, 2nd edn. Philadelphia, PA: Lippincott Williams & Wilkins, 2003: 137–56.

2. Singh JP, Evans JC, Levy D, *et al.* Prevalence and clinical determinants of mitral, tricuspid, and aortic regurgitation (the Framingham Heart Study). *Am J Cardiol* 1999; **83**: 897–902.

3. Klein AL, Burstow DJ, Tajik AJ, *et al.* Age-related prevalence of valvular regurgitation in normal subjects: a comprehensive color flow examination of 118 volunteers. *J Am Soc Echocardiogr* 1990; **3**: 54–63.

4. Cohen SR, Sell JE, McIntosh CL, Clark RE. Tricuspid regurgitation in patients with acquired, chronic, pure mitral regurgitation. I. Prevalence, diagnosis, and comparison of preoperative clinical and hemodynamic features in patients with and without tricuspid regurgitation. *J Thorac Cardiovasc Surg* 1987; **94**: 481–7.

5. Morrison DA, Ovitt T, Hammermeister KE. Functional tricuspid regurgitation and right ventricular dysfunction in pulmonary hypertension. *Am J Cardiol* 1988; **62**: 108–12.

6. Nath J, Foster E, Heidenreich PA. Impact of tricuspid regurgitation on long-term survival. *J Am Coll Cardiol* 2004; **43**: 405–9.

7. Dreyfus GD, Corbi PJ, Chan KM, Bahrami T. Secondary tricuspid regurgitation or dilatation: which should be the criteria for surgical repair? *Ann Thorac Surg* 2005; **79**: 127–32.

8. Colombo T, Russo C, Ciliberto GR, *et al.* Tricuspid regurgitation secondary to mitral valve disease: tricuspid annulus function as guide to tricuspid valve repair. *Cardiovasc Surg* 2001; **9**: 369–77.

9. Fukuda S, Gillinov AM, McCarthy PM, *et al.* Determinants of recurrent or residual functional tricuspid regurgitation after tricuspid annuloplasty. *Circulation* 2006; **114** (1 Suppl): I582–7.

10. Sadeghi HM, Kimura BJ, Raisinghani A, *et al.* Does lowering pulmonary arterial pressure eliminate severe functional tricuspid regurgitation? Insights from pulmonary thromboendarterectomy. *J Am Coll Cardiol* 2004; **44**: 126–32.

11. Pellikka PA, Tajik AJ, Khandheria BK, *et al.* Carcinoid heart disease: clinical and echocardiographic spectrum in 74 patients. *Circulation* 1993; **87**: 1188–96.

12. Moyssakis IE, Rallidis LS, Guida GF, Nihoyannopoulos PI. Incidence and evolution of carcinoid syndrome in the heart. *J Heart Valve Dis* 1997; **6**: 625–30.

13. Fox DJ, Khattar RS. Carcinoid heart disease: presentation, diagnosis, and management. *Heart.* 2004; **90**: 1224–8.

14. Yoong JK, Jaufeerally FR. Isolated tricuspid valve vegetations and steno-insufficiency in primary antiphospholipid syndrome *Singapore Med J* 2004; **45**: 127–9.

15. Rivera JM, Vandervoort PM, Vazquez de Prada JA, *et al.* Which physical factors determine tricuspid regurgitation jet area in the clinical setting? *Am J Cardiol* 1993; **72**: 1305–9.

16. Tribouilloy CM, Enriquez-Sarano M, Bailey KR, Tajik AJ, Seward JB. Quantification of tricuspid regurgitation by measuring the width of the vena contracta with Doppler color flow imaging: a clinical study. *J Am Coll Cardiol* 2000; **36**: 472–8.

17. Yock PG, Popp RL. Noninvasive estimation of right ventricular systolic pressure by Doppler ultrasound in patients with tricuspid regurgitation. *Circulation* 1984; **70**: 657–62.

18. Stephen B, Dalal P, Berger M, Schweitzer P, Hecht S. Noninvasive estimation of pulmonary artery diastolic pressure in patients with tricuspid regurgitation by Doppler echocardiography. *Chest* 1999; **116**: 73–7.

19. Lanzarini L, Fontana A, Campana C, Klersy C. Two simple echo-Doppler measurements can accurately identify pulmonary hypertension in the large majority of patients with chronic heart failure. *J Heart Lung Transplant* 2005; **24**: 745–54.

20. Choong CY, Abascal VM, Weyman J, *et al.* Prevalence of valvular regurgitation by Doppler echocardiography in patients with structurally normal hearts by two-dimensional echocardiography. *Am Heart J* 1989; **117**: 636–42.

21. Sloth E, Houlind KC, Pedersen EM, Hasenkam JM. Where to place the Doppler sample volume in the human main pulmonary artery: evaluated from magnetic resonance phase velocity maps. *Cardiovasc Res* 1997; **33**: 156–63.

22. Sloth E, Pedersen EM, Egeblad H, Hasenkam JM, Juhl B. Transesophageal multiplane imaging of the human pulmonary artery: a comparison of MRI and

multiplane transesophageal two-dimensional echocardiography. *Cardiovasc Res* 1997; **34**: 582–9.

23. Zoghbi WA, Enriquez-Sarano M, Foster E, *et al.* Recommendations for evaluation of the severity of native valvular regurgitation with two-dimensional and Doppler echocardiography. *J Am Soc Echocardiogr* 2003; **16**: 777–802.

24. Johnson GL, Kwan OL, Handshoe S, Noonan JA, DeMaria AN. Accuracy of combined two-dimensional echocardiography and continuous-wave Doppler recordings in the estimation of pressure gradient in right ventricular outlet obstruction. *J Am Coll Cardiol* 1984; **3**: 1013–18.

9

Left ventricular systolic and diastolic function

Fabio Guarracino

Introduction

Evaluation of left ventricular (LV) function is of major importance both in the cardiology clinic and in the perioperative setting. Cardiac ultrasound is particularly well suited for this purpose [1,2]. Transesophageal echocardiography (TEE) is a "semi-invasive" technique that can provide us with morphologic and functional information about the heart in the echo laboratory, the operating room, and the postoperative intensive care unit [3,4]. TEE provides high-quality real-time images of the beating heart by M-mode and two-dimensional (2D) echo, and qualitative and quantitative assessment of blood flow in the heart and vascular structures by Doppler technology. TEE has been shown to be an important tool for the evaluation of LV function in the management of critically ill patients, as a monitor of cardiac patients in cardiac and non-cardiac surgery, in ICU patients, and in a variety of specialized settings [2,5]. It may reveal causes of acute and chronic hemodynamic disturbance, and evaluate global and systolic function, preload, and diastolic function. Changes in regional contractility may enable us to identify acute myocardial ischemia in at-risk patients. TEE evaluation of the LV is based on a systematic study via M-mode, 2D, and Doppler flow investigation [6–8].

Systolic function

Whilst the term "contractility" is often used to describe systolic LV function, contractility refers more accurately to the inotropic state of the myocardium, that is the intrinsic power of the muscle fibers. This property depends on a variety of factors including the autonomic nervous system activity, arterial pH, and calcium release from the sarcoplasmic reticulum. A change in contractility is defined as an alteration of the inotropic state independent of preload, afterload, and heart rate. It is important to remember that most of the indices used in clinical practice to study LV per-

formance do not assess intrinsic myocardial contractility, being influenced also by heart rate and loading conditions.

Systolic evaluation in clinical practice

Evaluation of LV function using TEE requires that we consider the left ventricle to be a complex ellipsoid sphere [9]. This allows us to estimate LV function using methods based on the assessment of changes in diameters, areas, and volumes of the LV chamber both in systole and in diastole [10].

This evaluation is performed by obtaining LV images through standard views that can be easily obtained with modern omniplane transducers. The views routinely used are those recommended in practice guidelines by the American Society of Echocardiography and the Society of Cardiovascular Anesthesiologists [6,7,11]; they are shown in detail in Chapter 4.

Systolic function: changes in LV diameter

Based on observing the change in LV diameter, TEE allows us to measure fractional shortening (FS) [12]. This is obtained using the short-axis transgastric mid-papillary (mid-cavity) view of the LV, by M-mode measurement of the difference between end-diastolic and end-systolic diameters normalized for end-diastolic diameter (Fig. 9.1). The normal value is ≥ 30%.

Fractional shortening allows us to use simple linear dimensions as a method of estimating overall LV function. It is easy and quick to perform, but it also has important limitations. It assesses only the selected cross-section of the left ventricle, and therefore for FS to accurately reflect global LV function, there should be no alteration in regional LV contractility either at the apex or at the base. This may not be the case: for example, in the presence of basal hypokinesia or an apical aneurysm, mid-cavity FS would be a poor reflection of global LV systolic function. Other conditions

145

Core Topics in Transesophageal Echocardiography, ed. Robert Feneck, John Kneeshaw, and Marco Ranucci.
Published by Cambridge University Press. © Cambridge University Press 2010.

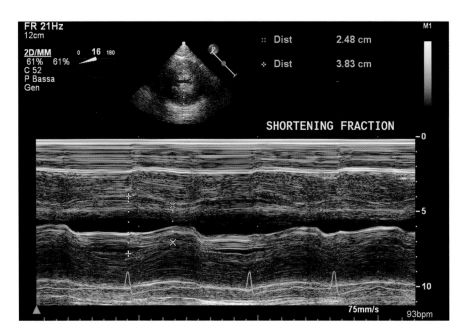

Figure 9.1. Measurement of fractional shortening (FS). Transgastric mid-papillary (mid-cavity) view of the LV, showing M-mode measurement of the difference between end-diastolic and end-systolic diameters normalized for end-diastolic diameter.

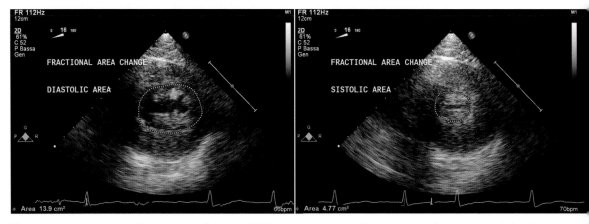

Figure 9.2. Measurement of fractional area of change (FAC). Transgastric mid-papillary (mid-cavity) short-axis view of the LV, showing 2D measurement of end-diastolic and end-systolic areas normalized for end-diastolic area.

that may adversely affect the uniform pattern of LV contraction include left bundle branch block and right ventricular dilation.

Systolic function: changes in LV area

LV systolic function may also be assessed by calculating the fractional area change (FAC). This is obtained in the mid-papillary (mid-cavity) transgastric short-axis view by 2D measurement of end-diastolic and end-systolic areas normalized for end-diastolic area (Fig. 9.2; Video 9.1). The normal value is ≥ 45%.

Approximately 70% of the LV stroke volume depends on contraction of the mid-papillary region of the LV. This is why FAC can provide a reasonable global estimate of LV function, and correlates well with ejection fraction. But, as with FS, this measurement also has limitations:

- FAC at mid-papillary level may not correlate with global function in patients with myocardial infarction or aneurysmal dilation in other areas of the LV that are not imaged through this view.
- Changes in loading conditions may also alter the FAC.

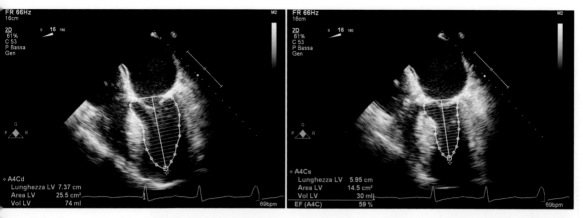

Figure 9.3. Measurement of ejection fraction (EF), obtained in long-axis views of the LV by measuring end-diastolic and end-systolic volumes normalized for end-diastolic volume.

The measurement of ventricular areas may be prone to user error, although it may be aided by automatic detection of the myocardial border, as with acoustic quantification (see *Automatic border detection*, below) [13].

Systolic function: changes in LV volume

Changes in LV chamber volumes allow us to assess LV function by measuring ejection fraction and stroke volume.

Ejection fraction

Ejection fraction (EF) is a well accepted and useful index of quantitative LV function, but it is influenced by changes in preload, afterload, and contractility. EF can be considered as a measurement of the interaction between preload, afterload, and contractility in determining ventricular performance. Thus it can be a good overall estimate of LV function [14].

EF calculation is obtained in long-axis views of the LV, by measuring end-diastolic and end-systolic volumes normalized for end-diastolic volume (Fig. 9.3). The normal value is ≥ 60%.

This measurement can be performed with two methods:

- **The area–length method.** The LV is assumed to be an ellipsoid sphere, and volumes are obtained by measuring LV areas and lengths at both end-diastole and end-systole [15]. The measurements require a long-axis view of the chamber without foreshortening of the LV. Such a view may be

> **Box 9.1. Technique for the measurement of ejection fraction (Fig. 9.5)**
>
> - Obtain the best long axis view you can by searching for the true apex without any foreshortening. In mid-esophageal long-axis views this often requires some retroflexion of the probe tip.
> - Adjust the settings in order to have the best detection of the endocardial border. By normal convention, the papillary muscles are included as part of the left ventricular cavity.
> - Always select appropriate sinus beats. End-diastole occurs at the peak of the R wave, and end-systole at the end of the T wave.
> - Take three heart cycles in sinus rhythm; average 9–10 cycles in atrial fibrillation.

difficult to obtain from the standard four-chamber mid-esophageal view (Fig. 9.4), and some retroflexion of the probe may be required to prevent foreshortening and thus visualize the true apex.

- **Simpson's rule.** This assumes that the LV volume can be obtained by summing the volumes of multiple slices of a known thickness that make up the left ventricle. Each slice is considered as an ellipsoid cylinder. The measurement requires two different long-axis views of the ventricular chamber. This method, known also as the "disk summation method," is integrated in the software of echo machines (Fig. 9.5). The technique is described in Box 9.1.

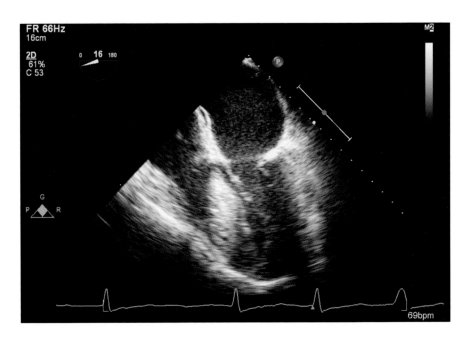

Figure 9.4. LV long axis. The true apex is not shown, and therefore calculation of EF in the long axis will be inaccurate.

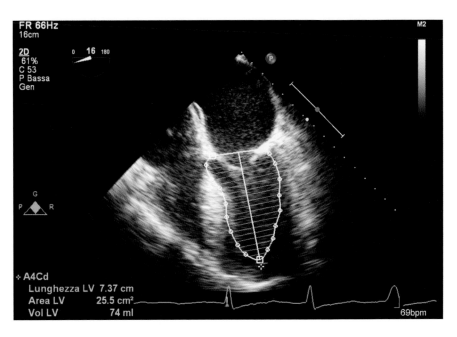

Figure 9.5. Simpson's method and disk summation for calculation of LV EF in the long axis (see Box 9.1).

Stroke volume

Stroke volume (SV) may be a useful index for evaluating a patient's hemodynamic status, and in assessing the response to therapy. It can be obtained with 2D TEE by measuring LV end-systolic and end-diastolic volumes, as described above for measuring EF. It may also be measured by using Doppler technology, which allows measurement of forward flow through any transverse sectional area within the heart, combined with a 2D echo measurement of an appropriate cross-sectional area (CSA).

Similar to EF, SV is influenced by loading conditions, contractility, and heart rate. SV is the difference between end-diastolic and end-systolic volumes, which are measured as part of the EF calculation. The normal value is 50–80 ml.

The technique required to calculate SV, using either the left ventricular outflow tract (LVOT) diameter or the aortic valve area, combined with pulsed-wave Doppler measurements at the LVOT or continuous-wave Doppler measurements, is described in detail in Chapter 13. However, the LVOT diameter and aortic valve area are relatively unchanging, and we can therefore use changes in the LVOT velocity–time integral or the aortic velocity–time integral as a means of rapidly monitoring changes in cardiac output in the intraoperative setting [16].

A change of velocity–time integral as a consequence of any treatment allows us to evaluate the response to therapy, thus influencing the patient's clinical management. This may be considered complementary to, rather than a replacement for, pulmonary artery catheterization [17].

Other indices of LV function include the following:

- isovolumic contraction time
- LV dP/dt
- maximal LV power
- peak aortic flow acceleration at early systole

These may be determined by TEE, but their use in everyday practice is limited by the complexity of the measurements and their time-consuming nature. They are also dependent on loading conditions and changes in inotropic state, and for LV dP/dt calculation mitral regurgitation needs to be present also.

End-systolic indices in LV function evaluation

A different approach to myocardial contractility is based on the investigation of the relationship of end-systolic indices. Such indices reflect the intrinsic inotropic state of the myocardium and are not influenced by loading conditions. The end-systolic volume to peak systolic pressure and the end-systolic area to peak systolic pressure are two of the relationships more widely studied in this field. The LV end-systolic pressure is read as the end-systolic arterial pressure at the dicrotic notch, while end-systolic volume, measured with methods described for EF calculation, and end-systolic area are obtained by TEE. By plotting end-systolic pressure and end-systolic area or volume, and then obtaining a new pressure–area or volume curve with manipulation of preload or afterload, it is possible to assess the inotropic state of the myocardium through the end-systolic pressure–volume relationship. These indices of myocardial performance are not currently

used in clinical TEE, and certainly accurate measurement of the dicrotic notch on the arterial waveform may be difficult. But future technological progress in this, and in the automation of such pressure–volume curves, may prove fruitful.

Regional contractility: the study of LV wall motion

Abnormal myocardial contractility and wall motion frequently occurs during episodes of myocardial ischemia or after myocardial infarction. Therefore a change in regional wall motion, as detected by echocardiography, is a reliable sign of myocardial ischemia [1,13]. Ultrasound is very sensitive in detecting myocardial ischemia, and TEE is reported to be more sensitive as a detector of ischemia than changes detected by either the ECG or pulmonary artery catheter [18].

However, certain limitations can make some assessments difficult. Assessment of regional wall motion abnormalities (RWMAs) is mostly subjective, and it takes a certain degree of experience to develop accuracy. Based on a semi-quantitative "eyeballing" evaluation, severity is graded from no RWMA (normal) to akinesia or dyskinesia. The appearance of a normally contracting LV wall on echo is characterized by motion and thickening. Description of the location and extent of RWMA requires a segmental model of the LV [19].

Based on the recommendations of the American Society of Echocardiography Standards Committee, the ASE/SCA guidelines for performing a TEE exam [6] suggest a division of the LV into three levels from base to apex (Fig. 9.6):

- basal level, extending from the mitral valve annulus to the tips of the papillary muscles
- mid-cavity level, extending from the tips to the bases of the papillary muscles
- apical level, representing the remaining part of the LV

The basal and mid-cavity levels are each divided into six segments, the apical level into four. Previously, the LV was divided into 16 segments, but the most recent reclassification has added a 17th segment – the apical cap (see Chapter 4, Fig. 4.4) [19]. This segmentation allows the evaluation of each single segment for motion and thickening during the systolic phase of the cardiac cycle. The 17 segments can be investigated

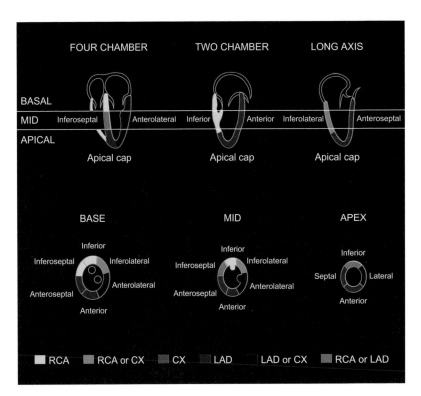

Figure 9.6. Diagram of LV segments long and short axis (new classification).

Table 9.1. Semi-quantitative analysis of LV wall motion

	% radial shortening	Thickening	Score
Normal	> 30	+++	1
Mild hypokinesis	10–30	++	2
Severe hypokinesis	< 10, > 0	+	3
Akynesis	0	0	4
Dyskinesis	Paradoxical	Thinning	5

through the four-chamber, two-chamber, and long axis views, and the transgastric basal and mid-papillary short-axis views (Fig. 9.6). A quantitative analysis of wall motion can be made using a scale for motion and thickening, which leads to a scoring system. The grading of motion is based on the evaluation of segmental radial shortening of the distance from the endocardium to the center of the LV cavity during systole. Thickening is graded on the increase in the distance between endocardial and epicardial border during systole. This increase is estimated visually on a scale from + to +++ (Table 9.1).

As previously stated, the evaluation of wall motion is highly dependent on the experience of the observer. Also, factors other than myofibril contraction may be responsible for LV wall movement.

The heart moves during respiration, and also undergoes rotational and translational movements. In the intraoperative setting other possible movements related to surgery may be present, and these may affect the evaluation [20–21]. Although based on an arbitrary estimation, systolic thickening is of great importance in the evaluation of wall motion because it is poorly influenced by rotational and translational movements, and has a high correlation with the extent of normally perfused myocardium [22,23].

For routine purposes, when monitoring myocardial ischemia, the transgastric mid-papillary short axis view is the most useful. It is easy to obtain and retain, thanks to the papillary muscle morphology. I allows good visualization of the myocardial region

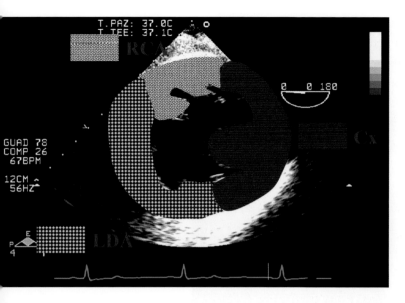

Figure 9.7. Distribution of LV coronary blood flow at mid-cavity (mid-papillary) level. RCA, right coronary artery; LDA, left anterior descending artery; Cx, circumflex artery.

supplied by all three main coronary arteries, so that any alteration in coronary blood flow may produce a predictable change in wall motion which can be readily identified and checked against any information from coronary angiogram (Fig. 9.7). Sensitivity and specificity for RWMA are very high at this level of the LV.

Based on RWMAs, the criteria for diagnosis of myocardial ischemia are as follows:

- the RWMA is a new finding (i.e. hypokinesis of a previously normally contracting myocardial segment, or akinesis of a previously hypokinetic area)
- it worsens by at least two scores
- it has a duration > 1 minute at least

Non-ischemic RWMA can occur due to normal regional heterogeneity, altered loading, tethering or systolic dysfunction, bundle branch block, and ventricular pacing. Also, causes related to coronary artery disease, such as infarction, stunning, and hibernating, can create RWMA (Videos 9.2–9.6).

New advances in global and regional LV evaluation

In recent years, progress in ultrasound technology has led to new advances in this field. Such advances include the automatic detection of tissue–blood interface [13] and measurement of myocardial tissue velocities [24].

Automatic border detection: acoustic quantification

In some echo machines software for automatic detection of the endocardial border is included. With this technology, called acoustic quantification, blood and tissue are clearly differentiated by integrated analysis of backscattered signals from the endocardium and blood [13]. A colored border indicator allows delineation of the endocardial borders. By drawing a region of interest (ROI) including the LV cavity, it is possible to get continuous, real-time determination of areas and volumes (Fig. 9.8; Video 9.7).

This method can reduce variability in border detection among operators, and is able to provide a real-time measurement of the LV areas and volumes, and therefore of FAC and EF. Accurate assessment, however, is strongly influenced by the quality of the images and the settings on the echo machine.

Color kinesis

This is based on acoustic quantification technology, of which it represents an extension. This technology tracks the motion of the endocardium in systole and provides color-coded images reflecting the magnitude and timing of endocardial motion photos [23–26]. The duration of the systolic phase of the cardiac cycle is divided into several segments. Each of these subphases is represented by a different color, starting from orange at isovolumic contraction, going through yellow during early ejection, then green, and finally

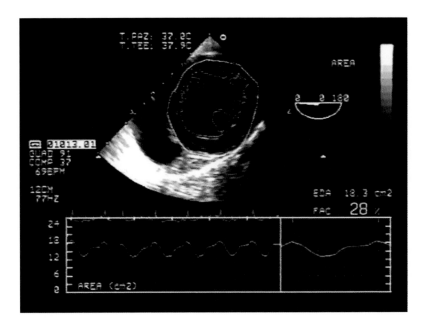

Figure 9.8. Automated border detection in a transgastric short-axis LV view.

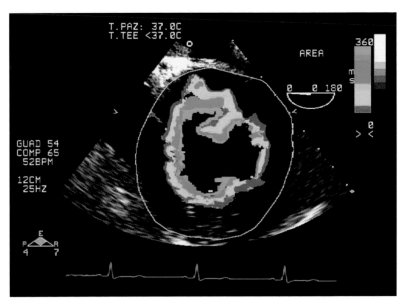

Figure 9.9. Border detection and LV wall motion evaluated by color kinesis. A transgastric short-axis view of the LV is shown.

blue at late systole. Each color corresponds to a different velocity of the endocardial wall towards the cavity. Normal segments show a full color pattern from orange to blue, reflecting an increase in velocity from 0 to 360 cm/s at end-systole. The color-coded image is very helpful in evaluating systolic movement of LV walls, so allowing a global and regional qualitative assessment of systolic LV function [25] (Fig. 9.9; Video 9.8).

Tissue Doppler imaging

Tissue Doppler imaging (TDI) is a recent application of Doppler technology designed to detect myocardial tissue velocity through the cardiac cycle. The Doppler technology is modified to detect low velocities from tissue movement: consecutive phase shifts of ultrasound reflected from the myocardium are detected, and intramural myocardial velocities are determined [24,26].

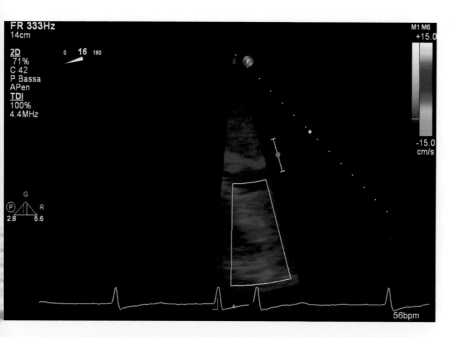

Figure 9.10. Myocardial movement represented by color Doppler.

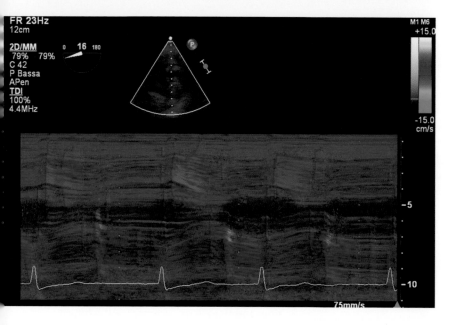

Figure 9.11. Tissue Doppler imaging showing color M-mode display.

Myocardial movement is represented with color Doppler by changes from blue to red according to standard pattern (Fig. 9.10; Video 9.9). No color is detected from akinetic segments.

The analysis can be performed with M-mode to assess myocardial velocities over time (Fig. 9.11). Pulsed-wave Doppler (PWD) application allows registration of myocardial velocities throughout the cardiac cycle, both in systole and in diastole (Fig. 9.12) [27].

PW-TDI provides a velocity map of the myocardial wall during both systole and diastole [25]. During systole a velocity (V_S) wave is recorded; the velocity of this wave is reduced during myocardial ischemia. The recording of V_S from ventricular segments leads to regional assessment of wall motion. Preliminary studies report high sensitivity and reproducibility, and indicate PW-TDI as a promising method to assess regional LV contractility [18,28].

153

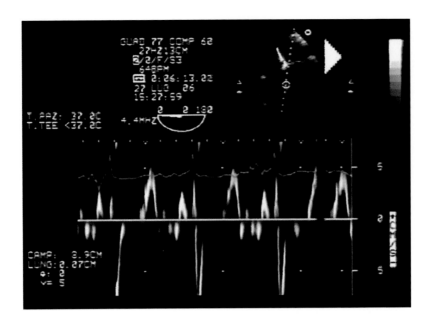

Figure 9.12. Pulsed tissue Doppler imaging showing registration of myocardial velocities (E′, A′, and S′ waves).

The usefulness of TDI examination may rely on the following:

- the ability to perform a complete evaluation of any segment of the LV wall
- the ability to obtain appropriate information on LV systolic function in those situations in which a standard 2D exam can be misleading, such as bundle branch block, patients with implanted pacemakers or pericardial abnormalities, and other situations that may cause apparent or true abnormal motion of LV segments

Clinical experience

The evaluation of regional myocardial contractility intraoperatively during off-pump coronary artery bypass, on-pump procedures, non-cardiac procedures in patients at risk for myocardial ischemia, and in the intensive care unit may be simply undertaken whenever myocardial ischemia is suspected [20,21,29]. Our routine evaluation is based on a 2D standard evaluation using the segmental model as described above, on color kinesis, and also on segmental evaluation of systolic myocardial velocities by TDI. In our experience this last method is particularly useful in those situations in which there is doubt about the performance of akinetic or severely hypokinetic segments at 2D exam. A TDI segmental evaluation allows us to evaluate the recovery after

coronary revascularization, to identify ischemia in a previously normal segment, and also to evaluate myocardial segments during ischemia for off-pump surgery. This last setting is particularly useful. Analysis of myocardial velocities during coronary occlusion by the surgeon facilitates an echo-guided policy of coronary shunting, using the shunt catheter only in those cases in which a reduction of velocities is registered after one minute of coronary artery occlusion [18,28,30].

Thus TEE evaluation of LV systolic function, both global and regional, provides insight into hemodynamic impairment in a variety of situations [2]. It requires a systematic approach, and a combination of 2D, M-mode, color Doppler, and spectral Doppler will allow us to obtain a qualitative and quantitative evaluation of systolic function. New technologies allow us to identify new indices of ventricular function, and these have promise for the future.

Diastolic function

Physiology of LV diastole

Diastolic function is essential for efficient systolic performance. Normal diastole allows adequate LV filling to occur under normal filling pressures. It is an energy-dependent process, and may therefore be adversely affected by pathological states, including myocardial ischemia.

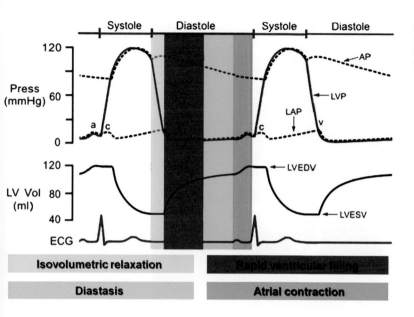

Figure 9.13. The physiology of LV diastole, showing isovolumic relaxation (IVR), rapid ventricular filling (RF), diastasis, and atrial contraction.

Several factors influence LV diastolic function, as shown in Table 9.2.

From a physiologic point of view, diastole is divided into four phases (Fig. 9.13):

- isovolumic relaxation (IVR)
- rapid ventricular filling (RF)
- diastasis
- atrial contraction

IVR is an active process during which a rapid fall of LV pressure occurs. IVR starts immediately following aortic valve closure. During this phase of diastole no filling of the LV cavity can be seen. When the IVR ends, and the LV pressure is below left atrial pressure, the mitral valve opens, allowing rapid filling of the LV by blood rushing from the left atrium (LV suction). During this time about 80% of LV fill-

ing occurs. A slower filling phase follows – diastasis. Then the atrium contracts, so completing the ventricular filling by adding about 15–20% of global filling volume.

Echo evaluation

Doppler echocardiography is the principal diagnostic tool to assess LV diastolic function non-invasively [31–33]. It allows us to analyze each phase through measurement of transmitral and pulmonary vein flows velocities. The transmitral flow velocity is related to the transmitral gradient, whereas pulmonary venous flow velocity reflects left atrial filling.

Color M-mode Doppler and TDI have also been introduced in the study of diastolic function in recent years [34,35]. They may be particularly useful, as they seem to be independent of conditions affecting mitral and pulmonary vein flow, such as loading conditions, age, and atrial fibrillation.

Mitral flow

The pulsed Doppler interrogation of the transmitral inflow velocity profile shows two distinct waves:

- an early wave, E wave, corresponding to the early rapid filling
- a second wave, the A wave, related to atrial contraction [36] (Fig. 9.14)

Diastasis, a short period with no atrioventricular gradient, occurs between the E and A waves.

Table 9.2. Factors affecting LV diastolic function

- Mitral valve function
- Gradient between left atrium and left ventricle
- State of left ventricular relaxation and compliance
- Left atrial function, and presence of sinus rhythm
- End-systolic (diastolic) volume or preload
- Afterload and heart rate
- Pericardium
- Right ventricular function

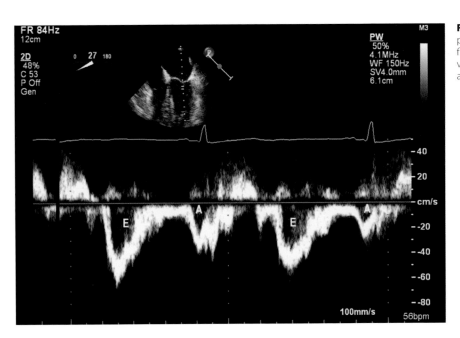

Figure 9.14. Pulsed-wave Doppler image of transmitral blood flow, showing an E wave (early ventricular filling – diastasis) and an A wave (atrial contraction).

Normally, the E wave has a higher peak velocity than the A wave, and a deceleration time (DT) between 160 and 240 ms. The normal ratio of E/A peak velocities is > 1.

Pulmonary vein flow

Pulsed Doppler sampling of flow from the pulmonary veins shows three waves:

- a systolic (S) wave
- a diastolic (D) wave, corresponding to rapid filling
- a reversed A (rA) wave, related to atrial contraction (Fig. 9.15)

Normally the S wave is higher than the D wave, with S/D peak velocity ratio > 1, and mitral A wave > pulmonary vein rA wave.

Similar to mitral flow, pulmonary vein flow is strongly affected by changes in loading conditions and by aging. Other clinical conditions affecting pulmonary venous flow velocities include impaired LV systolic function and mitral regurgitation. Thus it is difficult to evaluate diastole by examining pulmonary venous flow whenever systolic LV impairment and/or mitral regurgitation is present.

Color M-mode

The combination of color Doppler and M-mode technology facilitates the evaluation in space and time of blood flow entering the LV through the mitral valve towards the apex.

Color M-mode interrogation provides the spatio-temporal distribution of blood flow velocity within the LV across a vertical line. It provides a pattern with two waves: the first wave (E) propagating from the left atrium towards the LV apex, and a second wave (A) following atrial contraction (Fig. 9.16). This method allows us to study the propagation velocity (V_p) of the flow within the LV during the rapid and slow filling phases [37]. Early V_p is given by the slope of the color E wave. It is considered a useful index for the quantitative assessment of LV relaxation, and V_p seems to be independent of preload [38]. Its normal value is > 55 cm/s. In situations where ventricular relaxation is abnormal, V_p is reduced.

Tissue Doppler imaging: mitral annulus velocity

TDI quantifies the velocities of the myocardium during both systole and diastole [38,39]. A TDI pattern displays a systolic velocity signal (S_m), and two diastolic velocities, one during early (E_m) and the other during late (A_m) diastole. E_m sampled at the mitral annulus correlates with diastolic function, and seems to be independent of preload [40]. The analysis of mitral annulus velocity, obtained in the mid-esophageal long-axis four-chamber view at the mitral annulus, either at the lateral or septal annulus, has been proposed as a reliable method for

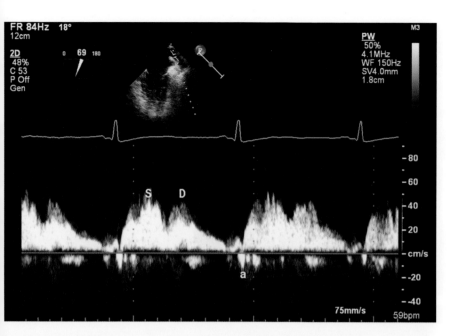

Figure 9.15. Normal Doppler pulmonary vein flow.

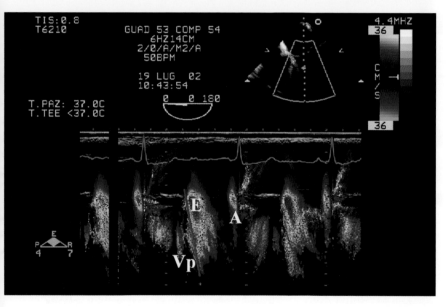

Figure 9.16. Color M-mode Doppler imaging, showing the first wave (E) propagating from the left atrium towards the LV apex, and a second wave (A) following atrial contraction. V_p is the propagation velocity of the flow within the LV during the rapid and slow filling phases, and early V_p is given by the slope of the color E wave.

assessing diastole (Fig. 9.17). The combination of annular velocity with E wave velocity from mitral inflow has been proposed as a better estimate of diastolic function [36,41,42].

Diastolic dysfunction

A certain degree of impaired diastole is typical of the aging process [43,44]. Diastolic dysfunction is commonly seen in chronic arterial hypertension and coronary artery disease. Cardiomyopathies, both restrictive and hypertrophic, show a pattern of altered diastole. Congestive heart failure, for example in dilated cardiomyopathy, is an example of concomitant systolic and diastolic dysfunction. Severe impairment of systolic LV function is often accompanied by diastolic dysfunction, whereas severe diastolic dysfunction can be found in the absence of systolic impairment [45,46].

157

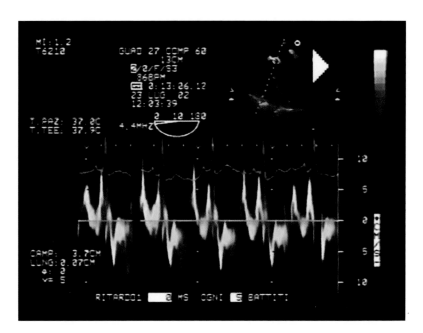

Figure 9.17. A tissue Doppler image showing two diastolic velocities, one during early (E_m) and the other during late (A_m) diastole, sampled at the mitral annulus.

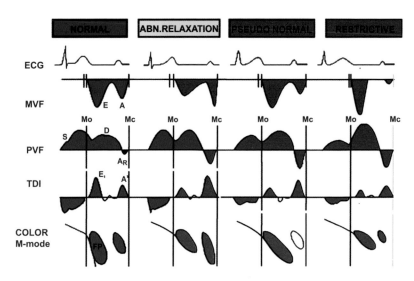

Figure 9.18. Findings of transmitral blood flow, pulmonary vein flow, tissue Doppler imaging, and color M-mode in different states of LV diastolic dysfunction. Green, normal patterns; red, abnormal.

Diastolic dysfunction occurs as a result of morphologic changes in cardiac structure. These may occur for a number of reasons, including the following:

- myopathies with hypertrophy
- increased myocardial mass or fibrosis
- following a reduction in myocardial perfusion, e.g. in coronary artery disease
- as a result of intra- and extravascular causes of obstruction to blood flow, e.g. pulmonary embolism and pericardial constraint and tamponade

On these bases a clinical classification of diastolic dysfunction is possible.

These clinical situations can be identified and evaluated by TEE with 2D and Doppler imaging, using a systematic and complete exam according to published guidelines [6,31]. Diastolic function, as evaluated by Doppler echocardiography [7], is classified into four stages, as follows (Fig. 9.18):

- normal filling
- stage I – abnormal relaxation
- stage II – pseudonormal pattern
- stage III – restricted advanced altered filling

Table 9.3. Summary of the Doppler findings of each diastolic pattern

Normal filling – LV filling occurs under normal filling pressures
Transmitral pulsed Doppler: E/A ratio > 1, DT < 220 ms
Pulmonary venous pulsed Doppler: S/D > 1
Color M-mode: V_p > 55 cm/s
Tissue Doppler echocardiography: E_m > 8–10 cm/s
Stage I: delayed relaxation – LV relaxation is reduced, compliance and filling pressures are normal
Transmitral pulsed Doppler: E/A ratio < 1, DT > 220 ms
Pulmonary venous pulsed Doppler: S/D > 1, high A wave
Color M-mode: V_p < 45 cm/s
Tissue Doppler echocardiography: E_m < 8 cm/s
Stage II: pseudonormal – LV relaxation and compliance are reduced, filling pressures are increased
Transmitral pulsed Doppler: high E wave, E/A ratio > 1, DT < 220 ms
Pulmonary venous pulsed Doppler: S/D < 1, high (> 35 cm/s) A wave > mitral A wave
Color M-mode: V_p < 45 cm/s
Tissue Doppler echocardiography: E_m < 8 cm/s
Stage III: restrictive pattern – severely reduced LV relaxation and compliance
Filling pressures are markedly increased, leading to earlier mitral valve opening and shorter IRT (< 70 ms)
Transmitral pulsed Doppler: high E wave, E/A ratio > 2, DT < 150 ms
A wave > mitral A wave
Pulmonary venous pulsed Doppler: S/D < 1
Color M-mode: V_p < 45 cm/s
Tissue Doppler echocardiography: E_m < 8 cm/s

These different patterns can follow each other during the natural history of diastolic dysfunction, going from normal to abnormal relaxation, to the restrictive pattern. Table 9.3 summarizes the Doppler findings of each different diastolic pattern.

Index of global myocardial performance

In 1995 Tei and coworkers described a new index of global systolic and diastolic LV performance [47]. This myocardial performance index (MPI) is expressed by the formula MPI = ICT + IRT / ET, where ICT is the isovolumic contraction time, IRT is the isovolumic relaxation time, and ET the ejection time. Such time intervals can all be obtained using Doppler echo. The normal value of the index is 0.4.

Systolic dysfunction causes a prolonged ICT and a reduction of ET, while diastolic impairment prolongs the IRT. In patients with heart failure the Tei index is > 0.5.

Clinical considerations

Evaluation of the diastolic phase is important for the management of critical patients in the perioperative period. If abnormal ventricular relaxation and compliance is found [48,49], drugs to increase diastolic time may be used, including β-blockers, and treatment to preserve atrial contraction may be useful also. In patients with a restrictive (stage III) pattern, measures to prolong diastolic filling would prove ineffective, and inotropic agents should be considered.

In our institution routine titration of drug effect on diastolic function is performed by sequential measurements of V_p and E_m. Also a combination of end-diastolic area by planimetry and wedge pressure measurement by pulmonary artery catheter is routinely performed in those cases in which small areas and high pressures are found, in order to facilitate the optimization of preload and cardiac output.

TEE facilitates a complete evaluation of diastolic LV function by assessing diastolic phases and elucidating structural causes of altered diastole. The use of this tool has relevant implications in the management of hemodynamic derangement due to impaired diastolic function, in vasoactive drugs titration, in the detection of myocardial ischemia, and in performing prognostic stratification.

References

1. Odell DH, Cahalan MK. Assessment of left ventricular global and segmental systolic function with transesophageal echocardiography. *Anesthesiol Clin* 2006; **24**: 755–62.

2. Douglas PS, Khandheria B, Stainback RF, Weissman NJ. ACCF/ASE/ACEP/ASNC/SCAI/SCCT/SCMR 2007 appropriateness criteria for transthoracic and transesophageal echocardiography. *J Am Soc Echocardiogr* 2007; **20**: 787–805.

3. Waller BF, Taliercio CP, Slack JD, *et al.* Tomographic views of normal and abnormal hearts: the anatomic basis for various cardiac imaging techniques, Part I. *Clin Cardiol* 1990; **13**: 804–12.

4. Waller BF, Taliercio CP, Slack JD, *et al.* Tomographic views of normal and abnormal hearts: the anatomic basis for various cardiac imaging techniques, Part II. *Clin Cardiol* 1990; **13**: 877–84.

5. Poelaert JI, Trouerbach J, De Buyzere M, Everaert J, Colardyn FA. Evaluation of transesophageal echocardiography as a diagnostic and therapeutic aid in a critical care setting. *Chest* 1995; **107**: 774–9.

6. Shanewise JS, Cheung AT, Aronson S, *et al.* ASE/SCA guidelines for performing a comprehensive intraoperative multiplane transoesophageal echocardiography examination: recommendations of the American Society of Echocardiography Council for Intraoperative Echocardiography and the Society of Cardiovascular Anesthesiologists Task Force for Certification in Perioperative Transesophageal Echocardiography. *J Am Soc Echocardiogr* 1999; **12**: 884–900.

7. Cheitlin MD, Armstrong WF, Aurigemma GP, *et al.* ACC/AHA/ASE 2003 guideline update for the clinical application of echocardiography: summary article. A report of the American College of Cardiology/American Heart Association Task Force on Practice Guidelines (ACC/AHA/ASE Committee to Update the 1997 Guidelines for the Clinical Application of Echocardiography). *Circulation* 2003; **108**: 1146–62.

8. Henry WL, DeMaria A, Gramiak R, *et al.* Report of the American Society of Echocardiography Committee on Nomenclature and Standards in Two-dimensional Echocardiography. *Circulation* 1980; **62**: 212–17.

9. Schiller NB, Shah PM, Crawford M, *et al.* Recommendations for quantitation of the left ventricle by two-dimensional echocardiography. *J Am Soc Echocardiogr* 1989; **2**: 358–67.

10. Lang RM, Bierig M, Devereux RB, *et al.* Recommendations for chamber quantification: a report from the American Society of Echocardiography's Guidelines and Standards Committee and the Chamber Quantification Writing Group, developed in conjunction with the European Association of Echocardiography, a branch of the European Society of Cardiology. *J Am Soc Echocardiogr* 2005; **18**: 1440–63.

11. Standardization of cardiac tomographic imaging. From the Committee on Advanced Cardiac Imaging and Technology, Council on Clinical Cardiology, American Heart Association; Cardiovascular Imaging Committee, American College of Cardiology; and Board of Directors, Cardiovascular Council, Society of Nuclear Medicine. *Circulation* 1992; **86**: 338–9.

12. Colombo PC, Municino A, Brofferio A, *et al.* Cross-sectional multiplane transesophageal echocardiographic measurements: comparison with standard transthoracic values obtained in the same setting. *Echocardiography* 2002; **19**: 383–90.

13. Siostrzonek P, Mundigler G, Hassan A, Zehetgruber M. Echocardiographic diagnosis of segmental wall motion abnormalities. *Acta Anaesthesiol Scand Suppl* 1997; **111**: 271–4.

14. Nahar T, Croft L, Shapiro R, *et al.* Comparison of four echocardiographic techniques for measuring left ventricular ejection fraction. *Am J Cardiol* 2000; **86**: 1358–62.

15. Hozumi T, Shakudo M, Shah PM. Quantitation of left ventricular volumes and ejection fraction by biplane transesophageal echocardiography. *Am J Cardiol* 1993; **72**: 356–9.

16. Guarracino F. [The role of transesophageal echocardiography in intraoperative hemodynamic monitoring] *Minerva Anestesiol* 2001; **67**: 320–4.

17. Jacka MJ, Cohen MM, To T, Devitt JH, Byrick R. The use of and preferences for the transesophageal echocardiogram and pulmonary artery catheter among cardiovascular anesthesiologists. *Anesth Analg* 2002; **94**: 1065–71.

18. Hameed AK, Gosal T, Fang T, *et al.* Clinical utility of tissue Doppler imaging in patients with acute myocardial infarction complicated by cardiogenic shock. *Cardiovasc Ultrasound* 2008; **6**: 11.

19. Cerqueira MD, Weissman NJ, Dilsizian V, *et al.* Standardized myocardial segmentation and

nomenclature for tomographic imaging of the heart. A statement for healthcare professionals from the Cardiac Imaging Committee of the Council on Clinical Cardiology of the American Heart Association. *Circulation* 2002; **105**: 539–42.

20. Hogue CW, Dávila-Román VG. Detection of myocardial ischemia by transesophageal echocardiographically determined changes in left ventricular area in patients undergoing coronary artery bypass surgery. *J Clin Anesth* 1997; **9**: 388–93.

21. Kolev N, Ihra G, Swanevelder J, *et al.* Biplane transoesophageal echocardiographic detection of myocardial ischaemia in patients with coronary artery disease undergoing non-cardiac surgery: segmental wall motion vs. electrocardiography and haemodynamic performance. *Eur J Anaesthesiol* 1997; **14**: 412–20.

22. Shanewise JS. How to reliably detect ischemia in the intensive care unit and operating room. *Semin Cardiothorac Vasc Anesth* 2006; **10**: 101–9.

23. Macieira-Coelho E, Dionísio I, Garcia-Alves M, *et al.* Comparison between dobutamine echocardiography and thallium-201 scintigraphy in detecting residual stenosis, ischemia, and necrosis in patients with prior myocardial infarction. *Clin Cardiol* 1997; **20**: 351–6.

24. Ng AC, Tran D, Newman M, *et al.* Comparison of myocardial tissue velocities measured by two-dimensional speckle tracking and tissue Doppler imaging. *Am J Cardiol* 2008; **102**: 784–9.

25. Mor-Avi V, Spencer K, Gorcsan J, *et al.* Normal values of regional left ventricular endocardial motion: multicenter color kinesis study. *Am J Physiol Heart Circ Physiol* 2000; **279**: H2464–76.

26. Garcia MJ, Rodriguez L, Ares M, *et al.* Myocardial wall velocity assessment by pulsed Doppler tissue imaging: characteristic findings in normal subjects. *Am Heart J* 1996; **132**: 648–56.

27. Batterham A, Shave R, Oxborough D, Whyte G, George K. Longitudinal plane colour tissue-Doppler myocardial velocities and their association with left ventricular length, volume, and mass in humans. *Eur J Echocardiogr* 2008; **9**: 542–6.

28. Olson JM, Samad BA, Alam M. Prognostic value of pulse-wave tissue Doppler parameters in patients with systolic heart failure. *Am J Cardiol* 2008; **102**: 722–5.

29. Minhaj M, Patel K, Muzic D, *et al.* The effect of routine intraoperative transesophageal echocardiography on surgical management. *J Cardiothorac Vasc Anesth.* 2007; **21**: 800–4.

30. Swaminathan M, Morris RW, De Meyts DD, *et al.* Deterioration of regional wall motion immediately after coronary artery bypass graft surgery is associated with long-term major adverse cardiac events. *Anesthesiology* 2007; **107**: 739–45.

31. Garcia MJ. Comprehensive echocardiographic assessment of diastolic function. *Heart Fail Clin* 2006; **2**: 163–78.

32. Garcia MJ, Thomas JD, Klein AL. New Doppler echocardiographic applications for the study of diastolic function. *J Am Coll Cardiol* 1998; **32**: 865–75.

33. Thomas JD, Weyman AE. Echocardiographic Doppler evaluation of left ventricular diastolic function: physics and physiology. *Circulation* 1991; **84**: 977–90.

34. Kasner M, Westermann D, Steendijk P, *et al.* Utility of Doppler echocardiography and tissue Doppler imaging in the estimation of diastolic function in heart failure with normal ejection fraction: a comparative Doppler-conductance catheterization study. *Circulation* 2007; **116**: 637–47.

35. Labovitz AJ, Pearson AC. Evaluation of left ventricular diastolic function: clinical relevance and recent Doppler echocardiographic insights. *Am Heart J* 1987; **114**: 836–51.

36. Mizuno H, Ohte N, Wakami K, *et al.* Peak mitral annular velocity during early diastole and propagation velocity of early diastolic filling flow are not interchangeable as the parameters of left ventricular early diastolic function. *Am J Cardiol* 2008; **101**: 1467–71.

37. Garcia MJ, Smedira NG, Greenberg NL, *et al.* Color M-mode Doppler flow propagation velocity is a preload insensitive index of left ventricular relaxation: animal and human validation. *J Am Coll Cardiol* 2000; **35**: 201–8.

38. Nagueh SF, Middleton KJ, Kopelen HA, Zoghbi WA, Quiñones MA. Doppler tissue imaging: a noninvasive technique for evaluation of left ventricular relaxation and estimation of filling pressures. *J Am Coll Cardiol* 1997; **30**: 1527–33.

39. Rakowski H, Appleton C, Chan KL, *et al.* Canadian consensus recommendations for the measurement and reporting of diastolic dysfunction by echocardiography: from the Investigators of Consensus on Diastolic Dysfunction by Echocardiography. *J Am Soc Echocardiogr* 1996; **9**: 736–60.

40. Wang M, Yip GW, Wang AY, *et al.* Peak early diastolic mitral annulus velocity by tissue Doppler imaging adds independent and incremental prognostic value. *J Am Coll Cardiol* 2003; **41**: 820–6.

41. Sohn DW, Chai IH, Lee DJ, *et al.* Assessment of mitral annulus velocity by Doppler tissue imaging in the evaluation of left ventricular diastolic function. *J Am Coll Cardiol* 1997; **30**: 474–80.

42. Palecek T, Linhart A, Bultas J, Aschermann M. Comparison of early diastolic mitral annular velocity and flow propagation velocity in detection of mild to moderate left ventricular diastolic dysfunction. *Eur J Echocardiogr* 2004; **5**: 196–204.

43. Bukachi F, Waldenström A, Mörner S, *et al.* Age dependency in the timing of mitral annular motion in relation to ventricular filling in healthy subjects: Umea General Population Heart Study. *Eur J Echocardiogr* 2008; **9**: 522–9.

44. Fukuta H, Little WC. Diagnosis of diastolic heart failure. *Curr Cardiol Rep* 2007; **9**: 224–8.

45. Arques S, Roux E, Luccioni R. Current clinical applications of spectral tissue Doppler echocardiography (E/E' ratio) as a noninvasive surrogate for left ventricular diastolic pressures in the diagnosis of heart failure with preserved left ventricular systolic function. *Cardiovasc Ultrasound* 2007; **5**: 16.

46. Zile MR, Lewinter MM. Left ventricular end-diastolic volume is normal in patients with heart failure and a normal ejection fraction: a renewed consensus in diastolic heart failure. *J Am Coll Cardiol* 2007; **49**: 982–5.

47. Tei C, Ling LH, Hodge DO, *et al.* New index of combined systolic and diastolic myocardial performance: a simple and reproducible measure of cardiac function: a study in normals and dilated cardiomyopathy. *J Cardiol* 1995; **26**: 357–66.

48. Guarracino F, Lapolla F, Danella A, *et al.* Reduced compliance of left ventricle. *Minerva Anestesiol* 2004; **70**: 225–8.

49. Voon WC, Su HM, Yen HW, *et al.* Validation of isovolumic relaxation flow propagation velocity as an index of ventricular relaxation. *Ultrasound Med Biol* 2007; **33**: 1098–103.

The right ventricle

Patrick Wouters

Introduction

As the role of the right ventricle (RV) in the maintenance of circulatory homeostasis has become recognized, clinical and scientific interest in the diagnosis,
pathophysiology, and treatment of RV failure has
expanded. RV failure has an independent effect on
clinical outcome in various cardiopulmonary disease
states including primary pulmonary hypertension,
advanced heart failure, and idiopathic dilated cardiomyopathy [1–5]. RV dysfunction also occurs frequently in patients with low output syndrome after
cardiac surgery and has a higher mortality than LV
failure in the perioperative setting [6–8].

The unique ability of transesophageal echocardiography (TEE) to discriminate right from left heart
failure and rapidly to detect life-threatening conditions where RV dysfunction predominates, for example in acute pulmonary hypertension and pulmonary
embolus, makes it a powerful diagnostic and monitoring tool in the perioperative setting. The echocardiographer should understand the important differences
in anatomy, function, and pathophysiology between
the left and right ventricle.

Anatomy

The shape of the RV is more complex than that of the
left ventricle (LV) and does not conform to any simple
geometrical model. In cross-section, the normal RV is
crescent-shaped, whereas the LV is circular. The interventricular septum (IVS) bows convex towards the RV
free wall. In a longitudinal section, the RV resembles a
triangle with its base at the tricuspid valve (Fig. 10.1).
The RV consists of an inflow part (sinus) and an outflow part (conus), with different embryological origins
and distinct anatomical and functional characteristics
(Fig. 10.2). The inflow part lies posteroinferiorly and
has a heavily trabeculated apical region (trabeculae
carnae). The outflow part is positioned anterosuperiorly and is smooth-walled. The distinct chambers are
anatomically separated by a semicircular arch of four

muscle bundles: the parietal band, the infundibular
septum, the septal band, and the moderator band. The
superior part of this arch composes the crista supraventricularis, which separates the atrioventricular valve
from the semilunar valve. The inferior part, termed
the trabecula septomarginalis, is continuous with the
moderator band which joins the base of the anterior
papillary muscle.

The following characteristics are unique to RV
morphology and are used to distinguish it from LV
morphology in complex congenital heart diseases:

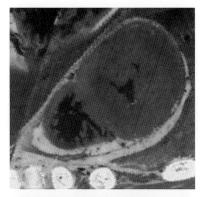
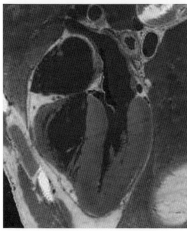

Figure 10.1. Right
ventricle in short-
and long-axis cross-
section. Note the
relative thickness of
the LV wall compared
to that of the RV.

163

Core Topics in Transesophageal Echocardiography, ed. Robert Feneck, John Kneeshaw, and Marco Ranucci.
Published by Cambridge University Press. © Cambridge University Press 2010.

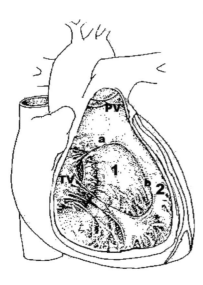

Figure 10.2. The right ventricular inflow (1, sinus) and outflow (2, conus) tracts. a, crista supraventricularis; b, trabecula septomarginalis; PV, pulmonary valve; TV, tricuspid valve.

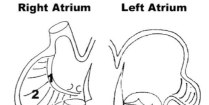

Figure 10.3. In the right atrium, a posterior smooth-walled part where the superior and inferior caval vein enter (1) is differentiated from the trabeculated anterolateral part, lined by the pectinate muscles that extend into the atrial appendage (2). The appendage of the right atrium is short and broad, while the left atrial appendage is long and narrow.

1. separation of the atrioventricular valve from the semilunar valve
2. the presence of abundant trabeculations in the apex
3. the presence of a septal band
4. a chordal insertion at the interventricular septum (IVS)
5. a more apical insertion of the atrioventricular valve

The normal RV contains only one-fifth to one-sixth the muscle mass of the LV, and its wall thickness is about half that of the LV (Fig. 10.1). The superficial layers of the RV sinus are continuous with those of the LV, and the deeper muscle bundles are continuous with the interventricular septum. The RV is predominantly supplied by branches of the right coronary artery, except for the anteroseptal wall and a small part of the mid and distal anterior free wall, which also receive blood from the left anterior descending coronary artery.

The right atrium (RA) is located above and medially from the RV. It consists of a posterior smooth-walled part where the superior and inferior caval vein enter, and a trabeculated anterolateral part, lined by the pectinate muscles that extend into the atrial appendage. The crista terminalis separates the trabeculated part from the smooth area. The RA is differentiated from the left atrium (LA) morphologically by the structure of its atrial appendage. The appendage of the right atrium is short and broad, whereas the left atrial appendage is long and narrow (Fig. 10.3). The Eustachian valve (valve of the inferior vena cava), the

Thebesian valve (valve of the coronary sinus), and the Chiari network (vestige of the right valve of the sinus venosus) are embryological remnants only found in a morphologic right atrium.

The tricuspid valve (TV) is always part of the right ventricle, and the bileaflet mitral valve is always part of the left ventricle.

2D visualization of the RV with TEE

Problems and artifacts

When imaging the heart from the esophagus, the anteriorly located RV is seen in the far field of the sector scan, where the resolution of ultrasound is lowest. Artifacts generated from interposed structures such as calcifications or valve prostheses can significantly degrade the RV image.

The long- and short-axis views of the RV are defined by the corresponding views of the LV, but these two standard echocardiographic imaging planes (mid-esophageal [ME] four-chamber and transgastric [TG] short-axis) often transect the RV in an oblique way. Coarse trabeculations, and particularly the moderator band, can easily be confused with an intraventricular thrombus (Fig. 10.4; Video 10.1). The use of different scanning angles, with attention to motion and thickening of such structures, is helpful in the differential diagnosis. Individual variations in the relative position of the heart with regard to the esophagus, or abnormal structures and anatomical configurations (e.g. a dilated ascending aorta, ventricular aneurysm, or hiatus hernia), may also prohibit optimal imaging of the RV with standard views. Discrete probe manipulations and the proper use of the multiplane capacity of TEE are often necessary to fully visualize the RV.

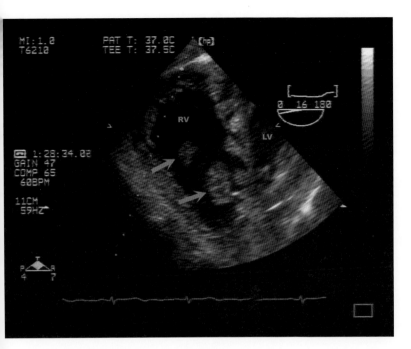

Figure 10.4. Coarse trabeculations and the moderator band mimicking intraventricular thrombus in the RV.

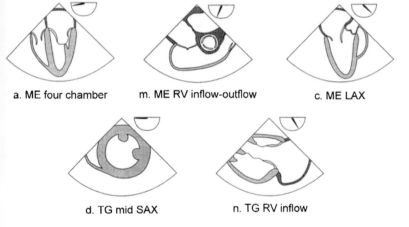

a. ME four chamber   m. ME RV inflow-outflow   c. ME LAX

d. TG mid SAX   n. TG RV inflow

Figure 10.5. Standard TEE views of the RV.

RV imaging planes

Given its complex anatomy, the RV should be studied from different viewing angles. The nomenclature and illustrations used here conform to the ASE/SCA guidelines [9]. Unclassified views will be illustrated separately. For the RV there are five classified views (Fig. 10.5). Starting with the ME four-chamber view, the RA, the interatrial septum (IAS), the TV (septal and anterior leaflets), the basal and apical segments of the RV, and the IVS are seen. Advancing the probe slightly deeper from this position shows the coronary sinus and the posterior TV leaflet. Particularly useful for examining the RV is the ME RV inflow–outflow view, obtained by clockwise rotation of the multiplane angle to 60–90°. This is also termed the "wrap around" view, since it appears to have the RA, RV, and pulmonary artery (PA) wrapped around the aortic valve (AV) and left atrium. It shows the posterior leaflet of the TV, the RV inferior free wall, the RV outflow tract, and the pulmonary valve (PV). The ME long-axis view is obtained with further rotation (120–140°) and shows a small portion of the RV outflow tract (RVOT)

165

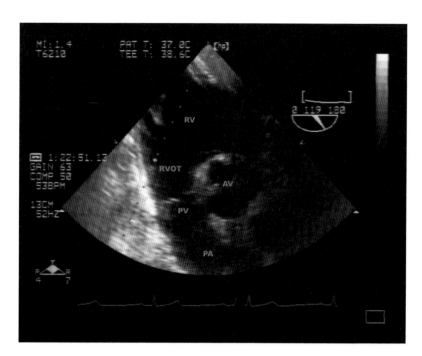

Figure 10.6. The non-standard TG RV outflow view shows the RV inflow and outflow tracts, the pulmonary valve, and the pulmonary artery. AV, aortic valve; PA, pulmonary artery; PV, pulmonary valve; RV, right ventricle; RVOT, right ventricular outflow tract.

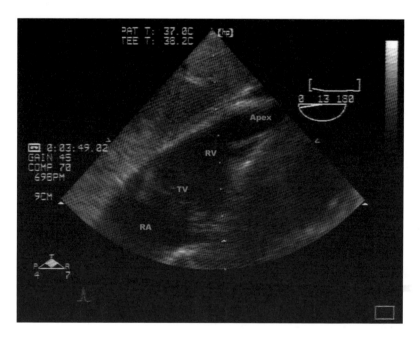

Figure 10.7. The non-standard deep TG RV apical view. RA, right atrium; RV, right ventricle; TV, tricuspid valve.

with a short-axis view of the PV lying anterior to the AV (Video 10.2).

When rotating the sector scan back to 0° and advancing the probe into the stomach, the TG mid short-axis view shows the typical crescent shape of the RV with the convex position of the IVS. When turning the probe to the right and rotating the multiplane sector to 90° a TG RV inflow view is obtained, revealing a long axis of the RV (the same process as for obtaining a TG long-axis view of the LV). It shows the RA and the TV (anterior and posterior leaflets), and is useful for examining the TV subvalvular apparatus and the anterior and inferior part of the RV free wall (Videos 10.3, 10.4). With rotation to 110–140° the

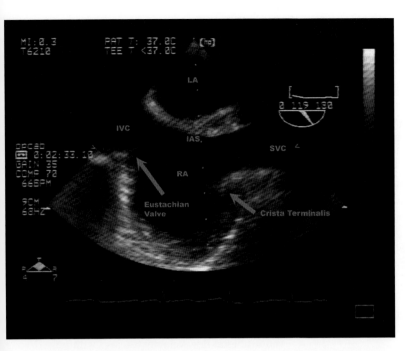

Figure 10.8. Bicaval view, showing the left (LA) and right (RA) atria, inferior (IVC) and superior (SVC) venae cavae, and inter-atrial septum (IAS).

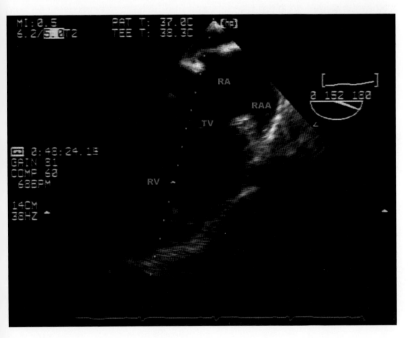

Figure 10.9. The modified RV long-axis view. RA, right atrium; RAA, right atrial appendage; RV, right ventricle; TV, tri-cuspid valve.

non-standard TG RV outflow view shows the inflow and outflow parts of the RV, and clockwise turning of the shaft allows complete inspection of the RV apex (Fig. 10.6). Finally the non-standard deep TG RV apical view (Fig. 10.7) is obtained by advancing the probe deep into the stomach with maximal anteflexion of the tip and turning it to the right. It is sometimes necessary to reduce the transducer frequency to allow better ultrasound penetration. This view is helpful when echogenic structures are interposed between the esophagus and the RV, and it brings the apex into the near field.

Right atrium

To inspect the right atrium and measure its dimensions, the ME four-chamber view and the bicaval view obtained in the upper mid-esophageal position at a 90° multiplane angle are complementary views that show the interatrial septum and fossa ovalis. The latter demonstrates the crista terminalis to the right of the screen (at the junction with the superior vena cava), and the Eustachian valve on the left side of the screen (at the junction with the inferior vena cava) (Fig. 10.8; Videos 10.5, 10.6). Turning the probe in a clockwise fashion shows the right branch of the PA in short axis. A view that is not classified but particularly helpful to inspect the right atrium and right atrial appendage is the modified RV long-axis view, obtained by further rotation to 160° (Fig. 10.9).

Doppler interrogation of the RV with TEE

For a thorough RV examination, the anatomic information obtained by imaging should be complemented by physiologic information obtained from interrogation with color, pulsed-wave, and continuous-wave Doppler.

Superposition of the **color Doppler imaging** mode on the 2D views allows for global inspection and semi-quantitative evaluation of abnormal flow velocities and direction. Non-laminar jet flows are always abnormal in the low-pressure right system except for a discrete red-colored systolic jet of tricuspid regurgitation

that is present in about 85% of the population. In the ME four-chamber view, attention is focused on any abnormal passage of blood over an interatrial and interventricular septum and the presence of severe tricuspid regurgitation. The bicaval view allows a more complete view of the interatrial septum in search of a patent foramen ovale with color Doppler, but contrast injection is ultimately required to definitely exclude this diagnosis.

Pulsed-wave Doppler is used to make quantitative measurements of lower blood velocities. Pulsed Doppler interrogation of diastolic tricuspid inflow is performed in a ME four-chamber view with the sample gate positioned at the tip of the leaflets. It shows an early (E) and late atrial (A) wave in normal sinus rhythm with slightly lower values than those reported for the mitral valve [10]. In the bicaval view, the sample gate can be positioned over an IAS defect to assess the direction of shunt flow (left-to-right or right-to-left shunt).

Multiplane TEE is also well suited to study hepatic venous blood flow velocity tracings with pulsed-wave Doppler. Adequate velocity signals can be obtained from the right and middle hepatic veins using 66° and 75° multiplane angles in nearly all patients [11]. Typical for the hepatic flow pattern is the presence of early diastolic flow reversal, which is not present in the normal pulmonary venous left-sided correlate. It may reflect more extensive diastolic recoil of the tricuspid annular ring as compared to the mitral annular ring (Fig. 10.10).

Continuous-wave Doppler plays an important role in the study of pathological conditions of the RV

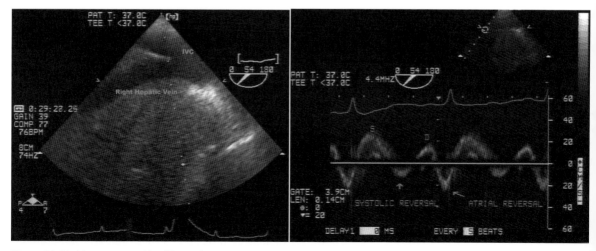

Figure 10.10. Hepatic venous blood flow velocity tracings with pulsed-wave Doppler.

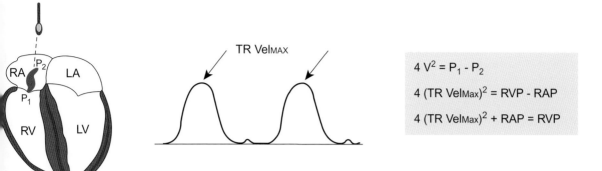

Figure 10.11. Calculation of RV systolic pressure from a regurgitant jet across the tricuspid valve.

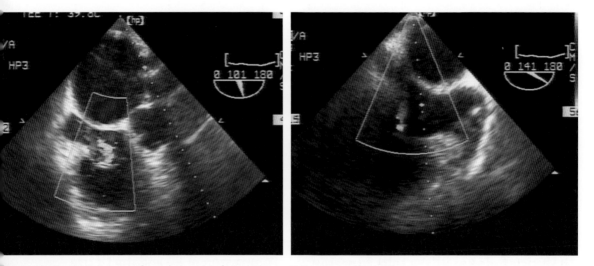

Figure 10.12. Alternative views for exploring a jet of tricuspid regurgitation. See text for details.

and pulmonary circulation. A crucial application is the measurement of RV pressures from the velocity signal of a tricuspid regurgitant (TR) jet. The peak velocity of a TR jet corresponds to the peak instantaneous pressure gradient between the RV and the RA. Summation of this pressure gradient with RA pressure provides an accurate estimation of peak RV pressures (Fig. 10.11). When no other mechanical obstructions within or distal to the RV outflow tract are present, this pressure corresponds with PA systolic pressure.

In addition, diastolic pulmonary artery pressure can be estimated with TR velocity analysis. Assuming that RV and PA pressures are equal immediately before the start of ejection (= isovolumic contraction), the TR velocity timed precisely to that moment

corresponds to diastolic PA pressure in the same way as peak systolic TR velocity corresponds to peak PA pressure [12].

The measurement of RV pressures should always be part of a routine TEE examination. Even when a PA catheter is available, it is worthwhile to practice this technique and gain confidence for its application in patients without such invasive catheters. In the ME four-chamber view, the TR jet may not be parallel to the insonating Doppler scan line, and complementary views are often necessary to avoid underestimating RV pressures. For example, starting from a bicaval view, turning the shaft counterclockwise and bringing the multiplane angle back from 90° to 70° until the TV appears on the lower left side of the screen often allows a better alignment with the TR jet. Alternatively, a

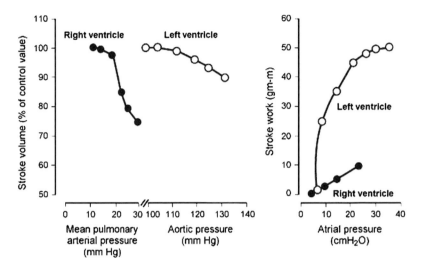

Figure 10.13. Comparison of right and left ventricular response to increasing filling (atrial pressure) and afterload (aortic and pulmonary artery pressure). Reproduced with permission from *Braunwald Heart Disease*, 5th edn. Philadelphia, PA: Saunders, 1997.

modified RV long-axis view or modified deep TG apical view should be explored (Fig. 10.12). Pressure measurements should be made from whichever window yields the highest velocity signal.

When an interventricular septal defect is present, whether as a congenital lesion or as a complication of an acute myocardial infarction, RV pressure can be estimated with continuous-wave Doppler interrogation of the left-to-right shunt. Substracting the peak instantaneous pressure gradient (apply modified Bernoulli to peak transseptal flow velocity) from LV peak systolic pressure (substituted by systolic blood pressure) provides RV systolic pressure.

Analysis of global RV systolic function

Phylogenetically, the right ventricle is a relative newcomer, dating back only 200 million years to the evolution of mammals, and served as an adaptation to air-breathing and land-living. Its function is to propel deoxygenated blood through a low-impedance pulmonary circulation with a resistance of only one-tenth that of the systemic circulation. As a consequence, the normal adult RV is a thin-walled, very compliant structure that is able to accommodate large blood volumes with a minimal rise of ventricular pressure. Its pumping action has been compared to that of a bellows working in series with a low-pressure circuit. Compared to the LV, the RV is less responsive to increased preload and is particularly sensitive to increased afterload (Fig. 10.13).

A number of techniques have been used to assess RV systolic function. These are shown in Table 10.1, and discussed below.

Table 10.1. Methods of assessing sysytolic right ventricular function

Comparison of RV and LV size
Abnormalities of intraventricular septum
Measurements of RV dimensions
Tricuspid annular plane systolic excursion (TAPSE)
The total ejection isovolume (TEI) index
Intraventricular pressure development (RV dP/dt_{max})
Tissue Doppler imaging
RV free-wall longitudinal motion

Comparison of RV and the LV size

The primary response of the RV to any hemodynamic disturbance, be it an inappropriate loading condition or a primary contractile failure, is dilation. Echocardiography is particularly suited to detect such a volume increase qualitatively by comparing the relative sizes of the RV and the LV in an ME four-chamber view. In normal conditions the RV occupies less than 60% of the LV area. Mild enlargement exists when RV area is 60–100% of the LV area, and severe enlargement is present when RV area exceeds LV area. With dilation, the RV also changes its shape from triangular to globular in the ME four-chamber view. In normal conditions, the RV long axis extends to only two-thirds the length of the LV, and the apex of the heart is always formed by the LV. Formation of the apex by the RV rather than the LV is an additional sign of severe volume increase. In the TG short-axis view the septal curvature, which normally is convex towards the crescent-shaped

RV cavity, flattens and the septum progressively deviates towards the LV, producing an elliptical or circular short-axis shape of the RV cavity (Videos 10.7, 10.8).

Abnormalities of the interventricular septum

Abnormalities in the shape and motion of the IVS reflect the altered pressure differences between the LV and RV. Analysis of the timing of these abnormalities with regard to the cardiac cycle may help to differentiate between pressure and volume overload of the RV. The normal IVS is curved towards the RV throughout the entire cardiac cycle. It moves towards the RV in diastole and towards the LV in systole. With volume overload, the IVS shows diastolic flattening and may even move towards the LV in end-diastole. This paradoxical diastolic motion is due to higher filling pressures in the RV. During early systole, restoration of the pressure differences results in a transient motion towards the RV.

With pressure overload, the IVS is flat throughout the entire cardiac cycle with a maximal distortion from end-systole to early diastole. In patients with chronic pressure overload and RV hypertrophy, the septum may even become convex towards the LV and move towards the RV in systole.

The interatrial septum normally is flat or curved towards the right atrium. If the IAS is curved towards

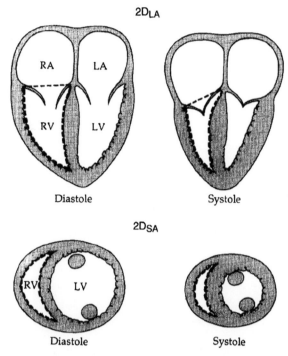

Figure 10.14. Quantitative measurements of RV dimensions in the long and short axis.

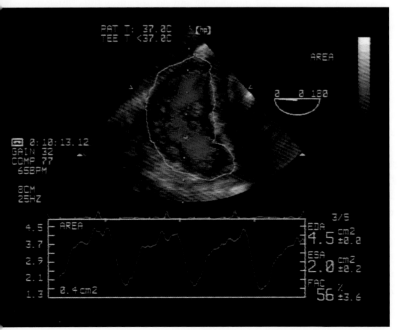

Figure 10.15. Automatic RV border detection with TEE in the transgastric view. End-systolic and end-diastolic areas, and fractional area of change, are shown.

171

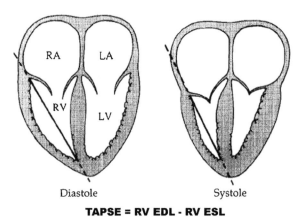

Diastole   Systole

TAPSE = RV EDL - RV ESL
RV EDL

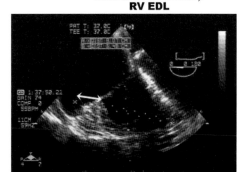

Figure 10.16. Calculation of tricuspid annular plane systolic excursion (TAPSE). EDL, end-disatolic length; ESL, end-systolic length.

the LA, it indicates that RA pressures exceed those of the LA, which is a common sign for imminent RV dysfunction in cardiac surgery.

Measurements of RV dimensions

These qualitative TEE approaches are simple and rapid techniques to detect abnormal RV performance and thus prompt a more detailed analysis and a search for a cause. Quantitative measurements of RV dimensions and areas are performed in the TG short-axis and ME four-chamber views (Fig. 10.14). By analogy with the LV, fractional shortening (100 × (EDD – ESD)/EDD) and fractional area change (FAC) (100 × (EDA – ESA)/EDA) can be calculated with standard formulae [13]. Automatic border detection with TEE even provides online RV cross-sectional areas, and close agreement between RV stroke volume and stroke area (max RV area – min RV area) in the ME four-chamber view has been reported with this technique [14] (Fig. 10.15). However, the standard views often transect the RV in

an oblique fashion, and the endocardial border of the RV may be difficult to trace due to trabeculations and poor image resolution. Contrast echocardiography significantly improves endocardial border visualization with TTE [15,16], but this is not routine practice in the operating room or ICU today.

Tricuspid annular plane systolic excursion (TAPSE)

Tricuspid annular plane systolic excursion corresponds to wall shortening of the RV free wall along its long axis. It quantifies the distance traveled by the lateral TV annulus from the base towards the apex during ejection. This measurement is straightforward and overcomes the limitations of geometric assumptions for volume calculations as well as the difficulty of tracing endocardial edges (Fig. 10.16). For the normal RV the total systolic excursion of the tricuspid annular plane is about 2.5 cm during spontaneous ventilation; this corresponds to a long-axis FS of about 30%. As long as 25 years ago, this measurement was shown to correlate well with angiographically determined RV ejection fraction [17]. The measurements mentioned above only consider the size and function of the sinus, i.e. the inflow part of the RV. While this is the largest and most dynamic part, approximately 20% of the RV is missed or neglected by omitting the conus or outflow part [18].

Ejection fraction and its surrogate variables are load-dependent and do not allow the clinician to distinguish between reduced contractile performance (e.g. ischemic or postischemic dysfunction) and inappropriate loading conditions (e.g. pulmonary hypertension) as possible causes of RV dysfunction. Such a differential diagnosis is crucial, however, if we are to select the proper therapy both for chronic and for acute RV failure, and it is generally acknowledged that a load-independent index of contractile performance is required. Experimental studies have shown that the load-independent indices for LV contractile performance such as preload recruitable stroke work (PRSW) and end-systolic pressure–volume relationship (ESPVR) are also applicable to the RV [19]. However, although perhaps feasible in clinical practice [20], such an analysis is too cumbersome and relies particularly on accurate volume estimation. Three-dimensional online echocardiography may solve this problem in the near future [21]. Alternatively, specific non-volumetric methods based on the use of 2D echocardiography and Doppler have been further developed.

Total ejection isovolume (TEI) index

The total ejection isovolume index or myocardial performance index, first described by Tei and coworkers in 1995, is a Doppler derived measurement combining systolic and diastolic time intervals as a parameter of global ventricular function. It is calculated as the sum of isovolumic contraction and relaxation time divided by ejection time [22] from blood velocity measurements in the pulmonary artery and tricuspid valve (Fig. 10.17). This index has been studied extensively and has been shown to correlate with symptoms and survival in a variety of disease states including primary pulmonary hypertension and amyloidosis [22,23] and in patients undergoing pulmonary thrombendarterectomy [24]. However, other investigators have reported load dependency of this index in the LV [25] and RV [26]. In addition, it has been demonstrated that the TEI index initially decreases with RV infarction but pseudonormalizes when RV infarctions become more extensive [27]. This complicates the interpretation of the index considerably, and its incremental value (as compared to ejection fraction) in acute perioperative settings remains to be established.

Intraventricular pressure development (RV dP/dt_{max})

The maximum rate of intraventricular pressure development (RV dP/dt_{max}), traditionally measured with intraventricular manometers, is one of the most popular and frequently used indices of ventricular performance in experimental settings, even though it is not load-independent either [28]. With echocardiography, RV dP/dt can be determined non-invasively with continuous-wave Doppler of the tricuspid regurgitant velocity. The maximum value of the first derivative of this velocity is estimated by measuring the time needed to achieve an increase from 0 to 2 m/s and corresponds to dP/dt_{max} [29]. At present, this measurement is not routinely used, probably because it is less accurate with increased atrial pressures [30]. Some of its limitations seem to be overcome by calculating the ratio of dP/dt to maximal pressure development dP/dt[31]. Although at this stage such measurements need significant processing, they may offer future potential for use with TEE.

Tissue velocity, strain, and strain rate

Tissue Doppler imaging and 2D strain analysis are increasingly being used to study RV myocardial motion and deformation. Analogous to the study of mitral annular descent as an index of LV function, systolic tricuspid annular velocity (S$_m$) has been reported to correlate with RV contractile performance [32] and is a significant independent predictor of survival in patients with symptomatic heart failure [33]. With color Doppler imaging it was shown that the RV has higher long-axis regional velocities, a greater excursion of its lateral atrioventricular valve ring, and reduced circumferential shortening velocities when compared to the left ventricle. RV longitudinal shortening is dominant over short-axis function in healthy young subjects, but this relationship changes with aging [34]. Ejection indices, including S$_m$ and maximum strain rate, are however also affected by changes in afterload.

RV isovolumic acceleration (IVA)

Recent measurements of isovolumic acceleration of RV free-wall longitudinal motion with tissue Doppler have demonstrated that it is a relatively load-independent index of RV contractility [35]. Although the precise physiological correlate of this index is not clear yet, clinical studies have suggested its potential in patients with repaired transposition of the great arteries [36]. It is important to note, however, that for Doppler-based techniques the use of the correct incident angle is crucial, and this is a significant limitation for TEE: the insonating angle is always oblique to the direction of motion of the RV annular ring and RV free wall.

The diversity of indices and approaches specifically developed to study RV function suggests that the ideal method is not yet available. For the perioperative

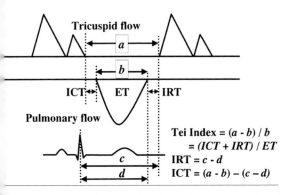

Figure 10.17. Calculation of the TEI (total ejection isovolume) index. ICT, isovolumic contraction time; ET, ejection time; IRT, isovolumic relaxation time.

clinician, however, the ongoing discussion on the use of a load-independent index of RV contractile performance may seem somewhat abstract, and a pragmatic approach can be much more relevant to evaluate the RV in acute heart failure. This consists of the following;

1. determination of RV size (semi-quantitative / quantitative)
2. assessment of RV pressure (TR jet and modified Bernoulli equation)
3. timing of septal displacement (shape and position of IVS and IAS)
4. measurement of ejection performance (FAC, FS, TAPSE)
5. interrogation of PA flow profile and PA pressure gradient.

The degree and direction of changes in these variables will provide a clue to the type of RV pathology (see *Acute and chronic RV dysfunction*, below).

Regional RV function

Wall motion and myocardial thickening may be more difficult to assess in the RV than in the LV. The RV wall is thinner and more irregular, the contractile amplitude is lower, and the contraction pattern is asynchronous [18]. Subtle regional dysfunction is therefore more difficult to diagnose. According to current guidelines on intraoperative TEE, it requires either

akinesia or dyskinesia to establish a clear diagnosis of regional dysfunction [9]. There is no standard topographic approach to describe regional RV function but, as for the LV, the free wall of the RV can be divided into basal, mid-, and apical segments. Reference to anterior and inferior segments and the RVOT may also be used to localize specific regions of the RV wall. Regional function of the IVS is described using the segmental model for the LV.

Quantitative assessment of regional RV function has been attempted using color kinesis, which provides regional information on the magnitude and timing of cardiac wall motion [37]. However, this technique is affected by translation and rotation of the heart and depends particularly on image quality and gain settings – a problem for TEE, where the RV is in the far field of the sector. Further studies are necessary to examine its potential. Strain rate imaging has also been proposed to analyze regional RV function. It provides excellent time resolution but its spatial resolution is rather low for the thin-walled RV, and clinical validation studies are needed [38]. Problems associated with an inappropriate insonating angle with Doppler techniques currently limit their applicability with TEE.

Diastolic RV function

Techniques to examine RV diastolic performance are based primarily on those developed to study LV diastolic function. Diastolic RV dysfunction can present with the same relative changes in E- and A-wave

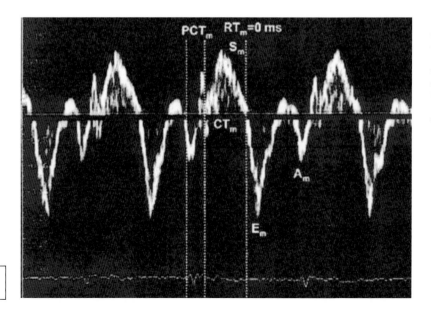

Figure 10.18. Tissue Doppler image of motion of the atrioventricular valve annular ring. A_m, diastolic annular motion due to atrial contraction; CT contraction time (systole); E_m, diastolic annular motion due to diastasis; PCT presystolic contraction time; RT, systolic relaxation time; S_m, systolic tricuspid annular velocity.

velocities, E/A wave ratios, and deceleration time as for transmitral inflow with impairment of LV relaxation and compliance [39]. Atrioventricular valve inflow characteristics not only depend on diastolic function but are influenced by loading conditions as well. The use of tissue Doppler to interrogate diastolic motion of the atrioventricular valve annular ring partially overcomes this limitation and may reveal more robust indicators of diastolic performance (Fig. 10.18) [40,41].

Additional information on systolic and diastolic function of the RV can be obtained by examining the hepatic flow pattern with TEE [42]. In general, systolic and diastolic forward flow and late diastolic flow reversal patterns reflect the inflow dynamics of the RA and resemble those observed in the pulmonary veins for the LV. The ratio of the total hepatic venous reverse flow integral to total forward flow integral increases with diastolic dysfunction [43]. In general, hepatic flow patterns are significantly affected by mechanical ventilation and changes in intra-abdominal pressure. The presence of tricuspid regurgitation also complicates interpretation of the hepatic flow signal with regard to diastolic RV performance.

The appearance of a late diastolic forward flow signal in the PA, coinciding with atrial contraction, has been reported to indicate restrictive RV filling in patients with tetralogy of Fallot [44,45].

Acute and chronic RV dysfunction

From a physiologic perspective, disorders of the right-sided circulation can be classified as diseases resulting in pressure overload, diseases resulting in volume overload, and diseases that interfere primarily with RV myocardial systolic and/or diastolic function. However, there is frequent overlap between these categories.

Acute pressure overload due to pulmonary hypertension or pulmonary embolus is an important cause of perioperative RV dysfunction. The most reliable TEE sign is an increased ratio of R/L end-diastolic area exceeding 0.6 [46]. In the early stage of disease, Doppler interrogation of the tricuspid regurgitant jet shows elevated RV pressures, but these may again decrease as RV function and cardiac output start to decline. There is almost always a considerable degree of tricuspid regurgitation. The PA velocity profile shows a shorter acceleration time (< 90 ms), the ratio of acceleration time to RV ejection time (RVET)

decreases (< 0.45), and the signal becomes triangular in shape. With severe pulmonary hypertension, a typical mid-systolic notch is seen (Fig. 10.19). Indirect signs of elevated right-sided pressures should also be looked for: an enlarged diameter of the coronary sinus (diameter > 1 cm), a flattened IVS with paradoxical motion, and an IAS that is curved towards the left atrium. It is particularly difficult to quantify RV function in the setting of pressure overload, since most indices of cardiac performance are load-dependent. With acute increases of afterload, the untrained RV is globally hypokinetic and is rarely able to generate mean pressures higher than 40 mmHg.

In pulmonary embolism, TEE inspection of the inferior vena cava (IVC), RA, and RV may show thrombi in transit or central emboli in the PA. Fresh thrombi usually have a protruding and elongated appearance. For many of the RV findings to be apparent, pulmonary emboli must produce an obstruction of ≥ 25% of the pulmonary vascular bed [47].

Chronic pressure overload due to pulmonary valve stenosis, chronic pulmonary hypertension, or chronic thromboembolic disease of the PA is associated with RV hypertrophy. TEE shows prominent trabeculations and the RV free-wall thickness exceeds 5 mm. Persistent RV pressure increases will eventually shift the center of the heart to the RV. The RV assumes a circular shape and the LV appears ellipsoid. The septum is concave on the right side and shows paradoxical motion throughout the cardiac cycle. Interrogation of the tricuspid regurgitant jet invariably shows high velocities indicative of elevated intra-cavity RV pressures.

Acute volume overload, when it occurs as an isolated defect, is better tolerated by the RV. When acute RV dysfunction does develop, it is mostly because the

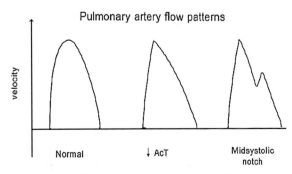

Figure 10.19. The pulmonary artery velocity profile, showing a shorter acceleration time (AcT) and typical mid-systolic notch in severe pulmonary hypertension.

causal event also induces a variable degree of pressure overload or LV failure. A typical example is an acute interventricular septal defect complicating myocardial infarction. TEE shows an enlarged RV with dynamic ejection parameters and an IVS that is flat and moving towards the LV at end-diastole.

Chronic volume overload occurs with persistent left-to-right shunts (e.g. atrial septal defect) and severe pulmonary or tricuspid valve regurgitation. Cardinal features of isolated volume overload are an increased ratio of RV to LV area and diastolic paradoxical IVS motion. Other TEE signs depend on the effect of chronic volume overload on the pulmonary vasculature and RV contractile performance. Isolated volume overload may be tolerated clinically for many years and present as an unexpected finding in the operating room.

RV ischemia is documented in nearly 50% of patients with acute inferoposterior myocardial infarction and is associated with a significantly increased early in-hospital morbidity and mortality [48,49]. The features of increased RV volume can be less reliable, depending on the degree of LV involvement in the ischemic process. Backward failure of the LV may also induce increased RV afterload, and the resultant effect on RV pressures is variable. FAC and TAPSE have been used to describe RV systolic functional decline in patients suffering acute RV infarction, and TAPSE lower than 1 cm was found to have a positive predictive value of 75%. In the setting of cardiac surgery, global dysfunction of the RV due to ischemia is a frequent problem: the right coronary artery is very susceptible to air emboli, and retrograde cardioplegia techniques may leave the RV poorly protected [50].

Cardiac tamponade

External compression of the RA or RV are particularly relevant in cardiac surgery. Intraoperatively, the retractors used during harvesting of the internal mammary arteries may directly compress the RV. Upon sternal closure, distended lungs may compromise RV function by reducing preload and increasing afterload. TEE shows reduced RV dimensions and enlarged cava veins. Tricuspid inflow velocities are typically lower and hepatic vein flow shows pronounced respiratory variation. In the postoperative setting, TEE is the preferred technique to detect cardiac tamponade, and it may show the compressive effect of localized blood collections around the RA and/or RV (Fig. 10.20).

RV tumors and systemic diseases

Tumors on the right side of the heart are rare, and occur more frequently in the atrium than in the ventricle. RA tumors are often benign unless they invade from outside (e.g. from renal carcinoma entering via the IVC), whereas RV tumors are frequently malignant. Echocardiographic signs of malignancy are pericardial effusions,

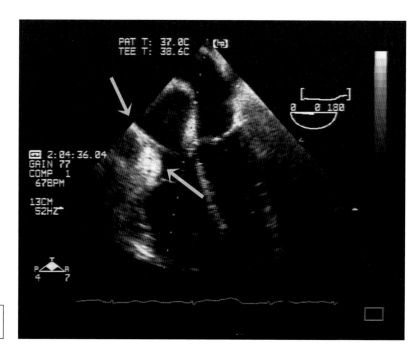

Figure 10.20. Arrows indicating compression of the RA and RV due to localized blood collections.

rregularity of the mass, and invasion. TEE can be useful to guide transvenous cardiac biopsy [51].

Systemic diseases such as sarcoidosis and amyloidosis cause restrictive cardiomyopathy and ventricular hypertrophy, which may also involve the RV. Carcinoid disease affects the heart in about 50% of patients and almost exclusively concerns the RV, with progressive destruction of the right-sided cardiac valves [52].

References

1. D'Alonzo GE, Barst RJ, Ayres SM, *et al.* Survival in patients with primary pulmonary hypertension. Results from a national prospective registry. *Ann Intern Med* 1991; **115**: 343–9.

2. Monchi M, Bellenfant F, Cariou A, *et al.* Early predictive factors of survival in the acute respiratory distress syndrome. A multivariate analysis. *Am J Respir Crit Care Med* 1998; **158**: 1076–81.

3. Gavazzi A, Berzuini C, Campana C, *et al.* Value of right ventricular ejection fraction in predicting short-term prognosis of patients with severe chronic heart failure. *J Heart Lung Transplant* 1997; **16**: 774–85.

4. Baker BJ, Wilen MM, Boyd CM, Dinh H, Franciosa JA. Relation of right ventricular ejection fraction to exercise capacity in chronic left ventricular failure. *Am J Cardiol* 1984; **54**: 596–9.

5. Ghio S, Gavazzi A, Campana C, *et al.* Independent and additive prognostic value of right ventricular systolic function and pulmonary artery pressure in patients with chronic heart failure. *J Am Coll Cardiol* 2001; **37**: 183–8.

6. Davila-Roman VG, Waggoner AD, Hopkins WE, Barzilai B. Right ventricular dysfunction in low output syndrome after cardiac operations: assessment by transesophageal echocardiography. *Ann Thorac Surg* 1995; **60**: 1081–6.

7. Reichert CL, Visser CA, van den Brink RB, *et al.* Prognostic value of biventricular function in hypotensive patients after cardiac surgery as assessed by transesophageal echocardiography. *J Cardiothorac Vasc Anesth* 1992; **6**: 429–32.

8. Maslow AD, Regan MM, Panzica P, *et al.* Precardiopulmonary bypass right ventricular function is associated with poor outcome after coronary artery bypass grafting in patients with severe left ventricular systolic dysfunction. *Anesth Analg* 2002; **95**: 1507–18.

9. Shanewise JS, Cheung AT, Aronson S, *et al.* ASE/SCA guidelines for performing a comprehensive intraoperative multiplane transesophageal echocardiography examination: recommendations of the ASE Council for intraoperative echocardiography and the SCA Task Force for certification in perioperative transesophageal echocardiography. *Anesth Analg* 1999; **89**: 870–84.

10. Yu CM, Sanderson JE, Chan S, *et al.* Right ventricular diastolic dysfunction in heart failure. *Circulation* 1996; **93**: 1509–14.

11. Meierhenric R, Gauss A, Georgieff M, Schutz W. Use of multi-plane transoesophageal echocardiography in visualization of the main hepatic veins and acquisition of Doppler sonography curves. Comparison with the transabdominal approach. *Br J Anaesth* 2001; **87**: 711–17.

12. Lanzarini L, Fontana A, Lucca E, Campana C, Klersy C. Noninvasive estimation of both systolic and diastolic pulmonary artery pressure from Doppler analysis of tricuspid regurgitant velocity spectrum in patients with chronic heart failure. *Am Heart J* 2002; **144**: 1087–94.

13. Rafferty T, Durkin M, Harris S, *et al.* Transesophageal two-dimensional echocardiographic analysis of right ventricular systolic performance indices during coronary artery bypass grafting. *J Cardiothorac Vasc Anesth* 1993; **7**: 160–6.

14. Ochiai Y, Morita S, Tanoue Y, *et al.* Use of transesophageal echocardiography for postoperative evaluation of right ventricular function. *Ann Thorac Surg* 1999; **67**: 146–52.

15. Tokgozoglu SL, Caner B, Kabakci G, Kes S. Measurement of right ventricular ejection fraction by contrast echocardiography. *Int J Cardiol* 1997; **59**: 71–4.

16. van den Bosch AE, Meijboom FJ, McGhie JS, *et al.* Enhanced visualisation of the right ventricle by contrast echocardiography in congenital heart disease. *Eur J Echocardiogr* 2004; **5**: 104–10.

17. Kaul S, Tei C, Hopkins JM, Shah PM. Assessment of right ventricular function using two-dimensional echocardiography. *Am Heart J* 1984; **107**: 526–31.

18. Geva T, Powell AJ, Crawford EC, Chung T, Colan SD. Evaluation of regional differences in right ventricular systolic function by acoustic quantification echocardiography and cine magnetic resonance imaging. *Circulation* 1998; **98**: 339–45.

19. Karunanithi MK, Michniewicz J, Copeland SE, Feneley MP. Right ventricular preload recruitable stroke work, end-systolic pressure-volume, and dP/dt_{max}-end-diastolic volume relations compared as indexes of right ventricular contractile performance in conscious dogs. *Circ Res* 1992; **70**: 1169–79.

20. Oe M, Gorcsan J, Mandarino WA, *et al.* Automated echocardiographic measures of right ventricular area as an index of volume and end-systolic pressure-area relations to assess right ventricular function. *Circulation* 1995; **92**: 1026–33.

21. Aebischer NM, Czegledy F. Determination of right ventricular volume by two-dimensional echocardiography with a crescentic model. *J Am Soc Echocardiogr* 1989; **2**: 110–18.

22. Tei C, Dujardin KS, Hodge DO, *et al.* Doppler echocardiographic index for assessment of global right ventricular function. *J Am Soc Echocardiogr* 1996; **9**: 838–47.

23. Tei C, Dujardin KS, Hodge DO, *et al.* Doppler index combining systolic and diastolic myocardial performance: clinical value in cardiac amyloidosis. *J Am Coll Cardiol* 1996; **28**: 658–64.

24. Menzel T, Kramm T, Mohr-Kahaly S, *et al.* Assessment of cardiac performance using Tei indices in patients undergoing pulmonary thromboendarterectomy. *Ann Thorac Surg* 2002; **73**: 762–6.

25. Lutz JT, Giebler R, Peters J. The "TEI-index" is preload dependent and can be measured by transoesophageal echocardiography during mechanical ventilation. *Eur J Anaesthesiol* 2003; **20**: 872–7.

26. Abd El Rahman MY, Abdul-Khaliq H, Vogel M, *et al.* Value of the new Doppler-derived myocardial performance index for the evaluation of right and left ventricular function following repair of tetralogy of fallot. *Pediatr Cardiol* 2002; **23**: 502–7.

27. Yoshifuku S, Otsuji Y, Takasaki K, *et al.* Pseudonormalized Doppler total ejection isovolume (Tei) index in patients with right ventricular acute myocardial infarction. *Am J Cardiol* 2003; **91**: 527–31.

28. Mason DT. Usefulness and limitations of the rate of rise of intraventricular pressure (dp/dt) in the evaluation of myocardial contractility in man. *Am J Cardiol* 1969; **23**: 516–27.

29. Anconina J, Danchin N, Selton-Suty C, *et al.* Noninvasive estimation of right ventricular dP/dt in patients with tricuspid valve regurgitation. *Am J Cardiol* 1993; **71**: 1495–7.

30. Imanishi T, Nakatani S, Yamada S, *et al.* Validation of continuous wave Doppler-determined right ventricular peak positive and negative dP/dt: effect of right atrial pressure on measurement. *J Am Coll Cardiol* 1994; **23**: 1638–43.

31. Kanzaki H, Nakatani S, Kawada T, *et al.* Right ventricular dP/dt/P(max), not dP/dt(max), noninvasively derived from tricuspid regurgitation velocity is a useful index of right ventricular contractility. *J Am Soc Echocardiogr* 2002; **15**: 136–42.

32. Alam M, Hedman A, Nordlander R, Samad B. Right ventricular function before and after an uncomplicated coronary artery bypass graft as assessed by pulsed wave Doppler tissue imaging of the tricuspid annulus. *Am Heart J* 2003; **146**: 520–6.

33. Meluzin J, Spinarova L, Dusek L, *et al.* Prognostic importance of the right ventricular function assessed by Doppler tissue imaging. *Eur J Echocardiogr* 2003; **4**: 262–71.

34. Kukulski T, Hubbert L, Arnold M, *et al.* Normal regional right ventricular function and its change with age: a Doppler myocardial imaging study. *J Am Soc Echocardiogr* 2000; **13**: 194–204.

35. Vogel M, Schmidt MR, Kristiansen SB, *et al.* Validation of myocardial acceleration during isovolumic contraction as a novel noninvasive index of right ventricular contractility: comparison with ventricular pressure-volume relations in an animal model. *Circulation* 2002; **105**: 1693–9.

36. Vogel M, Derrick G, White PA, *et al.* Systemic ventricular function in patients with transposition of the great arteries after atrial repair: a tissue Doppler and conductance catheter study. *J Am Coll Cardiol* 2004; **43**: 100–6.

37. Vignon P, Weinert L, Mor-Avi V, *et al.* Quantitative assessment of regional right ventricular function with color kinesis. *Am J Respir Crit Care Med* 1999; **159**: 1949–59.

38. Jamal F, Bergerot C, Argaud L, Loufouat J, Ovize M. Longitudinal strain quantitates regional right ventricular contractile function. *Am J Physiol Heart Circ Physiol* 2003; **285**: H2842–7.

39. Spencer KT, Weinert L, Lang RM. Effect of age, heart rate and tricuspid regurgitation on the Doppler echocardiographic evaluation of right ventricular diastolic function. *Cardiology* 1999; **92**: 59–64.

40. Yalcin F, Kaftan A, Muderrisoglu H, *et al.* Is Doppler tissue velocity during early left ventricular filling preload independent? *Heart* 2002; **87**: 336–9.

41. Cicala S, Galderisi M, Caso P, *et al.* Right ventricular diastolic dysfunction in arterial systemic hypertension: analysis by pulsed tissue Doppler. *Eur J Echocardiogr* 2002; **3**: 135–42.

42. Mishra M, Swaminathan M, Malhotra R, Mishra A, Trehan N. Evaluation of right ventricular function during CABG: transesophageal echocardiographic assessment of hepatic venous flow versus conventional right ventricular performance indices. *Echocardiography* 1998; **15**: 51–8.

43. Nomura T, Lebowitz L, Koide Y, Keehn L, Oka Y. Evaluation of hepatic venous flow using transesophageal echocardiography in coronary artery bypass surgery: an index of right ventricular function. *J Cardiothorac Vasc Anesth* 1995; **9**: 9–17.

44. Gatzoulis MA, Clark AL, Cullen S, Newman CG, Redington AN. Right ventricular diastolic function 15 to 35 years after repair of tetralogy of Fallot: restrictive physiology predicts superior exercise performance. *Circulation* 1995; **91**: 1775–81.

45. Helbing WA, Niezen RA, Le Cessie S, *et al.* Right ventricular diastolic function in children with pulmonary regurgitation after repair of tetralogy of Fallot: volumetric evaluation by magnetic resonance velocity mapping. *J Am Coll Cardiol* 1996; **28**: 1827–35.

46. Mansencal N, Joseph T, Vieillard-Baron A, *et al.* Comparison of different echocardiographic indexes secondary to right ventricular obstruction in acute pulmonary embolism. *Am J Cardiol* 2003; **92**: 116–19.

47. McIntyre KM, Sasahara AA. The hemodynamic response to pulmonary embolism in patients without prior cardiopulmonary disease. *Am J Cardiol* 1971; **28**: 288–94.

48. Zehender M, Kasper W, Kauder E, *et al.* Eligibility for and benefit of thrombolytic therapy in inferior myocardial infarction: focus on the prognostic importance of right ventricular infarction. *J Am Coll Cardiol* 1994; **24**: 362–9.

49. Bellamy GR, Rasmussen HH, Nasser FN, Wiseman JC, Cooper RA. Value of two-dimensional echocardiography, electrocardiography, and clinical signs in detecting right ventricular infarction. *Am Heart J* 1986; **112**: 304–9.

50. Baslaim GM, Huynh TT, Stewart JA, *et al.* Assessment of right ventricular function postretrograde cardioplegia by transesophageal echocardiography. *J Card Surg* 1998; **13**: 32–6.

51. Lynch M, Clements SD, Shanewise JS, Chen CC, Martin RP. Right-sided cardiac tumors detected by transesophageal echocardiography and its usefulness in differentiating the benign from the malignant ones. *Am J Cardiol* 1997; **79**: 781–4.

52. Pellikka PA, Tajik AJ, Khandheria BK, *et al.* Carcinoid heart disease: clinical and echocardiographic spectrum in 74 patients. *Circulation* 1993; **87**: 1188–96.

Cardiac masses and pericardial disease

Robert Feneck

Introduction

Transesophageal echocardiography (TEE) is a useful modality for imaging cardiac masses. A number of factors are responsible for this, including the proximity of the TEE probe to the heart, the higher frequencies available with modern TEE probes, and the comparatively poor echo windows often associated with transthoracic imaging (TTE). Masses in the right atrium (RA), left atrium (LA) and left atrial appendage (LAA), and aorta are particularly well imaged with TEE. TEE is also able to show the lesion with greater clarity; thus the echo-characteristic appearance of the mass, the presence and the nature of any attachment, and the anatomical relationship to surrounding structures can be easily identified [1,2].

TEE may be of significant value in establishing the primary diagnosis, particularly if the mass is causing mitral regurgitation or is a source of embolism [3]. Cardiac surgery for an intracardiac mass has been recognized as a Class IIa indication for TEE [4]. Intraoperative TEE may be performed to check on the preoperative findings, to evaluate the heart for any additional pathology, and for aiding the process of intraoperative decision making regarding the surgical management of the removal [5–7].

Although many cardiac masses are easily visible on TEE, some are more subtle, and confusion may arise if atypical normal variants are identified as abnormal pathology. An exhaustive list of such normal variants is beyond the scope of this chapter, but some common normal structures that are mistaken for a cardiac mass are shown in Table 11.1.

Intracardiac masses are an interesting challenge. Thrombi and vegetations are most commonly encountered, followed by a variety of uncommon cardiac neoplasms and, even more infrequently, foreign bodies. Extracardiac masses in close contact to the heart include congenital cysts, non-cardiac neoplasms, abscesses, and loculated fluid collections.

Cardiac tumors

Primary cardiac tumors are rare. Although it varies in different series, an incidence of approximately 0.15% has been reported [8]. In contrast, secondary (metastatic) tumors appear to be up to 20 times more common, although they are usually found as an incidental finding at postmortem examination in patients with disseminated disease.

The clinical features associated with cardiac tumors are features of embolization, obstruction including increased atrial pressure and reduced ventricular filling, and arrhythmia.

Primary cardiac tumors

Benign

Table 11.2 shows the incidence of different primary cardiac tumors. In adults, myxomas are most frequently encountered (45%), followed by lipomas and papillary fibroelastomas. In children, rhabdomyomas are the most commonly occurring benign neoplasm.

Atrial myxoma

Atrial myxomas are relatively slow-growing and therefore usually present in patients over 40 years of age. The main clinical features are those of left atrial and pulmonary venous obstruction, and hence increasing dyspnea may be seen. If the tumor is large enough to obstruct transmitral blood flow this may provoke

Table 11.1. Structures mistaken for intracardiac tumors

Large Eustachian valve
Crista terminalis
Chiari network
Moderator band (RV)
False tendons (LV)
Papillary muscles
Pectinate muscles (LAA, RA)

Core Topics in Transesophageal Echocardiography, ed. Robert Feneck, John Kneeshaw, and Marco Ranucci.
Published by Cambridge University Press. © Cambridge University press 2010.

Table 11.2. Frequency of primary intracardiac tumors in adults

Myxoma	45%
Lipoma	20%
Papillary fibroelastoma	15%
Angioma	5%
Hemangioma	5%
Fibroma	3%
Rhabdomyoma	1%

severe dyspnea on exertion. Alternatively, embolic phenomena may be noted, with the brain and splanchnic organs particularly vulnerable.

Atrial myxomas account for 90% of all cardiac tumors found at operation, and 50% of tumors found at autopsy. They are most usually found in the left atrium (> 80%), occasionally in the right atrium (< 10%), but have been described in any cardiac chamber. Multiple locations have been described in up to 3% of patients.

Atrial myxomas are usually attached to the interatrial septum (up to 90%), but may arise from other locations including the atrial free wall, near the atrial inflow orifices, the valvular annuli, or the atrial appendages. They are classically attached via a stalk or pedicle, although this may be more difficult to identify in larger broad-based tumors.

Detailed multiplane imaging may be required to identify the point of attachment and exclude multiple tumors. Multiple myxomas may be part of a "syndrome myxoma" characterized by a familial occurence, cutaneous lesions, endocrine tumors, and a high post-operative recurrence rate.

Myxomas have typical but not unitary characteristics on echo. Often, they are polypoid, gelatinous, and deformable throughout the cardiac cycle. Small cystic echolucencies may be apparent within the tumor mass, giving it a mottled appearance in contrast to thrombus and other cardiac masses. Gelatinous myxomas may fragment and embolize at any time, and this has been described in up to 40% of patients. Such tumors may also generate thrombus formation, which is also prone to embolization. Embolization is also particularly likely during surgery and manipulation of the heart. However, myxomas may also have a fibrous non-deformable contour, and though less likely to fragment, these may more commonly obstruct the atrioventricular valves. The degree of obstruction will be dependent on the size as well as the consistency of the tumor, and hard or even calcified myxomas may cause significant damage to the atrioventricular valve leaflets.

Tumor prolapse may obstruct transmitral blood flow, thus causing turbulent inflow and functional mitral stenosis. Turbulence may be seen by mosaic inflow signals on color-flow Doppler imaging, and a transmitral gradient may also be seen by continuous-wave Doppler (Videos 11.1–11.6).

Although the provisional diagnosis of myxoma will have been made before surgery, intraoperative TEE is valuable to identify any residual tumor and assess damage to the valve apparatus or interatrial septum that might have occurred either before or during surgery and needs subsequent repair. It should be remembered that imaging can only give a probable diagnosis, and that no matter how classical the appearance of the mass, the true diagnosis is made by histology.

Lipoma (including lipomatous hypertrophy of the interatrial septum)

Lipomas are the second most common benign cardiac tumor. Pericardial and epicardial lipomas may be very large, but myocardial lipomas are usually small, solitary, asymptomatic, well-encapsulated lesions within the subendocardium or subepicardium. In contrast to myxomas, they are not intracavity lesions and are without an attachment stalk or pedicle. They have a well-demarcated, echodense nodular appearance (Video 11.7).

Cardiac magnetic resonance imaging is usually particularly useful in establishing the diagnosis, owing to the unique appearance of fat with this imaging modality.

Lipomatous hypertrophy of the interatrial septum is not a true neoplastic process, since the fat deposition is neither homogenous nor encapsulated. It typically has an echodense dumbbell appearance, since the fat infiltrates the muscular interatrial septum but spares the membranous fossa ovalis. The maximal atrial septal thickness is often in excess of 15 mm. Cardiac magnetic resonance is rarely required to confirm the diagnosis, although it may be useful in other types of lipomatous infiltration including infiltration of the pulmonary veins, venae cavae, and coronary sinus (Fig. 11.1; Video 11.8).

Papillary fibroelastoma

Clinically, papillary fibroelastomas may be silent, or present as a result of embolization to the cerebral or coronary circulations.

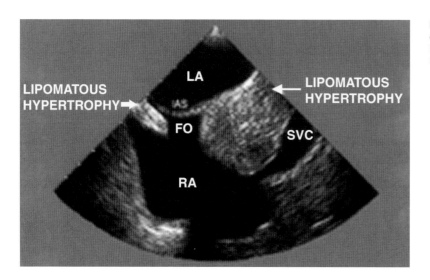

Figure 11.1. Lipomatous hypertrophy of the interatrial septum. The fossa ovalis is spared. FO, fossa ovalis; LA, left atrium; RA, right atrium; SVC, superior vena cava.

They are the most common tumors of cardiac valves, usually involving the mitral or aortic valves. More than 90% are solitary, and usually less than 1.5 cm long. The lesions have a characteristic shimmering mobility of a frond-like structure with circular masses, attached via a small pedicle. Prolapse across or through the valve orifice may occur.

Papillary fibroelastomas on the atrioventricular valves usually occur on the mid portion of the atrial side; on the aortic and pulmonary valves the lesions may occur anywhere, not restricted to either side of the valve. Rarely, the papillary muscles and chordae may become involved (Videos 11.9, 11.10).

Papillary fibroelastomas are different from Lambl's excrescences, which are small filamentous lesions that occur along the closure lines on the ventricular side of the valve. In contrast to papillary fibroelastomas [9], there is no evidence that Lambl's excrescences either embolize or cause stroke [10], although the incidence of both structures increases with age (Video 11.11). Another benign deformity of the valve leaflets consists of the nodules of Arantius, a leaflet-thickening deformity seen at the central portion of the aortic valve leaflets.

Finally, valvular lesions may be produced by systemic lupus erythematosus (SLE). These are seen after multiple episodes of lupus endocarditis, and are classically berry-shaped excrescences that are located on both the atrial and ventricular sides of the tricuspid valve, which differentiates them from rheumatic disease, in which the lesions appear only on the atrial side. In SLE the lesions may also occur on the chordae tendineae and papillary muscles, and these features,

along with the fact that papillary fibroelastoma most commonly occurs on the aortic valve, further help to differentiate the two (Video 11.12).

Cardiac rhabdomyoma and fibroma

These are most frequently seen in children. Cardiac rhabdomyomas are associated with tuberous sclerosis in which situation multiple tumors are often seen. The tumor itself has a well-circumscribed, echodense appearance. They are usually found in the ventricles in the ventricular septum or apex. They are rarely found in the atria and do not involve the valve (Fig. 11.2).

Cardiac fibromas are usually solitary, and are found in the ventricular myocardium, most commonly in the left ventricular (LV) free walls, less frequently in the interventricular septum or the right ventricle (RV). They generally have a homogenous, hyper-refractile appearance that easily demarcates the tumor from the surrounding myocardium.

Malignant primary cardiac tumors

The overwhelming majority of malignant primary cardiac tumors are sarcomas, with angiosarcoma being the most common of these. They are usually found in the right atrium, which is involved in 80% of cases. They may be polypoid, protruding into the RA cavity, or infiltrate along the epicardial or pericardial surface. They may involve either the right or left heart chambers, and may cause myocardial dysfunction and/or valve obstruction. Myxosarcomas usually arise in the left atrium, and they may involve the mitral valve.

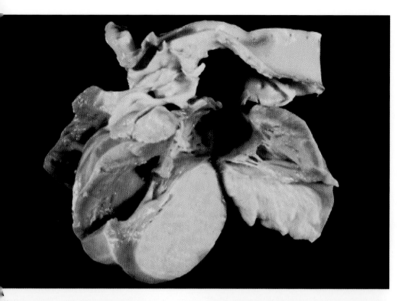

Figure 11.2. (A) Transection of a cardiac rhabdomyoma. (B) Four-chamber apical view in a third-trimester fetus with multiple cardiac rhabdomyomas. LA, left atrium; LV, left ventricle; RA, right atrium; RV, right ventricle; T, tumor.

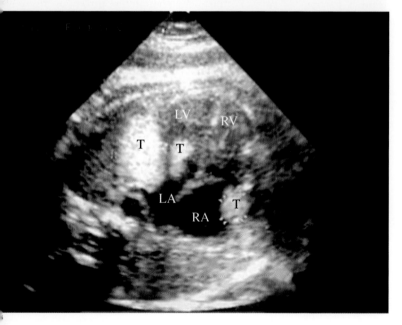

Lymphoma is the most common non-sarcomatous primary malignant lesion, but is nonetheless very rare. They appear as a large mass infiltrating the heart.

The differences between benign and malignant primary cardiac tumors are shown in Table 11.3.

Secondary cardiac neoplasms

Secondary cardiac tumors are much more common than primary tumors. Nearby primary tumors including bronchus, esophagus, and breast may spread either by direct extension or by lymphatic spread. Metastases to the heart will frequently involve the pericardium, and a pericardial effusion is common. Blood-borne metastases are commonly seen with renal cell carcinoma, hepatoma, Wilms' tumor, and uterine leiomyoma, as well as melanoma and leukemia. These lesions may cause either myocardial infiltration or large intracavity metastatic deposits, frequently on the right side of the heart. Such intracavity lesions have a significantly different appearance

Table 11.3. Differences between benign and malignant cardiac tumors

Benign	Malignant
Common	Rare
Usually in adults	Usually in children
Well circumscribed	Poorly demarcated
Often clear source of attachment	Immobile and fixed to adjoining cardiac structures
No direct extension/invasion of surrounding structures	Direct extension especially into venae cavae/pulmonary veins
Pericardial effusion rare	Pericardial effusion common

from e.g. myxoma, and may infiltrate the heart, causing the tissues to have a heterogenous appearance on echo.

It is rare to undertake perioperative TEE in these patients, but when it is done great care should be taken to avoid pharyngeal and esophageal trauma, particularly in patients with primary malignant disease of the mediastinum or esophagus.

Pericardial cysts

Pericardial cysts are frequently asymptomatic and may be an incidental finding. They are found more commonly in the right rather than the left cardiophrenic angle [11]. They usually have an echolucent unilocular cavity. The important differential diagnosis is a simple pleural effusion and, most importantly, a blood-containing structure such as a giant right atrium.

Mediastinal cysts, including bronchogenic and duplication cysts, may occur. These have a more echodense appearance on TEE, and may contain thicker mucilaginous material that may layer differently with postural change [12].

Anterior mediastinal tumors including thymoma, lymphoma, and teratoma, and posterior mediastinal tumors, may be imaged on TEE. These and other tumors may cause compression of surrounding structures.

Although TEE may be better than TTE, MRI and CT remain the most effective modalities for imaging these masses [13].

Thrombus

Thrombus has a characteristic echocardiographic appearance. It is usually homogenous and well demarcated, with variably increased echodensity compared to the surrounding myocardium, and is deposited with a laminated or layered appearance along the endocardial surface. It does not have a stalk or pedicular attachment, or evidence of tissue invasion or infiltration. Frequently a thin border of echolucency can be seen between the thrombus and the endocardial surface, thus demarcating the thrombus from the myocardium.

Left atrial

Thrombus in the left atrium is easily seen with TEE due to the close proximity between the esophagus and the LA. TEE has been recommended as being superior to TTE for detecting LA thrombus [14].

Factors promoting LA thrombus are associated with blood stasis, and include atrial fibrillation, significant LA enlargement which may be associated with left ventricular dysfunction, mitral stenosis, and mitral prosthesis. Mitral regurgitation is not commonly associated with LA thrombus, because of turbulence created by the high-velocity regurgitant jet.

Thrombus in the LA most frequently involves the LAA; indeed, it may be confined to it in up to 45% of cases. The LAA is easily seen using a mid-esophageal two-chamber view, although the transgastric long-axis view and the mid-esophageal short-axis view at the level of the aortic valve but with the probe slightly rotated to the left may also be useful (Figs. 11.3, 11.4 Videos 11.13, 11.14).

In these views, the LAA tapers to a discrete tip and often comb-like pectinate muscular ridges are evident. A truncated or blunt LAA tip should give rise to suspicion of thrombus, particularly in the presence of other risk factors. However, thrombus may be mistaken for LA tissue in the presence of two or more small additional lobes of the LAA, and for the ridge of tissue – the "coumadin ridge" – that separates the

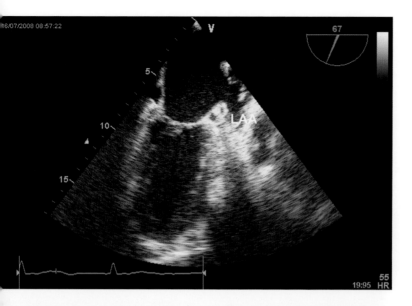

Figure 11.3. Mid-esophageal two-chamber view showing the left atrial appendage (LAA).

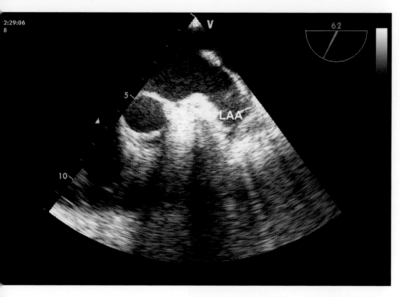

Figure 11.4. Mid-esophageal AV short-axis view turned to the left, showing the left atrial appendage (LAA).

LAA from the upper pulmonary vein (Figs. 11.5, 11.6; Video 11.15).

LA spontaneous echo contrast (SEC) has been associated with an enhanced risk of thrombus formation and hence systemic embolization, both in patients in atrial fibrillation and in sinus rhythm [15,16]. SEC results from protein-mediated red cell aggregation in circumstances of relative stasis. It has a characteristic appearance described as "smoke" (Videos 11.16–11.19). There is a relationship between the appearance of smoke and LA size, particularly in mitral valve disease, where SEC is much more prevalent if the LA diameter is greater than 60 mm. The presence of

"smoke" is also associated with LAA antegrade (emptying) blood flow velocity, which may be measured with pulsed-wave Doppler (Fig. 11.7). This in turn has been used a method of stratifying the risk of thrombus and thromboembolism.

Thus there is an important relationship between the appearance of SEC, atrial size, LAA velocity, and cardiac rhythm. The relationship between LAA velocity and the incidence of SEC in atrial fibrillation and sinus rhythm is shown in Table 11.4. Patients in sinus rhythm have higher LAA velocities, but the association between relatively low values and higher incidence of SEC remains.

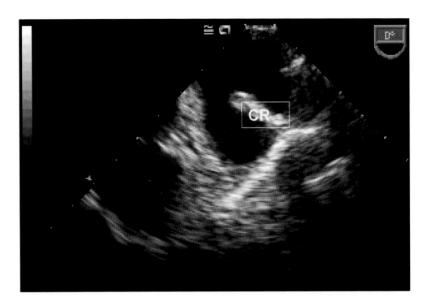

Figure 11.5. TEE view showing the coumadin ridge (CR).

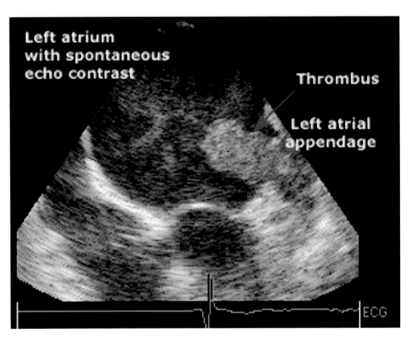

Figure 11.6. Thrombus in the left atrial appendage (LAA).

The appearance of SEC is important. Dense echo contrast is more predictive of thrombus than faint contrast, and those patients in AF with SEC have a much higher incidence of thrombus (89%) than those patients with SEC but in sinus rhythm, where the incidence of thrombus is 13%.

LA thrombus may also be present in the LA cavity. Some degree of thrombus mobility may be seen; rarely, the thrombus may be a free-floating "ball thrombus" retained in the LA by relative stenosis of the mitral valve but carrying a substantial risk of obstruction and embolization.

Left ventricular

Whereas left atrial thrombus is best seen using TEE, left ventricular thrombus is easily visualized using TTE, and TEE rarely adds to the diagnostic rate.

LV thrombus occurs in areas of blood stasis, most commonly associated with areas of severe hypokinesis or akinesis particularly associated with myocardial

Table 11.4. Relationship between blood flow velocity in the left atrial appendage (LAA), spontaneous echo contrast (SEC), thrombus, and cardiac rhythm

Cardiac rhythm	LAA velocity	SEC incidence	Thrombus incidence
Atrial fibrillation	< 20 cm/s	75%	89%
	> 20 cm/s	58%	
Sinus rhythm	< 40 cm/s	87%	13%
	> 40 cm/s	19%	

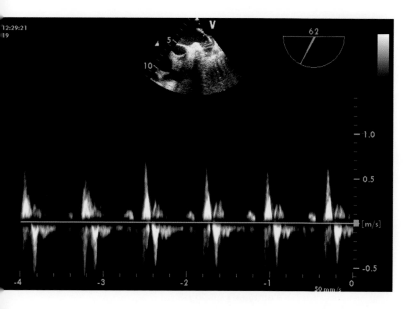

Figure 11.7. Pulsed-wave Doppler (PWD) signal of blood flow emptying from the left atrial appendage (LAA).

nfarction, or in LV aneurysm. The echocardiographic characteristics of LV thrombus are similar to those of LA thrombus, but the incidence of SEC is lower. The large majority of LV thrombi are apical. They are relatively easily seen in the apical four-chamber TTE window. In TEE, the LV apex is in the far field of the mid-esophageal long-axis views and may be subject to foreshortening, making visualization of the thrombus difficult. This may be overcome using the transgastric long-axis and deep transgastric views.

However, differentiation between the papillary muscles and thrombus in the transgastric short-axis view may be difficult.

Right heart

Right atrial thrombus may be seen following embolization from a deep venous thrombosis, or as thrombus that has formed on an indwelling RA catheter or pacing wire. RA thrombus may be mistaken for other structures, including the Eustachian valve, Chiari network, or crista terminalis. This last structure runs as a muscular ridge from the anterior portion of the superior vena cava orifice to the anterior portion of the inferior vena cava orifice and separates the anterior trabeculated portion of the RA from the posterior smooth part (Fig. 11.8).

Right ventricular thrombi are also usually apical in their location. They are again associated with blood stasis, usually following myocardial infarction, dilated cardiomyopathy, and RV failure due to lung disease, e.g. cor pulmonale. In contrast to the LV, the RV endocardium is markedly trabeculated. This and the presence of the moderator band, which runs as a muscle band from the free wall to the ventricular septum near the apex, may make thrombus identification difficult.

Sources of embolism

The heart is a significant source of emboli, and up to 75% of cardiac emboli lodge in the brain. Cardiac causes of embolization are therefore important, and echocardiography has a major role in screening for sources of embolization, which may be divided into direct and indirect sources (Table 11.5). Direct sources include intracardiac thrombus, intracardiac tumors especially atrial myxomas, valve vegetations in endocarditis, and mobile aortic plaque.

The importance of thrombus in the LA, LAA, and LV, and of LA myxoma, has been described above.

The atrial septum may act as a source of emboli in two ways. First, it may be a conduit for emboli via a patent foramen ovale. Second, an atrial septal aneurysm may act both as a source of embolism, due to stasis, and as a conduit, because they frequently have multiple fenestrations.

Recent studies have suggested that TEE is significantly better than TTE for screening for embolic causes of stroke [17–19], and it remains a primary indication for the technique (Table 11.6) [3]. In this situation, a goal-directed approach is recommended, incorporating a standardized protocol including adequate visualization of all cardiac structures with emphasis on both atria, LAA, interatrial septum, mitral valve apparatus, and thoracic aorta. If possible, the screening procedure should be done with minimal or no seda-

tion, since a Valsalva maneuver is an important part of the procedure. This maneuver, in conjunction with a contrast injection of agitated saline, may be useful to demonstrate a patent foramen ovale and right-to-left shunt. Screening for LA thrombus in patients who are about to undergo elective cardioversion has also been validated as a useful technique [20,21].

In patients who have suffered a neurological event, the indications for screening to identify a possible source are shown in Table 11.7.

Endocarditis

A number of studies have suggested that TEE is superior to TTE for detecting endocarditis with vegetations [22–24]. In patients with vegetations, the embolic risk appears to be related more to the size of the vegetation rather than to the presence of positive blood cultures [22]. Endocarditis is dealt with more fully in Chapter 18.

Aortic atheroma

The echocardiographic imaging of the aorta and the features of aortic atheroma are reviewed in Chapter 12. Although it would appear intuitive that atheroma in the descending aorta would embolize distally, diastolic flow reversal in the descending aorta may allow atheroma located just below the brachiocephalic vessels to embolize centrally.

Pulmonary embolism

The role of echocardiography in pulmonary embolism is to provide a rapid and accurate diagnosis rather

Table 11.5. Sources of emboli

Direct	Indirect
Thrombus	Valve disease
Tumor	Dilated cardiomypathy
Vegetation	Atrial septal aneurysm
Aortic atheroma	Atrial septal defect
	Patent foramen ovale

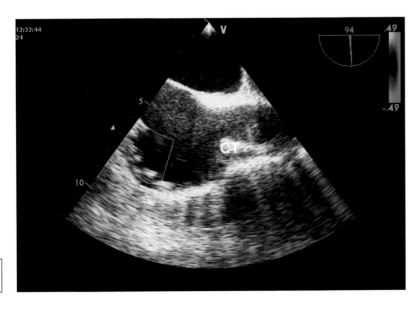

Figure 11.8. Mid-esophageal bicaval view showing the crista terminalis (CT).

Table 11.6. Transthoracic (TTE) versus transesophageal echocardiography (TEE) for detection of potential cardioembolic sources

Diagnosis by TTE [a]	Diagnosis by TEE (primarily or alone)
Mitral stenosis	Left atrial thrombus
Dilated cardiomyopathy	Left atrial spontaneous contrast
Left ventricular aneurysm	Atrial septal aneurysm
Left ventricular thrombus	Patent foramen ovale
Mitral valve prolapse	Aortic atheroma
Vegetation	
Atrial septal defect	

[a] TTE is sufficient; TEE may be additive but is not essential.

Table 11.7. Indications for echocardiography in patients with neurological events or other vascular occlusive events

	Class
1. Patients of any age with abrupt occlusion of a major peripheral or visceral artery	I
2. Younger patients (typically < 45 years) with cerebrovascular events	I
3. Older patients (typically > 45 years) with neurological events without evidence of cerebrovascular disease or other obvious cause	I
4. Patients for whom a clinical therapeutic decision (anticoagulation, etc.) will depend on the results of echocardiography	I
5. Patients with suspicion of embolic disease and with cerebrovascular disease of questionable significance	IIa
6. Patients with a neurological event and intrinsic cerebrovascular disease of a nature sufficient to cause the clinical event	IIb
7. Patients for whom the results of echocardiography will not impact a decision to institute anticoagulant therapy or otherwise alter the approach to diagnosis or treatment	III

than to reveal the source of the embolism, unless the source is itself contained within the right heart. This may result from thrombus, and rarely tumor, as discussed previously. Indwelling central venous catheters and pacing wires may act as a focus for thrombus formation. The thrombus itself may be seen as a mass in the pulmonary arterial tree. Location may be difficult, and the upper esophageal views need to be examined with care. Supportive features of pulmonary embolus will be those of increased RV volume and failure, including RV dilation, tricuspid regurgitation, reduced

LV volume and paradoxical septal motion. Increased RV and RA pressure may cause increased shunt potential through a patent foramen ovale (Video 11.19).

Pericardial disease

The pericardial cavity is a potential space between the visceral and parietal pericardium. It usually contains 20–30 mL of serous fluid. The visceral pericardium overlies the epicardial surface, and the parietal lining of the fibrous pericardium separates the heart other intrathoracic structures. The pericardium has the following attachments:

- superior attachments to the great arteries
- at atrial level, posterior attachments to the venae cavae and pulmonary veins

The superior attachments create the transverse sinus, and the posterior attachments create the pericardial sinus.

The pericardium may be congenitally absent, which is both rare and usually asymptomatic. It may also be partially absent, usually on the left side, with the potential for LV herniation. Patients with congenital absence of the pericardium may demonstrate exaggerated posterior LV wall motion, and paradoxical septal wall motion. The RV may also appear dilated. Although its function is not fully clear, the pericardium may protect against cardiac chamber dilation and excessive ventricular filling.

Effusions

The size and likely location of a pericardial effusion may vary, as shown in Table 11.8. Large effusions may be associated with horizontal counterclockwise rotation and marked anterior–posterior motion. Regional wall motion of the septum may be abnormal, and there may also be motion abnormalities of the tricuspid, mitral, and aortic valves.

Postoperative pericardial effusions are not uncommon in the cardiac surgical population, with a peak incidence on the 10th postoperative day [25]. The clinical symptoms are due to cardiac chamber compression, and although the largest effusions may be most likely to cause the greatest degree of compression, localization and loculation of the effusion may provoke severe symptoms in patients with relatively small effusions. Loculated posterior effusions causing LA compression may be particularly troublesome. Posterior effusions must be differentiated from a left pleural effusion and benign pericardial cysts. The

Table 11.8. Location and dimensions of pericardial effusions

Effusion	Location	Width (mm)	Volume (mL)
Small effusion	Behind posterior LV wall	< 10	< 100
Moderate effusion	Posterior, plus lateral, apical, and anterior expansion	10–15	100–500
Large effusion	Circumferential distribution, but largest posteriorly	> 15	> 500

former are common following surgery, but are easily excluded by TTE. Pericardial cysts will not occur de novo in the postoperative period. Anterior effusions are uncommon without any posterior fluid collection. Loculated anterior echo-free spaces are more suggestive of epicardial fat, particularly in obese, elderly, diabetic females.

The location of the effusion will often determine which TEE imaging planes are most useful. The transgastric short-axis view may be useful, although other views may be necessary to distinguish a pericardial fluid collection from a left pleural effusion.

Cardiac tamponade

Cardiac tamponade may be defined as the decompensated phase of cardiac compression resulting from increased intrapericardial pressure. It is characterized by pulsus paradoxus (reduction in systemic pressure on inspiration during spontaneous ventilation) and eventually a reduction in stroke volume and cardiac output.

Cardiac tamponade causes significant impairment to ventricular filling and may need urgent drainage. Postoperative cardiac tamponade is an acute surgical emergency and requires a speedy and accurate diagnosis. The clinical stigmata are peripheral cooling (or failure to rewarm) oligo-anuria, increased cardiac filling pressures and systemic hypotension. Classically there is a picture of increased chest tube drainage which has suddenly reduced or ceased altogether.

Unfortunately, this clinical picture is not diagnostic. The clinical stigmata mentioned above are also indicative of a developing low output state due to myocardial failure. Increased chest tube output will trigger blood or colloid transfusion, which together with LV failure may cause cardiac filling pressures to elevate markedly. Persistent systemic hypotension may be treated with inotropic vasopressor amines, which may also increase venous pressures whilst having little beneficial effect on urine output, peripheral temperature, and blood pressure.

An accurate diagnosis excluding cardiac tamponade would be enormously helpful in this situation. This is often difficult, because blood in the pericardium may exist both as fluid and as solid blood clot. Postoperative hemopericardium is much more difficult to identify than a pericardial effusion.

Signs of cardiac chamber compression may be valuable. Persistent invagination of the anterior RV free wall may be seen in diastole until atrial contraction. RA inversion may also be seen, and its significance is more marked if it is long-lasting, even into systole. However, elevated right heart pressures may prevent RA or RV diastolic collapse and therefore mask the compressive effects of the tamponade.

Other suggestive signs are a decrease in RA or RV size, abnormal motion of the ventricular septum, and a dilated inferior vena cava.

There are a number of respiratory changes that are often seen with cardiac tamponade in spontaneously breathing patients in two-dimensional, M-mode, and Doppler measurements. However, these are of less practical value in postoperative tamponade, since these patients are often still receiving intermittent positive pressure ventilation (IPPV). Thus the echocardiographic diagnosis rests with demonstrating compression and right heart filling impairment.

Constrictive pericarditis

Constrictive pericarditis is characterized by a fibrotic, inflamed, or calcified pericardial sac. The pericardium presents a significant restriction to cardiac filling, which is usually markedly reduced. RA pressure is increased, often to 20 mmHg or more. RV systolic and diastolic pressures are elevated, with a narrow pulse pressure. The cause of constrictive pericarditis is frequently following infection, although other causes include radiation therapy, metabolic and connective tissue disorders, and neoplasm.

Table 11.9. Echocardiographic findings associated with cardiac tamponade and constrictive pericarditis

Cardiac tamponade
Early diastolic collapse of RV
Atrial inversion (late diastole to early systole)
Decreased RA or RV size
Abnormal ventricular septal wall motion
Respiratory variation (ventricular chamber size, Doppler flows in pulmonary and hepatic veins, tricuspid/mitral valves)
Constrictive pericarditis
Normal ventricular size
Normal atrial size; reduced wall motion
Left shift of ventricular and atrial septum (spontaneous ventilation)
Paradoxical ventricular septal motion
Diastolic flattening of LV posteriorly

An early report suggested that up to 0.3% of cardiac surgical patients develop postoperative constrictive pericarditis, even though the pericardium is left widely open at the end of surgery [26].

There is frequently a thickened, highly echoreflective interface surrounding the heart, particularly seen anteriorly. A pericardial effusion may also be seen, and this may contain solid matter including thrombus or fibrin. Tricuspid regurgitation is a not uncommon finding.

The transmitral and pulmonary venous flow pattern, and the transtricuspid and hepatic vein flow pattern, seen in cardiac tamponade are also seen in constrictive pericarditis. An inspiratory/expiratory variation of mitral peak early (E wave) velocity of 25% is frequent, with increased diastolic hepatic flow reversal. Changes in LV compliance may mask the mitral inflow effect, and if the variation in E-wave velocity is not seen, reducing preload by sitting or reverse Trendelenburg may serve to unmask it.

These respiratory variations seen in spontaneously breathing patients will occur in the opposite direction in patients on IPPV. The change in respiratory variation seen during and after pericardectomy may serve as a useful predictive tool for surgical success.

The differentiation between constrictive pericarditis and restrictive cardiomyopathy is important. Both conditions may show the stigmata of decreased LV compliance, i.e. increased peak E-wave transmitral velocity and E/A ratio, reduced transmitral deceleration time, and a pulmonary venous systolic/diastolic ratio of < 1. However, in restrictive cardiomyopathy the respiratory variation is absent, in contrast to constrictive pericarditis. Furthermore, tissue Doppler may be valuable in differentiating between the two conditions, unless the constriction is more confined to the base as opposed to being evenly distributed. In these circumstances, the differentiation is best made using either color tissue Doppler, myocardial strain rate imaging, or other techniques able to quantify myocardial motion (Videos 11.25–11.27).

The echocardiographic findings associated with constrictive pericarditis are contrasted with those of cardiac tamponade in Table 11.9.

Conclusion

In patients with a suspected cardiac mass, transesophageal echocardiography is recommended for determining its nature, and for the assessment of sources of cardiac embolism. A suspected cardiac mass is a Class I or IIa indication for an intraoperative study. TEE also has a place as a screening test, for example in patients requiring elective cardioversion. The proximity of the atria and ease of imaging of the venae cavae may make the technique particularly suitable.

TEE has less to offer in the patient with pericardial disease, especially when compared to transthoracic imaging. However, it may be particularly useful in patients with loculated or trapped pericardial fluid, for example in the postoperative setting.

References

1. DeVille JB, Corley D, Jin BS, *et al.* Assessment of intracardiac masses by transesophageal echocardiography. *Tex Heart Inst J* 1995; **22**: 134–7.

2. Aru GM, Falchi S, Cardu G, *et al.* The role of transesophageal echocardiography in the monitoring of cardiac mass removal; a review of 17 cases. *J Card Surg* 1993; **8**: 554–7.

3. Flachskampf FA, Decoodt P, Fraser AG, *et al.* Working Group on Echocardiography of the European Society of Cardiology. Guidelines from the Working Group. Recommendations for performing transesophageal echocardiography. *Eur J Echocardiogr* 2001; **2**: 8–21.

4. Cheitlin MD, Armstrong WF, Aurigemma GP, *et al.* ACC/AHA/ASE 2003 guideline update for the clinical application of echocardiography: summary article. A report of the American College of

Cardiology/American Heart Association Task Force on Practice Guidelines (ACC/AHA/ASE Committee to Update the 1997 Guidelines for the Clinical Application of Echocardiography). *Circulation* 2003; **108**: 1146–62.

5. Dujardin KS, Click RL, Oh JK. The role of intraoperative transesophageal echocardiography in patients undergoing cardiac mass removal. *J Am Soc Echocardiogr* 2000; **13**: 1080–3.

6. Leslie D, Hall TS, Goldstein S, Shindler D. Mural left atrial thrombus: a hidden danger accompanying cardiac surgery. *J Card Surg* 1998; **39**: 649–50.

7. Schuetz WH, Welz A, Heymer B. A symptomatic papillary fibroelastoma of the left ventricle removed with the aid of transesophageal echocardiography. *Thorac Cardiovasc Surg* 1993; **41**: 258–60.

8. Salcedo EE, Cohen GI, White RD, Davison MB. Cardiac tumors: diagnosis and management. *Curr Probl Cardiol* 1992; **17**: 73–137.

9. Zurrú MC, Romano M, Patrucco L, Cristiano E, Milei J. Embolic stroke secondary to cardiac papillary fibroelastoma. *Neurologist* 2008; **14**: 128–30.

10. Goldman JH, Foster E. Transesophageal echocardiographic (TEE) evaluation of the aortic valve, left ventricular outflow tract, and pulmonary valve. *Cardiol Clin* 2000; **18**: 711–29.

11. Feigin DS, Fenoglio JJ, McAllister HA, Madewell JE. Pericardial cysts: a radiologic–pathologic correlation and review. *Radiology* 1977; **125**: 15–20.

12. Page JE, Wilson AG, de Belder MA. The value of transoesophageal ultrasonography in the management of a mediastinal foregut cyst. *Br J Radiol* 1989; **62**: 986–8.

13. Faletra F, Ravini M, Moreo A, *et al.* Transesophageal echocardiography in the evaluation of mediastinal masses. *J Am Soc Echocardiogr* 1992; **5**: 178–86.

14. DiNardo JA. Echocardiographic evaluation of intracardiac masses and septal defects. In: Konstadt SN, Shernan S, Oka Y, eds., *Clinical Transesophageal Echocardiography: a Problem-Oriented Approach*, 2nd edn. Philadelphia, PA: Lippincott Williams & Wilkins, 2003: 191–202.

15. Black IW. Spontaneous echo contrast: where there's smoke there's fire. *Echocardiography* 2000; **17**: 373–82.

16. Sadanandan S, Sherrid MV. Clinical and echocardiographic characteristics of left atrial spontaneous echo contrast in sinus rhythm. *J Am Coll Cardiol* 2000; **35**: 1932–8.

17. Gutterman DD, Ayres RW. Use of echocardiography in detecting cardiac sources of embolus. *Echocardiography* 1993; **10**: 311–20.

18. Reynolds HR, Jagen MA, Tunick PA, Kronzon I. Sensitivity of transthoracic versus transesophageal echocardiography for the detection of native valve vegetations in the modern era. *J Am Soc Echocardiogr* 2003; **16**: 67–70.

19. Walpot J, Pasteuning WH, Hoevenaar M, *et al.* Transesophageal echocardiography in patients with cryptogenic stroke: does it alter their management? A 3-year retrospective study in a single non-referral centre. *Acta Clin Belg* 2006; **61**: 243–8.

20. Klein AL, Grimm RA, Murray RD, *et al.* Use of transesophageal echocardiography to guide cardioversion in patients with atrial fibrillation. *N Engl J Med* 2001; **344**: 1411–20.

21. Klein AL, Grimm RA, Jasper SE, *et al.* ACUTE Steering and Publications Committee for the ACUTE Investigators. Efficacy of transesophageal echocardiography-guided cardioversion of patients with atrial fibrillation at 6 months: a randomized controlled trial. *Am Heart J* 2006; **151**: 380–9.

22. Blanchard DG, Ross RS, Dittrich HC. Nonbacterial thrombotic endocarditis: assessment by transesophageal echocardiography. *Chest* 1992; **102**: 954–6.

23. Stoddard MF, Dawkins PR, Longaker RA. Mobile strands are frequently attached to the St. Jude Medical mitral valve prosthesis as assessed by two-dimensional transesophageal echocardiography. *Am Heart J* 1992; **124**: 671–4.

24. Walz ET, Slivka AP, Tice FD, *et al.* Noninfective mitral valve vegetations identified by transesophageal echocardiography as a cause of stroke. *J Stroke Cerebrovasc Dis* 1998; **7**: 310–14.

25. Weitzman LB, Tinker WP, Kronzon I, *et al.* The incidence and natural history of pericardial effusion after cardiac surgery: an echocardiographic study. *Circulation* 1984; **69**: 506–11.

26. Cimino JJ, Kogan AD. Constrictive pericarditis after cardiac surgery: report of three cases and review of the literature. *Am Heart J* 1989; **118**: 1292–301.

The thoracic aorta

Robert Feneck, Andrzej Wielogorski

Introduction

Transesophageal echocardiography (TEE) is a valuable means of assessing diseases of the thoracic aorta. The close proximity between the esophagus and the aorta ensures that good-quality images are easily obtainable for most of its length. The exception is the area from the distal ascending aorta to the mid transverse aortic arch, which may be difficult to visualize because the trachea and right main bronchus are located between the esophagus and the ascending aorta.

TEE has a number of advantages in imaging the aorta, particularly in the emergency situation. The investigation is relatively low-cost, easily available at the bedside, and rapid, with a very high diagnostic pick-up rate. It may also be undertaken as part of a more generalized cardiac assessment which may reveal other relevant information. However, in common with other indications for TEE, it is operator-dependent, requiring skill and experience for the correct interpretation of images, and may be contraindicated in certain conditions, especially esophageal disease. In the emergency setting, trauma to the head and neck may also act as a contraindication.

Anatomy

The aortic wall (Fig. 12.1) consists of:

- an innermost intima lined by the vascular endothelium
- the media, interlaced elastic tissue and smooth muscle, comprising 80% of the arterial wall thickness
- the adventitia, the thin outermost layer composed of collagen, containing the vasa vasorum and aortic lymphatics

These layers are not usually distinguishable by echocardiography, although they may become so when disrupted by trauma or aortic dissection.

The thoracic aorta is conventionally divided into four regions, as shown in Figure 12.2. These are the aortic root, the ascending aorta, the aortic arch, and the descending thoracic aorta.

Aortic root

The aortic root begins at the aortic valve, includes the three sinuses of Valsalva, and terminates at the sinotubular junction. It lies within the pericardium, and so disruption of the aortic root may result in a hemopericardium. The structure of the sinuses of Valsalva is such that they permit full systolic opening of the aortic valve leaflets, and effective closing in diastole. The sinuses are also the weakest point in the aorta. Measurements of the aortic root may be useful not only in diagnosing the presence and severity of disease, but also in surgical planning. It is therefore necessary to be aware of the normal values. These are:

- aortic valve annulus diameter: 1.8–2.6 cm
- sinus of Valsalva diameter: 2.1–3.4 cm
- sinotubular junction diameter: 2.2–3.4 cm

Ascending aorta

The ascending aorta begins at the sinotubular junction and continues until the origin of the innominate (brachiocephalic) artery. It has no branches. Usually at least the most proximal four centimetres lie in the pericardial sac. Failure to image the distal ascending aorta is usual, and this may complicate surgical planning in patients with extensive aneurysmal dilation. The length of the aortic root and ascending aorta is 7.5–10 cm. The dimensions of the aorta at this level have been shown to evolve with age, particularly in subjects over the age of 40 years [1].

Aortic arch

The aortic arch extends from the innominate artery on the right to the subclavian artery at the level of the ligamentum arteriosum on the left. It gives off three

Core Topics in Transesophageal Echocardiography, ed. Robert Feneck, John Kneeshaw, and Marco Ranucci.
Published by Cambridge University Press. © Cambridge University Press 2010.

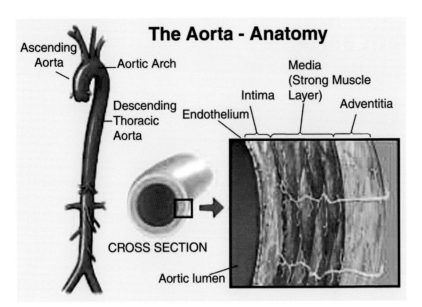

The Aorta - Anatomy

Ascending Aorta

Aortic Arch

Descending Thoracic Aorta

Intima

Endothelium

Media (Strong Muscle Layer)

Adventitia

CROSS SECTION

Aortic lumen

Figure 12.1. Anatomy of the aorta.

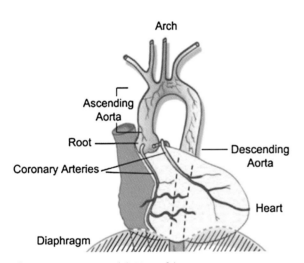

Arch

Ascending Aorta

Root

Coronary Arteries

Descending Aorta

Heart

Diaphragm

Figure 12.2. Anatomical divisions of the aorta.

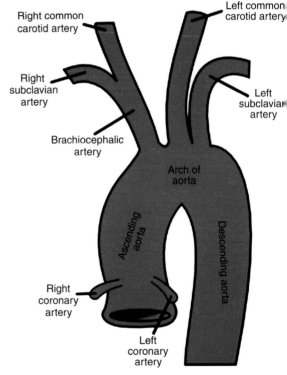

Right common carotid artery

Left common carotid artery

Right subclavian artery

Left subclavian artery

Brachiocephalic artery

Arch of aorta

Ascending aorta

Descending aorta

Right coronary artery

Left coronary artery

Figure 12.3. Branches of the thoracic aorta.

branches from its superior aspect: the innominate (brachiocephalic), the left common carotid, and the left subclavian artery (Fig. 12.3). The aortic arch is effectively shielded from the TEE probe by the trachea and right main bronchus, as described earlier, and echocardiographic measurements of the aortic arch dimensions are not usually available. However, other techniques including epiaortic scanning have been shown to be effective in scanning those areas of the ascending aorta and proximal aortic arch that are inaccessible to conventional TEE [2,3]. In addition, techniques have been developed to improve the visualization of these regions with conventional TEE [4].

Descending thoracic aorta

The descending aorta commences at the left subclavian. In contrast to the ascending aorta and aortic arch, the descending aorta is fixed to the thorax by the

Table 12.1. TEE views of the thoracic aorta

Mid-esophageal ascending aortic short-axis view Usual probe tip depth: 25–35 cm Transducer angle: 0–60°	**o. ME asc aortic SAX**
Mid-esophageal ascending aortic long-axis view Usual probe tip depth: 25–35 cm Transducer angle: 100–150°	**p. ME asc aortic LAX**
Descending aortic short-axis view Usual probe tip depth: 30–40 cm Transducer angle: 0°	**q. desc aortic SAX**
Descending aortic long-axis view Usual probe tip depth: 30–40 cm Transducer angle: 90–110°	**r. desc aortic LAX**
Upper esophageal aortic arch long-axis view Usual probe tip depth: 20–25 cm Transducer angle: 0°.	**s. UE aortic arch LAX**
Upper esophageal aortic arch short-axis view Usual probe tip depth: 20–25 cm Transducer angle: 90°	**t. UE aortic arch SAX**

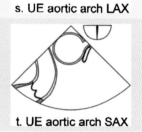

195

ligamentum arteriosum, and by the paired intercostal arteries along the thoracic spine. The portion of descending aorta between the left subclavian artery proximally and the ligamentum arteriosum distally is known as the aortic isthmus. This area is the most common location for coarctation, patent ductus arteriosus, and aortic rupture due to deceleration injuries. Initially the descending aorta runs caudally and close to the esophagus in the left thorax. The aorta runs progressively posteriorly to the esophagus and is directly posterior at the level of the diaphragm. The normal dimensions of the descending aorta are as follows:

- proximal descending aorta, immediately below aortic arch: diameter 1.4–3.0 cm
- descending aorta, at level of diaphragm: diameter 1.3–2.8 cm

TEE imaging of the aorta

A number of standard cross-sectional views have been described which are suitable for imaging the aorta. These views have been described in Chapter 4.

TEE imaging of the thoracic aorta is subject to the same considerations of safety and risk assessment as TEE imaging of any other structure. However, two considerations should be especially borne in mind. First, passage of a TEE probe can be a strong cardiovascular stimulus even in an anesthetized patient, resulting in a burst of severe hypertension. This may be dangerous for a patient with either an aneurym or a dissection and who is at risk of aortic rupture. Second, the aorta and the esophagus are in close proximity, and the aortic arch and esophagus cross at the level of T4/5. Weakness of the aorta due to aneurysmal dilation at this point may increase the risk of aortic rupture on passage of the probe. These considerations should be borne in mind whenever a TEE is performed for disease of the thoracic aorta.

Aortic views

The standard views for imaging the thoracic aorta are shown in Table 12.1 and Videos 12.1–12.8.

Structures and pathology within the aortic root and early ascending aorta may be identified with reference to other structures in close proximity. However, other areas are not near other easily recognizable structures, and therefore can be localized by their distance from the incisors. The following distances may be useful:

- 20–25 cm from incisors: distal aortic arch
- 30–35 cm from incisors: mid thoracic descending aorta

- 40–50 cm from incisors: distal thoracic aorta at the level of the diaphragm

Other possible ways of localizing lesions in the descending aorta are to use the distance from the left subclavian artery, or alternatively to rotate the probe through 90° and note the cardiac structures at the same level [5]. Localization may be difficult if the aorta itself is very tortuous in its course.

Imaging the branches of the aorta

A number of the branches of the aorta can be imaged using TEE. The coronary arteries may be imaged using the mid-esophageal aortic short-axis view as a starting point (Fig. 12.4; Video 12.9).

Frequently the probe will need small manipulations, and the transducer will need to be rotated slightly, in order to pursue the course of the relevant vessels. Usually, the left main stem can be seen easily arising from the region of the left coronary cusp. The right coronary artery is usually seen with more difficulty, originating from the region of the right coronary cusp.

The innominate and left carotid arteries are not usually visible due to being shaded by the trachea, but the left subclavian may be visible as described above.

Diseases of the aorta

A number of diseases of the aorta are amenable to TEE imaging (Table 12.2). These are discussed below. In addition, TEE may be used to monitor device placement, including endovascular stents in the thoracic aorta and intra-aortic balloon catheters. In cardiac surgery patients, the aortic cannula and the antegrade cardioplegia cannula may be seen, as well as endoaortic clamps. The newer techniques of transcatheter and transapical aortic valve replacement are discussed in Chapter 17.

Congenital aortic disease
Coarctation of the aorta

Coarctation of the aorta may present as a partial narrowing, or rarely a complete occlusion, of the aorta. It is usually located just distal to the left subclavian artery or the ligamentum arteriosum, at the aortic isthmus although preductal and ductal coarctation is also described (Fig. 12.5).

Accurate diagnosis using TEE may be very difficult. This region is not easy to image, and more than one imaging plane may be necessary to visualize the lesion. Although Doppler should be able to identify an

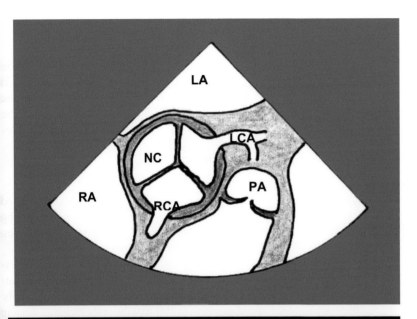

Figure 12.4. Short-axis view of the right and left coronary arteries. RA, right atrium; LA, left atrium; PA, pulmonary artery; LCA, left coronary artery; RCA, right coronary artery; NC, non-coronary cusp.

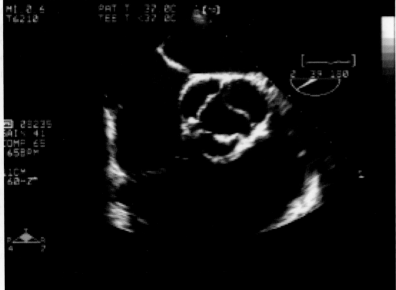

increase in turbulence and flow acceleration through the coarctation, in practice it may be difficult to orientate the Doppler beam in the direction of blood flow. For similar reasons, calculation of the pressure gradient across the lesion may not be possible.

TEE may however be valuable for detecting associated abnormalities. Approximately 80% of patients with coarctation of the aorta may also have a bicuspid aortic valve, possibly with associated aortic stenosis or regurgitation [6]. Other associated abnormalities may include left ventricular hypertrophy, aortic aneurysm,

dissection, or rupture, and endocarditis, particularly on an abnormal valve. There is a recognized association between coarctation, bicuspid aortic valve, and cystic medial necrosis [6,7].

Persistent ductus arteriosus

The ductus arteriosus connects the pulmonary artery to the aorta in the fetal circulation. Closure usually occurs within days after birth, but the defect may be more common in premature babies and

Table 12.2. Indications for TEE imaging of the thoracic aorta

Congenital aortic disease

- Coarctation of the aorta
- Patient ductus arteriosus
- Supravalvular aortic stenosis

Acquired aortic disease

- Dissection of the aorta
- Aortic aneurysm
- Aortic atherosclerosis
- Masses within the aorta

Traumatic injury

Localization of devices

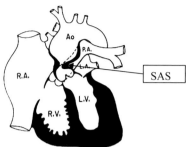

Figure 12.6. Supravalvular aortic stenosis (SAS). Ao, aorta; LA, left atrium; LV, left ventricle; PA, pulmonary artery; RA, right atrium; RV, right ventricle

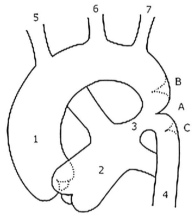

Figure 12.5. Locations of coarctation of the aorta. A, ductal coarctation; B, preductal coarctation; C, postductal coarctation. 1, ascending aorta; 2, pulmonary artery; 3, ductus arteriosus; 4, descending aorta; 5, brachiocephalic trunk; 6, left common carotid artery; 7, left subclavian artery.

Supravalvular aortic stenosis

Supravalvular aortic stenosis is a narrowing of the aorta usually at the level of the border of the sinus of Valsalva (Fig. 12.6).

The majority of cases are caused by hypoplasia of the aorta, although more rarely a membrane (10%) or narrowed segment (20%) may be responsible.

TEE imaging of this area of the aorta is usually straightforward, and the lesion is often imaged without difficulty. Doppler studies will be more dependent on the exact nature and location of the lesion.

Acquired aortic disease

Dissection of the aorta

Aortic dissection is a surgical emergency. Patients may present with a variety of features, but severe chest pain is usually a symptom. Back pain may also be present. Involvement of the innominate and/or carotid arteries may lead to focal neurological signs, which may be transient or permanent. Loss of consciousness is not uncommon.

Involvement of the aortic valve may produce severe aortic regurgitation leading to breathlessness and pulmonary edema. Rupture at the level of the sinuses of Valsalva will produce cardiac tamponade, and compression or hypoperfusion of the coronary arteries may lead to myocardial ischemia.

Involvement of the subclavian vessels may produce hypoperfusion of the upper limb. This may manifest itself either as a loss of the radial or brachial pulse, cooling of the limb, or frank ischemia of the upper limb. Aortic dissection may be extensive and involve the renal and mesenteric vessels and the blood supply to the lower limbs.

The dissection occurs as an initial tear in the aortic intima, the innermost layer of the aortic wall. Blood under systemic pressure then forces a passage

those with other congenital disorders. Following closure the ductus becomes fibrosed as the ligamentum arteriosum. A ductus that persists into adolescence or adulthood can be imaged using TEE. Flow through the ductus can be detected using color-flow Doppler imaging. A right-to-left shunt may be detected using contrast echocardiography, with absence of contrast in the ascending aorta. A simple calculation of pulmonary pressure may be obtained by detecting the pressure gradient and subtracting it from arterial, or aortic, pressure [8,9]. A persistent left-to-right shunt will eventually lead to pulmonary arterial hypertension and right ventricular hypertrophy, both of which may simply be demonstrated using TEE.

through the elastic tissue and muscle of the media. The tear may penetrate the partial or full circumference of the aorta, in the latter case leading to a "double-barreled" aorta. This may rarely lead to intussusception of the intimal flap into the vessel lumen [10,11]. If the outermost layer, the adventitia, is breached, then massive blood loss may occur, causing sudden cardiac tamponade if the tear is proximal, or hypotension and severe hemorrhage if the tear occurs more distally, i.e. outside the pericardiac sac, which extends to approximately the first 4 cm of the ascending aorta.

Diseases which cause degradation of the aortic media will be important causative factors. Age, systemic hypertension, and atherosclerosis may be contributory. With aging, degenerative changes lead to breakdown of collagen, elastin, and smooth muscle and an increase in basophilic ground substance. This condition is termed cystic medial necrosis. Atherosclerosis leading to occlusion of the vasa vasorum may also be implicated in the etiology. The histological changes of cystic medial necrosis have been noted in patients with abnormal elastic tissue including Marfan syndrome, Ehlers–Danlos syndrome, Turner syndrome, Noonan syndrome, Takayasu disease, osteogenesis imperfecta, and a family history of aortic dissection, all of which predispose to aortic dissection. Patients with coarctation have also been noted to have a high incidence of cystic medial necrosis, which may explain the formation of aneurysmal dilation at the site of balloon dilation of the coarctation [12,13].

Aortic dissection has also occurred as a complication of surgical aortic cannulation and retrograde femoral arterial perfusion, and following coronary angioplasty [14–16]. Conditions associated with transient but severe hypertension, including pregnancy, have been implicated also.

Aortic dissection usually occurs within 10 cm of the aortic valve or immediately distal to the left subclavian artery, presumably associated with the high shearing forces in these areas. However, in fact the dissection may occur anywhere in the aorta.

The two methods of classifying aortic dissection are shown in Figure 12.7. The most commonly used classification is the Stanford classification, especially since this is most easily associated with surgical decision making.

The diagnosis of aortic dissection is confirmed by imaging, and a number of modalities have been used.

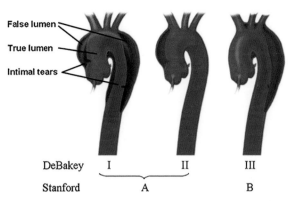

False lumen
True lumen
Intimal tears

DeBakey   I   II   III
Stanford   A   B

Figure 12.7. Classification of aortic dissection: DeBakey and Stanford systems.

Aortography, once commonly used, has now been largely displaced. The sensitivity of TEE has been shown to be significantly greater [17]. Magnetic resonance imaging (MRI) has been shown to have the greatest sensitivity and specificity for diagnosis [18], but the test itself is time-consuming, particularly for an ill patient, and may not be available in the referring community or general hospital. On the other hand, contrast-enhanced computed tomography (CT), particularly using a 64-slice machine or greater, will be able to demonstrate an aortic dissection almost as effectively as MRI and is an investigation that is more commonly available – and perhaps also more appropriate in the emergency setting [19,20].

TEE has long been recognized as having an important role [21]. Image quality is usually excellent, particularly in the most important area for the surgeon – that is, at the level or the aortic root and proximal ascending aorta. Difficulty in imaging the ascending aorta and aortic arch is a drawback.

A useful management protocol is to perform contrast-enhanced CT either at the referring hospital or at the surgical unit to establish the diagnosis and extent of the dissection, followed by TEE. In these circumstances, TEE is undertaken with the patient anesthetized and immediately before surgery in order to prevent a potentially dangerous burst of hypertension developing during the passage of the probe. The surgical team thence has TEE images available in real time.

Although TEE usually produces striking images of the dissection, this is not always the case. The identification of an intimal flap is diagnostic. This should be imaged in a number of views, in order to identify its exact anatomical location and to exclude confounding

199

artifacts. The flap typically moves synchronously with the cardiac cycle. Dissection at the level of the aortic root may produce severe aortic regurgitation. Rarely, the dissection flap may prolapse through the aortic valve, preventing regurgitation (Videos 12.10–12.20).

Short-axis views of the aorta may reveal the flap separating the true and false lumens. This is especially true of imaging the descending aorta, although one should take care to exclude a mirror artifact in the long-axis view. Color-flow Doppler may be particularly useful at establishing the true and false lumens, and also the site of the initial tear and re-entry site. Blood flow in the false lumen is decreased, and the true lumen can usually be seen to expand in systole. Thrombus may also become visible in the false lumen.

TEE may also be combined with surface imaging of the neck to detect extension of the dissection flap into the neck vessels. This can frequently be seen even with simple high-frequency scanners designed for use for central vein catheter insertion.

Accurate TEE imaging of aortic dissection may be confounded by a number of artifacts. These include reverberation or side-lobe artifacts masquerading as an intimal flap, and reverberation artifacts within the aortic lumen. Intravascular catheters and other devices may generate artifacts also, but these can usually simply be moved or removed.

In addition to conventional aortic dissection, a number of other pathologies may cause acute aortic syndrome (AAS), the acute presentation of patients with characteristic "aortic pain" caused by one of several life-threatening thoracic aortic pathologies. These include intramural hematoma (IMH), penetrating atherosclerotic ulcer, aneurysmal leak, and traumatic transection.

IMH may evolve to overt dissection or even rupture, and may occur suddenly or be heralded by ongoing acute aortic syndrome. IMH has no mechanisms of decompression by a re-entry tear but rather reveals intramural (intramedial) thickening or echolucent pockets of non-communicating blood with potential for rupture or, at times, regression and resorption of hematoma with time. As in overt dissection, widening of the mediastinum or the aortic shadow, pleural effusion and pain, aortic regurgitation, and pericardial effusion may emerge after initial IMH, whereas focal neurological signs or malperfusion syndrome are incidental.

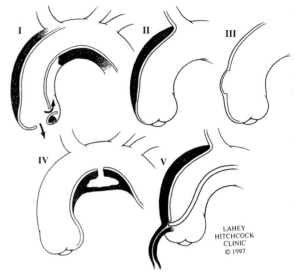

Fig 12.8. Variants of aortic dissection: I, classic dissection with flap between true and false aneurysm and clot in false lumen; II, intramural hematoma; III, limited intimal tear with eccentric bulge at tear site; IV, penetrating atherosclerotic ulcer with surrounding hematoma, usually subadventitial; V, iatrogenic or traumatic dissection illustrated by coronary catheter causing dissection. Reproduced with permission from from Svensson *et al.*, *Circulation* 1999; **99**: 1331–6 [24].)

TEE examination will usually reveal an aortic IMH of greater than 7 mm in the short-axis view, associated with a layered appearance of the aortic wall when viewed in the long axis extending for more than 1 cm, in the absence of an intimal flap. Frequently the aortic wall has an echo pattern similar to hematoma, with areas of the appearance of fresh blood [22,23]. It is important to be able to distinguish IMH from mural thrombus within the aortic lumen.

The appearance of an IMH and other variants of aortic dissection are shown in Figure 12.8.

Thus aortic dissection is a particularly strong indication for TEE, and one where safety and practicality combine to endorse the use of intraoperative TEE. Aortic dissection has been classified amongst those conditions designated as Class I indications for intraoperative TEE [25].

Aortic aneurysm

Aortic aneurysm may be defined as a true or false aneurysm. True aneurysms contain all three layers of the vessel wall in the aneurysm, whereas false aneurysms contain none and may be thought of as encapsulated areas of aortic rupture. In surgical patients they may develop at the site of aortic cannulation, but they may also occur as a result of infection, ruptured atheromatous plaque, or trauma [26].

The etiology of a true aortic aneurysm has much in common with aortic dissection. Atherosclerosis, often associated with hypertension and aging, and more rarely Marfan syndrome, Ehlers–Danloss syndrome, aortitis, and syphilis have all been implicated. Coarctation and bicuspid aortic valve have also been reported as associated conditions. Aortic aneurysm in patients with Marfan syndrome frequently has a characteristic appearance of a widely dilated aortic root and tapering aneurysmal dilation of the ascending aorta – the so-called "inverted pear" appearance (Fig. 12.9; Videos 12.21–12.26).

TEE may be extremely valuable in imaging an aortic aneurysm. Nonetheless there are safety issues that should be considered, particularly regarding the safe passage of the TEE probe. Patients with any evidence of aortic compression of surrounding structures, including the esophagus and major airways, may be at risk. In particular a history of dysphagia should be noted, and if any resistance to passage of the probe is encountered the procedure may have to be abandoned.

Each exam should be directed to assessing the location and size of the aneurysm, although the size may differ slightly from that shown by a CT or MRI assessment. The involvement of any other structures should be sought, particularly the aortic valve. The diameter of the aortic annulus, sinuses of Valsalva, and sinotubular junction can be assessed from the mid-esophageal aortic long-axis view as described in Chapter 6. The mid-esophageal short-axis view is also useful for assessing the aortic valve, particularly if there is annular dilation and regurgitation. This may enable surgical decision making to consider the need for either replacing, repairing, or resuspending the aortic valve.

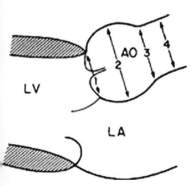

Fig 12.9. In Marfan syndrome, dilation usually starts at the sinuses of Valsalva. This measurement is critical in monitoring the early evolution of the condition. Diameters must be related to normal values for age and body surface area. AO, aorta; LA, left atrium; LV, left ventricle.

Aortic atherosclerosis

As the age of patients undergoing cardiac surgery increases, age-related risk factors assume greater importance as outcome determinants. Aortic atheroma is a major factor in determining outcome. The risk of stroke has been shown to be significantly higher in patients with atherosclerotic disease of the aorta [27], and intraoperative detection of atheroma by TEE has been associated with a higher incidence of early and late cerebral and peripheral embolic events [28–33].

The appearance of aortic atheroma may be variable, and this in turn may be related to its prognostic impact. TEE imaging may identify atheroma as bright spots due either to the thickness of the plaque or to calcification. Plaque thickness should be measured from the intimal surface perpendicularly to the outer edge of the vessel wall. Atheroma may be stratified in five grades, starting at normal and progressing to simple intimal thickening, then sessile atheroma (attached throughout its base, not mobile and not attached by a "stalk") of varying thickness, to protruding atheroma with mobile elements visible (Table 12.3).

A systematic approach to locating atheroma in the aorta has been described, employing a six-segment model consisting of a proximal, mid, and distal third of the ascending aorta (zones 1–3), a proximal and distal part of the aortic arch (zones 4–5), and a proximal segment of the descending aorta (zone 6). Further localization is aided by subdividing each segment into four quadrants: anterior, posterior, left, and right [34]. Identification of atheroma in the descending aorta during cardiac surgery is important, not simply because it may lead to peripheral embolization if it becomes detached for any reason, but also because it predicts atheroma both elsewhere in the aorta and in other vessels [35] and correlates with an increased incidence of stroke [36,37].

Ultrasound imaging has been shown to be superior to surgical digital palpation at detecting all types of atheroma apart from hard calcified plaque [38,39]. However, the distal ascending aorta and aortic arch are not routinely visible during TEE. An obturator has been described to circumvent this problem [4], but alternatively epivascular scanning has been shown to be more effective than TEE for imaging these areas [40] (Videos 12.27–12.30).

Masses within the aorta

True tumors of the aorta, including leiomyosarcoma, fibroelastoma, and epithelioma, are fortunately

Table 12.3. Grading the severity of atheroma [29]

Grade	Severity	Description
1	Normal	No intimal thickening
2	Mild	Intimal thickening 3 mm without irregularities
3	Moderate	Sessile atheroma > 3 mm with intimal irregularities
4	Severe	Sessile atheroma 5 mm
5	Severe	Atheroma protruding 5 mm with mobile components

extremely rare. Mostly, masses within the aorta are thrombus or atheroma, or a combination of the two. Areas of low flow may predispose to thrombus formation, for example within a true or especially false aneurysm. Vegetations due to bacterial endarteritis have been described [41]. In rare circumstances, tumor invasion of the thoracic aorta may occur also.

Traumatic injury

Traumatic injury to the aorta usually occurs as a result of rapid deceleration injury or blunt chest trauma. Motor vehicle accidents may be responsible for the majority of both, but blast injuries, falls, or crush injuries may also be involved.

Rapid deceleration may produce a transverse injury to the aorta, usually at the level of the aortic isthmus [42]. This area is immediately proximal to the immobile descending aorta, and immediately distal to the mobile aortic arch. It may occur as a full or partial thickness injury, involving the media and intima, or all three layers. A transection injury may occur, with the aorta held together by remnants of the adventitia. Most of these injuries prove immediately lethal, and early surgery may be indicated in many of the survivors.

TEE may provide an effective and rapid imaging technique for diagnosing traumatic injury to the aorta, and has the further benefit of providing a comprehensive imaging assessment of the heart and other vessels as well.

The inability of TEE to image the complete aorta has already been described. For this reason, and particularly in patients who are stable, contrast-enhanced CT may be an effective alternative imaging modality, with TEE reserved for intraoperative use in a protocol similar to that described for aortic dissection.

Localization of devices

As an imaging modality, TEE may have a role in detecting appropriate placement of endovascular

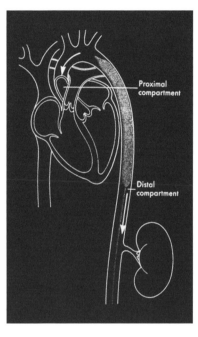

Fig 12.10. The correct positioning of an intra-aortic balloon.

devices, including endovascular stents and intra-aortic balloon pump (IABP) catheters. Endovascular stenting is frequently undertaken under x-ray screening, but TEE may have a role in assessing the aorta pre-procedure and in follow-up.

Accurate IABP catheter placement is important to ensure optimum counter-pulsation. The catheter tip should ideally be located 2 cm distal to the left subclavian artery, or several centimetres distal to the junction of the aortic arch and descending aorta (Fig. 12.10; Videos 12.30, 12.31).

If imaging these structure is difficult, an alternative is to image the aortic valve, identify the level of the aortic valve leaflets, and then rotate the probe through 180° to image the descending aorta, and position the IABP catheter tip at the level of the aortic leaflets.

Intraoperative TEE is valuable in locating and positioning devices for minimally invasive cardiac surgery, for example in positioning the endoaortic balloon clamp. The development of minimally invasive valve surgery has been facilitated by the TEE-aided positioning of the prosthetic aortic valve. This subject is dealt with more fully in Chapter 17.

Conclusion

Transesophageal echocardiography is a valuable imaging technique for assessing diseases of the aorta. In particular, it is valuable in assessing aortic aneurysm and aortic dissection, and in identifying the location and severity of aortic atheroma. This may have useful prognostic implications, and also be invaluable for guiding the use and positioning of intravascular devices located in the aorta or needing passage through the aorta to the cardiac chambers.

References

1. Garcier JM, Petitcolin V, Filaire M, *et al.* Normal diameter of the thoracic aorta in adults: a magnetic resonance imaging study. *Surg Radiol Anat* 2003; **25**: 322–9.

2. Rosenberger P, Shernan SK, Löffler M, *et al.* The influence of epiaortic ultrasonography on intraoperative surgical management in 6051 cardiac surgical patients *Ann Thorac Surg* 2008; **85**: 548–53.

3. Djaiani G, Ali M, Borger MA, *et al.* Epiaortic scanning modifies planned intraoperative surgical management but not cerebral embolic load during coronary artery bypass surgery. *Anesth Analg* 2008; **106**: 1611–18.

4. Li YL, Wong DT, Wei W, Liu J. A novel acoustic window for trans-oesophageal echocardiography by using a saline-filled endotracheal balloon. *Br J Anaesth* 2006; **97**: 624–9.

5. Pantin EJ, Cheung AT. Transesophageal echocardiographic evaluation of the aorta and pulmonary artery. In: Konstadt SN, Shernan S, Oka Y, eds., *Clinical Transesophageal Echocardiography: a Problem-Oriented Approach*, 2nd edn. Philadelphia, PA: Lippincott Williams & Wilkins, 2003: 215–44.

6. Warnes CA. Bicuspid aortic valve and coarctation: two villains part of a diffuse problem. *Heart* 2003; **89**: 965–6.

7. Fedak PW, Verma S, David TE, *et al.* Clinical and pathophysiological implications of a bicuspid aortic valve. *Circulation* 2002; **106**: 900–4.

8. Andrade A, Vargas-Barron J, Rijlaarsdam M, *et al.* Utility of transesophageal echocardiography in the examination of adult patients with patent ductus arteriosus. *Am Heart J* 1995; **130**: 543–6.

9. Shyu KG, Lai LP, Lin SC, Chang H, Chen JJ. Diagnostic accuracy of transesophageal echocardiography for detecting patent ductus arteriosus in adolescents and adults. *Chest* 1995; **108**: 1201–5.

10. Goldberg SP, Sanders C, Nanda NC, Holman WL. Aortic dissection with intimal intussusception: diagnosis and management. *J Cardiovasc Surg (Torino)* 2000; **41**: 613–15.

11. Ruvolo G, Voci P, Greco E, *et al.* Aortic intussusception: a rare presentation of type A aortic dissection evidenced by transesophageal echocardiography. *J Cardiovasc Surg (Torino)* 1993; **34**: 385–7.

12. Korkut AK, Cetin G, Saltik L. Management of a large pseudo-aneurysm secondary to balloon angioplasty for aortic coarctation. *Acta Chir Belg* 2006; **106**: 107–8.

13. Aydogan U, Dindar A, Gurgan L, Cantez T. Late development of dissecting aneurysm following balloon angioplasty of native aortic coarctation. *Cathet Cardiovasc Diagn* 1995; **36**: 226–9.

14. Miyatake T, Matsui Y, Suto Y, *et al.* A case of intraoperative acute aortic dissection caused by cannulation into an axillary artery. *J Cardiovasc Surg (Torino)* 2001; **42**: 809–11.

15. Alfonso F, Almería C, Fernández-Ortíz A, *et al.* Aortic dissection occurring during coronary angioplasty: angiographic and transesophageal echocardiographic findings. *Cathet Cardiovasc Diagn* 1997; **42**: 412–15.

16. Moles VP, Chappuis F, Simonet F, *et al.* Aortic dissection as complication of percutaneous transluminal coronary angioplasty. *Cathet Cardiovasc Diagn* 1992; **26**: 8–11.

17. Bansal RC, Chandrasekaran K, Ayala K, Smith DC. Frequency and explanation of false negative diagnosis of aortic dissection by aortography and transesophageal echocardiography. *J Am Coll Cardiol* 1995; **25**: 1393–401.

18. Nienaber CA, von Kodolitsch Y, Nicolas V, *et al.* The diagnosis of thoracic aortic dissection by noninvasive imaging procedures. *N Engl J Med* 1993; **328**: 1–9.

19. Smith AD, Schoenhagen P. CT imaging for acute aortic syndrome. *Cleve Clin J Med* 2008; **75**: 7–9, 12, 15–17, 23–4.

20. Chughtai A, Kazerooni EA. CT and MRI of acute thoracic cardiovascular emergencies. *Crit Care Clin* 2007; **23**: 835–53.

21. Adachi H, Omoto R, Kyo S, *et al.* Emergency surgical intervention of acute aortic dissection with the rapid diagnosis by transesophageal echocardiography. *Circulation* 1991; **84** (5 Suppl): III14–19.

22. Song JK. Diagnosis of intramural haematoma *Heart* 2004; **90**: 368–71.

23. Mohr-Kahaly S, Erbel R, Kearney P, Puth M, Meyer J. Aortic intramural hemorrhage visualized by transesophageal echocardiography: findings and prognostic implications. *J Am Coll Cardiol* 1994; **23**: 658–64.

24. Svensson LG, Labib SB, Eisenhauer AC, Butterly JR. Intimal tear without hematoma: an important variant of aortic dissection that can elude current imaging techniques. *Circulation* 1999; **99**: 1331–6.

25. Cheitlin MD, Armstrong WF, Aurigemma GP, *et al.* ACC/AHA/ASE 2003 guideline update for the clinical application of echocardiography: summary article. A report of the American College of Cardiology/ American Heart Association Task Force on Practice Guidelines (ACC/AHA/ASE Committee to Update the 1997 Guidelines for the Clinical Application of Echocardiography). *Circulation* 2003; **108**: 1146–62.

26. Kouchoukos NT, Dougenis D. Surgery of the thoracic aorta. *N Engl J Med* 1997; **336**: 1876–88.

27. Gardner TJ, Horneffer PJ, Manolio TA, *et al.* Stroke following coronary artery bypass grafting: a ten-year study. *Ann Thorac Surg* 1985; **40**: 574–81.

28. Coletti G, Torracca L, La Canna G, *et al.* Diagnosis and management of cerebral perfusion phenomenon during aortic dissection repair by transesophageal Doppler echocardiographic monitoring. *J Card Surg* 1996; **11**: 355–8.

29. Katz ES, Tunick PA, Rusinek H, *et al.* Protruding aortic atheromas predict stroke in elderly patients undergoing cardiopulmonary bypass: experience with intraoperative transesophageal echocardiography. *J Am Coll Cardiol* 1992: **20**: 70–7.

30. Jones EF, Kalman JM, Calafiore P, Tonkin AM, Donnan GA. Proximal aortic atheroma: an independent risk factor for cerebral ischemia. *Stroke* 1995; **26**: 218–24.

31. Amarenco P, Cohen A, Tzourio C, *et al.* Atherosclerotic disease of the aortic arch and risk of ischemic stroke. *N Engl J Med* 1994; **331**: 1474–9.

32. Tunick PA, Rosenzweig BP, Katz ES, *et al.* High risk for vascular events in patients with protruding aortic atheromas: a prospective study. *J Am Coll Cardiol* 1994; **23**: 1085–90.

33. The French Study of Aortic Plaques in Stroke Group. Atherosclerotic disease of the aortic arch as a risk factor for recurrent ischemic stroke. *N Engl J Med* 1996; **334**: 1216–21.

34. Royse C, Royse A, Blake D, Grigg L. Assessment of thoracic aortic atheroma by echocardiography: a new classification and estimation of risk of dislodging atheroma during three surgical techniques. *Ann Thorac Cardiovasc Surg* 1998; **4**: 72–7.

35. Konstadt SN, Reich DL, Kahn R, Viggiani RF. Transesophageal echocardiography can be used to screen for ascending aortic atherosclerosis. *Anesth Analg* 1995; **81**: 225–8.

36. Mizuno T, Toyama M, Tabuchi N, *et al.* Thickened intima of the aortic arch is a risk factor for stroke with coronary artery bypass grafting. *Ann Thorac Surg* 2000; **70**: 1565–70.

37. Kutz SM, Lee VS, Tunick PA, Krinsky GA, Kronzon I. Atheromas of the thoracic aorta: a comparison of transesophageal echocardiography and breath-hold gadolinium-enhanced 3-dimensional magnetic resonance angiography. *J Am Soc Echocardiogr* 1999; **12**: 853–8.

38. Machleder HI, Takiff H, Lois JF, Holburt E. Aortic mural thrombus: an occult source of arterial thrombo-embolism. *J Vasc Surg* 1986; **4**: 473–8.

39. Hartman GS, Yao FS, Bruefach M, *et al.* Severity of aortic atheromatous disease diagnosed by transesophageal echocardiography predicts stroke and other outcomes associated with coronary artery surgery: a prospective study. *Anesth Analg* 1996; **83**: 701–8.

40. Sylivris S, Calafiore P, Matalanis G, *et al.* The intraoperative assessment of ascending aortic atheroma; epiaortic imaging is superior to both transesophageal echocardiography and direct palpation. *J Cardiothorac Vasc Anesth* 1997; **11**: 704–7.

41. Bansal RC, Ashmeik K, Razzouk AJ. An unusual case of vegetative aortitis diagnosed by transesophageal echocardiography. *J Am Soc Echocardiogr* 2001; **14**: 237–9.

42. Pretre R, Chilcott M. Blunt trauma to the heart and great vessels. *N Engl J Med* 1997; **336**: 626–32.

Hemodynamic assessment

Marco Ranucci, Alfredo Pazzaglia

Introduction

The principles of reflection of sound waves from moving objects were established by Christian Doppler, an Austrian physicist, in 1842. The incorporation of Doppler technology into medical ultrasound has introduced a powerful tool for diagnosis and monitoring in sick patients. Transesophageal echocardiography (TEE) allows the physician to obtain both rapid and reliable information at the bedside, and may be particularly useful in those patients with a difficult acoustic window for transthoracic imaging [1–5]. The information obtained may often obviate the need for further invasive hemodynamic examination. In particular, with the routine introduction of echo-Doppler, it has become possible to perform hemodynamic calculations in a non-invasive manner [6]. The accuracy of the hemodynamic information is strongly dependent both on the quality of the study and on the proper application of the principles of Doppler echocardiography and flow dynamics [7,8]. The application of echo-Doppler to the study of valve function allows us to grade the severity of valve pathology [9], and to study the flow through different cardiac structures and calculate stroke volume (SV) and cardiac output (CO). Data obtained by TEE should be interpreted in the light of the clinical environment if we are to obtain an accurate evaluation of the cardiac patient. Adherence to the existing guidelines on performing a TEE examination should minimize errors and reduce the possibility of incorrect hemodynamic assessments [1–11].

Basic equations

Three main equations form the basis of hemodynamic calculations: the flow equation, the Bernoulli equation, and the continuity equation.

The flow equation

The flow equation states that flow is the product of the cross-sectional area (CSA) and the distance that a fluid moves in a given time (Fig. 13.1). In echocardiography, this distance equates to the distance a column of blood has traveled in one heartbeat, known as the stroke distance. This may be calculated by averaging the velocity of blood over one heartbeat, by mapping out the Doppler velocity signal integrated against time: the velocity–time integral (VTI) [6].

VTI is automatically calculated by all modern echo machines by tracing the profile of a pulsed-wave (PWD) or continuous-wave (CWD) Doppler signal (Figs. 13.2, 13.3). To assess the volume passing through an orifice, we can apply the equation:

$$\text{Volume (cm}^3\text{)} = \text{CSA (cm}^2\text{)} \times \text{VTI (cm)} \qquad (13.1)$$

The Bernoulli equation

The Bernoulli equation, in its complete form, determines the value of a pressure gradient created by flow passing through a restricted orifice [10]. It can be simplified as follows:

$$\Delta P = \tfrac{1}{2}\,\rho(V_b^2 - V_a^2) \qquad (13.2)$$

where

ρ is the *density* of blood ($1.06 \times 10^3\,\text{kg/m}^3$)

V_b is the velocity at point b (distal to the restriction)

V_a is the velocity at point a (proximal to the restriction)

Since V_a is comparatively very low, it can usually be omitted, and the final equation is

$$\Delta P = 4 \times V^2 \qquad (13.3)$$

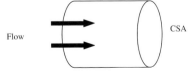

Flow

CSA

Flow = CSA x Velocity

Since volume is the product of flow and time, the above equation can be rewritten:

Volume = CSA x Velocity x Time

Figure 13.1. Determination of flow: the flow equation.

205

Core Topics in Transesophageal Echocardiography, ed. Robert Feneck, John Kneeshaw, and Marco Ranucci.
Published by Cambridge University Press. © Cambridge University Press 2010.

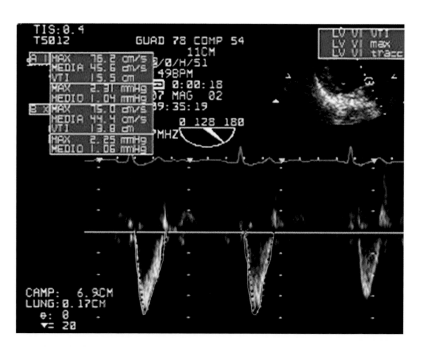

Figure 13.2. Stroke volume assessment using pulsed-wave Doppler (PWD). Two beats are examined and the velocity–time integral (VII) is calculated as the mean of the two (14.6 cm). If the LVOT diameter is 2 cm, the LVOT cross-sectional area (CSA) is 3.14 cm² and the stroke volume (SV) is 46 cm³.

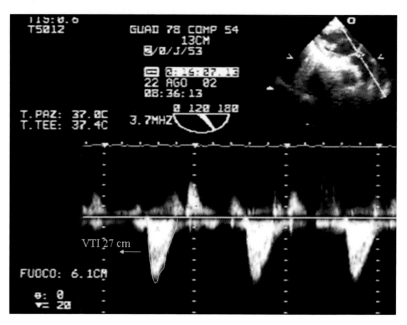

Figure 13.3. Stroke volume assessment using continuous-wave Doppler (CWD). The VTI is 27 cm. If the aortic valve area is 2 cm², the SV is 54 cm³.

The continuity equation

The continuity equation is used to calculate the area of a stenotic or regurgitant valve [11]. The principle of the formula relates to the "conservation of flow." The flow rate into a tube will equal the flow rate out of the same tube. If the CSA of one part of that tube is reduced the velocity of flow will increase in that part of the tube.

CSA and velocity (V) are inversely proportional (Fig. 13.4):

$$CSA \times V = \text{constant} \tag{13.4}$$

Stroke volume and cardiac output

To determine the stroke volume [2,12–17], Equation 13.1 is used [6].

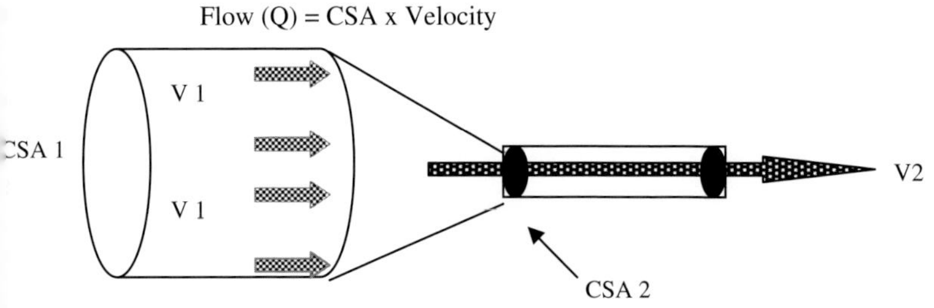

Flow (Q) = CSA x Velocity

Figure 13.4. The continuity equation.

Thus we can see that:

Q 1 = CSA 1 x V1

Q 2 = CSA2 x V2

But Q1 = Q2

Therefore : CSA 1 x V 1 = CSA 2 x V 2 (3)

CSA 2 = Q 1/ V2

In order to ensure accuracy it is essential to properly match the site of the Doppler signal to the correct anatomic measure of CSA. This is assessed as follows:

a. **Obtain VTI and CSA**

   i. Ensure that the Doppler beam is as parallel as possible to the direction of blood flow seen in the two-dimensional (2D) echo examination. The angle of incidence between the Doppler beam and the direction of blood flow should be not more than 20°. This will produce an error of 6% or less in the calculation (see Chapter 2). The best view is usually obtained using the transgastric views (long-axis transgastric view at 90–120°, or deep transgastric view at 0–20°: see Chapter 4).
   Obtain a PWD signal tracing by placing the sampling volume at the left ventricular outflow tract (LVOT) level, about 5 mm proximal to the aortic valve. The VTI is calculated by tracing the middle of the dense envelope of the spectral recording (Fig. 13.2; Video 13.1).

   ii. The CSA required for this calculation is the LVOT area. This is derived from the LVOT diameter measured in the 2D mid-esophageal long-axis view at 120°.
   M-mode is an accurate method of calculating this distance, but it should only be used if the angle of incidence to the aorta is 90°. The

measurement should be made at the level of the aortic annulus during systole (Fig. 13.5). From this diameter, and by assuming a circular section, the CSA is determined by the following equation:

$$CSA = D^2 \times 0.785 \qquad (13.5)$$

where

CSA = cross-sectional area of LVOT

D = diameter of LVOT

b. **Stroke volume** (SV) is calculated as CSA × VTI.
c. **Cardiac output** (CO) is SV × heart rate [12–14].

There is a second way to determine SV, based on a CWD signal instead of PWD [16]. In this case, there is no specific sampling point, and the CWD signal reflects the velocity of all the blood cells moving along the path of the sound beam (Fig. 13.3). The VTI obtained with a CWD signal is usually larger than the corresponding one obtained with PWD (Video 13.2). The relevant CSA must therefore be that cross-sectional area which is the smallest along the line of the Doppler beam. This is normally at the aortic valve. In order to measure the aortic valve CSA, one method requires using the 2D short-axis view of the aortic valve (mid-esophageal at 30–60°), and obtaining the CSA by planimetry: that is, tracing the edges of the aortic valve during systole (Fig. 13.6). This method may be subject to errors, particularly if the valve is severely abnormal.

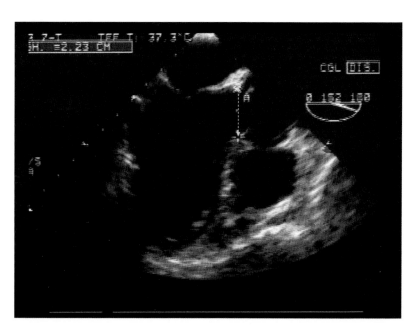

Figure 13.5. Measurement of the left ventricular outflow tract (LVOT) diameter in the mid-esophageal long axis view.

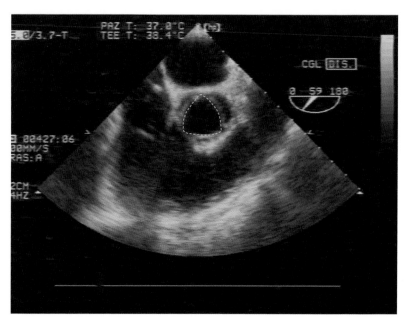

Figure 13.6. Planimetry of the aortic valve in the mid-esophageal short-axis view.

Greatest accuracy is achieved by considering the shape of the aortic valve orifice not at its largest point during systole, but as an equilateral triangle, which represents its average shape during systole [16]. The area of the aortic valve can then be calculated by using the formula for the area of an equilateral triangle:

$$\text{Area} = \frac{l^2 \times \sqrt{3}}{4} \qquad (13.6)$$

where l is the length of one side.

Theoretically, SV could be measured from transmitral flow rather than aortic flow. In this case the VTI of transmitral flow is assessed using the mid-esophageal four-chamber view at the 2D examination (Fig. 13.7). The sampling volume of the PWD should be positioned so that in diastole it is at the level of the annulus. Using the same view the mitral annulus diameter can be measured, tracing a line from the base of the posterior and anterior leaflets during early to mid-diastole, one frame

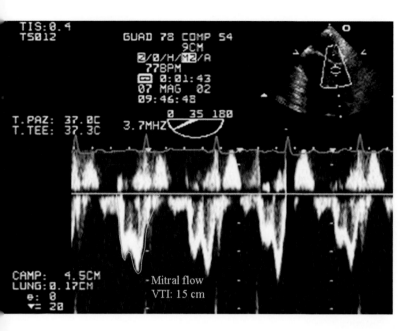

Figure 13.7. Stroke volume assessment using a PWD study of the mitral flow. The velocity–time integral (VTI) is 15 cm. If the mitral annulus diameter is 2.4 cm, the mitral valve area is 4.5 cm², and the SV is 67.5 cm³. Note the position of the PWD sampling volume.

after the leaflets begin to close after their initial opening.

The CSA can be assessed by measuring the diameter of the annulus and applying Equation 13.5. However, this method is much less accurate than the method described above for the LVOT, not least because the mitral annulus is not circular. Planimetry of the mitral valve in the basal short-axis view does not constitute a more accurate method, because of the funnel shape and plastic nature of the mitral valve.

Pressures and gradients

The pressure gradient across an orifice, for example a valvular stenosis, may be assessed using the modified Bernoulli equation (Equation 13.3) [17]. CWD is commonly employed when assessing aortic stenotic lesions, and PWD is used for the mitral valve [18–20].

Modern echo machines automatically calculate the pressure gradient from the Doppler signal waveform. The mean pressure gradient is calculated from a complete trace of the profile of the waveform, whereas the peak gradient may be identified simply by identifying the point of peak flow velocity.

For transaortic pressure gradients, the Doppler signal needs to be parallel to transaortic blood flow; this can be achieved using the standard transgastric views, as already described. Transmitral pressure gradients may be obtained in the standard four-chamber view. Gradients across the pulmonary valve are more difficult to obtain, because of the difficulty in aligning the Doppler beam parallel to the direction of blood flow across the valve. This may sometimes be obtained by using an upper esophageal 90° view.

Intracardiac pressures may be calculated with TEE providing that one or more cardiac valves is regurgitant. By measuring the peak velocity of the regurgitant flow, a pressure gradient can be established. The sum of the pressure gradient and the pressure in the chamber receiving the regurgitant flow is equal to the pressure in the chamber driving the regurgitant flow:

$$\text{Driving pressure} = \text{Pressure gradient} + \text{Pressure distal to the regurgitant flow} \quad (13.7)$$

Many pressures can be calculated in the presence of regurgitant flow. The most commonly measured pressures are:

a. **Systolic pulmonary artery pressure** (sPAP). This is calculated from the peak velocity, and hence peak pressure gradient, of a tricuspid regurgitation jet, and is usually determined with CWD (Fig. 13.8; Video 13.3). The pressure distal to the regurgitant flow is the right atrial pressure (RAP). The equation is:

$$\text{sPAP} = \text{Peak pressure gradient} + \text{RAP} \quad (13.8)$$

b. **Left atrial pressure** (LAP). This calculation requires mitral valve regurgitation. The peak velocity and the resulting pressure gradient are determined usually using a CWD signal. (NB: mitral regurgitation flow is often

209

Box 13.1. Are TEE-based SV and cardiac output determination reliable?

The theoretical basis of all the equations used is sound, but the main problem remains that both 2D and Doppler determinations are strongly operator-dependent. Potential sources of error include:

• Doppler beam more than 20° from the direction of blood flow
• inaccurate border tracing of the Doppler "envelope"
• inaccuracies in CSA determination.

Also, during intrathoracic intermittent positive pressure (IPPV) there is a considerable beat-to-beat variation of the stroke volume, which may be reflected by differences in VTI. In sinus rhythm, at least three beats should be chosen for measurement of VTI and the mean value taken for SV calculation. In atrial fibrillation, 7–10 beats should be measured.

TEE may be useful as a "trend monitor" of SV and cardiac output. Given that the CSA is relatively stable in the same patient, the serial changes in VTI may accurately reflect equivalent changes in SV. When serially monitoring VTI, CW Doppler measurement of flow through the aortic valve appears to have less variability than PW Doppler measurements either at the level of the aortic valve or the LVOT.

characterized by a very high peak velocity.) The driving pressure is the systolic systemic arterial pressure (sSAP). The equation is:

$$LAP = sSAP - \text{Peak pressure gradient} \quad (13.9)$$

c. **Left ventricular end-diastolic pressure** (LVEDP). This requires aortic valve regurgitation. The end-diastolic pressure gradient is calculated using a CWD signal. The driving pressure is the diastolic systemic arterial pressure (dSAP). The appropriate equation is:

$$LVEDP = dSAP - \text{End-diastolic pressure gradient} \quad (13.10)$$

Regurgitant volumes, fractions, regurgitant orifices, and stenotic valve areas

According to the continuity equation, the blood flow entering a cardiac chamber in diastole is equal to the blood flow leaving that chamber in systole. If we apply this concept to regurgitant valves, we can measure the

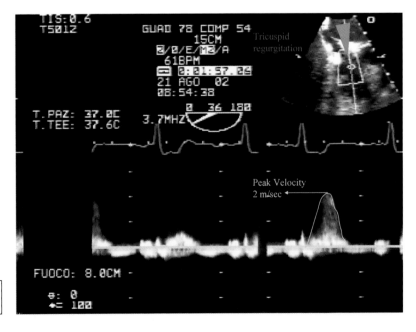

Figure 13.8. Systolic pulmonary pressure assessment. The peak velocity of the tricuspid regurgitation is 2 m/s (measured using CWD). According to the Bernoulli equation, the peak gradient is 16 mmHg. If the right atrial pressure is 10 mmHg, the systolic pulmonary pressure is 26 mmHg.

Box 13.2. Calculation of pressure gradients

Since the calculation of pressure gradients relies on the **square of velocity**, small errors in determining this last parameter are amplified. It is therefore very important to find the best parallel alignment of the Doppler signal with blood flow.

Once obtained, the measurement is reliable unless:

1. the velocity proximal to the stenosis exceeds 1.5 m/s
2. there are two stenotic lesions in the blood flow path (e.g. subaortic stenosis + aortic valve stenosis)
3. the stenotic lesion is very long, tunnel-like.

Box 13.3. Doppler estimations of pulmonary artery pressure and left atrial pressure

The assumption that RV systolic pressure is equal to pulmonary artery systolic pressure relies on the absence of pulmonary valve stenosis, and assumes that the systolic right ventricular pressure is equal to the systolic pulmonary artery pressure (sPAP) [18,19].

The assumption that LV systolic pressure is equal to aortic systolic pressure (systemic arterial pressure) relies on the absence of aortic valve stenosis. This measurement is difficult and prone to error. The driving pressure (sSAP) is very high, and a small error in the determination of the peak pressure gradient leads to an unacceptable error in LAP measurement. This is particlarly relevant, since accurate measurement of LAP may be important clinically [20].

volume of the regurgitant blood during the cardiac cycle [21–27].

Mitral regurgitation

The regurgitant volume (RV_{mitral}) is the difference between the volume entering the left ventricle during diastole (mitral inflow volume) and the volume leaving the left ventricle during systole through the aortic valve (aortic outflow volume):

$$RV_{mitral} = \text{Mitral inflow volume} - \text{Aortic outflow volume}$$
(13.11)

and the regurgitant fraction is:

$$\frac{RV_{mitral}}{\text{Mitral inflow volume}} \times 100$$
(13.12)

In order to solve the equations above, we need to know the transmitral inflow volume and the aortic outflow volume. Both are derived from Equation 13.1. The VTI of the mitral inflow and of the aortic outflow may be obtained according to the method described above for determining SV; the CSA of the mitral annulus and of the LVOT can be calculated with Equation 13.5 by measuring the annulus and LVOT diameters, as explained for the SV calculations.

However, as previously described, inaccuracies may occur owing to difficulties in calculating accurately the cross-sectional area of the mitral valve. This

technique should therefore be used with caution. The regurgitant volume of the mitral valve will be underestimated if there is concomitant aortic regurgitation.

Aortic regurgitation

The diastolic filling volume of the left ventricle is the sum of the aortic regurgitant volume and of the mitral inflow volume; according to the continuity equation it is equal to the aortic outflow volume. The aortic regurgitant volume (RV_{aortic}) is therefore:

$$RV_{aortic} = \text{Aortic outflow volume} - \text{Mitral inflow volume}$$
(13.13)

and the aortic regurgitant fraction is:

$$\frac{RV_{aortic}}{\text{Aortic outflow volume}} \times 100$$
(13.14)

The above equations may be solved with the same method applied for mitral regurgitation, although similar strong caveats apply regarding the estimation of transmitral volume. The regurgitant volume of the aortic valve will be underestimated if there is concomitant mitral regurgitation.

As a result of these difficulties, the severity of mitral and aortic valve regurgitation is not usually assessed by these techniques (see also Chapters 6 and 7).

Box 13.4. Measuring aortic stenosis by the continuity equation

Mitral and aortic regurgitant volumes and fractions are not usually estimated by the techniques described, because of inherent inaccuracies [21]. Mitral stenosis is most accurately assessed either by pressure half-time (PHT) or by proximal isovelocity surface area (PISA).

   Aortic stenosis, particulary in calcific aortic stenosis, is most accurately assessed by the continuity equation. However, there are potentially important sources of error.

   From the equation

$$AVA = \frac{LVOT\ area \times VTI_{LVOT}}{VTI_{aortic\ value}}$$

we need to measure the following:
- LVOT diameter, in order to calculate LVOT cross-sectional area
- pulsed-wave Doppler signal at the LVOT
- continuous-wave Doppler signal through the aortic valve

Typical values in aortic stenosis could be LVOT 2.1 cm, PWD VTI 12.1 cm, CWD VTI 50 cm. Thus:

$$AVA = \frac{(2.1)^2 \times 0.785 \times 12.1}{50} = 0.8\ cm^2$$

However, a 10% systematic error in the measurements could result in:

$$AVA = \frac{(2.3)^2 \times 0.785 \times 14}{45} = 1.3\ cm^2$$

Accuracy is essential. In particular:
- care in measuring the LVOT diameter
- optimal CWD beam alignment
- optimal PWD beam alignment, including care in avoiding the prestenotic flow acceleration region close to the stenotic valve [25].

Box 13.5. Aortic valve regurgitation pressure half-time

Aortic valve regurgitation PHT should be used with caution in the intraoperative setting. This index is strongly afterload-dependent, and the common changes in peripheral resistances that occur under general anesthesia may severely impair its reliability.

Mitral stenosis

Theoretically, the area of a stenotic mitral valve can be determined by planimetry using the basal transgastric view at the level of the mitral annulus. However, this measurement may be difficult in the presence of heavy calcification of the leaflets and/or annulus. Moreover, a small error in planimetry may result in a large underestimation of the valve area.

   Important information concerning mitral valve function and anatomy, and diastolic left ventricular function, may be obtained by the study of transmitral flow.

   Figure 13.9 shows a typical pattern of transmitral flow. Normally, it is composed of an E wave (passive rapid ventricular filling), and an A wave (atrial contraction). The E/A ratio is normally > 1, and decreases with age, reaching the value of 1 at about 60 years of age.

   Many parameters may be derived from the Doppler signal of mitral inflow. These include the transmitral pressure gradient, E/A peak velocities, and the deceleration time (DT). This latter is the time from the E-wave velocity peak to its intersection with the zero-velocity line (or extrapolation to the zero-velocity line). Its normal value is 140–200 ms, and it increases with age. The pressure half-time (PHT) is the time from the E-wave peak velocity to the time point at which the pressure gradient is halved (Fig. 13.10). The PHT strongly correlates with the mitral valve area (MVA), and can be calculated as follows:

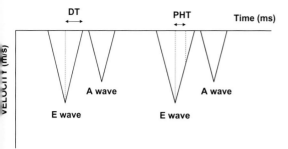

Figure 13.9. Normal transmitral flow.

$$MVA = 220/PHT \quad (13.15)$$

Although it is often reliable, potential errors with the PHT method may occur as a result of a rapid heart rate, the presence of aortic regurgitation, and alterations in compliance in the left atrium or left ventricle. In some patients the descending portion of the E wave is curvilinear rather than linear. In these circumstances the PHT should be calculated from the final, linear portion of the curve [6,22–24]. Estimations of mitral valve area based on PHT have not been validated immediately following mitral valve repair surgery, although PHT is often used in this way in clinical practice.

Finally, the MVA can be determined according to the continuity equation (Equation 13.4), based on the assumption that the volume entering the left ventricle during diastole (mitral inflow volume) is equal to the volume leaving the ventricle during systole (aortic outflow volume), assuming a steady state of ventricular performance. According to the equation used for the SV assessment:

$$MVA \times VTI_{mitral} = \text{Aortic outflow volume} \quad (13.16)$$

The aortic outflow volume is calculated with the equations used for the SV determination, and the mitral VTI is assessed from the transmitral flow profile. The MVA is:

$$MVA = \frac{SV_{aortic}}{VTI_{mitral}} \quad (13.17)$$

However, the use of the continuity equation for the determination of the MVA will be inaccurate in the presence of mitral and/or aortic regurgitation.

Aortic stenosis

The aortic valve area (AVA) may be determined with 2D planimetry using a mid-esophageal short-axis view as shown in Figure 13.6. However, planimetry may overestimate or underestimate aortic valve area [11], and therefore the AVA in aortic stenosis is usually determined using the continuity equation. The principle of measurement is that the flow through the LVOT is equal to the flow through the aortic valve.

Therefore:

$$AVA = \frac{LVOT\ area \times VTI_{LVOT}}{VTI_{aortic\ valve}} \quad (13.18)$$

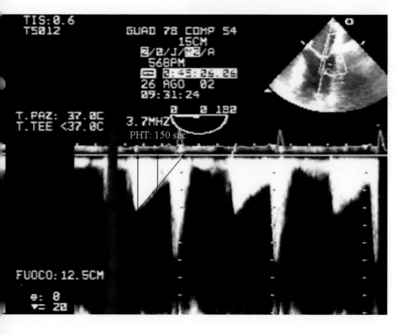

Figure 13.10. Mitral valve area assessment. The PHT is measured at 150 mmHg using CWD. The mitral valve area is 220/150 = 1.5 cm².

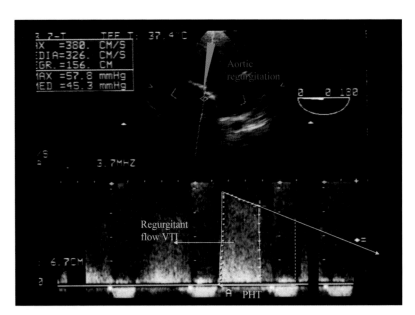

Figure 13.11. Pressure half-time (PHT) assessment of regurgitant aortic flow using CWD.

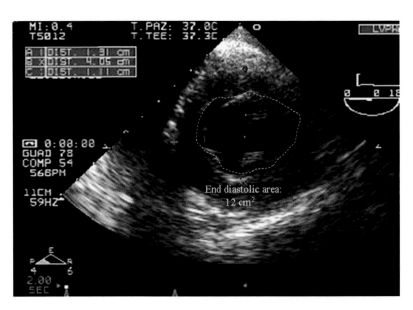

Figure 13.12. End-diastolic LV area assessment with a mid-papillary, transgastric view. End-diastolic diameters are measured.

In practice, the left ventricular outflow tract VTI (VTI_{LVOT}) should be determined at the level of the LVOT with a PWD signal, while the VTI of the aortic valve flow must be determined with a CWD signal.

Regurgitant valve lesions: effective regurgitant orifice area (EROA)

Both mitral valve and aortic valve regurgitant lesions may be quantified by applying the continuity equation (Equation 13.4), thus determining the regurgitant volume and the regurgitant fraction, as previously described. With the same equation it is possible to assess the EROA.

For a regurgitant valve, once we have determined the regurgitant volume, the EROA is:

$$EROA = \frac{\text{Regurgitant volume}}{\text{Regurgitant flow VTI}} \quad (13.19)$$

If we consider a regurgitant mitral valve, the regurgitant VTI is determined with a CWD signal of the

Table 13.1. Factors that influences left ventricular compliance

Myocardial ischemia
Restrictive cardiomyopathy
Right-to-left interventricular septal shift
Aortic stenosis
Cardiac tamponade
Myocardial fibrosis
Inotropic drug use
Hypertension

regurgitant flow. The same equation can be applied to a regurgitant aortic valve (Fig. 13.11) [26,27]. The analysis of a regurgitant aortic flow offers some more information about the aortic regurgitation severity.

The rate of velocity decline from its early peak to late diastole is proportional to the severity of the aortic regurgitation. This concept is expressed by the aortic regurgitation deceleration time (DT) and pressure half-time (PHT), which are analogous to the corresponding stenotic mitral valve values (see below). Usually, a PHT ≤ 250 ms is suggestive of severe aortic regurgitation.

Preload and fluid responsiveness assessment

These data are qualitative, but may be helpful in assessing some patients [28–50]. In clinical practice, left ventricular end-diastolic pressure (LVEDP) can be estimated using left atrial pressure or pulmonary artery wedge pressure (PAWP), but the relative invasiveness of the procedure, and in particular the difficulty of interpreting the data in chronically sick patients, have led to their value being questioned. Echocardiography may allow us to estimate left atrial pressure and LVEDP in a less invasive manner [28,29].

Two-dimensional imaging of the LV cavity allows the quantification of LV volumes. The calculations obtained correlate well with other techniques. The assessment of LV filling is routinely evaluated from the transgastric short-axis view at the level of the papillary muscles, since variations in volume are more easily seen in this plane than in the long axis. The end-diastolic area (Fig. 13.12) at the transgastric short-axis view has proved to be a more sensitive index of LV filling than PAWP during abdominal aortic aneurysmectomy [15]. An end-diastolic area ≤ 5 cm^2 per m^2 body surface area is accepted as the cutoff value for a hypovolemic state in hyperdynamic conditions (Videos 13.4 and 13.5).

The use of **mitral flow patterns** as a surrogate for LV pressure has some limitations, chiefly related to the influence of loading conditions and ventricular compliance (Table 13.1).

However, LVEDP can be estimated from the deceleration time (DT) of early diastolic mitral inflow using PWD. The sample volume (2 mm width) must be placed at the tips of the mitral leaflets and the DT must be measured on the early filling (E) wave, extrapolating

Figure 13.13. Pulmonary vein blood flow: pulsed-wave Doppler pattern.

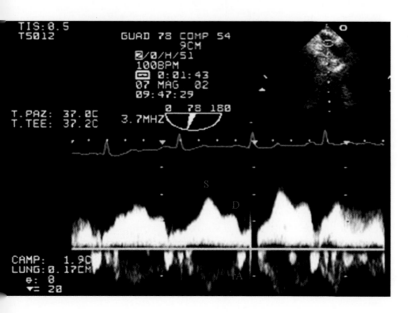

the descending slope to the baseline. This method correlates with pulmonary capillary wedge pressure (PCWP) in those patients with an ejection fraction less than 35%. The shorter the DT, the higher the PCWP. A DT $\geq$ 150 ms has a sensitivity of 93% and a specificity of 100% for predicting a PCWP $\leq$ 10 mmHg [30–35].

Pulmonary venous flow and especially the systolic/diastolic ratio strongly correlate with mean left atrial pressure, but this correlation depends on LV function and cardiac output. Pulmonary venous flow is examined by placing the PWD sample volume at least 1 cm into the pulmonary vein. Color-flow can often help to locate the ostium of the pulmonary veins (Video 13.6). Typically, pulmonary vein flow is composed of systolic (S), diastolic (D), and atrial reversal (rA) waves (Fig. 13.13). The S/D ratio and the velocity and duration of rA reflect ventricular compliance and ventricular filling pressure. In patients with preserved LV function the correlation is positive, so that a high left atrial pressure is represented by a high systolic wave. However, whenever LV contractility is depressed, high left atrial pressure is represented by an S wave of decreased amplitude [36–38].

Other modalities such as color M-mode and tissue Doppler imaging (TDI) have added other criteria for the evaluation of preload, and their use in combination with classical transmitral flow indices helps in the estimation of atrial pressure.

The flow velocity from the mitral inflow area towards the apex (from mitral valve plane to 4 cm distally into the LV cavity) can be measured using the transesophageal four-chamber view by placing an M-mode cursor in the center of the brightest color inflow. The information obtained by **color M-mode** is similar to the data obtained by simultaneously positioning more sample volumes at different levels from the mitral annulus to the apex of the LV. When the mitral valve opens, flow is initially propagated from the left atrium to the left ventricle. This corresponds to early filling (E wave in PWD study of mitral valve) followed by a second flow wave dependent on atrial contraction (A wave). Flow at the mitral valve clearly occurs earlier than at the LV apex. The transit time of flow from the mitral annulus to the apex is represented by the slope of the color wavefront. Adjusting the color Doppler setting to produce color aliasing, the slope of the first color alias, or of the color/non-color interface (black-to-red transition zone) during early filling, represents the flow propagation velocity (V_p) of

the blood flowing towards the apex [39–41]. Young healthy subjects typically have a $V_p \geq$ 55cm/s. Older patients, and those with LV hypertrophy and/or advanced diastolic dysfunction, have a lower V_p. The V_p has been shown to be correlated inversely with the time constant of LV isovolumic relaxation (τ) and to be relatively preload-independent. The ratio between the inflow velocity and the flow propagation velocity relates linearly to the mean left atrial pressure [42–44].

Tissue Doppler imaging (TDI) is a newer technique that records the systolic and diastolic velocities within the myocardium, often evaluated at the edge of the mitral annulus [45]. The Doppler signal arising from tissue motion differs from blood motion in two main respects:

1. Tissue velocities are lower (20 cm/s) than the velocities of red cells (20–100 cm/s).
2. The amplitude of the signal arising from cardiac structures (myocardium, mitral and tricuspid annulus) is significantly higher (approximately 100 times greater than blood cells).

Conventional blood-flow Doppler uses a high-pass filter to remove low velocities caused by wall motion. By rearranging the filter and the amplification (both gains and filter must be set low) the Doppler signal reflected by cardiac tissue can be displayed. The sample volume (5 mm) must be placed within the myocardium or at the mitral annulus (lateral or septal in the mid-esophageal four-chamber view), and a spectral recording of velocities is reproduced.

The spectral longitudinal velocity of the myocardium is represented by a systolic deflection (negative deflection), and two diastolic deflections (positive deflections) represent early filling (E_m) and atrial flow (A_m). The early diastolic wave at the mitral annulus reduces with age, and has been shown to be an index of LV relaxation that is relatively insensitive to left atrial pressure.

The ratio of transmitral E velocity to E_m has been recently demonstrated to correlate well with mean left atrial (or pulmonary capillary wedge) pressure in a number of clinical scenarios, including depressed or normal systolic LV function, hypertrophic cardiomyopathy, sinus tachycardia, and atrial fibrillation [46,47].

Doppler can be useful in assessing hemodynamic instability and hypotension caused by a reduction of biventricular preload (i.e. due to hemorrhage or pathologic fluid shifts) and in predicting the hemo-dynamic response to fluid loading. We may also need to take into account LV stroke volume variation as a result of the specific interactions of the heart and the lungs during intermittent positive pressure ventila-tion (IPPV) [48]. It is known that under these condi-tions variations in SV may be induced by the effects of IPPV on venous blood flow. These variations are more evident in patients with a reduced preload ("fluid responders"). This SV variation may be iden-tified with a CWD study of the aortic flow, and can be expressed in terms of aortic blood flow velocity variation. To measure this effect, more than one res-piratory cycle should be investigated. It may be use-ful to decrease the recording frequency in order to have as many aortic flow profiles as possible in the same screen. The maximal and minimal velocities should be measured, and the aortic blood velocity variation calculated; the difference between the two values divided by the mean value is the percentage variation. A value of about 12% has been demon-strated as a good cutoff for fluid responsiveness [49] (Fig. 13.14).

Doppler analysis of the transmitral flow has also been used as an index of fluid responsiveness. The ratio between the VTI of the E and A waves is an indicator of fluid responsiveness: the lower the val-ue, the more likely it is that the patient will benefit from fluid therapy, up to a ratio of 1.26 [50] (Fig. 13.15).

Semi-quantitative analysis of valve function

Semi-quantitative interpretation and analysis of blood flow proximal to and distal to the valve lesion, using Doppler (PWD, CWD) and color-flow Doppler are commonly used to evaluate the severity of heart valve disease. Several semi-quantitative classifications exist. These divide severity into three grades (mild, moder-ate, and severe) by assessing the pressure gradient across a stenotic valve, or with a regurgitant valve by assessing the area and maximum size of the regur-gitation jet signal into the relevant cardiac chamber [51,52].

In evaluating aortic stenosis, Doppler allows us to grade the severity by measuring the mean pressure gradient or by estimating the functional orifice area using the continuity equation.

However, the assessment of the severity of regur-gitant valves is more complex. The vena contracta, the area of the regurgitant jet, and the proximal isoveloc-ity surface area (PISA) method may be useful.

Vena contracta

The vena contracta is the narrowest part of the flow across the incompetent valve, just distal to the orifice. Its width, measured during color-flow Doppler exami-nation, can be used to evaluate the grade of the valve regurgitation [53–57].

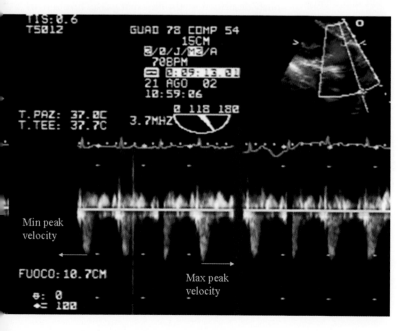

Figure 13.14. Aortic blood velocity variation measured with CWD in a long-axis transgastric view.

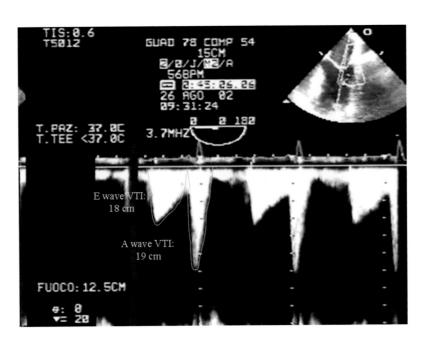

Figure 13.15. E/A wave VTI ratio for an indirect preload assessment. The ratio is 0.94, suggestive of fluid responsiveness of the patient.

Area of regurgitant jet

The area of the regurgitant jet may be proportional to the regurgitant volume, and may be considered as an index of the severity of a lesion. However, the spatial disposition of the jet may be affected by the geometry of the orifice, leading either to free flow into the center of the receiving chamber or to a small and narrow flow jet following a tissue surface, for example the left atrium. This is an example of the Coanda effect [58].

In this latter case a small visual color signal suggesting a small area of regurgitation is possibly a regurgitant jet with a high velocity secondary to a severe valvular lesion. The regurgitant jet area should therefore be used with caution when assessing severity of regurgitant lesions.

PISA

The proximal isovelocity surface area (PISA) method, which estimates regurgitation volume quantitatively, has been utilized for evaluating valve diseases [59–61]. It is another application of the continuity principle. The velocity of the flow increases symmetrically and progressively as it approaches a regurgitant or stenotic orifice (proximal convergence zone). In this zone the flow velocity appears organized into a series of shells of hemispherical shape. Each of these hemispheres is visible with color-flow Doppler at every point where aliasing occurs because the velocity exceeds the Nyquist limit. At the aliasing boundary there is a sharp color transition from bright blue to bright yellow. This aliasing point defines the radius of the isovelocity contour. In practice the aliasing boundary is often too close to the orifice, so the measurement of the radius can be imprecise. We can resolve this problem by creating the transition from blue to yellow at a lower velocity by reducing the color-flow scale setting (Nyquist limit). This will increase the PISA radius. This larger radius is easier to measure and allows more accurate flow calculations. From the principle of the conservation of mass, previously described, all the flow that passes through the area of any one of these hemispheres (CSA_{PISA}) is destined to pass through the regurgitant or stenotic orifice area ($CSA_{orifice}$). Thus a knowledge of the instantaneous flow at the isovelocity hemisphere enables us to calculate the orifice area. The area of a hemisphere can be calculated as $2\pi r^2$, where r is the radius from the orifice to the aliasing boundary. The instantaneous flow rate at that hemisphere (Q) is calculated by multiplying the area of the hemisphere ($2\pi r^2$) by the aliasing velocity (V_{PISA}).

Thus:

$$Q = 2\pi r^2\, V_{PISA} \qquad (13.20)$$

From the continuity equation:

Flow at orifice = Flow at PISA

$$CSA_{orifice} \times V_{max\text{-}orifice} = CSA_{PISA} \times V_{PISA}$$

$$CSA_{orifice} = \frac{CSA_{PISA} \times V_{PISA}}{V_{max\text{-}orifice}} \qquad (13.21)$$

The regurgitant volume can be estimated as $CSA_{orifice}$ multiplied by regurgitant VTI. The above calculations can be accurately performed only if the region of PISA appears hemispheric. To ensure this, the beam should be oriented parallel to flow and the color Doppler baseline shifted toward the direction of regurgitant flow until a semicircular area of PISA is easily visualized. This topic is further explored in Chapter 7.

Limitations of hemodynamic calculations

The accuracy of measuring blood flow velocity by Doppler depends on a parallel alignment of the ultrasound beam and the direction of blood flow. Thus the Doppler beam should be orientated as parallel as possible to the blood flow. Angle correction, although possible, is not recommended. If the difference between the angle of the Doppler beam and the direction of blood flow is $\leq 20°$ then the error in velocity measurement will be $\leq 10\%$. This is not important when investigating low-velocity jets, but in the case of a high-velocity jet a small error in the parallel orientation of the beam may be responsible for underestimating a pressure gradient because of the mathematical relationship between the velocity and the pressure gradient. Accurate flow measurements are best made where the cardiac dimensions are relatively constant throughout the cardiac cycle and thus an accurate measure of the cross-sectional area is possible. Similar considerations apply to other situations where difficulties may be encountered, e.g. annular or leaflet calcification, or prosthetic valves. It is

essential that where necessary the landmarks needed to measure the diameter of relevant structures (e.g. aortic valve annulus) are accurately visualized.

Conclusions

The quantification of hemodynamics by Doppler echocardiography using transesophageal windows may be useful in providing rapid information useful in the acute management of some patients. The data obtained should always be interpreted with caution and in association with data obtained from other modalities.

References

1. Practice guidelines for perioperative transesophageal echocardiography. A report by the American Society of Anesthesiologists and the Society of Cardiovascular Anesthesiologists Task Force on Transesophageal Echocardiography. *Anesthesiology* 1996; **84**: 986–1006.

2. Shanewise JS, Cheung AT, Aronson S, *et al*. ASE/SCA guidelines for performing a comprehensive intraoperative multiplane transesophageal echocardiography examination: recommendations of the ASE Council for intraoperative echocardiography and the SCA Task Force for certification in perioperative transesophageal echocardiography. *Anesth Analg* 1999; **89**: 870–84.

3. Cheitlin MD, Armstrong WF, Aurigemma GP, *et al*. ACC/AHA/ASE 2003 Guideline Update for the Clinical Application of Echocardiography: summary article. *J Am Soc Echocardiogr* 2003; **16**: 1091–110.

4. Cahalan MK, Abel M, Goldman M, *et al*. American Society of Echocardiography and Society of Cardiovascular Anesthesiologists task force guidelines for training in perioperative echocardiography. *Anesth Analg* 2002; **94**: 1384–8.

5. Quiñones MA, Douglas PS, Foster E, *et al*. ACC/AHA clinical competence statement on echocardiography: a report of the American College of Cardiology/ American Heart Association/ American College of Physicians – American Society of Internal Medicine Task Force on Clinical Competence. *J Am Coll Cardiol* 2003; **41**: 687–708.

6. Quiñones MA, Otto CM, Stoddard M, Waggoner A, Zoghbi WA. Recommendations for quantification of Doppler echocardiography: a report from the Doppler Quantification Task Force of the Nomenclature and Standards Committee of the American Society of Echocardiography. *J Am Soc Echocardiogr* 2002; **15**: 167–84.

7. Szokol JW, Murphy GS. Transesophageal echocardiographic monitoring of hemodynamics. *Int Anesthesiol Clin* 2004; **42**: 59–81.

8. Brown JM. Use of echocardiography for hemodynamic monitoring. *Crit Care Med* 2002; **30**: 1361–4.

9. Flachskampf FA, Decoodt P, Fraser AG, *et al*. Working Group on Echocardiography of the European Society of Cardiology. Guidelines from the Working Group. Recommendations for performing transesophageal echocardiography. *Eur J Echocardiogr* 2001; **2**: 8–21.

10. Currie PJ, Hagler DJ, Seward JB, *et al*. Instantaneous pressure gradient: a simultaneous Doppler and dual catheter correlative study. *J Am Coll Cardiol* 1986; **7**: 800–6.

11. Richards KL, Cannon SR, Miller JF, Crawford MH. Calculation of aortic valve area by Doppler echocardiography: a direct application of the continuity equation. *Circulation* 1986; **73**: 964–9.

12. Huntsman LL, Stewart DK, Barnes SR, *et al*. Noninvasive Doppler determination of cardiac output in man: clinical validation. *Circulation* 1983; **67**: 593–602.

13. Dittmann H, Voelker W, Karsch KR, Seipel L. Influence of sampling site and flow area on cardiac output measurements by Doppler echocardiography. *J Am Coll Cardiol* 1987; **10**: 818–23.

14. Muhiudeen IA, Kuecherer HF, Lee E, Cahalan MK, Schiller NB. Intraoperative estimation of cardiac output by transesophageal pulsed Doppler echocardiography. *Anesthesiology* 1991; **74**: 9–14.

15. Ryan T, Page R, Bouchier-Hayes D, Cunningham AJ. Transoesophageal pulsed wave Doppler measurement of cardiac output during major vascular surgery: comparison with the thermodilution technique. *Br J Anaesth* 1992; **69**: 101–4.

16. Darmon PL, Hillel Z, Mogtader A, Mindich B, Thys D. Cardiac output by transesophageal echocardiography using continuous-wave Doppler across the aortic valve. *Anesthesiology* 1994; **80**: 796–805.

17. Hatle L, Angelsen BA, Tromsdal A. Non-invasive assessment of aortic stenosis by Doppler ultrasound. *Br Heart J* 1980; **43**: 284–92.

18. Yock PG, Popp RL. Noninvasive estimation of right ventricular systolic pressure by Doppler ultrasound in patients with tricuspid regurgitation. *Circulation* 1984; **70**: 657–62.

19. Kircher BJ, Himelman RB, Schiller NB. Noninvasive estimation of right atrial pressure from the inspiratory collapse of the inferior vena cava. *Am J Cardiol* 1990; **66**: 493–6.

20. Ge ZM, Zhang Y, Fan DS, *et al*. Quantification of left-side intracardiac pressures and gradients using mitral and aortic regurgitant velocities by simultaneous left and right catheterization and continuous wave Doppler echocardiography. *Clin Cardiol* 1993; **16**: 863–70.

21. Rokey R, Sterling LL, Zoghbi WA, *et al*. Determination of regurgitant fraction in isolated mitral or aortic regurgitation by pulsed Doppler two-dimensional echocardiography. *J Am Coll Cardiol* 1986; **7**: 1273–8.

22. Hatle L, Brubakk A, Tromsdal A, Angelsen B. Noninvasive assesment of pressure drop in mitral stenosis by Doppler ultrasound. *Heart* 1978; **40**: 131–40.

23. Hatle L, Angelsen B, Tromsdal A. Noninvasive assessment of atrioventricular pressure half-time by Doppler ultrasound. *Circulation* 1979; **60**: 1096–104.

24. Loyd D, Ask P, Wranne B. Pressure half-time does not always predict mitral valve area correctly. *J Am Soc Echocardiogr* 1988; **1**: 313–21.

25. Skjaerpe T, Hegrenaes L, Hatle L. Noninvasive estimation of valve area in patients with aortic stenosis by Doppler ultrasound and two-dimensional echocardiography. *Circulation* 1985; **72**: 810–18.

26. Reimold SC, Ganz P, Bittl JA, *et al*. Effective aortic regurgitant orifice area: description of a method based on the conservation of mass. *J Am Coll Cardiol* 1991; **18**: 761–8.

27. Enriquez-Sarano M, Seward JB, Bailey KR, Tajik AJ. Effective regurgitant orifice area: a non-invasive Doppler development of an old hemodynamic concept. *J Am Coll Cardiol*. 1994; **23**: 443–51.

28. Rokey R, Kuo LC, Zoghbi WA, Limacher MC, Quiñones MA. Determination of parameters of left ventricular diastolic filling with pulsed Doppler echocardiography: comparison with cineangiography. *Circulation* 1985; **71**: 543–50.

29. Choong CY, Herrman HC, Weyman AE, Fifer MA. Preload dependence of Doppler-derived indexes of left ventricular diastolic function in humans. *J Am Coll Cardiol* 1987; **10**: 800–8.

30. Appleton CP, Hatle LK, Popp RL. Relation of transmitral flow velocity patterns to left ventricular diastolic function: new insights from a combined hemodynamic and Doppler echocardiographic study. *J Am Coll Cardiol* 1988; **12**: 426–40.

31. Vanoverschelde JL, Raphael DA, Robert AR, Cosyns JR. Left ventricular filling in dilated cardiomyopathy: relation to functional class and hemodynamics. *J Am Coll Cardiol* 1990; **15**: 1288–95.

32. Jaffe WM, Dewhurst TA, Otto CM, Pearlman AS. Influence of Doppler sample volume location on ventricular filling velocities. *Am J Cardiol* 1991; **68**: 550–2.

33. Benjamin EJ, Levy D, Anderson KM, *et al*. Determinants of Doppler indexes of left ventricular diastolic function in normal subjects (the Framingham Heart Study). *Am J Cardiol* 1992; **70**: 508–15.

34. Giannuzzi P, Imparato A, Temporelli PL, *et al.* Doppler-derived mitral deceleration time of early filling as a strong predictor of pulmonary capillary wedge pressure in postinfarction patients with left ventricular systolic dysfunction. *J Am Coll Cardiol* 1994; **23**: 1630–7.

35. Hurrell DG, Nishimura RA, Ilstrup DM, Appleton CP. Utility of preload alteration in assessment of left ventricular filling pressure by Doppler echocardiography: a simultaneous catheterization and Doppler echocardiographic study. *J Am Coll Cardiol* 1997; **30**: 459–67.

36. Nishimura RA, Abel MD, Hatle LK, Tajik AJ. Relation of pulmonary vein to mitral flow velocities by transesophageal Doppler echocardiography: effect of different loading conditions. *Circulation* 1990; **81**: 1488–97.

37. Kuecherer HF, Muhiudeen IA, Kusumoto FM, *et al.* Estimation of mean left atrial pressure from transesophageal pulsed Doppler echocardiography of pulmonary venous flow. *Circulation* 1990; **82**: 1127–39.

38. Hoit BD, Shao Y, Gabel M, Walsh RA. Influence of loading conditions and contractile state on pulmonary venous flow: validation of Doppler velocimetry. *Circulation* 1992; **86**: 651–9.

39. Steen T, Steen S. Filling of a model left ventricle studied by colour M mode Doppler. *Cardiovasc Res* 1994; **28**: 1821–7.

40. Barbier P, Grimaldi A, Alimento M, Berna G, Guazzi MD. Echocardiographic determinants of mitral early flow propagation velocity. *Am J Cardiol* 2002; **90**: 613–19.

41. Takatsuji H, Mikami T, Urasawa K, *et al.* A new approach for evaluation of left ventricular diastolic function: spatial and temporal analysis of left ventricular filling flow propagation by color M-mode Doppler echocardiography. *J Am Coll Cardiol* 1996; **27**: 365–71.

42. Stugaard M, Smiseth OA, Risoe C, Ihlen H. Intraventricular early diastolic filling during acute myocardial ischemia, assessment by multigated color M-mode Doppler echocardiography. *Circulation* 1993; **88**: 2705–13.

43. Stugaard M, Risoe C, Ihlen H, Smiseth OA. Intracavitary filling pattern in the failing left ventricle assessed by color M-mode Doppler echocardiography. *J Am Coll Cardiol* 1994; **24**: 663–70.

44. Garcia MJ, Palac RT, Malenka DJ, Terrell P, Plehn JF. Color M-mode Doppler flow propagation velocity is a relatively preload-independent index of left ventricular filling. *J Am Soc Echocardiogr* 1999; **2**: 129–37.

45. Rodriguez L, Garcia M, Ares M, *et al.* Assessment of mitral annular dynamics during diastole by Doppler tissue imaging: comparison with mitral Doppler inflow in subjects without heart disease and in patients with left ventricular hypertrophy. *Am Heart J* 1996; **131**: 982–7.

46. Oki T, Tabata T, Yamada H, *et al.* Clinical application of pulsed Doppler tissue imaging for assessing abnormal left ventricular relaxation. *Am J Cardiol* 1997; **79**: 921–8.

47. Nagueh SF, Middleton KJ, Kopelen HA, Zoghbi WA, Quiñones MA. Doppler tissue imaging: a noninvasive technique for evaluation of left ventricular relaxation and estimation of filling pressures. *J Am Coll Cardiol* 1997; **30**: 1527–33.

48. Reuter DA, Goetz AE, Peter K. Assessment of volume responsiveness in mechanically ventilated patients. *Anaesthesist* 2003; **52**: 1005–13.

49. Reuter DA, Felbinger TW, Schmidt C, *et al.* Stroke volume variations for assessment of cardiac responsiveness to volume loading in mechanically ventilated patients after cardiac surgery. *Intensive Care Med* 2002; **28**: 392–8.

50. Lattik R, Couture P, Denault AY, *et al.* Mitral Doppler indices are superior to two-dimensional echocardiographic and hemodynamic variables in predicting responsiveness of cardiac output to a rapid intravenous infusion of colloid. *Anesth Analg* 2002; **94**: 1092–9.

51. Perry GJ, Helmcke F, Nanda NC, Byard C, Soto B. Evaluation of aortic insufficiency by Doppler color flow mapping. *J Am Coll Cardiol* 1987; **9**: 952–9.

52. Miyatake K, Izumi S, Okamoto M, *et al.* Semiquantitative grading of severity of mitral regurgitation by real time two dimensional Doppler flow imaging technique. *J Am Coll Cardiol* 1986; **7**: 82–8.

53. Tribouilloy C, Shen WF, Quéré JP, *et al.* Assessment of severity of mitral regurgitation by measuring regurgitant jet width at its origin with transesophageal Doppler color flow imaging. *Circulation* 1992; **85**: 1248–53.

54. Fehske W, Omran H, Manz M, *et al.* Color-coded Doppler imaging of the vena contracta as a basis for quantification of pure mitral regurgitation. *Am J Cardiol* 1994; **73**: 268 –74.

55. Grayburn PA, Fehske W, Omran H, Brickner ME, Luderitz B. Multiplane transesophageal echocardiographic assessment of mitral regurgitation by Doppler color flow mapping of the vena contracta. *Am J Cardiol* 1994; **74**: 912–17.

56. Hall SA, Brickner ME, Willett DL, *et al.* Assessment of mitral regurgitation severity by Doppler color flow mapping of the vena contracta. *Circulation* 1997; **95**: 636–42.

221

57. Tribouilloy CM, Enriquez-Sarano M, Bailey KR, Seward JB, Tajik AJ. Assessment of severity of aortic regurgitation using the width of the vena contracta. *Circulation* 2000; **102**: 558–64.

58. Chao K, Moises VA, Shandas R, *et al.* Influence of the Coanda effect on color Doppler jet area and color encoding. In vitro studies using color Doppler flow mapping. *Circulation* 1992; **85**: 333–41.

59. Utsunomiya T, Doshi R, Patel D, *et al.* Calculation of volume flow rate by the proximal isovelocity surface area method: simplified approach using color Doppler zero baseline shift. *J Am Coll Cardiol* 1993; **22**: 277–82.

60. Enriquez-Sarano M, Miller FA, Hayes SN, *et al.* Effective mitral regurgitant orifice area: clinical use and pitfalls of the proximal isovelocity surface area method. *J Am Coll Cardiol* 1995; **25**: 703–9.

61. Tribouilloy CM, Enriquez-Sarano M, Fett SL, *et al.* Application of the proximal flow convergence method to calculate the effective regurgitant orifice area in aortic regurgitation. *J Am Coll Cardiol* 1998; **32**: 1032–9.

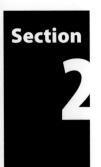

Practical issues in transesophageal echocardiography

14

Ischemic heart disease

Conventional myocardial revascularization

Patrick Wouters

Introduction

Several studies suggest that routine performance of transesophageal echocardiography (TEE) during coronary artery bypass grafting (CABG) is associated with improved outcomes, including a reduction in morbidity and mortality, and reduced duration of hospitalization [1–4].

However, the utilization of TEE for CABG surgery varies among different institutions and depends primarily on local protocols, the availability of trained staff, and resources. In 2003, guidelines for clinical application of echocardiography were published [5], including an intraoperative section based on previous recommendations [6]. CABG surgery patients may be considered to be at increased risk of myocardial ischemia, myocardial infarction (MI), or hemodynamic disturbances, which are considered a Class IIa indication for intraoperative TEE. However, acute hemodynamic disturbance may be considered a Class I indication. Clearly there is still some divergence of opinion about the usefulness and efficacy of TEE as a diagnostic and monitoring tool to improve outcome in CABG patients, although the trend seems to be moving strongly in favor of utilization.

It is important to recognize that the clinical utility of TEE in CABG is based on many factors and is not simply restricted to monitoring myocardial ischemia. It provides valuable information on the following:

- Other pathological conditions that are commonly present in patients with ischemic heart disease (IHD), e.g. the presence and extent of aortic atheromatous disease, which clearly has an impact on morbidity and mortality [7].
- An unexpected and previously undiagnosed defect may be found on routine TEE, necessitating a revision of the initial surgical plan or postoperative strategy [2].
- As a dynamic and integrated monitoring window on cardiac performance and an excellent guide to hemodynamic management [8–10].
- Earlier detection of procedure-related complications.

Although several of these aspects are also addressed in other chapters, this section of this chapter is directed towards an intervention-related analysis, combining all the utilities of TEE in a systematic approach towards the patient undergoing CABG surgery.

Detection and quantification of atheromatous aortic disease

Atherosclerosis of the thoracic aorta is a significant risk factor for perioperative cerebral injury and death after cardiac surgery [11–13]. Determination of the severity of aortic atheromatous disease with TEE has been considered a critical element in the management of CABG patients. Furthermore, it has been shown that the severity of descending aortic atheromatous disease, as assessed by TEE, predicted stroke and death associated with CABG surgery [14].

The degree [13] and localization [15] of aortic atherosclerosis can be assessed using a five-point scale previously described (see Chapter 12, Table 12.3). Localization of the lesions is based on a six-segment model, with each segment further divided into four quadrants. When examining the aorta, the depth settings should be turned down to 6 cm or lower, the gain decreased, and the highest ultrasound frequency used to improve image resolution (Fig. 14.1; Video 14.1). Although intraoperative TEE evaluation of aortic atheromatous disease is superior to surgical palpation, and was found to provide accurate and reproducible data [16], complete imaging of the thoracic aorta is not possible [17]. In particular, the mid-to-distal portion of the ascending aorta is not well visualized with

225

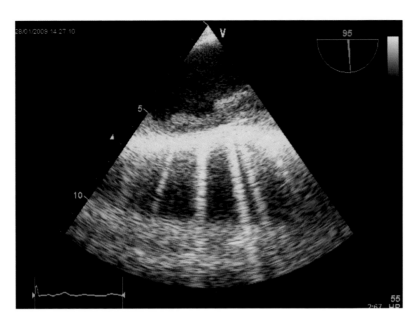

Figure 14.1. Atheroma in the descending aorta.

TEE due to interposition of the airways [18]. Since atheromatous disease can be focal and restricted to these segments, the utility of TEE in guiding surgical manipulations such as aortic cross-clamping has been questioned, and epiaortic scanning has been recommended instead [19,20]. A novel technique has been described to circumvent this problem, which may aid atheroma detection [21]. However, the detection of atheromata in the descending aorta with TEE has a positive predictive value for disease of the ascending aorta of 39% [15].

In clinical practice, the routine use of TEE may be valuable to screen for the presence of aortic atheromatous disease, since it is an important determinant of risk, particularly in patients older than 65 years. The consequence of detecting severe aortic disease should be the implementation of a strategy designed to deal with this diagnosis. Several solutions have been proposed to reduce the risk for thromboembolic complications in such patients. These include alternative sites for cannulation and proximal anastomoses, maximal use of arterial *in situ* grafts, the use of an intra-aortic filter [22–24], and a clampless proximal anastomosing device [25]. In addition, major interventions, including atherectomy or even replacement of the ascending aorta under deep hypothermic circulatory arrest, have been described [26]. Until recently, the results of such modifications have not been convincing [27]. Currently a promising solution is the use of off-pump CABG with complete arterial revascularization (OPCAB: see below).

Unexpected findings and associated disease in CABG surgery

A routine baseline TEE examination at the beginning of surgery may reveal a new and unexpected finding in 8–25% of patients. This may result in a primary or secondary interventional modification. The decision as to whether to alter the surgical plan is one of the most challenging dilemmas in cardiac surgery, and must be based on a number of aspects, including:

- the nature and severity of the newly diagnosed lesion
- its natural progression
- the risk profile and life expectancy of the patient
- the risk of the modified surgical intervention as compared to the originally planned procedure

Informed consent cannot be obtained from the anesthetized patient, and the available scientific evidence is often limited to case reports or small-scale studies. For the anesthesiologist involved in this decision, it is a prerequisite to have an advanced level of training in perioperative echocardiography. However, it is wise to be able to consult more widely and seek a specialist cardiological opinion when appropriate.

Patent foramen ovale (PFO)

PFO is the most frequently reported new diagnosis [3] (Fig. 14.2; Video 14.2). It is a common observation in about 25% of postmortem studies, and TEE is able to

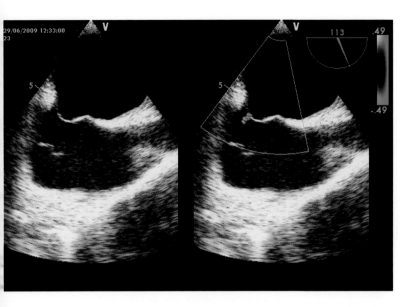

Figure 14.2. Color-flow Doppler reveals a small atrial septal defect with left-to-right shunt.

detect it with about the same frequency in the clinical setting. There is no clear answer as to whether a PFO should be repaired during CABG surgery. While PFO is usually a benign and asymptomatic defect, the peri-operative setting may expose the patient to increased risk for paradoxical embolism and cyanosis with right-to-left shunting [28].

An association has been reported between PFO and new-onset atrial fibrillation after conventional CABG, suggesting that pre-emptive therapy could be considered when PFO is diagnosed [29].

Atrial thrombus

TEE is a highly accurate method for identifying atrial thrombus [30–32]. It should be suspected whenever a patient presents with a history of atrial fibrillation, and when spontaneous echo contrast ("smoke") or enlarged atriae are seen on TEE examination. The diagnosis of atrial thrombus directs the surgical plan towards atriotomy and removal, or ligation of the atrial appendage.

Aortic valve disease

With aging of the CABG population, a substantial number of patients present with asymptomatic mild to moderate aortic stenosis or regurgitation, which is usually detected during angiography or preoperative transthoracic echo (TTE). Symptomatic severe aortic stenosis (AS) has long been recognized as an indication for aortic valve replacement. The management of asymptomatic patients with severe AS who are not undergoing other cardiac surgery is constantly under review [33]. However, in patients who are scheduled

for CABG surgery, aortic valve replacement (AVR) is recommended for those with either severe or moderate AS, but not for those with mild AS unless there is significant suspicion of an accelerating stenotic process such as significant calcification [34].

Similarly, the patient with low-gradient/low-flow AS may present a significant management problem. Although the level of evidence is currently weak, both American and European guidelines currently give strong consideration to the advisability of AVR in such patients who are already undergoing CABG surgery [34,35].

Proponents of AVR at the time of CABG argue that it will avoid the need for re-operation when or if the patient becomes symptomatic, and that one should not miss an optimal "window of opportunity" before left ventricular (LV) dysfunction appears. Opponents will point to the increased risk of a combined procedure, to the late morbidity, including endocarditis, embolism, and hemorrhage, and to the mortality associated with valve prostheses.

The immediate operative risk has been reported to increase from 1–3% with isolated CABG [36] to 6–7% with combined AVR and CABG [34]. The progression of aortic stenosis is about 0.1 cm^2 decrease of aortic valve area per year, or an increase of 5–10 mmHg in transvalvular gradient per year [33]. This progression is faster in older patients, when the valve is calcified, when leaflet mobility is restricted, and when the gradient at the time of diagnosis is higher than 25 mmHg mean [33,37]. However, if the main defect is restricted leaflet mobility in the presence of IHD, the rate of progress of the valve stenosis is much less clear.

The dilemma for the intraoperative echocardiographer is evident when the diagnosis of mild or moderate AS is only revealed for the first time under surgery. This requires expert evaluation of the aortic valve, and careful and focused decision making as to the best operative procedure. The dilemma is always best avoided by good preoperative assessment.

Aortic regurgitation is common, occurring in up to 53% of apparently healthy individuals above 60 years of age [38]. Unforeseen AR requiring valve replacement is rare, but even mild AR may complicate surgery if it is associated with inadequate delivery of antegrade cardioplegia [39].

Mitral valve disease

In most patients scheduled to undergo elective CABG surgery, the presence of mitral valve (MV) disease is well documented. Occasionally the intraoperative findings do not match the preoperative record, particularly in emergencies. There is consensus that mild mitral regurgitation (MR) (grade 1–2) requires no treatment and severe MR (grade 4) should be treated at the time of CABG. Recent practice guidelines suggest that if there is a structural abnormality such as prolapse or flail, the valve should be repaired or replaced [34]. However, this is a more challenging decision if off-pump surgical revascularization (OPCAB) was planned specifically to avoid the potential adverse effects of cardiopulmonary bypass.

Patients with severe ischemic MR should undergo MV repair or MV replacement, and the presence of symptomatic heart failure at the time of CABG surgery would support a decision to correct MR [34,40]. However, controversy exists as to whether patients having CABG surgery with moderate or mild MR should undergo MV surgery. In patients with moderate MR, early data suggest that the addition of corrective MV surgery to planned CABG may confer no additional benefit [41,42]. However, recent data suggest that long-term outcomes, both mortality and quality of life, appear to be better if MR is corrected at the time of CABG [43–47].

It is important to recognize that intraoperative TEE underestimates the severity of MR, because of more favorable hemodynamic conditions under general anesthesia [34,48]. An accurate assessment of true MR is more difficult intraoperatively, but the likelihood is that the degree of MR will be underestimated, and this should be borne in mind when considering the place of concomitant MV surgery.

Intraoperative monitoring with TEE during CABG surgery

General hemodynamics

TEE is used intraoperatively as a monitor of ventricular function and volume. An assessment of the accuracy of real-time interpretation of TEE information on hemodynamics using biplane echoprobes in CABG patients suggested that, in 75% of the analyses, the quantification of ejection fraction area and volume surrogates performed intraoperatively with TEE was within 10% of values obtained in offline analysis [49]. In a subsequent paper, the authors found TEE to be most influential on intraoperative decision making in about 20% of instances. Most of these comprised volume corrections and 3% were surgical interventions [9]. Others observed a similar pattern, with a predominant role for TEE in guiding clinical interventions in 25% of the cases studied [4,8].

Myocardial ischemia

The hallmark of myocardial ischemia is regional heterogeneity in the extent and time course of systolic wall motion. Alterations in regional function appear almost instantly when subendocardial blood flow is reduced, even before ST-segment changes occur. The sensitivity of TEE for myocardial ischemia is higher than sensitivity using ECG analysis, but its specificity is lower: regional wall motion abnormalities (RWMAs) can also be evoked by other mechanisms, for example by changes in loading conditions and by conduction delays or ventricular pacing [50,51] (Videos 14.3–14.6). Global diastolic function is also sensitive to myocardial ischemia, and acute changes in LV filling patterns occur early in the course of myocardial ischemia. Only when more than 40% of the muscle is involved does global ventricular systolic function deteriorate.

TEE is used to describe the presence of RWMAs in terms of severity and location. A complete mapping of the heart with preferably digital storage of the images is mandatory to allow comparison with the status after revascularization.

Topography

Multiplane echocardiography allows us to locate the area of dysfunction and identify the supplying coronary

A

Left Ventricular Segmentation

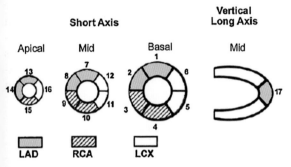

1. basal anterior
2. basal anteroseptal
3. basal inferoseptal
4. basal inferior
5. basal inferolateral
6. basal anterolateral

7. mid anterior
8. mid anteroseptal
9. mid inferoseptal
10. mid inferior
11. mid inferolateral
12. mid anterolateral

13. apical anterior
14. apical septal
15. apical inferior
16. apical lateral
17. apex

B

Coronary Artery Territories

Figure 14 3. (A) Topography related to perfusion territories of the major coronary branches. (B) Segmental numbers correspond to those shown in (A). LAD, left anterior descending; RCA, right coronary artery; LCX, circumflex coronary artery. Reproduced with permission from Cerqueira *et al.*, *Circulation* 2002; **105**: 539–42 [53].

artery. The original 16-segment model described to enable a framework for the assessment and classification of RWMAs [52] has recently been updated to a 17-segment model [53]. This now complies with the nomenclature used for other types of imaging in clinical practice (Fig. 14. 3). All the segments may be visualized with the views shown in Figure 9.6, with the exception of the apical cap, which is not usually seen by TEE.

The epicardial coronary arteries can also be seen at their origin from the aortic root (Fig. 14.4). The left and right coronary ostia are visualized with a mid-esophageal short-axis view (20–40°). Immediately above the sinus of Valsalva the left ostium is located at 2–3 o'clock, and the right coronary ostium is at 7 o'clock. The left main CA can be traced to a variable extent up to its branching into the circumflex and left anterior descending coronary arteries. Although calcifications and coronary plaques can be identified here with TEE,

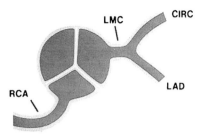

Figure 14.4. Schematic diagram of the aortic valve and coronary ostia. CIRC, circumflex coronary artery; LAD, left anterior descending coronary artery; LMC, left main coronary artery; RCA, right coronary artery.

they have little diagnostic value, as correlations with the degree of flow obstruction are poor. In acute aortic dissection it is possible to determine the involvement of the coronary ostia and look for the presence of color Doppler flow in the main coronary branches.

Quantification of regional contractile dysfunction

In clinical practice, wall motion is evaluated and scored using a semi-quantitative system that appears to correlate well with quantitative measures of coronary perfusion in patients with prior myocardial infarction (Table 14.1) [54]. Scoring is based on a visual analysis of inward wall motion signifying endocardial excursion and/or myocardial thickening as shown by the change in distance from the epicardium to the endocardium.

Wall thickening is a more reliable sign than endocardial movement, since akinetic segments may appear to move inward due to tethering from adjacent normal or hyperkinetic myocardium. Owing to the translational and rotational movements of the heart, endocardial excursion does not uniformly occur towards a single center on a fixed axis, and the use of a floating axis does not fully solve this problem. This may result is "pseudothickening," a visible phenomenon that occurs when the heart moves laterally through the imaging plane, creating the illusion of a change in wall thickness [55].

Suboptimal alignment of the probe along the axis of the heart may also result in changing cross-sections during systole and diastole with subsequent over- or underestimation of endocardial excursion (e.g. apical foreshortening).

Wall thickening measurements require an optimal endo- and epicardial border delineation. In clinical practice this is often complicated by image degradation or dropout at the lateral borders of the sector. In addition, the temporal resolution of the human eye is low,

Table 14.1. Semi-quantitative system for assessing left ventricular wall motion

Semi-quantitative	Endocardial excursion	Wall thickening	Score
Normal	> 30%	+++	1
Mild hypokinesis	10–30%	++	2
Severe hypokinesis	>0 but <10%	+	3
Akinesia	0	0	4
Dyskinesia	Systolic bulging	–	5

and subtle alterations in the timing of wall motion during the cardiac cycle (e.g. postsystolic wall thickening which does not contribute to ejection) are difficult to detect. M-mode echocardiography has the best temporal resolution but can only be applied to a limited number of segments.

Myocardial strain rate imaging, a technique based on color Doppler measurement of differential tissue velocities, is a promising new technique that attempts to overcome the majority of these limitations (Fig. 14.5). Strain rate imaging enables the measurement of longitudinal deformation, in addition to radial and circumferential motion. Endocardial fibers, which are most sensitive to ischemia, are arranged predominantly in the long axis of the heart. Color Doppler tissue imaging requires a perfect alignment of the interrogation beam with the heart, and this may be difficult to achieve with TEE [57]. Two-dimensional myocardial strain imaging overcomes this limitation but is not (yet) able to operate at the high temporal resolution obtained with tissue Doppler imaging techniques. Color kinesis, another method to quantify wall motion, is based on acoustic quantification and provides a color-coded image of the timing and magnitude of systolic endocardial excursion in real time [58] (Video 14.7). Unfortunately, this method does not overcome the artifacts induced by translation and rotation of the heart.

Pathophysiology of RWMAs

Regional myocardial dysfunction can indicate the presence of new-onset ischemia, but equally it may result from an old myocardial infarction, myocardial stunning, or hibernation, and routine TEE analysis of RWMAs does not allow discrimination between these distinct pathophysiological conditions. Since they have entirely different consequences in terms of prognosis and treatment, several tools have been examined to better define the underlying cause of RWMAs with echocardiography. Some pathophysiological characteristics unique for each condition can be examined with perfusion imaging and stress echocardiography. For example, myocardial stunning refers to a condition of reduced wall motion that persists after ischemia and reperfusion and ultimately – after hours or even days – reverts to normal function. RWMAs due to stunning are often less pronounced than ischemic RWMAs, they show gradual improvement with time, they occur in the absence of perfusion abnormalities, and they respond positively to inotropic stimulation

Perfusion imaging techniques with contrast agents have been used to study the extent of myocardial perfusion as well as the efficacy of myocardial protection

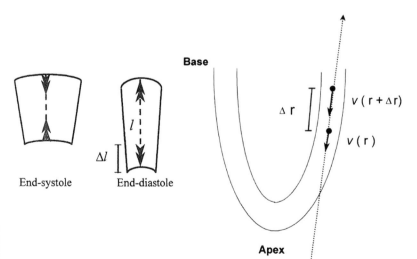

Figure 14.5. Principles of strain rate imaging. Schematic of how strain rate of tissue segment (Δr) is estimated from tissue velocity (V). Dashed line indicates orientation of ultrasound beam. Length is denoted l, and distance along beam as r. Strain rate is calculated by subtracting $V(r + \Delta r)$ from $V(r)$ over distance Δr between these two points. When velocities are equal, strain rate is zero and there is no compression or expansion. If $V(r + \Delta r) > V(r)$, strain rate is negative and there is compression. If $V(r) > V(r + \Delta r)$, strain rate is positive, indicating expansion. Reproduced with permission from Urheim et al., Circulation 2000; **102**: 1158–64 [56].

Base

Δr

$V(r + \Delta r)$

$V(r)$

l

Δl

End-systole

End-diastole

Apex

in patients undergoing CABG. These systems include an external ultrasound unit and an internal tracer which reflect the ultrasonic beam and may provide information on the matching between regional perfusion and function. RWMAs in normally perfused myocardium (e.g. stunned artifact conduction abnormalities) clearly have a different prognosis when compared to hypoperfused (i.e. ischemic, hibernating, or infarcted) dysfunctional areas [55].

Stress echocardiography examines the contractile reserve of dysfunctional myocardium. The regional wall motion of stunned myocardium shows improvement with dobutamine, while RWMAs due to myocardial ischemia worsen during pharmacological stress. Infarcted myocardium is akinetic or dyskinetic and by definition shows no contractile reserve. Intraoperative low-dose dobutamine has been shown to predict myocardial functional reserve and to determine functional recovery expected after coronary revascularization. Hibernating myocardium, a condition of chronic dysfunction in viable myocardium, shows a biphasic response to positive inotropic stress, with improved performance following low-dose dobutamine and deterioration after higher doses of dobutamine. A biphasic response to stress echocardiography has been associated with functional improvement following revascularization [57].

Monitoring of intraoperative surgical complications

During aortic cross-clamping/declamping

Aortic dissection and severe intramural hematoma have been noted as complications following CABG. The diagnosis of these complications can be quickly and easily made with intraoperative TEE, and routine use of TEE may allow for rapid treatment and the avoidance of potentially lethal outcomes [59].

Monitoring for intracardiac air

This is mainly an issue in open-chamber cardiotomy operations, but it also may occur in CABG [60] (Video 14.8). It occurs predominantly in the period between cross-clamp removal and termination of cardiopulmonary bypass (CPB). Air originates either from the pulmonary veins or from the aortic root. The main concern is gas microembolism into either the right coronary artery or the cerebral circulation. CO_2 embolism with endoscopic saphenous vein harvesting using

CO_2 insufflation in CABG patients has also been reported [61,62]. Monitoring with TEE is more sensitive than end-tidal CO_2 and pulmonary artery (PA) pressure monitoring [63].

Complications related to ischemic heart disease

Acute mitral regurgitation

New mitral insufficiency or worsening of existing MR can occur as a result of acute or chronic IHD. Papillary muscle dysfunction may occur in up to 50% of patients with anterior-wall MI. Annular mitral dilation and even chordal or papillary muscle rupture, especially with inferior-wall MI, should also be suspected as potential mechanisms (see Chapter 16).

Ventricular septal defect

Ventricular septal defect (VSD) is an infrequent complication of MI, but carries a high mortality. The VSD will produce a left-to-right shunt with pressure and volume overload of the right ventricle, which is usually acutely dilated. LV function is usually poor. Two-dimensional imaging may reveal the defect, and the use of color-flow Doppler along the interventricular septum shows a left-to-right shunt. The septal defect is often easier to visualize with TTE (Fig. 14.6; Video 14.9).

Ventricular pseudoaneurysm

Ventricular pseudoaneurysm is an alarming finding with a high risk of free cardiac wall rupture. It is characterized by its narrow base, and the wall is composed of thrombus. It differs from **ventricular aneurysm**, which has a broad base with a wall composed of dyskinetic or akinetic myocardium. The risk of rupture with a true aneurysm is lower (see *Left ventricular reconstruction*, below).

Intraventricular thrombus

Most often, thrombus formation complicates an acute MI in patients with low ejection fraction, in apical dyskinesis, or in the presence of a true LV aneurysm. Visualization may be enhanced with echocontrast agents. Intraventricular thrombus may be confused with trabeculations, muscle bands particularly in the right ventricle, and artifacts such as apical foreshortening.

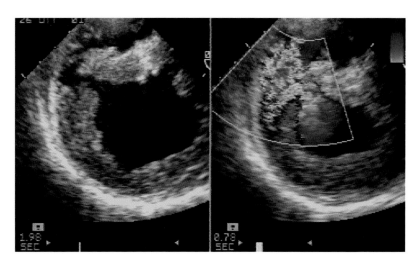

Figure 14.6. Short-axis transgastric view showing a post-infarction ventricular septal defect.

Off-pump (OPCAB) cardiac surgery

Sean Bennett

Introduction and terminology

Two approaches to myocardial revascularization without cardiopulmonary bypass (CPB) have been described. These are:

- **Minimally invasive direct coronary artery bypass (MIDCAB).** Usually this requires a surgical approach to the left anterior descending coronary artery via a modified left anterior thoracotomy. MIDCAB surgery is limited to patients with single-vessel coronary disease, and its use is not widespread. There may be some future with robotic surgery with this approach, using transesophageal echocardiography (TEE) to monitor myocardial ischemia, but recent results have been disappointing [64].
- **Off-pump coronary artery bypass (OPCAB).** The surgical approach is via a median sternotomy with the patient supine. OPCAB can be used to bypass any of the coronary arteries, and is therefore practical in a much larger patient population. OPCAB surgery has spawned the development of heart-stabilizing devices which allow multiple vessels to be grafted. These devices usually contain suction pads and tissue stabilizers, thus allowing the heart to be rotated and stabilized whilst still maintaining an effective cardiac output. Examples of such devices include the Medtronic Octopus and Starfish (Fig. 14.7).

Rationale for OPCAB

OPCAB surgery needs to achieve the following goals:

- the ability to graft all diseased vessels with a quality of anastomosis comparable to that achieved using CPB
- maintenance of the patient's circulation and avoidance of ischemic or hypoxic damage to vital organs

TEE may be invaluable in facilitating these goals. Firstly, TEE can help detect early evidence of myocardial ischemia and thus provide evidence for the quality of the anastomosis. Secondly, beat-to-beat cardiac output can be estimated, thereby monitoring the circulation. Displacement of the heart during the distal anastomosis may cause significant hemodynamic disturbance. If this is excessive it may effectively limit the number and quality of the anastomoses [65]. Thirdly, the direct imaging of regional wall motion, ventricular function, volume loading, and valve competence serves as an effective intraoperative monitor.

Retrospective studies suggest that off-pump surgery is associated with a lower incidence of stroke [66], and that it lowers overall morbidity and mortality in patients with severe atheromatous aortic disease [67,68].

Other aspects of recovery from cardiac surgery are improved in OPCAB patients in contrast to patients undergoing CABG on pump, and hence OPCAB surgery may be most appropriate in high-risk patients [69,70].

TEE during OPCAB

There are no randomized studies comparing OPCAB surgery with and without TEE. Guidelines regarding the use of intraoperative TEE have suggested that

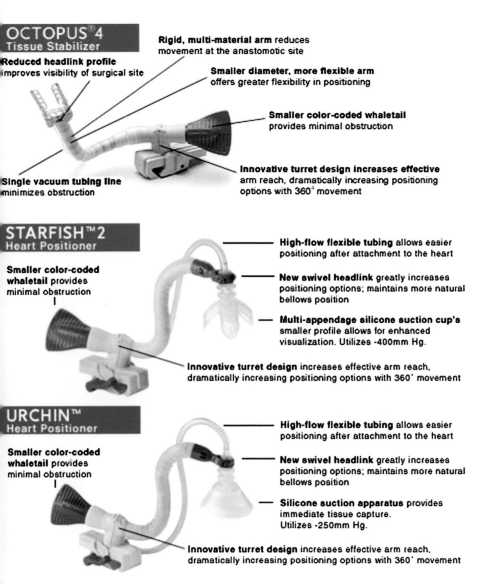

OCTOPUS®4
Tissue Stabilizer

Reduced headlink profile
improves visibility of surgical site

Rigid, multi-material arm reduces movement at the anastomotic site

Smaller diameter, more flexible arm offers greater flexibility in positioning

Smaller color-coded whaletail provides minimal obstruction

Single vacuum tubing line minimizes obstruction

Innovative turret design increases effective arm reach, dramatically increasing positioning options with 360° movement

STARFISH™2
Heart Positioner

Smaller color-coded whaletail provides minimal obstruction

High-flow flexible tubing allows easier positioning after attachment to the heart

New swivel headlink greatly increases positioning options; maintains more natural bellows position

Multi-appendage silicone suction cup's smaller profile allows for enhanced visualization. Utilizes -400mm Hg.

Innovative turret design increases effective arm reach, dramatically increasing positioning options with 360° movement

URCHIN™
Heart Positioner

Smaller color-coded whaletail provides minimal obstruction

High-flow flexible tubing allows easier positioning after attachment to the heart

New swivel headlink greatly increases positioning options; maintains more natural bellows position

Silicone suction apparatus provides immediate tissue capture. Utilizes -250mm Hg.

Innovative turret design increases effective arm reach, dramatically increasing positioning options with 360° movement

Figure 14.7. OPCAB tissue stabilizers: the Medtronic Octopus 4, Starfish 2, and Urchin. From www.medtronic.com.

OPCAB surgery is a Class IIb indication for intraoperative TEE [18], although currently there is generally little evidence. Future work may clarify this situation.

TEE may be valuable in OPCAB patients for the following reasons:

evaluation of left ventricular (LV) function, including diastolic function and preload
identification of regional wall motion abnormalities (RWMAs)
identification of other pathology that may contraindicate, complicate, or promote OPCAB over conventional CABG surgery

A full TEE examination before surgery should be undertaken, specifically noting ventricular function and chamber size. This may guide pharmacological and volume management, and alert the surgical team to the need for an intra-aortic balloon pump [71].

The ability to use TEE as a rapid-response monitor may be valuable, but TEE should not be regarded as a replacement for conventional monitoring. TEE offers valuable additional information, but its role and limitations must be clearly understood.

Pre-existing RWMAs should also be noted. Interpretation of views may be difficult because the cardiac distortion during grafting may produce apparent RWMAs that are not caused by ischemia. Also, cardiac displacement means that the standard transgastric short-axis view is rarely obtainable. The mid-esophageal views are more likely available, and from these we may be able to identify the relevant LV wall segments and assess their perfusion. RWMAs that persist after release of the tissue stabilizer may be associated with myocardial ischemia, as in conventional bypass [70].

TEE may be important in identifying other factors that may complicate OPCAB surgery or lead to conversion to on-pump CABG. These include the presence of intracardiac thrombus, intracardiac shunts, and mitral disease, which would bias the surgeon against OPCAB. Aortic atheroma, on the other hand, may favor OPCAB [72].

Left ventricular function

The standard techniques used to assess LV function (fractional area change, fractional shortening, etc.) are not possible when the heart is in an abnormal position. More reliance is placed on direct visual assessment of contractility and wall motion in 2D views. These must be interpreted in association with other data derived from invasive monitoring, primarily systemic arterial and atrial pressures.

During OPCAB the hemodynamic disturbance is most marked during grafting of the circumflex artery (Cx) or the inferolateral wall, next during right coronary artery (RCA) or inferior wall grafting, and least marked during left anterior descending (LAD) or anterior wall grafting. If grafting has been successful there is a return to baseline hemodynamics at the end of the procedure.

Cardiac index (CI) may vary according to the vessel. Typical values are CI > 2.8 L/min for LAD, CI > 2.4 L/min for RCA and CI > 2 L/min for Cx. It is worth noting that at the same time pulmonary capillary wedge pressure (PCWP), central venous pressure (CVP), and mean arterial pressure (MAP) also vary predictably. Pulmonary artery catheters (PACs) are particularly recommended in multivessel OPCAB [73].

The ability of TEE to monitor LV performance during the grafting procedure depends solely on the LV views available. During grafting of the circumflex artery the heart is lifted, apex up, rendering transgastric views useless and long-axis views poor. With experience some degree of monitoring remains possible. Placing a fluid-filled bag or gel cushion under the heart significantly improves imaging quality (Video 14.10).

However, quantification methods such as tissue Doppler imaging are not reliable, since correct angulation of the ultrasound beam with respect to the heart motion cannot be guaranteed. The echocardiographer will make a direct visual assessment of ventricular movement and size. Impaired movement combined with a fall in MAP should be considered in the context of LV diameter. The combination of decreased movement with a reduced LV end-diastolic diameter (LVEDD) will indicate the need for volume loading and checking on right and left inflow. For example twisting the heart to the patient's left can cause compression of the pulmonary artery, which can severely reduce LV filling. This is easily detected by TEE, and can quickly be resolved. Another common difficulty is caused by turning the heart up and to the right obstructing the venous inflow; this may be resolved by opening the right pleural cavity, allowing more room for the heart to be displaced without putting tension on the venous inflow vessels. The picture of reduced LV movement with an increased LVEDD should prompt repositioning of the heart, as this indicates regional or global ischemia which may develop into myocardial infarction. In this situation it is worth examining the mitral valve, as the development of mitral regurgitation is a poor prognostic sign.

Diastolic function

Myocardial ischemia is thought to impact on diastolic function before systolic function and hemodynamic changes [74]. Indicators of diastolic dysfunction include E and A wave velocity, E/A wave ratio, and mitral deceleration time. More accurate guidance can be obtained by combining these with measurement of the pulmonary vein inflow, but these are more time consuming. Typical data suggesting early diastolic dysfunction as "impaired relaxation" are an E wave velocity < 0.7 m/s, an A wave > 0.7 m/s, E/A ratio < 1 plus a deceleration time > 240 milliseconds. Diastolic dysfunction has been shown to occur during circumflex artery grafting with recovery afterwards [75].

Diastolic measurements can be made by studying the mitral inflow patterns and are described in more detail elsewhere in the book. Both E and A waves are obtainable during OPCAB surgery even when the heart is lifted and twisted. The reason for this is that although the left and right ventricles are lifted off the pericardium the basal structure of the heart remains in contact with the pericardium and can be visualized from the esophagus.

However, the association between measurable diastolic dysfunction and early ischemia in this setting remains unproven. There seem to be several reasons for this:

- The mechanical distortion of the heart due to the displacement and the clamp may well cause inflow abnormalities that are not due to new diastolic dysfunction. Indeed, mitral inflow velocities are affected by preload changes. Diastolic dysfunction may exist but not be due to ischemia.
- Brief episodes of ischemia may not be significant.

Correct angulation of the ultrasound beam with respect to the direction of mitral inflow is uncertain when the heart is displaced. So far, a reproducible diastolic marker for ischemia during OPCAB surgery remains elusive.

Regional wall motion abnormalities

Intraoperative identification of ischemic RWMAs is an interesting prospect but is fraught with difficulty.

Firstly, the position of the heart may make it impossible to clearly identify all the segments during grafting. At best 80% of relevant segments can be visualized [76]. Secondly, ischemia may be caused by the grafting of a snared vessel, dependent on the pre-existing flow in the native vessel, the use of intracoronary shunts, and the time required to complete the anastomosis. Thirdly, tissue stabilizers may cause a type of RWMA which is indistinguishable from early ischemic changes [77]. Thus the decision to continue with a graft in the presence of a new RWMA is not simple, and TEE will only offer part of the information required. Fortunately, RWMAs that occur during grafting tend to resolve once the graft is complete and the heart is returned to a normal position. RWMAs are seen in up to 53% of grafts. RWMAs that persist after the heart is replaced are less frequent but more significant. Faced with a persistent RWMA in the operating room the TEE and other relevant information should be made clear, and the resultant action will then depend on the surgeon's view of the quality of the anastomosis, the graft, and the vessel itself.

The use of intraoperative TEE may therefore serve to detect RWMAs, but not to prevent them.

Recent data suggest that RWMAs may be identified in a number of segments during OPCAB surgery, and have served to validate the use of TEE for ischemia detection during OPCAB.

Using the earlier 16-segment model, Wang *et al.* found that more than 14 segments could be interrogated even when the heart was displaced [76]. They used the standard mid-esophageal views, which can be used throughout most of the surgery, and defined the segments relating to the different coronary arteries. Ischemia was defined by a change of two or more grades on the standard scoring system, in at least two segments, taking into account both wall thickening and motion. A high incidence of wall motion abnormalities suggestive of ischemia was found, but placing the epicardial stabilizer produced RWMAs in 23% of patients, compared to 40% incidence during grafting. Approximately 5% of patients were converted to CPB due to instability; nine patients had RWMAs that persisted for longer than six months, and six of these episodes had been detected at the time the epicardial stabilizer was placed.

Preload

TEE is able to give a more direct measure of preload, either as LV end-diastolic volume or more simply as end-diastolic area/diameter, measured in the transgastric view. When the heart is displaced LVEDD may be measured in the mid-esophageal two-chamber view, using the mid-cavity dimension of the LV. This may be valuable in assessing volume loading during OPCAB. Typically, patients will require more volume than they might prior to CPB, as the heart seems better able to cope with manipulation if it is well filled but not failing.

Diagnostic use of TEE during OPCAB

The value of TEE in OPCAB surgery as a hemodynamic monitor has been discussed above. However, a TEE examination before surgery will identify findings which might complicate or contraindicate the OPCAB procedure. This situation is virtually unique in cardiac surgery, because OPCAB surgery is undertaken without CPB, whereas almost all other procedures will necessitate the use of CPB. This will markedly alter the surgical plan.

Valve lesions

Occasionally, significant valve lesions will be revealed de novo during OPCAB surgery. These have been dealt with in the earlier section of this chapter. However, the presence of mitral regurgitation may be particularly relevant, and even mild degrees of regurgitation can cause hemodynamic disturbance when the heart is dislocated. This may occur particularly during grafting of the circumflex or distal right coronary territory. The elevation of the LV whilst the atria are relatively fixed has a tendency to cause mitral valve distortion and regurgitation. Patients in whom the valve is already incompetent may experience sudden deterioration, and the patient may become too unstable to proceed with OPCAB. Mitral regurgitation will be a contributing factor to the off-pump to on-pump conversion rates currently quoted [78].

Intracardiac shunts

In the adult population small patent foramen ovale defects with little or no flow are quite commonly detected. However, the physical displacement of the heart during OPCAB may lead to the development of a right-to-left shunt. This may be resolved simply by repositioning the heart. TEE is useful both to detect and to resolve this situation.

Intracardiac masses or thrombus

The detection of any mass in the cardiac chambers would serve as a contraindication to OPCAB surgery, since the mass may obstruct or fragment and embolize during cardiac displacement. Whilst TEE is invaluable in detecting masses, the most likely potential problem is thrombus.

Thrombus in the left atrium is relatively easy to detect (see Chapter 11), but small thrombi in the LV are much more difficult to detect, particularly at the LV apex. This may occur particularly in patients with poor LV function and/or aneurysmal dilation of the ventricle.

Aortic atheroma

The diagnostic difficulties and prognostic importance of aortic atheroma have been discussed above. Although epiaortic scanning is superior to TEE in diagnosing atheroma in the ascending aorta, there is a strong association between plaque in the descending and/or proximal ascending aorta and the distal ascending aorta (see Chapter 12). TEE can be used to alert the operator to the embolic risk in the area of cannulation. Minimal interference to the ascending aorta has been shown to improve neurological outcome in the elderly and is a positive indication for OPCAB surgery [79,80].

Conclusion

There is clear evidence that OPCAB surgery reduces the adverse consequences of on-pump CABG surgery, although some doubts persist about the quality of revascularization. However, the extent to which TEE contributes to successful OPCAB surgery is not clear. By conducting a systematic TEE examination, given adequate experience in the use of non-standard views, it seems likely that the small number of complications can be further reduced.

Left ventricular reconstruction

Marco Ranucci, Serenella Castelvecchio, Marisa Di Donato

Introduction

Following myocardial infarction (MI), the left ventricle (LV) may experience changes in size and shape. These have been defined as "ventricular remodeling." The natural history of LV remodeling includes changes occurring in the acute period, in the early period following myocardial infarction, and throughout the whole late post-infarction period. During the acute and early period after MI, the infarcted area is more susceptible to distorting forces, while the late modifications in size and shape are due to a complex interaction of forces involving both the infarcted and non-infarcted areas [81].

Dilation of the left ventricle allows the chamber to eject an adequate stroke volume (SV) despite a depression of LV contractility. However, the increased radius of the remodeled ventricle induces an increase in workload and wall tension, according to Laplace's law:

$$\text{Tension (within the myocardial walls)} = \text{Pressure (transmural)} \times \text{Radius} / \text{Thickness (wall)} \quad (14.1)$$

A model of the natural history of LV remodeling was proposed in 1997 by Dor and Di Donato [81] (Fig. 14.8)

At its most extreme, the LV remodeling process leads to the formation of a true aneurysm, with a well defined area of dyskinesia. However, aggressive early reperfusion treatment has changed the natural history of LV remodeling following MI. Early reperfusion

(a) NORMAL   (b) NECROSIS   (c) SLIMMING

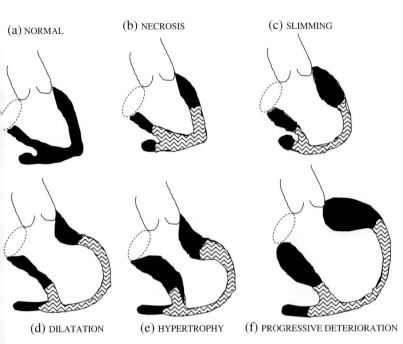

Figure 14.8. The natural history of post-MI LV remodeling. From Dor & Di Donato, *Curr Opin Cardiol* 1997; **12**: 533–7 [81].

(d) DILATATION   (e) HYPERTROPHY   (f) PROGRESSIVE DETERIORATION

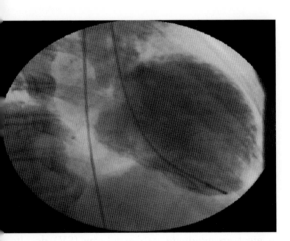

Figure 14.9. Cineangiography of a round-shaped LV following myocardial infarction.

results in a sparing of the epicardium and occasionally the middle shell of the myocardium, but with no effect on the endocardial layer. The resultant LV remodeling results in a dilated and rounded shape, resembling a non-ischemic cardiomyopathy rather than an ischemic, dyskinetic aneurysm [82] (Fig. 14.9).

In addition, acute MI may lead to a third entity changing the shape of the LV: the **pseudoaneurysm**. Rupture of the free wall of the myocardium is a severe complication of acute MI. Often this is fatal even if promptly treated surgically. Occasionally, however, the ruptured free wall may be enclosed by the adjacent pericardial tissue, and a pseudoaneurysm is formed (Fig. 14.10). Two-dimensional (2D) echo allows us to differentiate between pseudoaneurysm and true aneurysm [83] (Fig. 14.11). When the free-wall rupture spares the epicardial layer, a **subepicardial aneurysm** is formed, with a morphological pattern similar to the pseudoaneurysm [84] (Fig. 14.12).

The first surgical approach to LV remodeling was mainly utilized in patients with a dyskinetic aneurysm [85]. Subsequently, different techniques were introduced, and surgical treatment is now possible even for dilated ischemic cardiomyopathy [86–93]. The surgical approach can be divided into three categories: the linear suture [85–89], the circular external suture [86,90], and the endoventricular patch plasty, or Dor operation [86,90–92].

Regardless of the specific technical aspects, the surgical approach should be directed to the following [82]:

a. **Relieve ischemia.** Comprehensive coronary revascularization should be undertaken, with particular emphasis on the left anterior descending coronary artery.

b. **Reduce ventricular volume.** The septal and anterior components are particularly important. To control the reduction in LV volume following resection, the use of an intraventricular balloon filled to a volume of 60–70 mL/m^2 body surface area has been recommended [94].

237

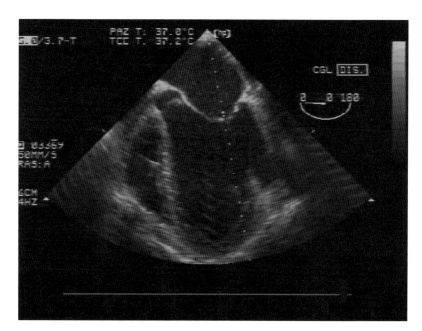

Figure 14.10. LV pseudoaneurysm.

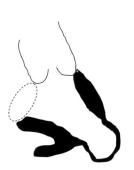 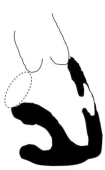

Figure 14.11. Discriminating criteria between LV true aneurysm and pseudoaneurysm.

TRUE ANEURYSM	PSEUDOANEURYSM
Wide neck (ratio between entry diameter and maximal diameter> 0.5)	Small neck (ratiobetween entry diameter and maximal diameter< 0.5)
Akinesia/dyskinesia	To-and-fro blood flow
Low rupture incidence	High rupture incidence
Possible thrombi formation	Very frequent thrombus formation

c. **Restore geometric shape**. Surgery is aimed at restoring effective geometry of the LV, through a proportional reduction of both the long and short axes.

d. **Repair mitral regurgitation**. In patients with mitral regurgitation, mitral valve repair may improve the quality of early and late outcomes following surgery. The repair may be performed through a left atrial approach, or via an intraventricular approach without the use of a prosthetic mitral ring [94] (Video14.11).

Intraoperative TEE monitoring is valuable for each of the above steps, and should be considered essential for surgery to restore the LV as described.

TEE and hemodynamics

Due to the underlying pathology, the majority of patients undergoing surgical LV restoration have moderate to severely decreased LV contractility, and many suffer from associated right ventricular (RV) dysfunction also (Fig. 14.13).

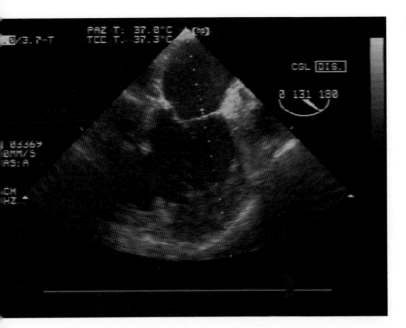

Figure 14.12. Subepicardial LV aneurysm.

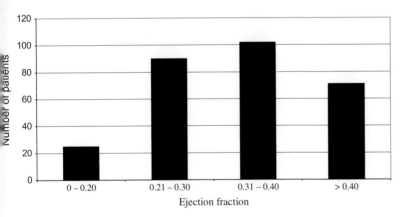

Figure 14.13. Distribution of patients undergoing LV reconstructive surgery according to LV ejection fraction.

There is a place for both pulmonary artery catheter (PAC) and TEE monitoring in these patients, particularly for weaning the patient from cardiopulmonary bypass. The altered LV size and shape make the process of assessing adequate LV filling particularly challenging. Pre-load assessment using the LV cross-sectional area at the mid-papillary level in the transgastric view may not be accurate in these patients. An estimate of adequate filling volume should be matched with the corresponding filling pressure (i.e. the pulmonary artery occlusion pressure) before and after surgery.

Moreover, TEE may provide useful information about the effects of inotropic drugs, and valuable information about RV function.

In fact, the majority of patients need inotropic support immediately after cardiopulmonary bypass and in the early postoperative period. The use of an intra-aortic balloon pump (IABP) may also be required. TEE may be useful in screening the aorta for atheroma, and to ensure correct positioning of the balloon.

TEE and LV size

Patients undergoing LV restoration surgery will need extensive preoperative preparation. The LV dimensions are generally known on the basis of the preoperative 2D echo study and cineangiography. Cardiac magnetic resonance may also be useful to define LV dimensions. Despite this, some additional information may be provided by intraoperative TEE. Using standard techniques, assessment of LV size may be valuable, especially if the preoperative study has been performed with the transthoracic approach in patients with a poor acoustic window. Cross-sectional areas at different levels of the LV (basal, mid-papillary, apex) may be calculated with standard transgastric views at end-diastole and end-systole, and the corresponding diameters may be assessed by 2D examination in the mid-esophageal view or using an M-mode Doppler in the transgastric, long-axis view.

This baseline information will be compared to the same variables collected after surgical LV restoration, in order to check whether the desired LV size has been achieved.

TEE and LV reshaping

The first surgical approaches to LV aneurysm were aimed only at removing the dyskinetic scar. In recent years the concept of "reshaping" the LV has become more important as a part of the surgical plan. In a round-shaped LV, the aim is to reduce both the long and the short axes, restoring a correct short-to-long axis ratio, or sphericity index.

The extent of the LV resection and the position of the ventricular patch both determine the new short-to-long axis ratio. To restore a correct shape to the LV, the ventricular patch should be directed towards the LV outflow tract, with an oblique orientation.

From a biomechanical point of view, the surgical aim is to change the shape from a "Roman arch" to "Gothic arch," by correctly positioning the LV apex, by reducing both the short and long axes, and by restoring the elliptical shape of the LV (Fig. 14.14). For a given longitudinal force, this new reshaped LV will suffer lower lateral force, thus increasing its functional capacity and limiting the tendency to further dilation.

Moreover, in a round-shaped LV the papillary muscles are laterally displaced, the posterior leaflet is retracted, and the mitral annulus is dilated: as a consequence, the mitral valve becomes incompetent.

TEE and mitral regurgitation repair

Mitral regurgitation in the situation of LV remodeling following myocardial infarction should be considered as a subset of the ischemic mitral regurgitation pattern. The ischemic regurgitant mitral valve is usually structurally normal. The main mechanism of mitral regurgitation is lack of coaptation due to mitral valve "tenting" in systole. This results from lateral papillary muscle displacement inducing a "tethering" mechanism [95]. Annular dilation seems less important as a mechanism for mitral regurgitation [96,97]. The tethering mechanism can be symmetric or asymmetric, resulting in different directions of the regurgitant jet [95]. Important information for grading the severity of the tethering mechanism can be obtained from the height (h) of the tent, and the tenting area (a) (Fig. 14.15). The best TEE view for measuring

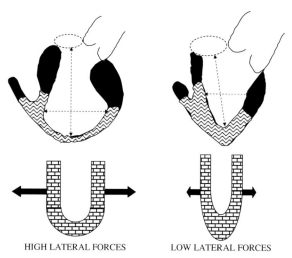

HIGH LATERAL FORCES   LOW LATERAL FORCES

Figure 14.14. The "Roman arch" shape of the remodeled LV results in higher lateral forces than the "Gothic arch" shape after a successful surgery.

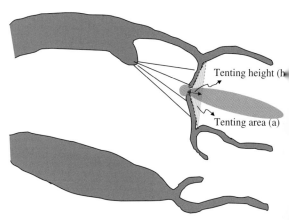

Tenting height (h)

Tenting area (a)

Figure 14.15. The mechanism of ischemic mitral valve regurgitation: the tethering mechanism and the consequent "tented" mitral valve behavior, with the tenting height (h) and area (a) measurements.

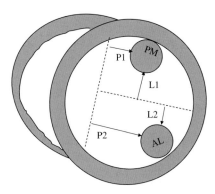

Figure 14.16. The transgastric short-axis view of the LV at mid-papillary level. P1 and P2, posterior displacements of the postero-medial (PM) and anterolateral (AL) papillary muscles; L1 and L2, lateral displacements of the PM and AL papillary muscles. L1 + L2 = interpapillary distance [95,97].

both these parameters is the transgastric, 90° long-axis view.

The tenting parameters have been identified as major determinants of functional mitral regurgitation, while global LV size, the sphericity index, and systolic LV function are poorly correlated with the degree of mitral regurgitation [95]. The severity of mitral valve regurgitation may be assessed using other parameters indicative of the papillary muscle displacement. Posterior and lateral displacement, and the interpapillary muscle distance, may be measured using TTE or TEE [95,97]. When using TEE, the transgastric short-axis view at mid-papillary level can be used (Fig. 14.16).

Intraoperative TEE is required for mitral valve repair during LV restoration surgery, but caution should be exercised in grading the severity of mitral valve regurgitation. This is more reliably achieved at the preoperative examination. Nor should it be used to guide the surgical choice of whether or not to repair the valve. Its role is to define the mechanism of the mitral regurgitation and, most importantly, to assess the quality of the surgical repair.

Postoperative diastolic function

There are few data available on LV diastolic function in patients following surgical ventricular reconstruction. Ventricular remodeling following an acute myocardial infarction is accompanied by changes in LV diastolic function due to scar formation, which in turn increases chamber stiffness, and compensatory hypertrophy of the remote zone, which is responsible for delayed relaxation [98]. Increases in LV filling

pressure may be responsible for LV dilation. Experimental studies have suggested an adverse effect on diastolic function induced by surgical LV volume reduction [99,100]. Both the changes in geometry and the LV volume reduction may theoretically be responsible.

Recent data suggest that following surgical ventricular reconstruction the LV filling pattern was unchanged in the majority of patients, the remainder showing either an improvement or a worsening pattern [101]. Based on univariate analysis, the preoperative conicity index and the end-diastolic volume difference before and after surgery (the result of surgical volume reduction) were associated with a worsening diastolic pattern. Globally dilated LV cavities are more likely to worsen in diastolic function, compared with LV cavities that are equally dilated but where the dilation mostly occurs at the apical level, due to the presence of a dyskinetic scar.

The surgical treatment of end-stage cardiac failure is currently a matter of significant controversy. The increasing number of patients affected, and the declining option of alternatives including cardiac transplantation, has increased interest in surgical LV reconstruction as an alternative to medical treatment. TEE will no doubt continue to play an important role in this area.

References

1. Savage RM, Lytle BW, Aronson S, *et al.* Intraoperative echocardiography is indicated in high-risk coronary artery bypass grafting. *Ann Thorac Surg* 1997; **64**: 368–74.

2. Mishra M, Chauhan R, Sharma KK, *et al.* Real-time intraoperative transesophageal echocardiography: how useful? Experience of 5,016 cases. *J Cardiothorac Vasc Anesth* 1998; **12**: 625–32.

3. Click R, Abel M, Schaff HV. Intraoperative transesophageal echocardiography: 5-year prospective review of impact on surgical management. *Mayo Clin Proc* 2000; **75**: 241–7.

4. Qaddoura FE, Abel MD, Mecklenburg KL, *et al.* Role of intraoperative transesophageal echocardiography in patients having coronary artery bypass graft surgery *Ann Thorac Surg* 2004; **78**: 1586–90.

5. Cheitlin MD, Armstrong WF, Aurigemma GP, *et al.* ACC/AHA/ASE 2003 guideline update for the clinical application of echocardiography: summary article. A report of the American College of Cardiology/American Heart Association Task Force on Practice Guidelines (ACC/AHA/ASE Committee to Update the

241

1997 Guidelines for the Clinical Application of Echocardiography). *Circulation* 2003; **108**: 1146–62.

6. Practice guidelines for perioperative transesophageal echocardiography. A report by the American Society of Anesthesiologists and the Society of Cardiovascular Anesthesiologists Task Force on Transesophageal Echocardiography. *Anesthesiology* 1996; **84**: 986–1006.

7. Grossi EA, Bizekis CS, Sharony R, *et al.* Routine intraoperative transesophageal echocardiography identifies patients with atheromatous aortas: impact on "off-pump" coronary artery bypass and perioperative stroke. *J Am Soc Echocardiogr* 2003; **16**: 751–5.

8. Kolev N, Brase R, Swanevelder J, *et al.* The influence of transoesophageal echocardiography on intra-operative decision making. A European multicentre study. European Perioperative TOE Research Group. *Anaesthesia* 1998; **53**: 767–73.

9. Bergquist BD, Bellows WH, Leung JM. Transesophageal echocardiography in myocardial revascularization: II. Influence on intraoperative decision making. *Anesth Analg* 1996; **82**: 1139–45.

10. Kneeshaw JD. Transoesophageal echocardiography (TOE) in the operating room. *Br J Anaesth* 2006; **97**: 77–84.

11. Roach GW, Kanchuger M, Mangano CM, *et al.* Adverse cerebral outcomes after coronary bypass surgery. Multicenter Study of Perioperative Ischemia Research Group and the Ischemia Research and Education Foundation Investigators. *N Engl J Med* 1996; **335**: 1857–63.

12. Newman MF, Wolman R, Kanchuger M, *et al.* Multicenter preoperative stroke risk index for patients undergoing coronary artery bypass graft surgery. Multicenter Study of Perioperative Ischemia (McSPI) Research Group. *Circulation* 1996; **94** (9 Suppl): II74–80.

13. Katz ES, Tunick PA, Rusinek H, *et al.* Protruding aortic atheromas predict stroke in elderly patients undergoing cardiopulmonary bypass: experience with intraoperative transesophageal echocardiography *J Am Coll Cardiol* 1992: **20**: 70–7.

14. Hartman GS, Yao FF, Bruefach M, *et al.* Severity of aortic atheromatous disease diagnosed by transesophageal echocardiography predicts stroke and other outcomes associated with coronary artery surgery: a prospective study. *Anesth Analg* 1996; **83**: 701–8.

15. Royse C, Royse A, Blake D, Grigg L. Assessment of thoracic aortic atheroma by echocardiography: a new classification and estimation of risk of dislodging atheroma during three surgical techniques. *Ann Thorac Cardiovasc Surg* 1998; **4**: 72–7.

16. Hartman GS, Peterson J, Konstadt SN, *et al.* High reproducibility in the interpretation of intraoperative transesophageal echocardiographic evaluation of aortic atheromatous disease. *Anesth Analg* 1996; **82**: 539–43.

17. Konstadt SN, Reich DL, Quintana C, Levy M. The ascending aorta: how much does transesophageal echocardiography see? *Anesth Analg* 1994; **78**: 240–4.

18. Dávila-Román VG, Phillips KJ, Daily BB, *et al.* Intraoperative transesophageal echocardiography and epiaortic ultrasound for assessment of atherosclerosis of the thoracic aorta. *J Am Coll Cardiol* 1996; **28**: 942–7.

19. Sylivris S, Calafiore P, Matalanis P, *et al.* The intraoperative assessment of ascending aortic atheroma; epiaortic imaging is superior to both transesophageal echocardiography and direct palpation. *J Cardiothorac Vasc Anesth* 1997; **11**: 704–7.

20. Glas KE, Swaminathan M, Reeves ST, *et al.* Council for Intraoperative Echocardiography of the American Society of Echocardiography; Society of Cardiovascular Anesthesiologists. Guidelines for the performance of a comprehensive intraoperative epiaortic ultrasonographic examination: recommendations of the American Society of Echocardiography and the Society of Cardiovascular Anesthesiologists; endorsed by the Society of T horacic Surgeons. *J Am Soc Echocardiogr* 2007; **20**: 1227–35.

21. Li YL, Wong DT, Wei W, Liu J. A novel acoustic window for trans-oesophageal echocardiography by using a saline-filled endotracheal balloon. *Br J Anaesth* 2006; **97**: 624–9.

22. Harringer W. Capture of particulate emboli during cardiac procedures in which aortic cross-clamp is used. International Council of Emboli Management Study Group. *Ann Thorac Surg* 2000; **70**: 1119–23.

23. Banbury MK, Kouchoukos NT, Allen KB, *et al.* Emboli capture using the Embol-X intraaortic filter in cardiac surgery: a multicentered randomized trial of 1,289 patients. *Ann Thorac Surg* 2003; **76**: 508–15.

24. Christenson JT, Vala DL, Licker M, *et al.* Intra-aortic filtration: capturing particulate emboli during aortic cross-clamping. *Tex Heart Inst J* 2005; **32**: 515–21.

25. Medalion B, Meirson D, Hauptman E, Sasson L, Schachner A. Initial experience with the Heartstring proximal anastomotic system. *J Thorac Cardiovasc Surg* 2004; **128**: 273–7.

26. Trehan N, Mishra M, Kasliwal RR, Mishra A. Surgical strategies in patients at high risk for stroke undergoing coronary artery bypass grafting. *Thorac Surg* 2000; **70**: 1037–45.

27. Rakowski H, Pearlman AS. Preventing perioperative stroke: look, but don't touch! *Am Heart J* 1999; **138**: 609–11.

28. Sukernik MR, Mets B, Kachulis B, *et al.* The impact of newly diagnosed patent foramen ovale in patients undergoing off-pump coronary artery bypass grafting: case series of eleven patients. *Anesth Analg* 2002; **95**: 1142–6.

29. Djaiani G, Phillips-Bute B, Podgoreanu M, *et al.* The association of patent foramen ovale and atrial fibrillation after coronary artery bypass graft surgery. *Anesth Analg* 2004; **98**: 585–9.

30. Manning WJ, Weintraub RM, Waksmonski CA, *et al.* Accuracy of transesophageal echocardiography for identifying left atrial thrombi: a prospective, intraoperative study. *Ann Intern Med* 1995; **123**: 817–22.

31. Koca V, Bozat T, Akkaya V, *et al.* Left atrial thrombus detection with multiplane transesophageal echocardiography: an echocardiographic study with surgical verification. *J Heart Valve Dis* 1999; **8**: 63–6.

32. Omran H, Jung W, Rabahieh R, *et al.* Imaging of thrombi and assessment of left atrial appendage function: a prospective study comparing transthoracic and transoesophageal echocardiography. *Heart* 1999; **81**: 192–8.

33. Dal-Bianco JP, Khanderia BK, Mookadam F, *et al.* Management of asymptomatic severe aortic stenosis. *J Am Coll Cardiol* 2008; **52**; 1279–92.

34. Bonow RO, Carabello BA, Chatterjee K, *et al.* 2008 Focused update incorporated into the ACC/AHA 2006 guidelines for the management of patients with valvular heart disease. A Report of the ACC/AHA Task Force on Practice Guidelines. *Circulation* 2008; **118**: e523–661.

35. Vahanian A, Baumgartner H, Bax J, *et al.* Guidelines on the management of valvular heart disease: the Task Force on the Management of Valvular Heart Disease of the European Society of Cardiology. *Eur Heart J* 2007; **28**: 230–68.

36. Society of Cardiothoracic Surgeons of Great Britain and Ireland. *National Adult Cardiac Surgical Database Report.* Henley-on-Thames: Dendrite Clinical Systems, 2001.

37. Filsoufi F, Aklog L, Adams DH, Byrne JG. Management of mild to moderate aortic stenosis at the time of coronary artery bypass grafting. *J Heart Valve Dis* 2002; **11** (Suppl. 1): S45–9.

38. Akasaka T, Yoshikawa J, Yoshida K, *et al.* Age-related valvular regurgitation: a study by pulsed Doppler echocardiography. *Circulation* 1987; **76**: 262–5.

39. Moisa RB, Zeldis SM, Alper SA, Scott WC. Aortic regurgitation in coronary artery bypass grafting: implications for cardioplegia administration. *Ann Thorac Surg* 1995; **60**: 665–8.

40. Harris KM, Sundt TM, Aeppli D, Sharma R, Barzilai B. Can late survival of patients with moderate ischemic mitral regurgitation be impacted by intervention on the valve? *Ann Thorac Surg* 2002; **74**: 1468–75.

41. Connolly MW, Gelbfish JS, Jacobowitz IJ, *et al.* Surgical results for mitral regurgitation from coronary artery disease. *J Thorac Cardiovasc Surg* 1986; **91**: 379–88.

42. Duarte IG, Shen Y, MacDonald MJ, *et al.* Treatment of moderate mitral regurgitation and coronary disease by coronary bypass alone: late results. *Ann Thorac Surg* 1999; **68**: 426–30.

43. Mallidi HR, Pelletier MP, Lamb J, *et al.* Late outcomes in patients with uncorrected mild to moderate mitral regurgitation at the time of isolated coronary artery bypass grafting. *J Thorac Cardiovasc Surg* 2004; **127**: 636–44.

44. Di Mauro M, Di Giammarco G, Vitolla G, *et al.* Impact of no-to-moderate mitral regurgitation on late results after isolated coronary artery bypass grafting in patients with ischemic cardiomyopathy. *Ann Thorac Surg* 2006; **81**: 2128–34.

45. Prifti E, Bonacchi M, Frati G, *et al.* Should mild-to-moderate and moderate ischemic mitral regurgitation be corrected in patients with impaired left ventricular function undergoing simultaneous coronary revascularization? *J Card Surg* 2001; **16**: 473–83.

46. Di Donato M, Frigiola A, Menicanti L, *et al.* Moderate ischemic mitral regurgitation and coronary artery bypass surgery: effect of mitral repair on clinical outcome. *J Heart Valve Dis* 2003; **12**: 272–9.

47. Filsoufi F, Aklog L, Byrne JG, *et al.* Current results of combined coronary artery bypass grafting and mitral annuloplasty in patients with moderate ischemic mitral regurgitation. *J Heart Valve Dis* 2004; **13**: 747–53.

48. Aklog L, Filsoufi F, Flores KQ, *et al.* Does coronary artery bypass grafting alone correct moderate ischemic mitral regurgitation? *Circulation* 2001; **104** (12 Suppl. 1): I68–75.

49. Bergquist BD, Leung JM, Bellows WH. Transesophageal echocardiography in myocardial revascularization: I. Accuracy of intraoperative real-time interpretation. *Anesth Analg* 1996; **82**: 1132–8.

50. Comunale ME, Body SC, Ley C, *et al.* The concordance of intraoperative left ventricular wall-motion abnormalities and electrocardiographic S–T segment changes: association with outcome after coronary revascularization. Multicenter Study of Perioperative Ischemia (McSPI) Research Group. *Anesthesiology* 1998; **88**: 945–54.

51. Seeberger MD, Cahalan MK, Rouine-Rapp K, *et al.* Acute hypovolemia may cause segmental wall motion abnormalities in the absence of myocardial ischemia. *Anesth Analg* 1997; **85**: 1252–7.

52. Shanewise JS, Cheung AT, Aronson S, *et al.* ASE/SCA guidelines for performing a comprehensive intraoperative multiplane transesophageal echocardiography examination: recommendations of the ASE Council for intraoperative echocardiography and the SCA Task Force for certification in perioperative transesophageal echocardiography. *Anesth Analg* 1999; **89**: 870–84.

53. Cerqueira MD, Weissman NJ, Dilsizian V, *et al.* Standardized myocardial segmentation and nomenclature for tomographic imaging of the heart: a statement for healthcare professionals from the Cardiac Imaging Committee of the Council on Clinical Cardiology of the American Heart Association. *Circulation* 2002; **105**: 539–42.

54. Stratton JR, Speck SM, Caldwell JH, *et al.* Relation of global and regional left ventricular function to tomographic thallium-201 myocardial perfusion in patients with prior myocardial infarction. *J Am Coll Cardiol* 1988; **12**: 71–7.

55. Heller LB, Aronson S. Assessment of regional ventricular function. In: Savage RM, Aronson S, eds., *Comprehensive Textbook of Intraoperative Transesophageal Echocardiography.* Philadelphia, PA: Lippincott Williams & Wilkins, 2005: 157–69.

56. Urheim S, Edvardsen T, Torp H, Angelsen B, Smiseth OA. Myocardial strain by Doppler echocardiography. Validation of a new method to quantify regional myocardial function. *Circulation* 2000; **102**: 1158–64.

57. Simmons LA, Weidemann F, Sutherland GR, *et al.* Doppler tissue velocity, strain, and strain rate imaging with transesophageal echocardiography in the operating room: a feasibility study. *J Am Soc Echocardiogr* 2002; **15**: 768–76.

58. Hartmann T, Kolev N, Blaicher A, Spiss C, Zimpfer M. Validity of acoustic quantification colour kinesis for detection of left ventricular regional wall motion abnormalities: a transoesophageal echocardiographic study. *Br J Anaesth* 1997; **79**: 482–7.

59. Cottrell DJ, Cornett ES, Seifer MS, *et al.* Diagnosis of an intraoperative aortic dissection by transesophageal echocardiography during routine coronary artery bypass grafting surgery. *Anesth Analg* 2003; **97**: 1254–6.

60. Tingleff J, Joyce FS, Pettersson G. Intraoperative echocardiographic study of air embolism during cardiac operations. *Ann Thorac Surg* 1995; **60**: 673–7.

61. Lin TY, Chiu KM, Wan, MJ, Chu SH. Carbon dioxide embolism during endoscopic saphenous vein harvesting in coronary artery bypass surgery. *J Thorac Cardiovasc Surg* 2003; **126**: 2011–15.

62. Chavanon O, Tremblay I, Delay D, *et al.* Carbon dioxide embolism during endoscopic saphenectomy for coronary artery bypass surgery. *J Thorac Cardiovasc Surg* 1999; **118**: 557–8.

63. Martineau A, Arcand G, Couture P, *et al.* Transesophageal echocardiographic diagnosis of carbon dioxide embolism during minimally invasive saphenous vein harvesting and treatment with inhaled epoprostenol. *Anesth Analg* 2003; **96**: 962–4.

64. Mierdl S, Byhahn C, Lischke V, *et al.* Segmental myocardial wall motion during minimally invasive coronary artery bypass grafting using open and endoscopic surgical techniques. *Anesth Analg* 2005; **100**: 306–14.

65. Khan NE, De Souza A, Mister R, *et al.* A randomized comparison of off-pump and on-pump multivessel coronary-artery bypass surgery. *N Eng J Med* 2004; **350**: 21–8.

66. Bucerius J, Gummert JF, Borger MA, *et al.* Stroke after cardiac surgery: a risk factor analysis of 16,184 consecutive adult patients. *Ann Thorac Surg* 2003; **75**: 472–8.

67. Sharony R, Grossi EA, Saunders PC, *et al.* Propensity case-matched analysis of off-pump coronary artery bypass grafting in patients with atheromatous aortic disease. *J Thorac Cardiovasc Surg* 2004; **127**: 406–13.

68. Trehan N, Mishra M, Kasliwal RR, Mishra A. Reduced neurological injury during CABG in patients with mobile aortic atheromas: a five-year follow-up study. *Ann Thorac Surg* 2000; **70**: 1558–64.

69. Plomondon ME, Cleveland JC, Ludwig ST, *et al.* Off-pump coronary artery bypass is associated with improved risk adjusted outcomes. *Ann Thorac Surg* 2001; **72**: 114–19.

70. Moises VA, Mesquita CB, Campos O, *et al.* Importance of intraoperative transoesophageal echocardiography during coronary artery bypass surgery without cardiopulmonary bypass. *J Am Soc Echocardiogr* 1998; **11**: 1139–44.

71. Kim KB, Lim C, Ahn H, Yang JK. Intraaortic balloon pump therapy facilitates posterior vessel off-pump coronary artery bypass grafting in high risk patients. *Ann Thorac Surg* 2001; **71**: 1964–8.

72. Chassot PG, van der Linden P, Zaugg M, *et al.* Off-pump coronary artery bypass surgery: physiology and anaesthetic management. *Br J Anaesth* 2004; **92**: 400–13.

73. Resano FG, Stamou SC, Lowery RC, Corso PJ. Complete myocardial revascularization on the beating heart with epicardial stabilisation: anesthetic considerations. *J Cardiothorac Vasc Anesth* 2000; **14**: 534–9.

74. Labovitz AJ, Lewen MK, Kern M, *et al.* Evaluation of left ventricular systolic and diastolic dysfunction during transient myocardial ischemia produced by angioplasty. *J Am Coll Cardiol* 1987; **10**: 748–5.

75. Biswas S, Clements F, Diodato L, *et al.* Changes in systolic and diastolic function during multivessel

off-pump coronary bypass grafting. *Eur J Cardiothorac Surg* 2001; **20**: 913–17.

76. Wang J, Filipovic M, Rudzitis A, *et al.* Transesophageal echocardiography for monitoring segmental wall motion during off-pump coronary artery bypass surgery. *Anesth Analg* 2004; **99**: 965–73.

77. Shiga T, Terajima K, Matsumura J, Sakamoto A, Ogawa R. Local cardiac wall stabilization influences the reproducibility of regional wall motion during off-pump coronary artery bypass surgery. *J Clin Monit Comput* 2000; **16**: 25–31.

78. Omae T, Kakihana Y, Mastunaga A, *et al.* Hemodynamic changes during off-pump coronary artery bypass anastomosis in patients with coexisting mitral regurgitation: improvement with milrinone. *Anesth Analg* 2005; **101**: 2–8.

79. Lev-Ran O, Loberman D, Matsa M, *et al.* Reduced strokes in the elderly: the benefits of untouched aorta off-pump coronary surgery. *Ann Thorac Surg* 2004; **77**: 102–7.

80. Grossi EA, Bizekis CS, Sharony R, *et al.* Routine intraoperative transesophageal echocardiography identifies patients with atheromatous aortas: impact on "off-pump" coronary artery bypass and perioperative stroke. *J Am Soc Echocardiogr* 2003; **16**: 751–5.

81. Dor V, Di Donato M. Ventricular remodeling in coronary artery disease. *Curr Opin Cardiol* 1997; **12**: 533–7.

82. Menicanti L, Di Donato M. The Dor procedure: what has changed after fifteen years of clinical practice? *J Thorac Cardiovasc Surg* 2002; **124**: 886–90.

83. Oh JK, Seward JB, Tajik AJ. Coronary artery disease. In: *The Echo Manual*. Philadelphia, PA: Lippincott Williams & Wilkins, 1999.

84. Yamamura Y, Yoshikawa J, Yoshida K, Akasaka T. Echocardiographic findings of subepicardial aneurysm of the left ventricle. *Am Heart J* 1994; **127**: 211–14.

85. Cooley DA, Collins HA, Morris GC, Chapman DW. Ventricular aneurysm after myocardial infarction: surgical excision with the use of temporary cardiopulmonary bypass. *J Am Med Assoc* 1958; **167**: 557–60.

86. Jatène AD. Left ventricular aneurysmectomy: resection or reconstruction. *J Thorac Cardiovasc Surg* 1985; **89**: 321–31.

87. Dor V, Kreitmann P, Jourdan J, *et al.* Interest of physiological closure (circumferential plasty on contractive areas) of left ventricle after resection and endocardectomy for aneurysm or akinetic zone: comparison with classical technique about a series of

209 left ventricular resections (abstract). *J Cardiovasc Surg* 1985; **26**: 73.

88. Elefteriades J, Solomon L, Salazar A, *et al.* Linear left ventricular aneurysmectomy: modern imaging studies reveal improved morphology and function. *Ann Thorac Surg* 1993; **56**: 242–52.

89. Kesler F, Fiore A, Naunheim K, *et al.* Anterior wall left ventricular aneurysm repair. *J Thorac Cardiovasc Surg* 1992; **103**: 841–8.

90. Mickleborough L, Maruyama H, Liu P, Mohamed S. Results of left ventricular aneurysmectomy with a tailored scar excision and primary closure technique. *J Thorac Cardiovasc Surg* 1994; **107**: 690–8.

91. Grossi E, Chimitz L, Galloway A, *et al.* Endoventricular remodeling of left ventricular aneurysm: functional, clinical and electrophysiological results. *Circulation* 1995; **92** (Suppl II): 98–100.

92. Shapira O, Davudoff R, Hilkert R, *et al.* Repair of left ventricular aneurysm: long-term results of linear repair versus endoaneurysmectorraphy. *Ann Thorac Surg* 1997; **63**: 401–5.

93. Cooley D. Management of left ventricular aneurysm by intracavity repair. *Operative Tech Thorac Surg* 1997; **2**: 151–60.

94. Menicanti L, Di Donato M, Frigiola A, *et al.* Ischemic mitral regurgitation: intraventricular papillary muscle imbrication without mitral ring during left ventricular restoration. *J Thorac Cardiovasc Surg* 2002; **123**: 1041–50.

95. Agricola E, Oppizzi M, Maisano F, *et al.* Echocardiographic classification of chronic ischemic mitral regurgitation caused by restricted motion according to tethering pattern. *Eur J Echocardiography* 2004; **5**: 326–34.

96. Otsuji Y, Kumanohoso T, Yoshifuku S, *et al.* Isolated annular dilatation does not usually cause important functional mitral regurgitation: comparison between patients with lone atrial fibrillation and those with idiopathic or ischemic cardiomyopathy. *J Am Coll Cardiol* 2002; **39**: 1651–6.

97. Yiu SF, Enriquez-Sarano M, Tribouilloy C, *et al.* Determinants of the degree of functional mitral regurgitation in patients with systolic left ventricular dysfunction: a quantitative clinical study. *Circulation* 2000; **102**: 1400–6.

98. Raya T, Gay R, Lancaster L, *et al.* Serial changes in left ventricular relaxation and chamber stiffness after large myocardial infarction in rats. *Circulation* 1988; **77**: 1424–31.

99. Dickstein ML, Spotnitz HM, Rose EA, Burkhoff D. Heart reduction surgery: an analysis of the impact on cardiac function. *J Thorac Cardiovasc Surg* 1997; **113**: 1032–40.

100. Ratcliffe MB, Wallace AW, Salahieh A, *et al.* Ventricular volume, chamber stiffness, and function after anteroapical aneurysm plication in the s heep. *J Thorac Cardiovasc Surg* 2000; **119**: 115–24.

101. Castelvecchio S, Menicanti L, Ranucci M, Di Donato M. Impact of surgical ventricular restoration on diastolic function: implications of shape and residual ventricular size. *Ann Thorac Surg* 2008; **86**: 1849–54.

Cardiomyopathies

Alexander Ng, Justiaan Swanevelder

Introduction

Cardiomyopathies comprise a heterogeneous group of diseases of the myocardium. They have been defined by the American Heart Association and the European Society of Cardiology.

The American Heart Association has proposed that cardiomyopathies are myocardial diseases associated with mechanical and/or electrical dysfunction that usually (but not invariably) exhibit inappropriate ventricular hypertrophy or dilation and are due to a variety of causes that are frequently genetic. Cardiomyopathies may be confined to the heart or may be part of generalized systemic disorders, often leading to death or progressive heart-failure-related disability [1].

The European Society of Cardiology has defined cardiomyopathy as a myocardial disease in which the heart muscle is structurally and functionally abnormal, in the absence of coronary artery disease, hypertension, valvular heart disease, and congenital heart disease, sufficient to cause the observed myocardial abnormality [2].

Echocardiography is the imaging modality of choice for investigating and monitoring cardiomyopathies. Patients with cardiomyopathy may require invasive cardiological intervention, cardiac surgery, and electrical management of arrhythmias. Echocardiography plays an important role in all of these therapeutic procedures.

This chapter describes the classic types of cardiomyopathy and highlights their echocardiographic anatomical features.

Classification

Historically, cardiomyopathies were classified by the World Health Organization and International Federation of Cardiology Task Force in 1980 and again in 1995 [3]. The main categories were hypertrophic cardiomyopathy, dilated cardiomyopathy, restrictive cardiomyopathy, and arrhythmogenic right ventricular cardiomyopathy. Other categories included unclassified cardiomyopathies (e.g. non-compaction cardiomyopathy, mitochondrial cardiomyopathy) and specific cardiomyopathies, e.g. ischemic, valvular, hypertensive, inflammatory, and metabolic.

The classification of cardiomyopathies is confusing for four reasons. Firstly, patients in one category may also have features of another category: for example, patients with hypertrophic cardiomyopathy may have restrictive physiology. Secondly, patients with proven genetic mutations for one category may not have the quintessential structural or functional features of that category: for example, hypertrophic cardiomyopathy without left ventricular (LV) hypertrophy. Thirdly, there are insufficient categories, as new cardiomyopathies have been proposed: e.g. ion channel cardiomyopathies. These are electrical rather than structural diseases of the myocardium. Fourthly, some categories should not be considered as cardiomyopathies. Heart muscle diseases attributable to hypertension, valve disease, and ischemia should not be considered as cardiomyopathies, because they are not primary diseases of the myocardium.

The American Heart Association has recently proposed a more detailed classification, taking into account the multiplicity of organ involvement, genetics, structural changes, cellular events, and physiological abnormalities. This classification separates disease involving predominantly the heart (primary cardiomyopathies) from secondary cardiomyopathies, in which myocardial disease is part of a large number of generalized systemic multiorgan disorders [1].

The European classification of cardiomyopathies differs from the American classification, consisting of the following main categories [2]:

- hypertrophic cardiomyopathy (HCM)
- dilated cardiomyopathy (DCM)
- restrictive cardiomyopathy (RCM)

247

Core Topics in Transesophageal Echocardiography, ed. Robert Feneck, John Kneeshaw, and Marco Ranucci.
Published by Cambridge University Press. © Cambridge University Press 2010.

- arrhythmogenic right ventricular cardiomyopathy (ARVC)
- unclassified, e.g. LV non-compaction

The categories are further subdivided by genetics and subtypes.

It is evident that there is no ideal classification for cardiomyopathies. It is likely that the classification will continue to be modified and refined over time in the light of new evidence. However, from an echocardiographic point of view, a simplified classification based on structure and function is probably the most useful. Accordingly, this chapter will describe the classic cardiomyopathies: hypertrophic cardiomyopathy, dilated cardiomyopathy, restrictive cardiomyopathy, arrhythmogenic right ventricular cardiomyopathy, and LV non-compaction.

Principles of echocardiographic assessment

Echocardiography is one component of a complete assessment of patients with cardiomyopathy. The patient's medical history, as well as a general medical examination, should also be reviewed. The echocardiographic examination should include:

- LV chamber dimensions and morphology
- LV wall thickness
- LV systolic function, including regional wall motion abnormalities
- mitral valve disease, aortic valve disease
- LV diastolic function, including left atrial (LA) size
- pulmonary arterial hypertension
- right ventricle (RV) chamber size and morphology
- tricuspid and pulmonary valve abnormalities
- right atrium (RA) size

Hypertrophic cardiomyopathy

Hypertrophic cardiomyopathy is a disease of the sarcomere, presenting at any age. It has an even gender distribution and occurs in all races worldwide. Many patients are asymptomatic, whilst others may experience dyspnea, syncope, chest pain, and atrial fibrillation [4]. Hypertrophic cardiomyopathy is a common cause of sudden death in the young adult.

Mutations of genes coding for several proteins have been identified. The age of onset of disease, degree of hypertrophy, risk of sudden cardiac death, and life expectancy have been shown to be associated with specific mutations in the β-myosin heavy chain and cardiac troponin T genes [5].

Echocardiographic features of hypertrophic cardiomyopathy

Patients with hypertrophic cardiomyopathy have a histological appearance of hypertrophy, sarcomeric disarray, and interstitial fibrosis. Hypertrophic cardiomyopathy is emerging to be a disease of energy utilization, involving excessive energy use, inadequate energy production, and aberrant signaling of energy deficiency [6]. These abnormalities of structure and function may, in part, be detected by echocardiography. The characteristic features of hypertrophic cardiomyopathy are LV hypertrophy, LV outflow tract obstruction, and diastolic dysfunction. It is important to try to differentiate hypertrophic cardiomyopathy from the LV hypertrophy found in hypertension or in trained athletes.

LV hypertrophy

Patients with hypertrophic cardiomyopathy demonstrate LV hypertrophy (Figs. 15.1, 15.2, 15.3) in the absence of systemic disease such as hypertension and aortic stenosis. Usually LV hypertrophy occurs in the septum, and it may extend into the ventricular free wall (Video 15.1) [7]. From an echocardiographic perspective, three important points should be investigated:

1. **Magnitude of hypertrophy**. LV wall thickness is variable in hypertrophic cardiomyopathy, but an end-diastolic value of 15 mm is characteristic [8]. Maximal wall thickness of ≥ 30 mm is a risk factor for sudden cardiac death [4].

2. **Distribution of hypertrophy**. There is much structural heterogeneity in hypertrophic cardiomyopathy, but four patterns of LV hypertrophy may be recognized:

   Type 1: anterior septal hypertrophy
   Type 2: anterior and posterior septal hypertrophy
   Type 3: extensive hypertrophy sparing the posterior basal wall
   Type 4: apical hypertrophy, especially in Japanese people

3. **Absence of LV hypertrophy**. Patients with mutations for hypertrophic cardiomyopathy may not have LV hypertrophy. However, it may still be

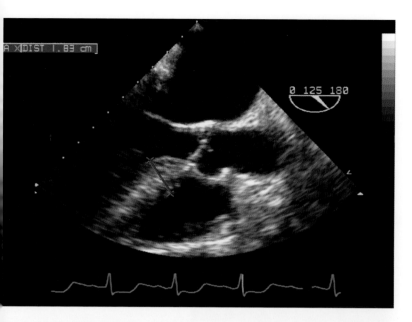

Figure 15.1. HCM: mid-esophageal long-axis view showing anteroseptal LV hypertrophy.

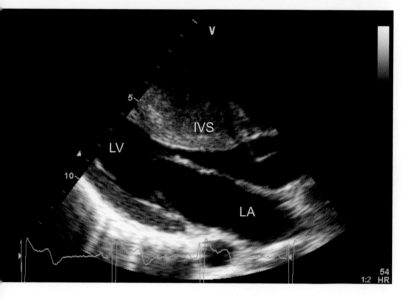

Figure 15.2. HCM: parasternal long-axis view (by transthoracic echo) showing anteroseptal LV hypertrophy.

possible to detect hypertrophic cardiomyopathy using echocardiography. For example, it has been shown that patients without LV hypertrophy but with mutations for hypertrophic cardiomyopathy had significantly lower systolic and early diastolic lateral and septal mitral annular velocities than controls. Septal mitral annual systolic velocity < 12 cm/s and early diastolic velocity < 13 cm/s were 100% sensitive and 90% specific for distinguishing mutation-positive patients from controls [9]. These results were confirmed by a study of patients with hypertrophic cardiomyopathy mutations over time. Over a two-year period, features of hypertrophic cardiomyopathy developed in the mutation-positive patients but not in the control group [10].

LV outflow obstruction

Echocardiography is useful for assessing obstruction to LV outflow, which may occur in the subaortic area

249

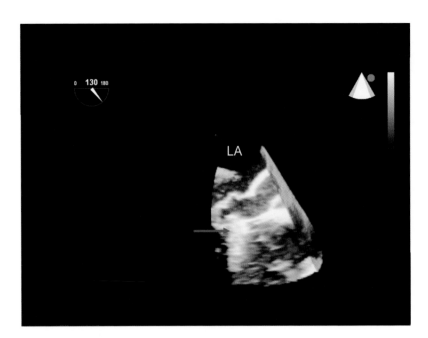

Figure 15.3. HCM: 3D transesophageal dataset showing anteroseptal LV hypertrophy (arrow).

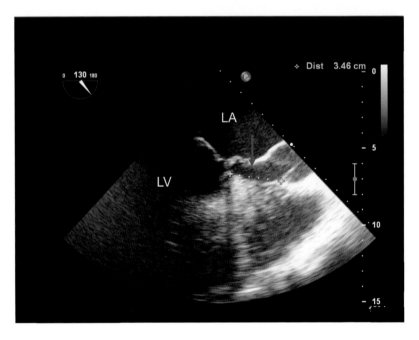

Figure 15.4. HCM: mid-esophageal long-axis view showing a narrow LV outflow tract (arrow).

(Figs. 15.4, 15.5), or occasionally in the mid LV cavity. When there is subaortic flow obstruction, there may be:

- Anterior movement of the mitral valve in systole (Figs. 15.6, 15.7; Video 15.2). A Venturi effect is thought to be responsible for dragging the anterior mitral leaflet into the LV outflow tract.
- A pressure gradient across the outflow tract (Fig. 15.8). This gradient may be variable, because

obstruction is dynamic. It is important to measure the subaortic gradient. A value of 30 mmHg or greater has physiological and therapeutic consequences. A large gradient is associated with hypertrophic cardiomyopathy-related death, progression to NYHA Class III and IV, and death from heart failure or stroke especially in patients aged 40 years or more [11].

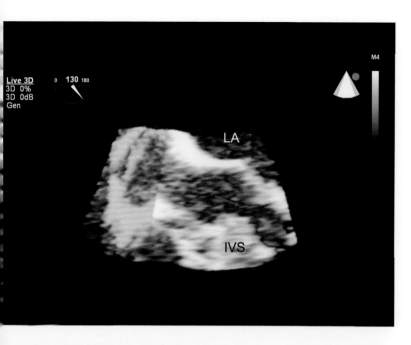

Figure 15.5. HCM: 3D transesophageal dataset showing a narrowed LV outflow tract (arrow).

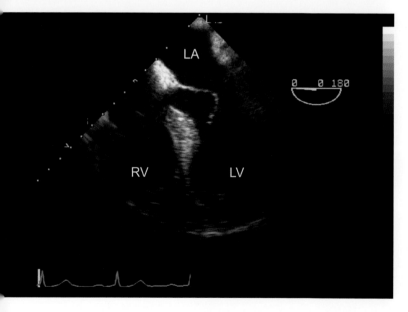

Figure 15.6. HCM: mid-esophageal five-chamber view showing anterior movement of the mitral valve in systole.

In addition, an abnormal blood pressure response during upright exercise in patients older than 40 years is a risk factor for sudden cardiac death.

- Dynamic mitral regurgitation, in which the regurgitant jet is usually posteriorly directed. An anterior or central jet may occur if there are other abnormalities with the mitral valve apparatus (Fig. 15.9). There may be degeneration, myxomatous disease, papillary muscle disease, restriction of the chords and leaflets, and long leaflets (Videos 15.3, 15.4) [12].
- Early closure of the aortic valve with fluttering of its cusps, visualized in M-mode.

In addition, mid-cavity obstruction may occur due to muscular apposition in a small LV cavity. There may be excessive hypertrophy of the mid-ventricle and papillary muscles.

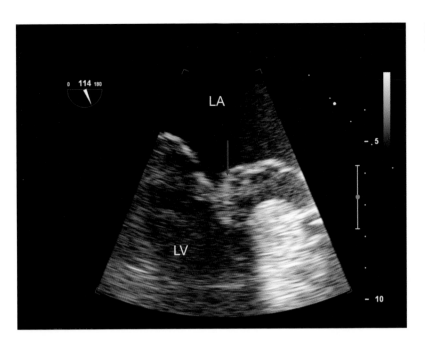

Figure 15.7. HCM: mid-esophageal long-axis view showing anterior movement of the mitral valve in systole.

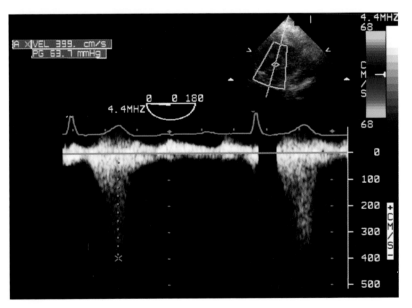

Figure 15.8. HCM: deep transgastric view with continuous-wave Doppler, showing increased flow velocity in the LV outflow tract.

Diastolic dysfunction

Patients with hypertrophic cardiomyopathy have diastolic dysfunction caused by impaired relaxation and reduced LV compliance. There are concomitant elevations in LV and LA pressures. Diastolic dysfunction is assessed by analysis of both transmitral spectral Doppler flow velocity (E) and mitral annular velocity (E′). Transmitral blood flow is represented by an early E wave and a late A wave, on pulsed-wave Doppler echocardiography. Unfortunately, in hypertrophic cardiomyopa-

thy, the E wave varies with preload and does not correlate well with LV hypertrophy, exercise capacity, and LA pressure. It is difficult to distinguish between a pseudo-normalized and normal transmitral E- and A-wave pattern. Further details may be found in Chapter 9.

Tissue Doppler measurement of mitral annular velocity (i.e. myocardial velocity rather than velocity of blood) allows for more accurate evaluation of diastolic dysfunction in patients with this cardiomyopathy. It has been shown that early diastolic mitral annular

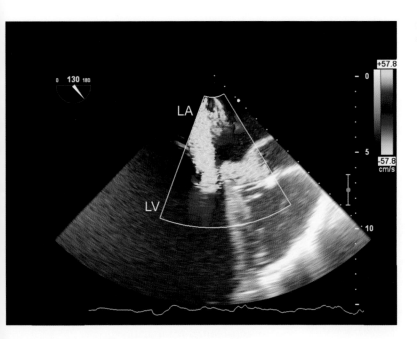

Figure 15.9. HCM: mid-esophageal long-axis view with color Doppler, showing mitral regurgitation and flow acceleration in the LV outflow tract.

velocities are significantly reduced in hypertrophic cardiomyopathy compared with controls. In addition, the ratio of transmitral velocity and mitral annular velocity (E/E') appears to correlate with NYHA functional class. Patients in NYHA Class III had significantly higher E/E' ratios than those in Class II or Class I [13].

Quantification of the severity of diastolic dysfunction is important because it has prognostic implications. Severe dysfunction in hypertrophic cardiomyopathy is uncommon, but it is associated with cardiovascular events such as death, cardiac transplantation, and implantable defibrillator discharge [14]. Also, in a regression analysis of 80 prospectively selected children with hypertrophic cardiomyopathy, a high transmitral E to septal E' ratio was found to be predictive not only of cardiac symptoms but also of death, cardiac arrest, and ventricular tachycardia [15].

Left atrial imaging may help to evaluate diastolic dysfunction. The LA may be enlarged, and this finding has been found to be associated with paroxysmal atrial fibrillation in patients with hypertrophic cardiomyopathy.

Additional echocardiographic features

Other findings may be recognized on echocardiography. These include:

- premature mitral annular calcification [16]
- dilated LV, at end stage, in non-obstructed hypertrophic cardiomyopathy
- apical aneurysm of the LV; this is a rare feature of hypertrophic cardiomyopathy and may be

unrecognized. It has been shown to be associated with thromboembolic stroke, progressive heart failure, and death [17].

Hypertrophic cardiomyopathy versus hypertensive LV hypertrophy

It may be difficult to distinguish, by echocardiography, between non-obstructive hypertrophic cardiomyopathy and LV hypertrophy due to hypertension. LV hypertrophy in hypertrophic cardiomyopathy is characteristically asymmetrical, whereas that of LV hypertrophy caused by hypertension has a concentric appearance. There is some evidence to suggest that the ratio of the interventricular septal thickness to posterior wall thickness (IVST/PWT) on 2D echocardiography, and systolic strain obtained by tissue Doppler imaging or regional myocardial function, are useful discriminators. Compared with hypertensive LV hypertrophy, IVST is expected to be increased, whereas the magnitude of systolic strain may be reduced in patients with hypertrophic cardiomyopathy [18].

Hypertrophic cardiomyopathy versus LV hypertrophy in athletes

Physiologically there are two forms of exercise in athletes [19]:

- Endurance exercise such as long-distance running, which imposes a volume load on the heart. There is a marked increase in LV size and a mild increase in wall thickness.

- Strength exercise such as weight lifting, which places a pressure load on the heart. There is expected to be an increase in wall thickness but only a mild increase in LV size.

Generally, the heart is exposed to a combination of the two types of exercise in athletes, and hence there is a spectrum of appearance of LV cavity size and wall thickness.

Hearts that have a thick wall but are not dilated may be physiologically adapted to exercise, or it may indicate hypertrophic cardiomyopathy. The following criteria may be utilized to support the diagnosis of pathological hypertrophy rather than physiological hypertrophy due to exercise [20]:

- LV outflow tract obstruction caused by systolic anterior motion of the mitral valve
- impaired diastolic function
- enlarged LA (> 50 mm in adult athletes)
- family history of hypertrophic cardiomyopathy in first-degree relatives
- left bundle branch block
- ST segment depression or deep T-wave inversion in two contiguous leads, except in V_1 and V_2 in athletes younger than 16 years

Echocardiography to monitor treatment of hypertrophic cardiomyopathy

In addition to pharmacological methods such as β-blockers and genetic testing in families, the man-agement of hypertrophic cardiomyopathy may include surgical septal myectomy or percutaneous alcohol septal ablation. Echocardiography has a major role during these interventions [13].

Septal myectomy

Septal myectomy is indicated in severe disease, i.e. symptomatic patients with LV outflow tract gradient of 50 mmHg. The procedure involves resection of septal muscle proximal to the aortic valve. In addition, mitral valve replacement or mitral valvuloplasty, and reduction of tethering of the anterior leaflet by the anterolateral papillary muscle, may be required (Figs. 15.10, 15.11). Further dissection is required in cases of mid-cavity obstruction. Intraoperative echocardiography is used to check for:

- residual gradient across the LV outflow tract
- iatrogenic ventricular septal defect
- systolic anterior motion of the mitral valve
- residual mitral regurgitation

In addition to a reduction in maximal instantaneous pressure across the LV outflow tract, septal myectomy has been shown to lead to improvements in other echocardiographic variables: reduction in LA volume index, E/A and E/E′ ratios [21].

Percutaneous alcohol septal ablation

Outflow tract obstruction may be reduced non-surgically by alcoholic septal infarction. This technique is based on the principle that infarction of the upper

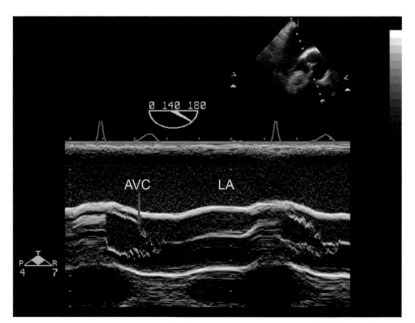

Figure 15.10. HCM: mid-esophageal long-axis view with M-mode across the aortic valve, showing fluttering and early closure of the aortic cusps. AVC, aortic valve closure.

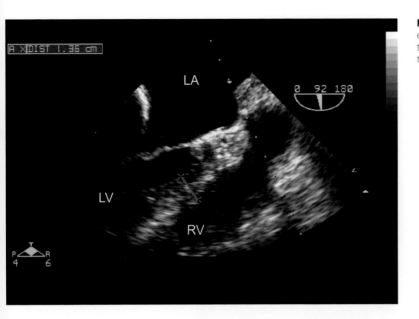

Figure 15.11. HCM: intraoperative mid-esophageal long-axis view post myectomy, demonstrating reduction in septal thickness.

septum leads to resolution of LV outflow obstruction and LV hypertrophy, and improvement of diastolic function.

Following coronary angiography, myocardial contrast echocardiography is required to identify the area of the septum that is supplied by the appropriate septal perforator artery. Complications may also be identified by echocardiography, including:

- mitral regurgitation due to papillary muscle infarction
- left or right ventricular free wall infarction
- cardiac tamponade due to perforation by a temporary pacemaker lead
- LV pump failure due to extensive septal necrosis [22]

After successful alcoholic septal ablation, there is an initial reduction in resting outflow gradient, with further decrease in the following year. Follow-up echocardiography should assess:

- LVOT gradient, using continuous-wave Doppler (CWD)
- the degree of LVH, i.e. LV wall thickness of selected segments, end-diastolic myocardial areas, and LV mass

It has been shown that septal ablation leads to a reduction in outflow gradient and LV wall thickness, as well as an increase in LV end-diastolic and LV end-systolic dimensions [23]. Although alcohol septal ablation is efficacious, its combined procedural complication rate of 27% has been found to be higher than the 5% rate following surgical myectomy [24].

Dilated cardiomyopathy

Dilated cardiomyopathy is a cytoskeletal cardiomyopathy [25]. There is impaired cytoskeletal force transmission and mechanotransduction [6]. Patients present with symptoms of heart failure and, at end stage, they may be referred for cardiac transplantation. In some cases, dilated cardiomyopathy with diffuse interstitial fibrosis is associated with sudden death [26].

Dilated cardiomyopathy is understood to be the final consequence of a variety of pathways such as hypertension, ischemia, toxins, and infection. In the absence of these etiological factors, dilated cardiomyopathy may still occur as a result of gene mutations [27].

Echocardiographic features of dilated cardiomyopathy

The following are echocardiographic features of dilated cardiomyopathy:

- **Ventricular dilation** (Figs. 15.12, 15.13, 15.14), shown by an increase in end-diastolic volume (Videos 15.5, 15.6). The LV is considered to be dilated if its end-diastolic volume is more than 117% of the predicted value for corrected age and body surface area [27].

255

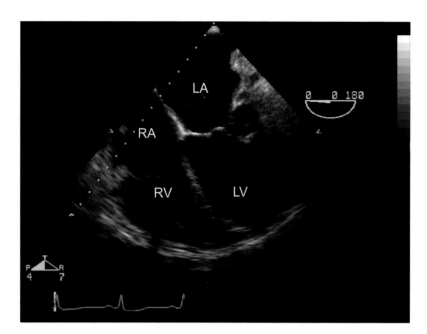

Figure 15.12. DCM: mid-esophageal four-chamber view showing LV and RV dilation.

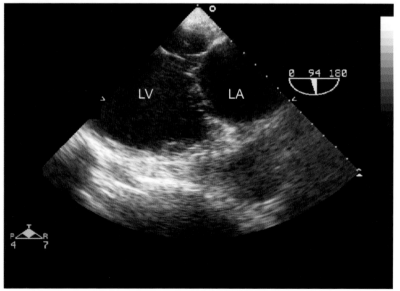

Figure 15.13. DCM: transgastric two-chamber view showing LV dilation. LV end-diastolic diameter may be measured in this view.

- **Severe ventricular systolic dysfunction** (Fig. 15.15). Typically, LV fractional shortening is < 20% and LV ejection fraction is < 35% [28].
- **Functional mitral regurgitation**, with a central jet (Fig. 15.16; Video 15.7) [29].
- **Dilation of the mitral annulus** and hence an increase in the annular dimensions (Fig. 15.17).
- **Tethering of both mitral leaflets** by displaced papillary muscles. The degree of tethering in

mid-systole is reflected in the angle between each leaflet and the annular plane, the height between the annular plane and leaflet point of coaptation, and the tenting area bordered by the annular plane and the two leaflets [29].

- **Functional tricuspid regurgitation** (Fig. 15.18).

It is desirable to differentiate dilated cardiomyopathy from two other conditions, ischemic heart disease and mitral valve disease.

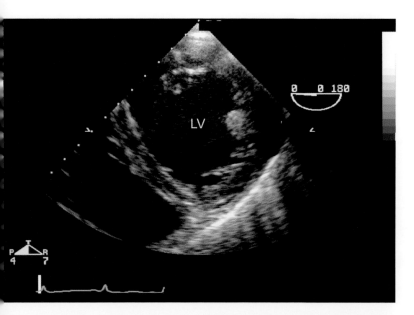

Figure 15.14. DCM: transgastric short-axis view showing LV dilation at the mid-papillary level.

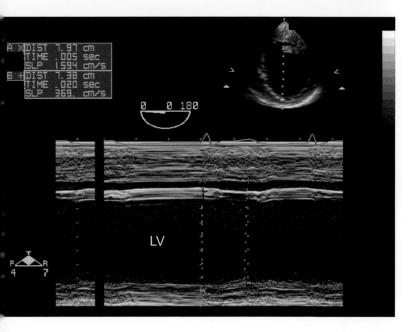

Figure 15.15. DCM: transgastric short-axis view with M-mode, showing poor fractional shortening.

Dilated cardiomyopathy versus LV end-stage ischemic heart disease

Both conditions have similar characteristics: low ejection fraction and elevation of pulmonary artery pressure. In contrast to LV dysfunction caused by ischemia, patients with dilated cardiomyopathy may have the following distinguishing features:

- absence of severe coronary artery disease
- absence of regional wall motion abnormalities

- presence of RV dysfunction, i.e. biventricular dysfunction (Fig. 15.19)

Dilated cardiomyopathy versus LV dysfunction caused by primary mitral valve disease

In both conditions there is low ejection fraction, elevation of pulmonary artery pressure, at least moderate mitral regurgitation, and absence of regional wall motion abnormalities. However, in contrast to LV dysfunction caused by mitral leaflet disease, patients

257

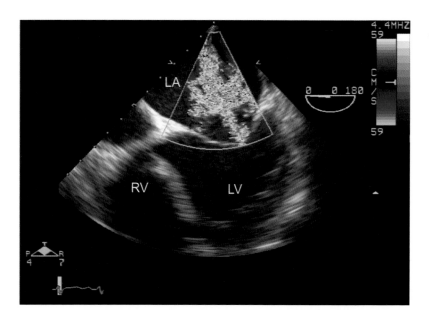

Figure 15.16. DCM: mid-esophageal four-chamber view with color Doppler, showing central mitral regurgitation.

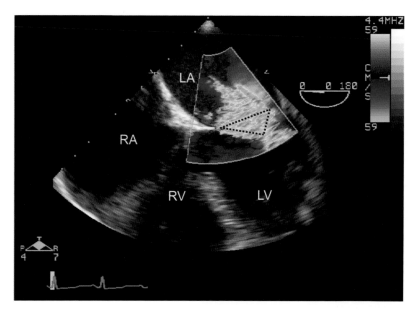

Figure 15.17. DCM: mid-esophageal four-chamber view with color Doppler, showing the tented area bordered by the annular plane and both mitral leaflets.

with dilated cardiomyopathy have the following distinguishing features:

- dilated mitral annulus
- abnormal papillary muscle angle
- leaflet tethering
- absence of severe leaflet pathology, e.g. rheumatic disease, flail, prolapse

Apart from assessment for cardiac transplantation, perioperative echocardiography has a number of roles in the management of patients with dilated cardiomyopathy. These roles include:

- Left ventricular assist device insertion and explantation [30].
- Positioning of intra-aortic balloon pump.
- Guiding left ventriculoplasty. This operation may involve partial left ventriculectomy, mitral valve repair, mitral valve replacement, and tricuspid valve repair [31].

Restrictive cardiomyopathy

Restrictive cardiomyopathy is a sarcomeric cardiomyopathy. Patients may have cardiomegaly, pulmonary

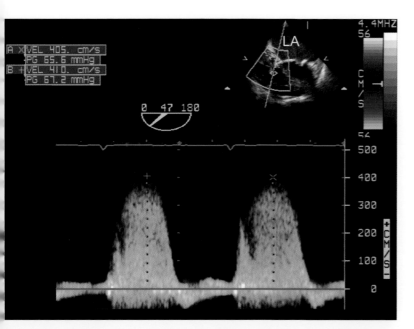

Figure 15.18. DCM: mid-esophageal view with continuous-wave Doppler, showing tricuspid regurgitation.

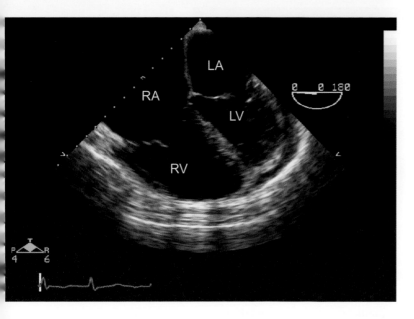

Figure 15.19. DCM: mid-esophageal four-chamber view, showing biventricular dilation and dysfunction.

venous congestion, pleural effusions, and atrial fibrillation. There is diastolic dysfunction with an elevation in filling pressures. Early end-diastolic pressure equalization between the atria and corresponding ventricles may occur, with the characteristic square root sign in transvalvular spectral Doppler [32].

The occurrence of idiopathic restrictive cardiomyopathy is associated with mutations to several genes [33,34]. Restrictive cardiomyopathy may occur in families and the mode of inheritance is autosomal

dominance [35]. Endomyocardial histology shows that patients with idiopathic restrictive cardiomyopathy have myocyte hypertrophy, as well as fibrosis in pericellular, perivascular, and endocardial areas.

Echocardiographic features of restrictive cardiomyopathy

Patients with this condition have the following echocardiographic features:

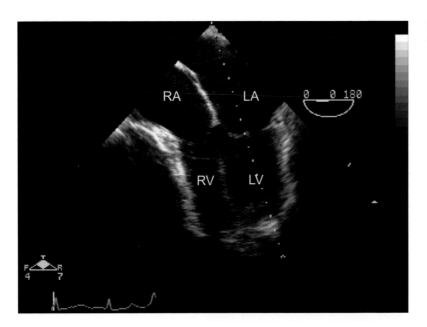

Figure 15.20. RCM: mid-esophageal four-chamber view, showing LA and RA dilation.

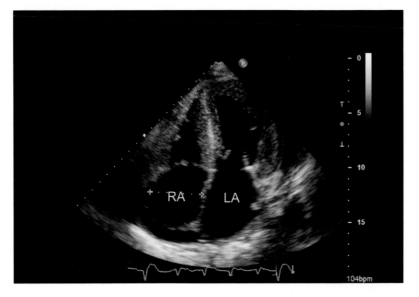

Figure 15.21. RCM: apical four-chamber view (by transthoracic echo), showing LA and RA dilation.

- dilation of both atria because of high filling pressures (Figs. 15.20, 15.21, 15.22; Video 15.8)
- ventricles that are neither hypertrophied nor dilated, in contrast to hypertrophic cardiomyopathy and dilated cardiomyopathy
- mild to moderate mitral and tricuspid valve regurgitation
- moderately elevated pulmonary pressures
- preserved systolic function
- pulmonary venous flow showing a blunted S wave, but pronounced diastolic and atrial

waves in patients in sinus rhythm (Fig. 15.23)
- a restrictive filling pattern, as transmitral velocity is increased, leading to an E/A ratio > 2 (Fig. 15.24). Deceleration time of the E wave is shortened to < 150 ms [32].

The transmitral flow velocity may not be a reliable guide to the elevated filling pressures present in restrictive cardiomyopathy. Transmitral velocity is determined not only by LV relaxation but also by LA pressure. In the early stages of restrictive cardiomy-

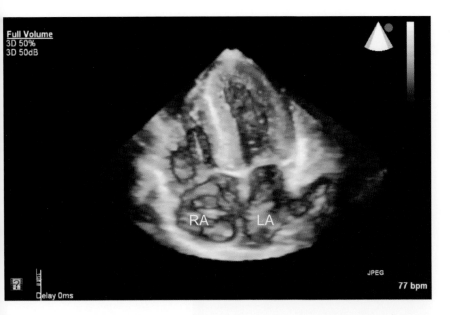

Figure 15.22. RCM: 3D transthoracic dataset, showing LA and RA dilation.

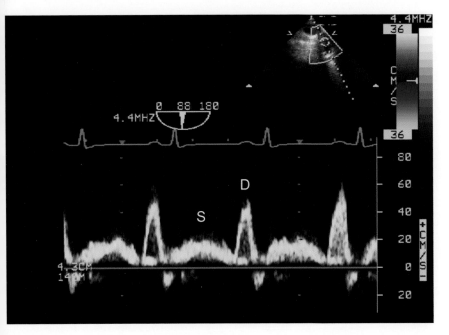

Figure 15.23. RCM: mid-esophageal transducer position with PWD in the left upper pulmonary vein showing blunted S wave.

opathy, transmitral velocity is reduced. However, with disease progression, compliance of the heart decreases and the increase in LA pressure becomes dominant, leading to the pseudonormalization of transmitral velocity. As described in the case of hypertrophic cardiomyopathy, E/E′ may be a more reliable guide to LV filling pressure, as this ratio increases with severity of disease.

Restrictive cardiomyopathy versus constrictive pericarditis

Restrictive cardiomyopathy shares some echocardiographic characteristics with constrictive pericarditis. In both conditions there is elevation of filling pressures and restriction of LV filling. In restrictive cardiomyopathy, there is stiffness due to myocardial disease,

261

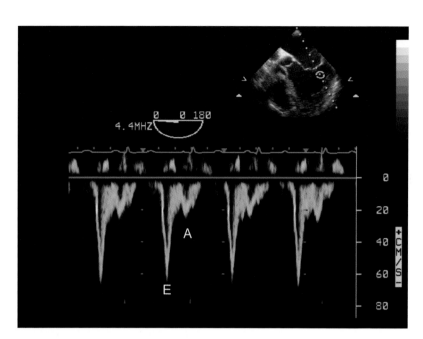

Figure 15.24. RCM: mid-esophageal five-chamber view with PWD at the mitral leaflet tips, showing a restrictive filling pattern.

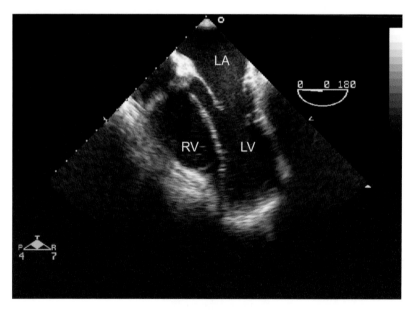

Figure 15.25. Constrictive pericarditis: mid-esophageal four-chamber view showing interventricular septal shift to the LV.

but in constrictive pericarditis stiffness is caused by pericardial disease. Two important echocardiographic techniques, mitral tissue Doppler velocity (E′) and assessment of interventricular septal dependence with respiration, may be used to distinguish between these two conditions.

Early mitral tissue Doppler velocity

Early mitral tissue Doppler velocity (E′) is preserved in constrictive pericarditis but blunted in patients with restrictive cardiomyopathy [36,37]. This reduction in myocardial annular velocity is consistent with the pathological finding that restrictive cardiomyopathy is a disease of the myocardium. In contrast, constrictive pericarditis is primarily a problem of relaxation due to a tight pericardium, and so myocardial tissue velocities are preserved. Thus, with progression of disease and elevation in LV filling pressure, the E/E′ ratio is increased in restrictive cardiomyopathy but not in constrictive pericarditis [38]. Similar findings have been obtained from the myocardial velocity gradient, which is a reflection of the rate of change of wall thickness. It has been shown that the Doppler myocardial velocity gradient across the posterior ventricular wall is reduced in restrictive cardiomyopathy but not in constrictive pericarditis [39].

Interventricular septal dependence with respiration

In constrictive pericarditis, but not in restrictive cardiomyopathy, there is interventricular septal dependence caused by reciprocal changes in filling of the LV and RV, with respiration. This occurrence has been studied in spontaneously breathing patients and may be explained by consideration of intrathoracic pressure, LA pressure, and LV pressure. In patients without constrictive pericarditis, intrathoracic pressure becomes negative during inspiration, with a concomitant decrease in both LA and LV pressure. Compared with expiration, there is little change in the pressure gradient between the LA and the LV in inspiration. Thus transmitral E velocity in inspiration is effectively similar to that in expiration. When there is pericardial constriction, intrathoracic pressure falls in inspiration without significant transmission to the heart and hence without reduction in LV pressure. Thus there is a reduction in gradient between the LA and the LV, and so transmitral blood flow velocity in inspiration may also decrease, to at least 25% lower than in expiration. However, transmitral blood velocity may not always vary with respiration in the supine position, and it may be necessary to decrease preload by adopting a head-up tilt to observe this change in a patient with constrictive pericarditis [40].

Whilst there is a decrease in LV filling and hence a reduction in transmitral blood flow velocity in inspiration, there is an increase in RV filling with an increase in transtricuspid blood flow velocity. The interventricular septum may be shifted towards the LV (Fig. 15.25), demonstrating interventricular dependence [41]. In expiration, the opposite happens: transmitral blood flow velocity increases and transtricuspid blood flow velocity decreases, compared with those detected in inspiration. Changes in blood flow with respiration may also be seen in other vessels – the pulmonary veins for the left side of the heart and the hepatic veins for the right side of the heart. Over the course of several respiratory cycles, in patients with constrictive pericarditis, the interventricular septum is seen to oscillate abnormally with respiration.

In addition, to facilitate diagnosis of restrictive cardiomyopathy and to distinguish it from constrictive pericarditis, other modalities such as computer tomography and magnetic resonance imaging may be necessary [42]. These investigations may be useful in the detection of pericardial thickening and calcification.

Arrhythmogenic right ventricular cardiomyopathy

Arrhythmogenic right ventricular cardiomyopathy is a cytoskeletal cardiomyopathy [25]. Patients with arrhythmogenic right ventricular cardiomyopathy may present with ventricular ectopics, sustained and non-sustained ventricular tachycardia, cardiac failure, and sudden death, especially in adolescence.

Arrhythmogenic right ventricular cardiomyopathy is a genetic cardiac disease involving mutations of genes coding for several proteins. The mode of inheritance is often autosomal dominance [6].

Echocardiographic features of arrhythmogenic right ventricular cardiomyopathy

In arrhythmogenic right ventricular cardiomyopathy there is loss of anchoring of intermediate filaments to the cytoplasmic membranes in adjoining cells, leading to myocyte detachment and death [6]. Replacement of the myocardium with fat and fibrous tissue occurs in all layers except the subendocardium [43]. Primarily there is thinning of the right ventricle, and in some cases this pathological process occurs also in the left ventricle (Figs.15.26, 15.27) [44].

In 1994 a joint task force of the European Society of Cardiology and the International Society and Federation of Cardiology published guidelines on the minimal diagnostic criteria for ARVC [45].

From an echocardiographic view point, early diagnosis is difficult, particularly because of the irregular shape and trabeculation of the normal right ventricle. Magnetic resonance imaging showing intramyocardial fatty infiltration is pathognomonic. However, a number of echocardiographic features have been shown to be suggestive of arrhythmogenic RV cardiomyopathy; these include [46]:

- trabecular derangement
- hyperreflexive moderator band
- sacculations

263

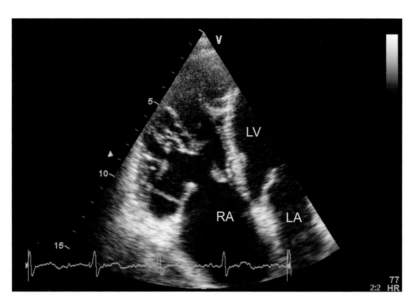

Figure 15.26. Apical four-chamber view (by transthoracic echo), showing RV dilation and abnormal morphology of RV free wall, suggestive of ARVC. There are excessive trabeculations.

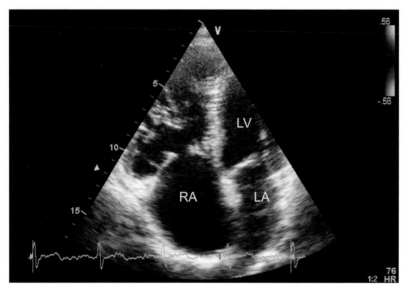

Figure 15.27. ARVC: apical four-chamber view (by transthoracic echo), showing a normal LV appearance.

- RV outflow tract dilation, diameter > 30 mm
- RV regional wall motion abnormality, affecting mainly the apex and anterior wall
- global RV dysfunction in severe disease, fractional shortening < 32%

Owing to the severe implications of arrhythmogenic right ventricular cardiomyopathy, sudden death in adolescence and its familial implications, early diagnosis would be ideal because of the possibility of improved risk stratification and treatment. An international registry has been set up in North America,

with the expectation that it may go some way to improve management of patients with arrhythmogenic right ventricular cardiomyopathy [47].

LV non-compaction

LV non-compaction is a sarcomeric cardiomyopathy affecting children and adults. The presenting features include heart failure, arrhythmias, and thromboembolism [16,48].

There are sporadic and familial cases of LV non-compaction; in the latter the mode of transmission is

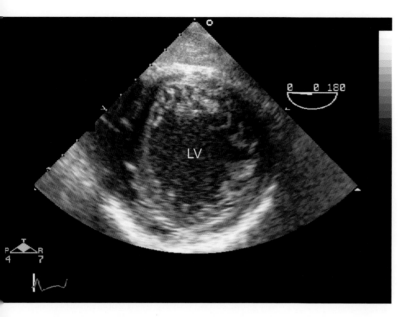

Figure 15.28. LV non-compaction: transgastric short-axis view of the LV showing a compacted layer and non-compacted layer.

utosomal dominance or, rarely, X-linkage [49]. Mutations in genes coding for several proteins have been identified in LV non-compaction [50]. Mutation of the α-cardiac actin gene has been shown to occur both in patients with LV non-compaction and in those with the apical form of hypertrophic cardiomyopathy [51].

Echocardiographic features of LV non-compaction

The following may be identified in patients with LV non-compaction:

- ventricular myocardium comprising a non-compacted layer and a compacted layer (Fig. 15.28), with a ratio ≥ 2
- multiple ventricular trabeculations, prominent in the middle and apical segments
- multiple deep intratrabecular recesses communicating with the ventricular cavity: appearance may be enhanced by color Doppler
- systolic dysfunction
- usually LV involvement

Conclusion

Although echocardiography forms only one part of the assessment of a patient with a cardiomyopathy, it is a valuable tool in discriminating between the various cardiomyopathies. In some cardiomyopathies the information acquired may allow the progress of the

diseases, the effect of therapy, and the prognosis to be elucidated.

References

1. Maron BJ, Towbin JA, Thiene G, *et al.* Contemporary definitions and classification of the cardiomyopathies: an American Heart Association Scientific Statement from the Council on Clinical Cardiology, Heart Failure and Transplantation Committee; Quality of Care and Outcomes Research and Functional Genomics and Translational Biology Interdisciplinary Working Groups; and Council on Epidemiology and Prevention. *Circulation* 2006; **113**: 1807–16.

2. Elliott P, Andersson B, Arbustini E, *et al.* Classification of the cardiomyopathies: a position statement from the European Society of Cardiology Working Group on myocardial and pericardial diseases. *Eur Heart J* 2008; **29**: 270–6.

3. Richardson P, Rapporteur MW, Bristow M, *et al.* Report of the 1995 World Health Organization/ International Society and Federation of Cardiology Task Force on the Definition and Classification of Cardiomyopathies. *Circulation* 1996; **93**: 841–2.

4. Maron BJ. Hypertrophic cardiomyopathy: a systematic review. *JAMA* 2002; **287**: 1308–20.

5. Roberts R, Sigwart U. New concepts in hypertrophic cardiomyopathies, part 1. *Circulation* 2001; **104**: 2113–6.

6. Ashrafian H, Watkins H. Reviews of translational medicine and genomics in cardiovascular disease: new disease taxonomy and therapeutic implications. *J Am Coll Cardiol* 2007; **49**: 1251–64.

7. Roberts R, Sigwart U. New concepts in hypertrophic cardiomyopathies, part 2. *Circulation* 2001; **104**: 2249–52.

8. Elliott PM, Poloniecki J, Dickie S, *et al.* Sudden death in hypertrophic cardiomyopathy: identification of high risk patients. *J Am Coll Cardiol* 2000; **36**: 2212–8.

9. Nagueh SF, Bachinski LL, Meyer D, *et al.* Tissue Doppler imaging consistently detects myocardial abnormalities in patients with cardiomyopathy and provides a novel means for an early diagnosis before and independently of hypertrophy. *Circulation* 2001; **104**: 128–30.

10. Nagueh SF, McFalls J, Meyer D, *et al.* Tissue Doppler imaging predicts the development of hypertrophic cardiomyopathy in subjects with subclinical disease. *Circulation* 2003; **108**: 395–8.

11. Maron BJ, McKenna WJ, Danielson GK, *et al.* ACC/ESC clinical expert consensus document on hypertrophic cardiomyopathy: a report of the American College of Cardiology Task Force on Clinical Expert Consensus Documents and the European Society of Cardiology Committee for Practice Guidelines (Committee to develop an expert consensus document on hypertrophic cardiomyopathy). *Eur Heart J* 2003; **24**: 1965–91.

12. Kaple RK, Murphy RT, DiPaola LM, *et al.* Mitral valve abnormalities in hypertrophic cardiomyopathy: echocardiographic features and surgical outcomes. *Ann Thor Surg* 2008; **85**: 1527–35.

13. Maron MS, Olivotto I, Betocchi S, *et al.* Effect of left ventricular outflow tract obstruction on clinical outcome in hypertrophic cardiomyopathy. *N Eng J Med* 2003; **348**: 295–303.

14. Kubo T, Gimeno JR, Bahl A, *et al.* Prevalence, clinical significance and genetic basis of hypertrophic cardiomyopathy with restrictive phenotype. *J Am Coll Cardiol* 2007; **49**: 2419–26.

15. McMahon CJ, Nagueh SF, Pignatelli RH, *et al.* Characterization of left ventricular diastolic function by tissue Doppler imaging and clinical status in children with hypertrophic cardiomyopathy. *Circulation* 2004; **109**: 1756–62.

16. Alizad A, Seward JB. Echocardiographic features of genetic diseases: part 1. *Cardiomyopathy. J Am Soc Echocardiogr* 2000; **13**: 73–86.

17. Maron MS, Finley JJ, Bos M, *et al.* Prevalence, clinical significance and natural history of left ventricular apical aneurysms in hypertrophic cardiomyopathy. *Circulation* 2008; **118**: 1541–9.

18. Kato TS, Noda A, Izawa H, *et al.* Discrimination of nonobstructive hypertrophic cardiomyopathy from hypertensive left ventricular hypertrophy on the basis of strain rate imaging by tissue Doppler ultrasonography. *Circulation* 2004; **110**: 3808–14.

19. Khamis RY, Mayet J. Echocardiographic assessment of left ventricular hypertrophy in elite athletes. *Heart* 2008; **94**: 1254–55.

20. Basavarajaiah S, Boraita A, Whyte G, *et al.* Ethnic differences in left ventricular remodeling in highly-trained athletes. *J Am Coll Cardiol* 2008; **51**: 2256–62.

21. Menon SC, Ackerman MJ, Ommen SR, *et al.* Impact of septal myectomy on left atrial volume and left ventricular diastolic filling patterns: an echocardiographic study on young patients with obstructive hypertrophic cardiomyopathy. *J Am Soc Echocardiogr* 2008; **21**: 684–8.

22. Faber L, Seggewiss H, Welge D, *et al.* Echo-guided percutaneous septal ablation for symptomatic hypertrophic obstructive cardiomyopathy: 7 years of experience. *Eur J Echocardiogr* 2004; **5**: 347–55.

23. Mazur W, Nagueh SF, Lakkis NM, *et al.* Regression of left ventricular hypertrophy after nonsurgical septal reduction therapy for hypertrophic obstructive cardiomyopathy. *Circulation* 2001; **103**: 1492–6.

24. Sorajja P, Valeti U, Nishimura RA, *et al.* Outcome of alcohol septal ablation for obstructive hypertrophic cardiomyopathy. *Circulation* 2008; **118**: 131–9.

25. Thiene G, Corrado D, Basso C. Cardiomyopathies: is it time for a molecular classification? *Eur Heart J* 2004; **25**: 1772–5.

26. Ellinor PT, Sasse-Klaassen S, Probst S, *et al.* A novel locus for dilated cardiomyopathy, diffuse myocardial fibrosis, and sudden death on chromosome 10q25–26. *J Am Coll Cardiol* 2006; **48**: 106–11.

27. Mestroni L, Rocco C, Gregori D, *et al.* Familial dilated cardiomyopathy: evidence for genetic and phenotypic heterogeneity. *J Am Coll Cardiol* 1999; **34**: 181–90.

28. Paraskevaidis IA, Dodouras T, Adamopoulos S, Kremastinos DT. Left atrial functional reserve in patients with nonischemic dilated cardiomyopathy: an echocardiographic dobutamine study. *Chest* 2002; **122**: 1340–7.

29. Kwan J, Shiota T, Agler D, *et al.* Geometric differences of the mitral valve apparatus between ischemic and dilated cardiomyopathy with significant mitral regurgitation: real-time three-dimensional echocardiography. *Circulation* 2003; **107**: 1135–40.

30. Dandel M, Weng Y, Siniawski H, *et al.* Prediction of cardiac stability after weaning from left ventricular assist devices in patients with idiopathic dilated cardiomyopathy. *Circulation* 2008; **118** (Suppl 1): S94–105.

31. Suma H, Tanabe H, Uejima T, *et al.* Selected ventriculoplasty for idiopathic dilated cardiomyopathy with advanced congestive heart failure: midterm results and risk analysis. *Eur J Cardiothorac Surg* 2007; **32**: 912–16.

32. Ammash NM, Seward JB, Bailey KR, *et al*. Clinical profile and outcome of idiopathic restrictive cardiomyopathy. *Circulation* 2000; **101**: 2490–6.

33. Kaski JP, Syrris P, Burch M, *et al*. Idiopathic restrictive cardiomyopathy in children is caused by mutations in cardiac sarcomeric protein genes. *Heart* 2008; **94**: 1478–84.

34. Mogensen J, Kubo T, Duque M, *et al*. Idiopathic restrictive cardiomyopathy is part of the clinical expression of cardiac troponin I mutations. *J Clin Invest* 2003; **111**: 209–16.

35. Zhang J, Kumar A, Kaplan L, *et al*. Genetic linkage of a novel autosomal dominant restrictive cardiomyopathy locus. *J Med Genet* 2005; **42**: 663–5.

36. Garcia MJ, Rodriguez L, Ares M, *et al*. Differentiation of constrictive pericarditis from restrictive cardiomyopathy: assessment of left ventricular diastolic velocities in longitudinal axis by Doppler tissue imaging. *J Am Coll Cardiol* 1996; **27**: 108–14.

37. Gorcsan J. Tissue Doppler echocardiography. *Curr Opin Cardiol* 2000; **15**: 323–9.

38. Ha JW, Oh JK, Ling LH, *et al*. Annulus paradoxus: transmitral flow velocity to mitral annular velocity ratio is inversely proportional to pulmonary capillary wedge pressure in patients with constrictive pericarditis. *Circulation* 2001; **104**: 976–8.

39. Palka P, Lange A, Donnelly JE, Nihoyannopoulos P. Differentiation between restrictive cardiomyopathy and constrictive pericarditis by early diastolic Doppler myocardial velocity gradient at the posterior wall. *Circulation* 2000; **102**: 655–62.

40. Oh JK, Tajik AJ, Appleton CP, *et al*. Preload reduction to unmask the characteristic Doppler features of constrictive pericarditis. *Circulation* 1997; **95**: 796–9.

41. Hurrell DG, Nishimura RA, Higano ST, *et al*. Value of dynamic respiratory changes in left and right ventricular pressures for the diagnosis of constrictive pericarditis. *Circulation* 1996; **93**: 2007–13.

42. Di Cesare E. MRI of cardiomyopathies. *Eur J Radiol* 2001; **38**; 179–84.

43. Fontaine G, Gallais Y, Fornes P, Hébert JL, Frank R. Arrhythmogenic right ventricular dysplasia/cardiomyopathy. *Anesthesiology* 2001; **95**: 250–4.

44. McCrohon JA, John AS, Lorenz CH, Davies SW, Pennell DJ. Left ventricular involvement in arrhythmogenic right ventricular cardiomyopathy. *Circulation* 2002; **105**: 1394.

45. McKenna WJ, Thiene G, Nava A, *et al*. Diagnosis of arrhythmogenic right ventricular dysplasia/cardiomyopathy. *Br Heart J* 1994; **71**: 215–18.

46. Yoerger DM, Marcus F, Sherrill D, *et al*. Echocardiographic findings in patients meeting task force criteria for arrhythmogenic right ventricular dysplasia. *J Am Coll Cardiol* 2005; **45**: 860–5.

47. Marcus F, Towbin JA, Zareba W, *et al*. Arrhythmogenic right ventricular dysplasia/cardiomyopathy (ARVD/C): a multidisciplinary study: design and protocol. *Circulation* 2003; **107**: 2975–8.

48. Maltagliati A, Pepi M. Isolated noncompaction of the myocardium: multiplane transesophageal echocardiography diagnosis in an adult. *J Am Soc Echocardiogr* 2000; **13**: 1047–9.

49. Markiewicz-Loskot G, Moric-Janiszewska E, Loskot M, *et al*. Isolated ventricular non-compaction: clinical study and genetic review. *Europace* 2006; **8**: 1064–7.

50. Klaassen S, Probst S, Oechslin E, *et al*. Mutations in sarcomere protein genes in left ventricular noncompaction. *Circulation* 2008; **117**: 2893–901.

51. Monserrat L, Hermida-Prieto M, Fernandez X, *et al*. Mutation in the alpha-cardiac actin gene associated with apical hypertrophic cardiomyopathy, left ventricular non-compaction and septal defects. *Eur Heart J* 2007; **28**: 1953–61.

Mitral valve repair

Fabio Guarracino

Introduction

In recent years the emphasis in surgery for mitral regurgitation has changed from valve replacement to valve conservation and repair [1–3]. This change is supported by evidence of better outcomes [4,5]. Mitral valve repair offers the advantage of lower perioperative morbidity and mortality, preservation of ventricular–mitral continuity by sparing the subvalvular apparatus, no requirement for anticoagulant therapy, and longer cardiac event-free life for the patient [6,7]. In many institutions, mitral repair surgery can be offered to almost every patient suffering from mitral regurgitation. Many different surgical approaches have been attempted, based on the mechanism of the disease and on the surgical philosophy [8–10]. In all of these approaches the aim is to completely eliminate the regurgitation [11].

Transesophageal echocardiography (TEE) has emerged as a valuable tool in mitral valve repair, with a role both in surgical decision making and in improving patient outcomes [12,13]. Intraoperative TEE provides real-time information about valve anatomy and function and should elucidate the mechanism of valvular dysfunction, and hence help the surgeon to plan the procedure [14,15]. In particular, the outcome is determined by the quality of the repair, and the adequacy of the repair is assessed by TEE in the operating room.

Intraoperative pre-bypass examination of the mitral valve

Intraoperative TEE is frequently performed under hemodynamic conditions that are very different from those of awake TEE. The effect of the relative vasodilation and hypotension produced in the anesthetized supine patient makes accurate assessment of the severity of mitral regurgitation more difficult. The degree of regurgitation is always reduced by anesthesia, and this must be taken into account when grading the severity

of mitral regurgitation [16]. In the cardiac surgical operating room it is possible to manipulate the blood pressure and heart rate to ensure that assessment of the valve is undertaken under hemodynamic conditions that mimic the awake state [17].

Intraoperative evaluation of the regurgitant mitral valve apparatus is perfomed twice, once before cardiopulmonary bypass and again after weaning from cardiopulmonary bypass [18,19].

The pre-bypass examination aims to refine the preoperative diagnosis in the following areas:

- examining the morphology and function of the mitral valve apparatus
- determining the mechanism of regurgitation
- assessing the severity of regurgitation (n.b. the hemodynamic effects of anesthesia – see above.)
- assessing the feasibility of repair
- checking for other cardiac structural and functional abnormalities

There should be a systematic examination of the entire mitral valve apparatus. This comprises both leaflets, the annulus, the subvalvular apparatus (including chordae and papillary muscles), and the left ventricle (LV) [20]. The anatomy and function is examined with 2D echo, followed by color Doppler evaluation of the regurgitant jet(s) [21,22]. The examination is performed following the standard views described in Chapter 5.

Particular attention should be paid to both apposition and coaptation. Apposition refers to the relationship of the edges of the leaflets to one another, and their relationship to the annulus. In normal apposition both leaflets lie on the same plane at annular level (Fig. 16.1). Coaptation refers to the way the leaflets touch one another along the entire closure line of the mitral valve. Good coaptation is essential for valvular competence.

Leaflet mobility may be described using the terminology introduced by Carpentier in the 1970s, which

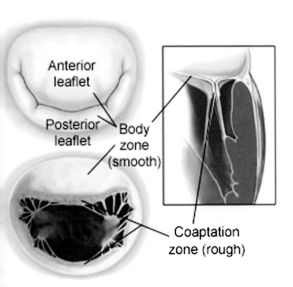

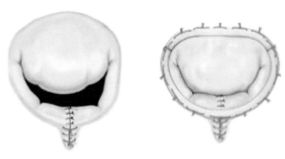

Figure 16.2. Persistent dilation of posterior annulus (circular shape) despite posterior resection. This is resolved by an annuplasty ring.

Figure 16.1. Normal coaptation zone of the mitral valve.

describes the function of mitral leaflets with regard to their relationship to the annular plane [23] (see also Chapter 7). Color Doppler evaluation adds further important information. The precise origin of the regurgitant jet from the closure line and the direction of the jet itself helps to determine the mechanism of the dysfunction (Fig. 7.20). Carpentier Class I mitral regurgitation is usually associated with central regurgitant jets going back into the left atrium (Video 16.1). Class II disease produces jets which flow away from the pathological leaflet. These may be very eccentric to the valve and may run around the left atrial wall (Coanda effect) (Videos 16.2–16.4). In Class IIIB, the regurgitant jet may be central or eccentric depending on the mechanism of the loss of coaptation (see 'ischemic mitral regurgitation, below). If the jet is eccentric it usually flows towards the affected leaflet, unlike the jet of a Class II lesion (Video 16.5).

Evaluation of leaflet dimensions is also helpful. In a normal valve the ratio of anterior to posterior leaflet height is 3/1, and the ratio of the anterior leaflet length to the anteroposterior annulus diameter is 2/3. Measurement of these dimensions is helpful in the pre-bypass assessment. In our experience an anterior leaflet with reduced height often predicts unsuccessful repair with annuloplasty alone in patients with Class I and IIIB lesions (annular dilation or ventricular dysfunction).

Annulus

The anterior part of the mitral annulus has a fibrous structure which is part of the aortic valve and the two trigones. The posterior annulus contains very little tissue other than cardiac muscle and is not supported by any fibrous structures. This may explain why annular dilation always occurs at the posterior part of the mitral annulus.

It is important to measure the anteroposterior diameter of the annulus and to describe its shape and motion [24]. The description should include the presence of calcification, which is more frequently seen in the posterior part of the annulus than in the anterior.

The measurement of the anteroposterior diameter, the most important measurement for the surgeon approaching a repair, is best performed in views which interrogate the anteroposterior axis of the valve (usually the mid-esophageal view at about 120°). The commissural diameter can be measured at around 60°, and this can be compared to the anteroposterior diameter to demonstrate the annular shape. This should normally be oval in a ratio of 2/3 with the shortest diameter in the anteroposterior plane. If both diameters are approaching the same value, the annulus will have dilated posteriorly to become circular in shape (Fig. 16.2).

The annulus shortens by about 30% of its length during systole. Periannular myocardial fibers contract during systole, and this dynamic behavior is important in maintaining mitral competence. The contraction occurs mainly in the posterior part of the annulus. This systolic movement can be evaluated by measuring the diameter both in systole and in diastole, or by sampling the annulus with tissue Doppler (Video 16.6). This evaluation is helpful in the setting of ischemic mitral regurgitation, and may help to decide whether moderate mitral regurgitation will benefit from annuloplasty combined with revascularization, or from revascularization alone.

Subvalvular apparatus

Evaluation of chordae tendineae is possible in the mid-esophageal views and in the transgastric long-axis view. This last view is often the best to visualize the chordae (Video 16.7). These views may demonstrate elongated, shortened, or ruptured chordae (Videos 16.8–16.10). Remember that both papillary muscles provide both leaflets with cords. The posteromedial papillary muscle provides cords to the middle to anterior parts of both leaflets, and cords from the anterolateral papillary muscle go to the middle and anterior parts of both leaflets (Fig. 16.3) [25]. Hence rupture of a primary cord from posteromedial papillary muscle may result in a flail lesion of either leaflet. The same views may allow other abnormalities of the papillary muscles to be seen (fibrosis, calcification, or rupture) (Videos 16.11, 16.12) [26].

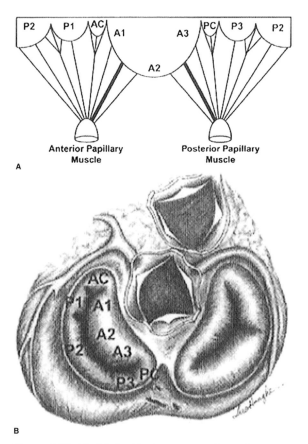

Figure 16.3. (A) Relationship between anterior and posterior papillary muscles, mitral valve scallops, and chordae tendineae. (B) Cross-section at the base of the heart showing the location of the segments and scallops of the mitral valve.

Ventricle

Evaluation of the LV completes the systematic assessment of the mitral apparatus. Attention should be paid to the papillary muscle attachments and the basal segments to look for wall motion abnormalities or aneurysmal muscle, which may be responsible for mitral regurgitation due to altered ventricular geometry in ischemic disease (Video 16.13) [27].

Ischemic mitral regurgitation

In patients with coronary artery disease and mitral regurgitation the valve is usually morphologically normal [28]. The regurgitation is caused by ventricular dysfunction, often associated with changes in LV geometry [29].

Such changes can be divided into those occurring at the basal level and those affecting the geometry of the mid and apical parts of the LV. The former involve the periannular region of the ventricle, and consist of akinesia and/or dilation of posterior annulus with a resulting increase in the anteroposterior annular diameter (Fig. 16.4). This may be seen fairly commonly in patients with moderate mitral regurgitation resulting from inferior myocardial infarction [30]. It is important to measure this diameter in the appropriate view, and to assess annular motion (see above). Annular contractility may be further assessed using low-dose dobutamine or atrial pacing with epicardial electrodes [31,32]. Under such stress condition annular systolic shortening and the myocardial velocities in the annular region are assessed. Annular shortening by one-third and an increase in systolic velocity indicate the presence of viable myocardium and predict recovery after revascularization. In this case the patient may be treated by revascularization without annuloplasty [33]. If no systolic shortening and no increase of systolic velocity is produced by dobutamine or atrial pacing, a negative predictive value can be attributed to the echo information. This suggests the need for revascularization plus annuloplasty. In ischemic mitral regurgitation a basal anteroposterior annulus diameter greater than 35 mm has a similar negative predictive value, and stress testing is unnecessary.

In chronic ischemic cardiomyopathy LV geometry is frequently altered in the middle to distal region of the ventricle, where the wall supports the papillary muscles [34]. The remodeling of the infarcted wall of the LV causes outward papillary muscle displacement

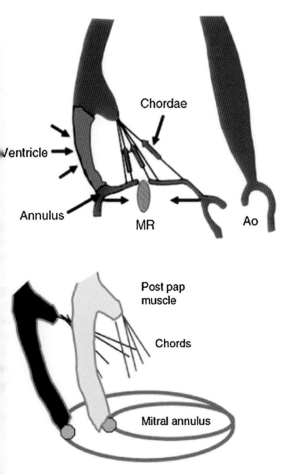

Figure 16.4. Schematic diagram of pathogenesis of ischemic MR. The mitral annulus dilates after ventricular dilaton and papillary muscle displacement. Since the chordal length remains fixed, greater annular dilation causes greater leaflet tethering. The tenting of leaflets is in proportion to papillary muscle displacement

This causes an increase of tethering forces on the edges of the leaflets and repositions the coaptation point well below the annular plane in the LV cavity. This leads to restricted motion of involved leaflets and to the tenting phenomenon.

TEE in these patients shows characteristically restricted leaflet movement, outward displacement of the papillary muscles, and downward displacement of the coaptation point [35]. It is possible to measure the tenting area below the annular plane by planimetry, and to measure the coaptation depth. Measurement of the tenting area and of the coaptation depth (the distance from the annular plane to the coaptation point) allows a grading of the severity of the tethering pattern. A tenting area greater than 4 cm^2 and a coaptation depth greater than 1.1 cm are considered to be severe, and in many centers these are contraindications to annuloplasty and may indicate a need for surgical LV reconstruction (see Chapter 14).

It should also be possible to distinguish between symmetric and asymmetric tethering. In symmetric tethering apical displacement of both leaflets is seen on 2D echo, and there is a centrally originating and centrally directed regurgitant jet. It is important not to mistake the central jet of symmetric tethering for one caused by annular dilation in a Class I lesion. This is important for surgical planning.

In asymmetric tethering there is predominantly posterior tethering of the two leaflets, and the regurgitant jet may originate centrally or come from the posterior commissures (Videos 16.14, 16.15). This jet is usually posteriorly directed. In asymmetric tethering a wall motion abnormality of the inferior wall is usually seen, whereas in the symmetric pattern it is often possible to detect an akinetic anterior wall or global LV dysfunction.

These data help identify the underlying mechanism of the ischemic mitral regurgitation, and guide surgical decision making [36,37].

Feasibility of repair

The feasibility of mitral valve repair depends on valve function and morphology [18]. These are assessed by TEE during pre-bypass. The final decision about the feasibility of repair is made by the operating surgeon based on the data provided by the TEE, in the context of the patient's clinical state [38]. The factors influencing this decision are different in organic and ischemic mitral insufficiency [39,40]. In current clinical practice the only remaining contraindication to repair of a mitral valve with organic, as opposed to functional, regurgitation is extensive annular and/or leaflet calcification. In the setting of ischemic regurgitation, the limiting factor is severe LV dysfunction with inadequate viable myocardium [41].

Post-bypass assessment of the repair

It is essential that the valve is assessed after the repair [42]. This evaluation requires the same systematic approach as the pre-bypass examination and involves TEE exploration of the mitral valve through the standard views to detect any residual regurgitant jet. The examination is performed after complete weaning from cardiopulmonary bypass, and only after preload and afterload have been stabilized. The post-bypass examination is directed to:

- assessing the success of the surgical procedure
- evaluating ventricular function
- detecting complications

The aim of the repair is to make the valve completely competent. If there is any mitral regurgitation after the procedure, two questions need to be answered:

1. How severe is the regurgitation?
2. What is the mechanism of the residual regurgitation?

These questions should be addressed in the light of the nature of the repair (was it simple or complex?) and the clinical state of the patient (is he or she at high risk if a second period of cardiopulmonary bypass is instituted?).

Any residual jet should be compared with the pre-bypass evaluation to assess its severity. It is important to grade the insufficiency correctly (Videos 16.16, 16.17) [43]. The hemodynamic conditions immediately after cardiopulmonary bypass are often not ideal. There may be low blood pressure, low cardiac output, and relative anemia. These lead to an underestimation of the severity of regurgitation, and should be corrected before any decision on grading of the severity of regurgitation is undertaken [44]. If the residual regurgitation is more than mild, a decision has to be taken to either accept the result, to perform a second repair, or to replace the valve. The mechanism of dysfunction will relate to the repair performed. For example, in a case of leaflet flail repaired with artificial cords, residual prolapse with regurgitation may be due to the artificial cords being too long [45]; or in a Barlow type valve treated with quadrangular resection and annuloplasty, a residual jet could be due to an incomplete annuloplasty [46].

When a complex repair has been performed and moderate residual regurgitation is detected, it is very important to consider the risk of a second pump run [47]. This is particularly so after complex repairs for ischemic mitral regurgitation, when a new repair may be difficult and a second pump run may present a very high risk in the presence of severe LV dysfunction.

Complications of mitral valve repair

The post-bypass TEE may identify:

- residual regurgitation (discussed above)
- systolic anterior motion (SAM) of the leaflets with dynamic LV outflow tract (LVOT) obstruction

- mitral stenosis
- coronary artery damage
- annular avulsion
- aortic valve damage

SAM with LVOT obstruction is associated with elongated anterior and/or posterior leaflet and a small LV cavity (Videos 16.18, 16.19). It may be precipitated by hypovolemia, afterload reduction due to vasodilators or anesthetics, or the use of inotropic drugs. Often the SAM can be resolved by medical therapy: withdrawing inotropic drugs, giving vasopressors (norepinephrine), β-blockers, and volume loading [48]. Sometimes it requires a second bypass run to correct the problem, either with a further repair or valve replacement.

Mitral stenosis is a rare consequence of edge-to-edge techniques. Annular avulsion can occur due to debridement of annular calcification (Video 16.20).

Wall motion abnormalities in the circumflex coronary artery territory can be a consequence of coronary interruption during annuloplasty.

Aortic regurgitation can be caused by trauma to the non-coronary cusp (note the continuity between aortic valve and anterior mitral leaflet).

Conclusion

Intraoperative transesophageal echocardiography has an important role in mitral valve repair. It can demonstrate functional valve anatomy and help to elucidate the mechanism of valve dysfunction. It is the only tool available for the immediate assessment of the repair. TEE promotes better outcomes. It is reported that patients with no residual regurgitation have better long-term symptoms and survival. In this respect TEE can be considered a safety net for ensuring the adequacy of surgical repair.

References

1. Bonow RO, Carabello BA, Kanu C, et al. ACC/AHA 2006 guidelines for the management of patients with valvular heart disease: a report of the American College of Cardiology/American Heart Association task force on practice guidelines. Circulation 2006; 114: e84–231.

2. Carabello BA. What is new in the 2006 ACC/AHA guidelines on valvular heart disease? Curr Cardiol Rep 2008; 10: 85–90.

3. Salem DN, O'Gara PT, Madias C et al. Valvular and structural heart disease: American College of Chest Physicians Evidence-Based Clinical Practice

Guidelines (8th Edition). *Chest* 2008; **133** (6 Suppl): 593S–629S.

4. Kouris N, Ikonomidis I, Kontogianni D, Smith P, Nihoyannopoulos P. Mitral valve repair versus replacement for isolated non-ischemic mitral regurgitation in patients with preoperative left ventricular dysfunction. A long-term follow-up echocardiography study. *Eur J Echocardiogr* 2005; **6**: 435–42.

5. Daimon M, Fukuda S, Adams DH, *et al.* Mitral valve repair with Carpentier-McCarthy-Adams IMR ETlogix annuloplasty ring for ischemic mitral regurgitation: early echocardiographic results from a multi-center study. *Circulation* 2006; **114** (1 Suppl): I588–93.

6. Gillinov AM, Blackstone EH, Nowicki ER, *et al.* Valve repair versus valve replacement for degenerative mitral valve disease. *J Thorac Cardiovasc Surg* 2008; **135**: 885–93.

7. Ailawadi G, Swenson BR, Girotti ME, *et al.* Is mitral valve repair superior to replacement in elderly patients? *Ann Thorac Surg* 2008; **86**: 77–85.

8. Schaff HV, Suri RM, Enriquez-Sarano M. Indications for surgery in degenerative mitral valve disease. *Semin Thorac Cardiovasc Surg* 2007; **19**: 97–102.

9. Carabello BA. Indications for mitral valve surgery. *J Cardiovasc Surg (Torino)* 2004; **45**: 407–18.

10. Adams DH, Anyanwu AC, Sugeng L, Lang RM. Degenerative mitral valve regurgitation: surgical echocardiography. *Curr Cardiol Rep* 2008; **10**: 226–32.

11. Braunberger E, Deloche A, Berrebi A, *et al.* Very long-term results (more than 20 years) of valve repair with Carpentier's techniques in non-rheumatic mitral valve insufficiency. *Circulation* 2001; **104** (12 Suppl. 1): I8–11.

12. Troianos CA, Konstadt S. Evaluation of mitral regurgitation. *Semin Cardiothorac Vasc Anesth* 2006; **10**: 67–71.

13. Kawano H, Mizoguchi T, Aoyagi S. Intraoperative transesophageal echocardiography for evaluation of mitral valve repair. *J Heart Valve Dis* 1999; **8**: 287–93.

14. Shernan SK. Perioperative transesophageal echocardiographic evaluation of the native mitral valve. *Crit Care Med* 2007; **35** (8 Suppl): S372–83.

15. Gallet B. Use of echocardiography in mitral regurgitation for the assessment of its mechanism and etiology for the morphological analysis of the mitral valve. *Ann Cardiol Angeiol (Paris)* 2003; **52**: 70–7.

16. Grewal KS, Malkowski MJ, Piracha AR, *et al.* Effect of general anesthesia on the severity of mitral regurgitation by transesophageal echocardiography. *J Cardiol* 2000; **85**: 199–203.

17. Gisbert A, Soulière V, Denault AY, *et al.* Dynamic quantitative echocardiographic evaluation of mitral regurgitation in the operating department. *J Am Soc Echocardiogr* 2006; **19**: 140–6.

18. Iglesias I. Intraoperative TEE assessment during mitral valve repair for degenerative and ischemic mitral valve regurgitation. *Semin Cardiothorac Vasc Anesth* 2007; **11**: 301–5.

19. Minhaj M, Patel K, Muzic D, *et al.* The effect of routine intraoperative transesophageal echocardiography on surgical management. *J Cardiothorac Vasc Anesth* 2007; **21**: 800–4.

20. Lambert AS, Miller JP, Merrick SH, *et al.* Improved evaluation of the location and mechanism of mitral valve regurgitation with a systematic transesophageal echocardiography examination. *Anesth Analg* 1999; **88**: 1205–12.

21. Colombo PC, Wu RH, Weiner S, *et al.* Value of quantitative analysis of mitral regurgitation jet eccentricity by color flow Doppler for identification of flail leaflet. *Am J Cardiol* 2001; **88**: 534–40.

22. Aikat S, Lewis JF. Role of echocardiography in the diagnosis and prognosis of patients with mitral regurgitation. *Curr Opin Cardiol* 2003; **18**: 334–9.

23. Radermecker MA, Limet R. Carpentier's functional classification of mitral valve dysfunction. *Rev Med Liege* 1995; **50**: 292–4.

24. Langer F, Rodriguez F, Cheng A, *et al.* Posterior mitral leaflet extension: an adjunctive repair option for ischemic mitral regurgitation? *J Thorac Cardiovasc Surg* 2006; **131**: 868–77.

25. Nielsen SL, Nygaard H, Fontaine AA, *et al.* Chordal force distribution determines systolic mitral leaflet configuration and severity of functional mitral regurgitation. *J Am Coll Cardiol* 1999; **33**: 843–53.

26. Nordblom P, Bech-Hanssen O. Reference values describing the normal mitral valve and the position of the papillary muscles. *Echocardiography* 2007; **24**: 665–72.

27. Stanley AW, Athanasuleas CL, Buckberg GD; RESTORE Group. Left ventricular remodeling and functional mitral regurgitation: mechanisms and therapy. *Semin Thorac Cardiovasc Surg* 2001; **13**: 486–95.

28. Agricola E, Oppizzi M, Pisani M, *et al.* Ischemic mitral regurgitation: mechanisms and echocardiographic classification. *Eur J Echocardiogr* 2008; **9**: 207–21.

29. Donal E, Levy F, Tribouilloy C. Chronic ischemic mitral regurgitation. *J Heart Valve Dis* 2006; **15**: 149–57.

30. Kumanohoso T, Otsuji Y, Yoshifuku S, *et al.* Mechanism of higher incidence of ischemic mitral regurgitation in patients with inferior myocardial

infarction: quantitative analysis of left ventricular and mitral valve geometry in 103 patients with prior myocardial infarction. *Thorac Cardiovasc Surg* 2003; **125**: 135–43.

31. Mahmood F, Lerner AB, Matyal R, Karthik S, Maslow AD. Dobutamine stress echocardiography and intraoperative assessment of mitral valve. *J Cardiothorac Vasc Anesth* 2006; **20**: 867–71.

32. Roshanali F, Mandegar MH, Yousefnia MA, Alaeddini F, Wann S. Low-dose dobutamine stress echocardiography to predict reversibility of mitral regurgitation with CABG. *Echocardiography* 2006; **23**: 31–7.

33. Aklog L, Filsoufi F, Flores KQ, *et al.* Does coronary artery bypass grafting alone correct moderate ischemic mitral regurgitation? *Circulation* 2001; **104** (12 Suppl. 1): I68–75.

34. Chaput M, Handschumacher MD, Tournoux F, *et al.* Mitral leaflet adaptation to ventricular remodeling: occurrence and adequacy in patients with functional mitral regurgitation. *Circulation* 2008; **118**: 845–52.

35. Otsuji Y, Gilon D, Jiang L, *et al.* Restricted diastolic opening of the mitral leaflets in patients with left ventricular dysfunction: evidence for increased valve tethering. *J Am Coll Cardiol* 1998; **32**: 398–404.

36. Kim YH, Czer LS, Soukiasian HJ, *et al.* Ischemic mitral regurgitation: revascularization alone versus revascularization and mitral valve repair. *Ann Thorac Surg* 2005; **79**: 1895–901.

37. Tibayan FA, Rodriguez F, Zasio MK, *et al.* Geometric distortions of the mitral valvular-ventricular complex in chronic ischemic mitral regurgitation. *Circulation* 2003; **108** (Suppl. 1): II116–21.

38. Omran AS, Woo A, David TE, *et al.* Intraoperative transesophageal echocardiography accurately predicts mitral valve anatomy and suitability for repair. *J Am Soc Echocardiogr* 2002; **15**: 950–7.

39. Chaudhry FA, Upadya SP, Singh VP, *et al.* Identifying patients with degenerative mitral regurgitation for mitral valve repair and replacement: a transesophageal

echocardiographic study. *J Am Soc Echocardiogr* 2004; **17**: 988–94.

40. Gazoni LM, Kern JA, Swenson BR, *et al.* A change in perspective: results for ischemic mitral valve repair are similar to mitral valve repair for degenerative disease. *Ann Thorac Surg* 2007; **84**: 750–7.

41. Akar AR, Doukas G, Szafranek A, *et al.* Mitral valve repair and revascularization for ischemic mitral regurgitation: predictors of operative mortality and survival. *J Heart Valve Dis* 2002; **11**: 793–800.

42. Okada Y, Nasu M, Takahashi Y, *et al.* Late results of mitral valve repair for mitral regurgitation. *Jpn J Thorac Cardiovasc Surg* 2003; **51**: 282–8.

43. Rizza A, Sulcaj L, Glauber M, *et al.* Predictive value of less than moderate residual mitral regurgitation as assessed by transesophageal echocardiography for the short-term outcomes of patients with mitral regurgitation treated with mitral valve repair. *Cardiovasc Ultrasound* 2007; **5**: 25.

44. Shiran A, Merdler A, Ismir E, *et al.* Intraoperative transesophageal echocardiography using a quantitative dynamic loading test for the evaluation of ischemic mitral regurgitation. *Am Soc Echocardiogr* 2007; **20**: 690–7.

45. Dreyfus GD, Souza Neto O, Aubert S. Papillary muscle repositioning for repair of anterior leaflet prolapse caused by chordal elongation. *J Thorac Cardiovasc Surg* 2006; **132**: 578–84.

46. Agricola E, Oppizzi M, Maisano F, *et al.* Detection of mechanisms of immediate failure by transesophageal echocardiography in quadrangular resection mitral valve repair technique for severe mitral regurgitation. *Am J Cardiol* 2003; **91**: 175–9.

47. Cerfolio RJ, Orzulak TA, Pluth JR, Harmsen WS, Schaff HV. Reoperation after valve repair for mitral regurgitation: early and intermediate results. *J Thorac Cardiovasc Surg* 1996; **111**: 1177–83.

48. Brown ML, Abel MD, Click RL, *et al.* Systolic anterior motion after mitral valve repair: is surgical intervention necessary? *J Thorac Cardiovasc Surg* 2007; **133**: 136–43.

Aortic valve surgery

Open aortic valve surgery

Justiaan Swanevelder, Alison Parnell

Introduction

Intraoperative transesophageal echocardiography (TEE) assessment of the patient with aortic valve (AV) disease provides up-to-date real-time information to the surgical and anesthetic teams. In a patient presenting for AV surgery, it yields valuable information on the structure of the aortic root and ascending aorta. It confirms the preoperative diagnosis, provides detail on mechanisms of pathology, and determines the feasibility of attempting a repair procedure. If repair is not possible, echocardiography provides measurements to plan the size and type of valve to be placed. Not only is continuous intraoperative echocardiography screening important for surgical decision making, but it is also valuable as a diagnostic monitor to the anesthetist. It guides perioperative patient management and identifies unexpected complications around the cardiopulmonary bypass period [1].

The routine use of intraoperative TEE in patients undergoing valve replacement for aortic stenosis (AS) and regurgitation (AR) has been validated. A retrospective study of 383 AS patients for aortic valve replacement (AVR) showed the influence of intraoperative TEE [2]. Echocardiography led to a change of surgical procedure in 49 patients (13%), including six in whom mitral valve replacement or repair was performed on the evidence of the intraoperative examination, although not originally planned, and 25 patients for whom the mitral procedure was cancelled because of intraoperative findings. The clinical impact and cost-saving implications of routine intraoperative echocardiography during valve replacement operations has also been confirmed in a prospective study [3]. Other authors have highly recommended intraoperative post-pump TEE as an integral diagnostic tool contributing valuable information in valve replacement surgery [4,5].

Pre-bypass

A critical TEE assessment of the morphology of valve leaflets, root, and ascending aorta will clarify mechanisms of pathology and guide the surgical procedure. Many patients will have both AS and AR, which complicates their assessment. Severe calcification of the annulus may affect valve choice and the presence of postoperative paravalvular leaks. The value of planimetry of the aortic valve area (AVA) in the mid-esophageal short-axis (ME AV SAX) view is limited in the setting of very calcified or bicuspid valves [6,7]. In the mid-esophageal long-axis (ME AV LAX) view it is easy to measure the diameter of the annulus, sinuses of Valsalva, sinotubular junction, and ascending aorta (Fig. 17.1). Although annular size does not change significantly during the cardiac cycle, it is good practice to make the measurement with the aortic valve open. The pressure in the left ventricular outflow tract (LVOT), and therefore annular diameter, will be at its maximum during this phase.

Effect of anesthesia on loading conditions and hemodynamic measurements

Intraoperative quantification of the severity of AV disease is usually not necessary in the patient whose diagnosis is well established preoperatively, but is included in a comprehensive examination (see Chapter 6). This is to confirm the original diagnosis and to provide an up-to-date baseline for future reference [8]. It will also diagnose previously unknown AV pathology in patients initially scheduled for other cardiac procedures. It is important to remember that the systemic vascular resistance has an influence on flow across a stenotic valve, and intraoperative hypotension will therefore increase the transvalvular pressure gradient in the anesthetized, off-loaded patient. On the other hand, systemic hypertension in a patient with AS may lead to a decrease in left ventricular (LV) output and thus a reduction in the transvalvular pressure gradient [9–13].

275

Core Topics in Transesophageal Echocardiography, ed. Robert Feneck, John Kneeshaw, and Marco Ranucci.
Published by Cambridge University Press. © Cambridge University Press 2010.

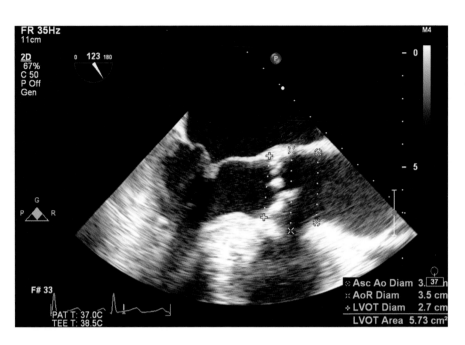

Figure 17.1. ME AV LAX view with measurements of aortic root: annulus 27mm, sinuses of Valsalva 35mm, sinotubular junction 32mm.

When grading aortic valve pathology by means of TEE under anesthesia, one should therefore consider the effect of altered loading conditions on the circulation and the indices used to grade stenosis and regurgitation. Reduction in ventricular filling, systemic vascular resistance, and blood pressure typically occur in the anesthetized patient and can reduce the apparent degree of pathology compared to preoperative assessments. Arrhythmias including atrial fibrillation are quite common in the intraoperative setting, and Doppler measurements should be carefully obtained and repeated to avoid inaccurate information. Peak and mean Doppler flow velocities and pressure gradients may be significantly affected intraoperatively in patients with AS. Using the continuity equation to calculate AVA may also have several pitfalls with TEE. The LVOT diameter can be difficult to accurately measure pre- and post-AVR due to poor image quality. Also, when the ultrasound beam is not parallel to the direction of blood flow, Doppler measurements will be inaccurate. Another cause of misinterpretation of findings in AS may be due to a mitral regurgitation (MR) jet. When attempting evaluation of the aortic valve in transgastric views, the continuous-wave Doppler beam may accidentally cross the MR flow. The orientation and high velocity of a possible MR jet will be similar to that of a high-velocity AS jet, resulting in an inaccurate calculation of AVA. The Doppler velocity index, dimensionless severity index, and double-envelope technique (see Chapter 6) (Fig. 17.2) are all similar in principle and use the continuity equation to find the ratio of LVOT to AV velocity [14–16]. These are fairly simple to obtain and provide a reasonably reliable estimation of the degree of AS under anesthesia [14]. Neither the effect of anesthesia nor the presence of AR will influence continuity equation calculations, because the decrease or increase in systolic flow affects Doppler measurements across the LVOT and AV equally. Epicardial echocardiography has been shown to be a valuable alternative, and complements TEE for quantitative intraoperative assessment of the AV [17]. This may be particularly important when TEE is contraindicated or not possible. In AV repair procedures in small children intraoperative epicardial 3D imaging has been shown to provide additional information over 2D TEE [18].

Pressure half-time, deceleration time, and effective regurgitant orifice area (EROA) calculated using the PISA method, may also be inaccurate intraoperatively in a patient with AR. Special care must be taken in the presence of an aortic aneurysm, when the PISA technique may overestimate EROA and regurgitant volume (Fig. 17.3). The PISA method is also less accurate with eccentric AR jets [19]. It has been shown that actual measurement of PISA with real-time 3D color Doppler yields more accurate regurgitant volumes than those calculated by the 2D color Doppler PISA technique [20]. The vena contracta, which is less flow/load-dependent, jet width/LVOT ratio, and holodiastolic flow reversal in the descending aorta, are much easier and more reliable parameters to obtain under the fast changing conditions of the operating theatre [21–24].

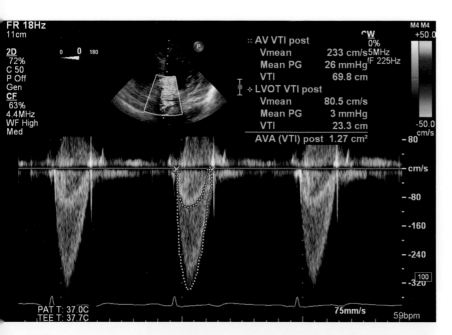

Figure 17.2. The "double-envelope" continuity equation technique to measure flow velocities across the AV and LVOT on a single Doppler signal.

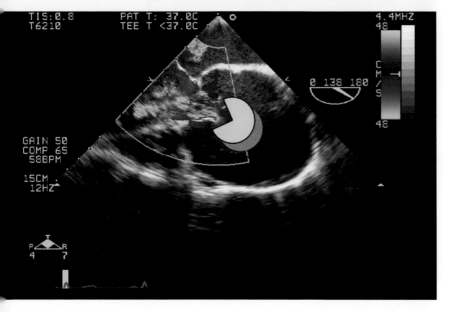

Figure 17.3. In a patient with an ascending aortic aneurysm the PISA technique is inaccurate and will overestimate effective regurgitant orifice area and regurgitant volume.

In order to gain more reliable information it may be necessary to simulate awake loading conditions by increasing afterload through administration of a vasopressor in cases of AR. On the other hand, in AS, low-dose dobutamine (inodilator) can be used to distinguish between pseudostenosis (low-output, low-gradient) and fixed stenosis [25]. Dobutamine stress echocardiography is well tolerated under general anesthesia, with fewer than 10% of patients experiencing any adverse event [26].

A complete examination is useful to identify any unexpected coexisting pathology. Evaluation of global and regional ventricular function, together with inspection of the mitral and tricuspid valves, is very important. Although patients should be fully investigated before embarking on surgery, it is fairly common to find the presence of an undiagnosed patent foramen ovale, additional mitral regurgitation more severe than expected, or an incompetent tricuspid valve. The presence of mitral stenosis will cause

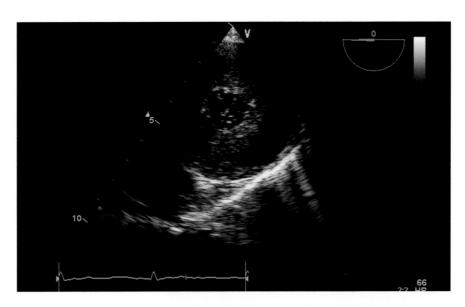

Figure 17.4. Aortic stenosis with compensatory left ventricular hypertrophy, which may result in impaired relaxation.

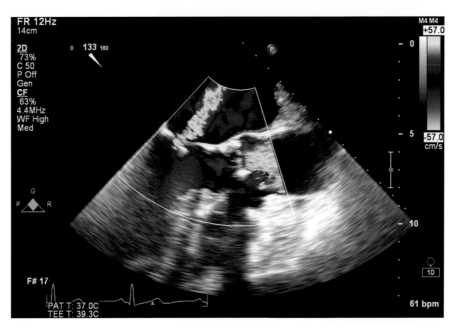

Figure 17.5. Functional mitral regurgitation secondary to raised systolic LV pressure from severe AS, as seen in this image is common, and may improve after AV replacement.

underestimation of an AS pressure gradient because of the fixed cardiac output and therefore decreased flow across the AV. Any extra procedures or on-the-table change of surgical plan will have serious implications for the patient. In an ideal situation the surgical and anesthetic team should be able to interpret and integrate any new echocardiography information in close cooperation with the cardiologist, and make a decision in the patient's best interest.

A common coexisting finding associated with AS is LV concentric hypertrophy with diastolic dysfunc-tion in the form of impaired relaxation (Fig. 17.4; Video 17.1). This is a response to the continuous high afterload at the level of the diseased AV. The decreased LV compliance means that filling pressures are no reliable indicators of volume loading. In chronic AR the LV usually responds with dilation due to long standing volume overload. It also experiences a high afterload and undergoes both eccentric and concentric hypertrophy. The LV is fairly tolerant to this volume overload, and systolic function is preserved till relatively late in the disease. The onset of LV systolic

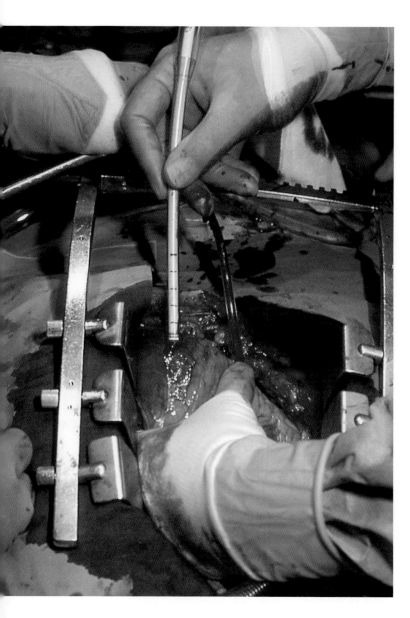

Figure 17.6. TEE is valuable in aortic dissection when placing the arterial cannula via the transapical approach through the AV into the ascending aorta, to ensure antegrade delivery of bypass blood into the true lumen.

dysfunction indicates progressive disease and is usually not reversible. Early operation will therefore improve long-term survival in a patient with chronic AR [27].

CABG and AS

The perioperative clinician may be faced with the dilemma of a patient for coronary artery bypass grafting (CABG) surgery in whom moderate aortic stenosis is discovered during intraoperative TEE. Quantification of aortic valve disease and the decision when to perform a combined CABG and AVR procedure can be difficult, especially when LV function is compromised.

Evidence shows that a subsequent AVR after a previous CABG has a higher mortality than a single combined procedure [28,29]. The degree of stenosis and calcification is important, because even in the asymptomatic patient progression of the disease process may be rapid. It is therefore recommended that valve replacement should be considered with even moderate AS at the time of the primary CABG procedure [28,30].

AVR and MR

Functional mitral regurgitation secondary to raised LV pressures from AS is common and may improve after aortic valve replacement (Fig. 17.5). However, data supporting this assumption are sparse. When the functional MR in an AS patient is graded more than 2+, with a left atrial diameter more than 5 cm and preoperative AV gradient less than 60 mmHg, or atrial fibrillation, there is a significantly higher risk of heart failure and persistent MR after AVR than in other AS patients [31]. If there is intrinsic mitral valve disease with abnormal anatomy of the leaflets, an additional procedure to the mitral valve should be considered straight away.

The ascending aorta, choice of cannulation site, and cardioplegia

Patients with severe AS and coexisting coronary artery disease have more extensive arteriosclerotic changes in the thoracic aorta compared to those with AS alone or patients without AV pathology [32]. Evaluation of the ascending aorta may demonstrate atheromatous disease, and influence surgical cannulation site and cross-clamp techniques. Dilation of the aortic root and ascending aorta is also a common finding in a patient with aortic stenosis or regurgitation. This may be post-stenotic dilation due to the long-term turbulent flow pattern distal to the lesion in AS. In AR it may be secondary to an intrinsic weakness of the aortic wall, such as that seen in a patient with a bicuspid aortic valve (congenital abnormality) or Marfan syndrome (connective tissue disorder). Weakness of the aortic tissue may require surgical intervention. In patients with dissection of the aorta, transapical transventricular placement of the arterial cannula across the AV into the ascending aorta is one of several possible techniques of arterial cannulation. This is the only technique that assures antegrade delivery of bypass blood flow into the true aortic lumen [33]. TEE is vital to ensure correct placement of this cannula across the AV (Fig. 17.6).

The presence of aortic regurgitation will influence the choice of cardioplegia administration technique for myocardial protection during valve surgery. With severe AR, cardioplegia cannot be administered through the cardioplegia cannula into the aortic root, as usually performed with a competent valve, because it will not reach the coronary arteries. Instead it will cause LV dilation through the regurgitant valve and an increase in LV wall tension, and suboptimal myocardial protection. Cardioplegia may therefore be administered using a special cannula (DLP or DeBakey) through each individual coronary artery, and/or via a retrograde cardioplegia cannula. Correct placement of the retrograde cardioplegia cannula into the coronary sinus could be confirmed with TEE.

Post-bypass
De-airing
TEE can confirm successful de-airing after any open-heart procedure [34]. This is usually done just before final separation from the cardiopulmonary bypass machine. Even small air bubbles can cause severe postoperative instability if they enter one of the coronary arteries. With the patient in the supine position, air will preferentially enter the right coronary artery originating from the anterior sinus of Valsalva. This may lead to acute biventricular failure and arrhythmias.

Ventricular filling and function, LVOT obstruction
During the period immediately after termination of cardiopulmonary bypass, TEE provides valuable information on ventricular filling and function, and is very helpful in guiding hemodynamic manipulation. The patient with chronic AV disease and LV hypertrophy or dilation has inherently poor LV compliance. This increased wall thickness reduces wall tension, as evidenced by Laplace's law. The implication in these patients is that the filling pressure is not a reliable index of preload. They may require intravenous fluid administration in the immediate post-bypass period, in spite of high filling pressures. With severe concentric hypertrophy the LV cavity can almost become obliterated (Fig. 17.7; Video 17.2). After valve replacement these patients may sometimes experience systolic anterior motion of the anterior leaflet of the mitral valve [35]. This is due to an acute reduction in afterload in the presence of an underfilled, hypertrophic LV. Positive inotropic agents are contraindicated, but appropriate volume loading, a vasoconstrictor (phenylephrine) and sometimes even β-blockade (negative inotropy, negative chronotropy) may be successful.

Assessment of valve function and position
Intraoperative TEE is very useful for immediate evaluation of the function and position of newly implanted heart valves. Any paravalvular leak should be critically examined and its long-term impact considered against the risks of a second bypass period. Abnormalities

identified in the operating theatre may require immediate surgical correction.

All prosthetic valves, even when they function normally, are to some extent obstructive to blood flow. A more accurate assessment of valve function can be made if the type of valve prosthesis is known. Patient–prosthesis mismatch may lead to a high flow velocity [36,37]. This occurs when the effective orifice area (EOA) of the valve prosthesis is smaller than expected in relation to the patient's body surface area. This phenomenon is discussed in more detail in Chapter 19. The normal values of gradients, pressure half-time, and EOA depend on valve type and size [38]. An unusually high peak velocity through a new valve must

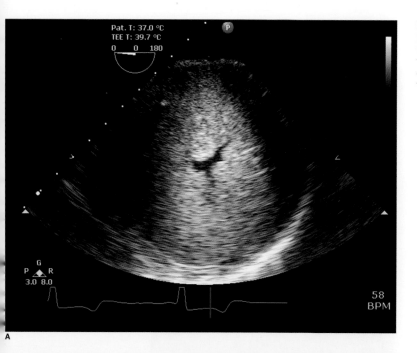

A

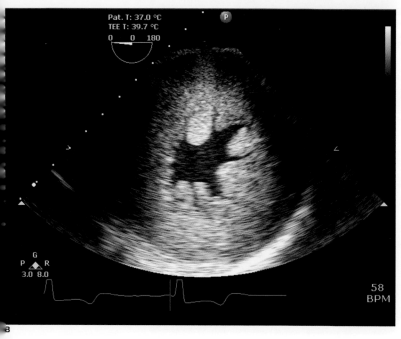

B

Figures 17.7. With severe AS the compensatory concentric hypertrophy of the LV (scanning depth 11cm, diastolic wall thickness 2.1cm) can lead to diastolic dysfunction and almost obliteration of the cavity: (A) systole; (B) diastole.

281

raise suspicion of prosthesis malfunction. In case of a bileaflet or tilting-disk mechanical prosthesis it is important to visualize the full excursion of the leaflets. This is often difficult because of echo shadowing and dropout due to metal in the valve. The transgastric (TG) view of the outflow tract and deep TG view are usually best to avoid artifacts and obtain a reliable Doppler evaluation of velocities across the AV. The use of real-time 3D provides additional information and the ability to assess both mechanical and bioprosthetic

prostheses from all angles (Fig. 17.8) [39,40]. Prosthesis malfunction with a leaflet or disk stuck in either the open or closed position can lead to serious perioperative morbidity. If there are concerns, and it is not possible to see leaflet motion clearly, fluoroscopy is indicated to confirm normal function of the valve.

The measurement of a high Doppler flow velocity across a newly implanted mechanical or bioprosthetic aortic valve immediately after the cessation of cardiopulmonary bypass can be misleading. Several factors

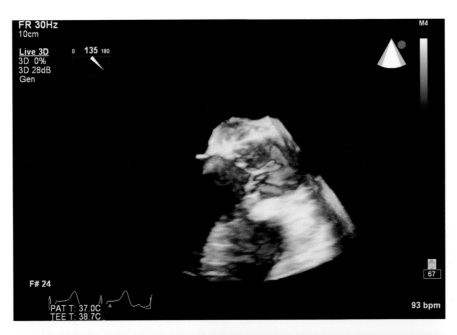

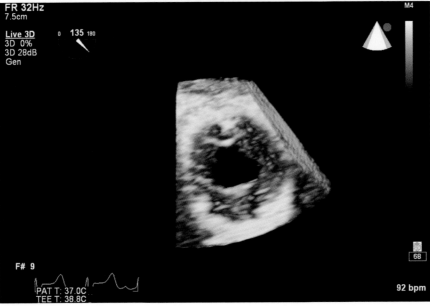

Figure 17.8. The use of real-time 3D echocardiography provides additional information and the ability to assess this bioprosthetic AV prosthesis from all angles.

may contribute to an increased velocity [37,41]. A Doppler measurement made through the smaller central orifice of a bileaflet prosthesis will demonstrate a higher peak velocity than through the larger side orifices. Making several measurements can decrease this error. Changes in stroke volume and cardiac output, which occur in the anesthetized, underfilled, patient can significantly affect "pressure gradients." Immediately after bypass, patients may require inotropic support and will therefore be in a hyperdynamic state with

a relatively low afterload. This functional "afterload mismatch" tends to normalize after a period of time. When a stentless bioprosthesis or homograft is implanted it is quite common to find an increased flow velocity across the valve immediately post-bypass [42]. An AS patient with concentric LV hypertrophy may demonstrate a subvalvular/LVOT gradient post-replacement without evidence of anatomic subvalvular obstruction. This happens because the hypertrophic LV experiences a relatively "low" filling pressure. After

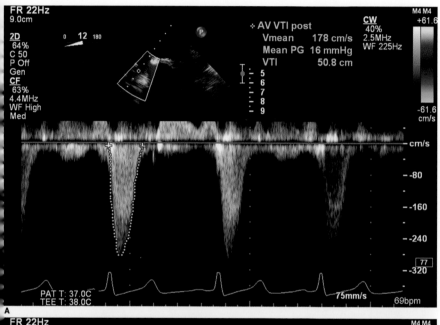

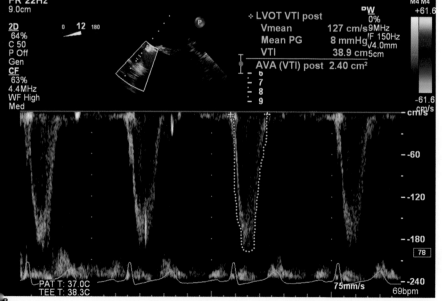

Figure 17.9. These post-AVR images show the value of intraoperative dimensionless severity index (DSI). (A) is a CWD measurement across the newly implanted AV and demonstrates a moderately raised peak flow velocity of 2.5 m/s, which calculates a peak pressure drop of 25 mmHg, mean of 16 mmHg and a VTI of 50.8 cm. The PWD evaluation of the LVOT in (B), however, demonstrates a mean pressure drop of 8 mmHg and VTI of 38.9 cm. This will give a DSI of 38.9/50.8 = 0.76, which means there is increased flow across both LVOT and new AV prosthesis. This is therefore not a pathological increase in gradient.

cardiopulmonary bypass the patient will also have a low hematocrit due to hemodilution from the bypass prime fluid. Blood viscosity is considered in the Bernoulli equation, and hemodilution may therefore affect calculation of the pressure gradient across the valve. The pressure recovery phenomenon (see Chapter 6) should always be considered when evaluating prosthetic valve function, especially if a small prosthesis (19, 21 mm) has been placed and the proximal ascending aorta is also small [43–45].

All of the above factors therefore make it important to calculate valve orifice area using the continuity equation. The Doppler velocity index (DVI) and dimensionless severity index (DSI) are practical methods for the reliable assessment of valves placed in the aortic position [15]. The DVI is the ratio of the peak velocity in the LVOT to the peak velocity across the AV, being proportional to the cross-sectional area of both of these structures. The DSI is similar in that it uses the ratio of the velocity–time integral (VTI) across the LVOT to the VTI across the AV. With both DVI and DSI a ratio of 0.25 or less suggests severe obstruction at valve level, while more than 0.5 means that flow is increased equally across the LVOT and AV (Fig. 17.9). Depth of anesthesia or a hyperdynamic circulation will therefore not influence the assessment, because decrease or increase in systolic flow affects Doppler measurements across both the LVOT and AV equally.

Moderate gradients therefore do not necessarily indicate imperfect surgical placement, and intraoperative TEE is able to discriminate between patients with functional phenomena and those with malfunction of the prosthesis.

Role of TEE in surgical decision making: specific procedures

AV replacement: stentless/homograft

A homograft is a cadaver valve, and it has many desirable characteristics. It has been shown to be durable and resistant to infections. It is therefore ideal in young patients and in the presence of infective endocarditis. However, its shelf availability in all sizes is variable between different centers. There are also several types of stentless bioprostheses available, produced from either porcine valves or bovine pericardium (Fig. 17.10). Every type has its own characteristics, advantages, and disadvantages, but the choice of prosthesis is outside the scope of this chapter. In both homograft and stentless bioprostheses the absence of

the stent allows for a larger EOA and superior hemodynamic profile compared to a similar-size mechanical or stented bioprosthetic valve. This is especially important in the patient with a smaller annular size, where prosthesis–patient mismatch may be a potential problem. Other advantages of both homografts and bioprosthetic valves are the lack of lifetime anticoagulation therapy, and superior remodeling and recovery of LV function.

These prostheses are technically more difficult to place, requiring both surgical experience and accurate

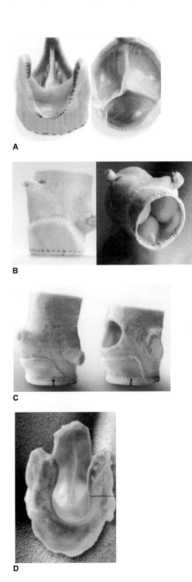

Figure 17.10. Examples of four different types of stentless AV bioprostheses: (A) St Jude Toronto Stentless Porcine Valve; (B) Medtronic Freestyle Heart Valve; (C) Edwards Prima Plus Stentless Bioprosthesis; (D) CryoLife O'Brien Stentless Aortic Bioprosthesis.

intraoperative TEE support [46]. Precise diameter measurements of the AV annulus, sinuses of Valsalva, sinotubular junction, and ascending aorta should be obtained. An experienced surgeon may choose the valve size based on personal assessment of the size of the annulus after opening the aorta, but will be guided by the pre-bypass echocardiographic annulus diameter. That way the exact choice of valve type and planning of procedure can be done in advance. Ideally the sinotubular junction measurement should be not more than 2 mm different to the annulus measurement. Discrepancy between these measurements due to dilation of the sinotubular junction or ascending aorta may lead to tethering and splaying of the stentless prosthesis leaflets after implantation. This distortion will result in AR. Considering these variations in pathology, the surgeon will then have to replace or remodel the sinotubular junction and/or part of the ascending aorta. The origin of the coronary ostia is important information, and this will also influence the surgeon's choice of prosthesis type (Fig. 17.11).

After AV replacement with a homograft or stentless valve, immediate post-bypass TEE is used to evaluate leaflet mobility and coaptation. The prosthesis inside the native root will have the appearance of a "tube within a tube" (Fig. 17.12). The aortic root wall may appear thicker, often with a potential space where the different layers of sinus of Valsalva wall and prosthesis overlap. Any turbulent flow pattern on color Doppler may indicate valve malposition due to improper sizing or implantation technique. High transvalvular pressure gradients are often measured under these hyperdynamic conditions, for reasons explained earlier, and should be interpreted in perspective [42].

Aortic valve repair

In complex aortic valve surgery, such as AV repair with or without root involvement, and whenever the ascending aorta is involved, the use of intraoperative TEE is essential [47]. The more complex the attempted procedure, the more important it is for the echocardiographer to understand the surgical procedure. The vast majority of aortic valves suitable for repair have regurgitant rather than stenotic lesions. Although severity of AR is certainly a consideration, diagnosing the mechanism of AR weighs more heavily in distinguishing those valves suitable for AV repair from the chronic abnormalities requiring replacement [48]. A functional classification for AR has been described to determine the mechanism of disease and assist in AV repair procedures [49]. The AV is viewed as a functional unit comprising the annulus, three cusps, sinuses of Valsalva, commissures, and sinotubular junction. Competence of the valve unit depends on the integrity of all its components, and abnormalities are shown in Table 17.1. Functional aortic annulus dilation does always appear to be present when there is AR, no matter what the lesion is [49].

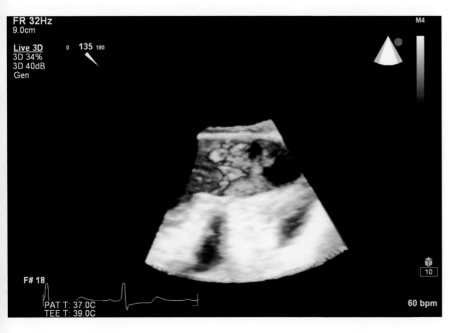

Figure 17.11. A 3D image of the aortic root in a patient with severe AS demonstrates the origin of the left main stem coronary artery clearly.

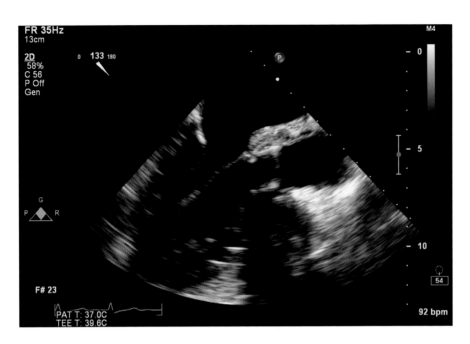

FR 35Hz
13cm

2D
58%
C 56
P Off
Gen

133

G

P   R

F# 23

PAT T: 37.0C
TEE T: 39.6C

92 bpm

Figure 17.12. A stentless aortic valve bioprosthesis may have the appearance of a "tube within a tube."

Table 17.1 Classification of the mechanisms of aortic regurgitation [50]

Type I	Normal-appearing cusps with functional aortic annulus dilation
	Ia: Distal ascending aorta dilation (sinotubular junction)
	Ib: Proximal (Valsalva sinuses) and sinotubular junction dilation
	Ic: Isolated functional aortic annulus dilation
	Id: Cusp perforation and functional aortic annulus dilation
Type II	Cusp prolapse: excess of cusp tissue or commissural disruption
Type III	Cusp retraction and thickening

A full discussion on surgical repair techniques of the aortic valve is outside the scope of this chapter; it has been reviewed thoroughly elsewhere [50–52].

An AV-sparing procedure is relatively easy to perform in the patient with aortic dissection without additional leaflet pathology, and involves resuspension of the cusps. Five potential mechanisms of AR in a patient with acute type A aortic dissection have been described [53] (see Chapter 6, Table 6.2).

The first three of these mechanisms can also occur in a patient without aortic dissection. Some patients can have more than one mechanism of AR. In aortic dissection the intimal flap prolapsing through the valve may keep the leaflets in the open position, causing severe AR, and this may severely impair ventricular function. Alternatively, the flap may act as

a valve during diastole, with remarkably little AR although the leaflets are open. In such a case, LV function may be preserved, leading to more stable hemodynamics.

The quality of an AV repair procedure can be assessed early, even during cardiopulmonary bypass soon after the aortic cross-clamp has been removed. The high aortic pressures due to non-pulsatile flow in the arterial cannula of the bypass circuit will indicate an unsuccessful procedure in the form of a continuous regurgitant jet. The presence of any residual aortic regurgitation after a repair procedure is a poor prognostic indicator of long-term outcome and should not be accepted. In such a case a second bypass run and replacement of the valve is indicated.

Ross procedure

The Ross procedure involves the replacement of a diseased aortic valve, usually in the younger age group, with the patient's own pulmonary autograft [54]. The pulmonary valve is then replaced with a cryopreserved homograft. The potential for valve "growth" and annular enlargement, together with avoiding permanent anticoagulation, makes this an attractive option in the growing patient [55]. It is also associated with lower rates of endocarditis, thromboembolism, and degeneration. Although technically demanding, in good surgical hands this procedure has been shown to provide excellent hemodynamic results and low morbidity and mortality rates in children and young adults [56]. Accurate assessment of the aortic and pulmonary anatomy is important for these procedures (Fig. 17.13). The diameters of the AV annulus, sinotubular junction, and ascending aorta should be measured. Severe dilation of the AV annulus (> 30 mm) or the ascending aorta indicates a connective tissue disorder with a risk of future regurgitation of the autograft and is therefore a contraindication to this procedure.

Due to its anterior location, the pulmonary valve is often better visualized by epicardial echocardiography rather than by the transesophageal option. The pulmonary valve should be tricuspid and without any degree of regurgitation or stenosis. The diameters of the pulmonary valve annulus and sinotubular junction should also be measured. The pulmonary artery sinotubular junction should match the aortic valve annulus. These measurements should be within 2 mm of each other to avoid distortion and subsequent regurgitation [57]. At the end of the procedure the function of both aortic autograft and pulmonary allograft

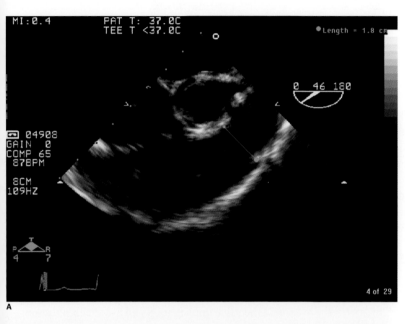

A

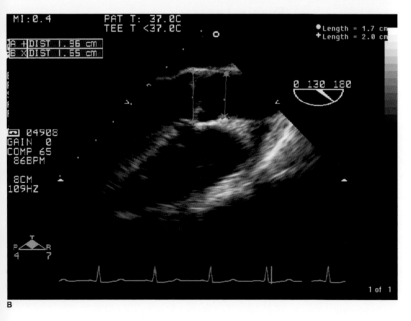

B

Figure 17.13. For a Ross procedure, accurate assessment of aortic and pulmonary anatomy is important. In this patient, (A) pulmonary valve annulus was measured at 18mm, with (B) aortic valve annulus at 17 mm and ST junction at 20 mm. A Ross procedure was therefore performed.

should be assessed. Any regurgitation of either graft indicates possible distortion during implantation and needs an immediate revision of the procedure. Narrowing of the anastomosis sites would leave a high risk for future complications. LV contractility and regional wall function should be carefully evaluated for any sign of ischemia or dysfunction in the immediate postoperative period. The first septal perforator branch of the left anterior descending coronary artery supplies the important basal anteroseptal segment of the LV. It is in close proximity to the pulmonary valve and at risk during harvesting of the valve.

Conclusion

For echocardiography to influence the success of AV surgery it must be performed at the highest diagnostic level. Those performing intraoperative TEE must have appropriate equipment, skills, and knowledge. Systematic examination, with accurate recording and reporting, and appropriate professional supervision, is essential to a high-level intraoperative service and improved patient outcome.

According to the 1996 guidelines of the American Society of Anesthesiologists (ASA) and the Society of Cardiovascular Anesthesiologists (SCA), valve replacement is a Category II indication for the use of perioperative TEE [58], meaning that there is lesser research evidence, but expert consensus, that TEE may influence the outcome of these procedures. In 2003 the American College of Cardiology (ACC), American Heart Association (AHA), and American Society of Echocardiograhy (ASE) published updated guidelines for the clinical applications of echocardiography [59]. In stentless bioprosthesis, homograft, the Ross procedure, and AV repair surgery, intraoperative TEE is recognized to play a valuable role, and these procedures are in the new Class I indication group. Endocarditis and acute, persistent, and life-threatening hemodynamic disturbances, as often seen after cardiopulmonary bypass, are also in Class I. Standard valve replacements, de-airing after cardiotomy, and patients at risk of ischemia or hemodynamic disturbances, however, fall within Class IIa. This means the weight of evidence/opinion is in favor of the usefulness of TEE in these procedures, although there is a divergence of opinion about its efficacy. Wide use and increasing experience of intraoperative TEE in AV surgery has established its place as a hemodynamic monitoring and diagnostic tool [60].

Transcatheter aortic valve implantation

Joerg Ender, Chirojit Mukherjee

Introduction

Transcatheter aortic valve implantation is an emerging technique that has been performed in elderly, high-risk patients with severe, symptomatic aortic stenosis [61,62].

As these patients have many associated comorbidities, efforts are made to provide safe, reliable anesthesia and early extubation [63]. A minimally invasive approach to valve implantation is preferable, and two methods are presently in use:

- the antegrade route using the transapical approach [64]
- the retrograde route using the transfemoral approach [65]

Both these methods have the potential advantage of avoiding sternotomy and cardiopulmonary bypass (CPB), thereby avoiding cardiac arrest [66]. Since these high-risk procedures are being performed under beating heart conditions, transoesophageal echocardiography (TEE) has a major role in guiding the implantation of the valve, especially for the transapical approach. A standardized method is recommended in order to facilitate the valve implantation and avoid complications.

Surgical procedure

The transapical approach

The principle behind this approach is to use the short distance and a relatively straight pathway between the left ventricular apex and the AV. Femoral vessels are prepared in case emergency CPB is required. A 6 French femoral arterial sheath is placed and an aortic root pigtail catheter is used for angiographic visualization. After these measures are adopted, an anterolateral minithoracotomy is performed through the left fifth intercostal space. The pericardium is retained with stay sutures, and purse-string sutures are applied to the LV apex, taking care to avoid the coronary arteries. The apex of the heart is then punctured using a soft guidewire, followed with a super-stiff guidewire. A 20 mm balloon catheter is positioned to facilitate valvuloplasty under rapid ventricular pacing (180–200 beats/minute). After successful balloon valvuloplasty, the catheter is replaced by a 33 French valve delivery system. The heart is de-aired and, once correct positioning is confirmed, the valve is deployed through the applicator device, again under rapid ventricular pacing. After implantation of the valve, the delivery system is removed and the LV apex is closed with purse-string sutures. The incision is closed conventionally and femoral vessels are decannulated [61].

The transfemoral approach

The percutaneous balloon-expandable AV is considered in patients in whom the anatomy of the iliac vessels is favorable for the passage of the delivery system. Femoral access is achieved and a 6 French sheath is introduced. A pigtail catheter is placed in the abdominal aorta for continuous arterial monitoring and angiographic demonstration of the anatomy of ileofemoral vessels. A temporary pacing lead may be inserted via the internal jugular or the femoral vein. After guidewire insertion, a 14 French sheath is introduced. A J-tipped guidewire is directed to cross the valve and then replaced with a super-stiff 260 cm long guidewire. Balloon valvuloplasty is then performed under rapid ventricular pacing. The Retroflex delivery system along with the crimped valve is directed towards the annulus of the native valve using fluoroscopic guidance. After satisfactory central and coaxial positioning, the valve is deployed. Aortic root angiography is used to confirm the correct position, and transaortic pressure gradients may be measured using TEE. After satisfactory implantation of the valve, the delivery system and guidewire are withdrawn and the femoral access is closed and pressure bandage is applied [66].

Echocardiographic implications

Both of these minimally invasive procedures are performed in patients with end-stage AV disease, and a step-by-step echocardiographic evaluation is recommended. After induction of anesthesia, a comprehensive TEE examination should be performed, in accordance with published guidelines [67]. In addition, there are some elements specific to transcatheter valve implantation. The TEE examination is performed as outlined below.

Annulus measurement: the concept of oversizing

As the valve is a sutureless balloon-expandable pericardial xenograft (Edwards Sapien®) or a self-expand-

able xenograft (CoreValve®), a valve size larger than the native annulus is required for safe fixation of the implanted valve. A valve 2–3 mm larger than the annulus measured by TEE is selected. Presently only two valve sizes are available for the transapical approach (23 mm and 26 mm; Edwards Lifesciences, Irvine, CA, USA). An aortic annulus of more than 25 mm is an exclusion criterion for transapical valve implantation. In contrast, the percutaneous approach allows implantation in an annulus measuring 27 mm with a 29 mm valve.

The preoperative TEE measurement of the annulus is therefore critically important, and care should be taken to measure the aortic annulus in the true long axis. We recommend starting with the ME AV SAX view. Visualization of all three commissures of the valve ensures that the echocardiographer is in the correct plane (except for bicuspid valves). From this short-axis view rotation of the plane to 90° enables a correct long-axis view (Video 17.3). The use of a 3D TEE probe with an x-plane mode is helpful, because it allows visualization of both views (SAX and LAX) (Video 17.4).

Measurements of the annulus, the sinuses, the sinotubular junction, and the ascending aorta are made in systole.

Guidewire for cardiopulmonary bypass

The bicaval view is used to confirm correct placement of the transfemoral venous guide wire.

Positioning of the valvuloplasty balloon

Surgical introduction of the guidewire transapically may be aided by echocardiographic guidance using the ME AV LAX view. Without this guidance there is a significant risk of affecting chords or leaflets of the mitral valve (Video 17.5). For the percutaneous approach, placement of the J catheter in the ascending aorta is confirmed (Video 17.6).

Balloon valvuloplasty

Using the ME AV SAX view, the balloon should be positioned in the center of the native valve to guarantee symmetric dilation (Video 17.7). Again, x-plane with the 3D probe is very helpful (Video 17.8).

After valvuloplasty

The ME AV LAX is used with color Doppler to detect the degree of aortic regurgitation due to balloon valvuloplasty (Video 17.9).

Positioning of the valve

For correct positioning of the valve prosthesis the ME LV LAX view is required. When using the transapical approach, correct placement is identified with the distal end of the nitinol cage not extending beyond the cusps of the native valve (Video 17.10). For the percutaneous approach, the cusps of the implanted valve are at a supra-annular position (Video 17.11). For both types of valve, it is important that the implantation is not too deep, so that motion of the anterior leaflet of the mitral valve is not compromised. If this occurs, perforation of the anterior mitral valve leaflet may result (Video 17.12).

Postoperative monitoring

The immediate postoperative period is an important recovery phase after a period of hemodynamic instability. The development of regional wall motion abnormalities may be assessed using the transgastric short axis (TG mid SAX) view (Video 17.13). The ME AV SAX and ME AV LAX views should be examined for paravalvular leaks (Videos 17.14, 17.15). Since the valves are sutureless, a degree of aortic regurgitation is inevitable. Moreover, repeated dilation or a repeat "valve-in-valve" implantation may be associated with considerable risks (Video 17.16). Hence the post-procedure evaluation should pay attention to grading the severity of aortic regurgitation in the existing hemodynamic state. A full assessment should include the normal criteria for aortic regurgitation, including pressure half-time calculation, measurement of jet width in relation to the width of the left ventricular outflow tract and in relation to total circumference of the AV. The transvalvular gradients are usually very low, because of the nature of the valves. The gradients are measured routinely in the transgastric long-axis (TG LAX) and deep transgastric (deep TG LAX) views. Any paravalvular leak can also be visualized in this view (Video 17.17). Proper movement of all three leaflets should be confirmed postoperatively, as there may be restriction related to technical difficulties or complications of the procedure itself (Videos 17.18a, 17.18b) leading to severe aortic regurgitation. Visualization of flow through the left and right coronary ostia should be sought in the ME AV SAX and ME AV LAX views.

These immediate postoperative measurements serve as a baseline marker for further comparison before postoperative discharge of the patient.

Real-time 3D TEE for transcatheter valve implantation

For transcatheter AV implantation, real-time 3D TEE may be of benefit to the surgeon and the echocardiographer. The x-plane mode allows two simultaneous 2D views of the structure with one perpendicular to the other, with a frame rate equivalent to conventional 2D technology. In transapical AV implantation, x-plane enables the echocardiographer to simultaneously visualize the AV in the short- and long-axis views. It is particularly useful for accurately measuring the aortic annulus and hence determining the valve size, as described above (Video 17.19). For the percutaneous retrograde approach, 3D is used to exclude the presence of major atheromatous plaques in the aorta (Video 17.20). Since it is real-time mode, surgical insertion of the guidewire and delivery system can be guided using the "live 3D mode" as well as the "thick Slice" mode for better visualization (Videos 17.21a, 17.21b). Visualization of the coronary ostia in the ME LAX view of the AV with the live 3D mode is possible, and may help to avoid compromise of the ostia (see above).

Limitations of TEE and general considerations

Transesophageal echocardiography is a useful tool in transcatheter AV implantation, but it has limitations. Fluoroscopy plays a major role during these procedures. The transfemoral procedure is often performed under local anesthesia, and in view of the comorbidities of these patients there is an increasing movement towards performing transapical valve implantations under high thoracic epidural anesthesia. In both of these situations TEE is not feasible in the awake patient. Fluoroscopic guidance is presently the gold standard for implantation and deployment of the valve. In the future, real-time 3D may be used to avoid repeated x-ray exposure, especially in patients with renal disease, but these techniques are at present at a relatively early stage.

Conclusion

Transcatheter valve implantation is a rapidly developing technique in the search for a minimally invasive approach for high-risk patients with symptomatic aortic valve disease [68]. Although the technique is clearly feasible, paravalvular regurgitation following valve implantation still seems to be a problem.

Nonetheless, both the number of procedures and the number of institutions undertaking them are growing rapidly [66]. Transesophageal echocardiography has a major role to play in the procedure. A systematic and structured TEE examination is helpful, both to prevent complications and to ensure proper deployment of the valve.

References

1. Qizilbash B, Couture P, Denault A. Impact of perioperative transesophageal echocardiography in aortic valve replacement. *Semin Cardiothorac Vasc Anaesth* 2007; **11**: 288–300.

2. Nowrangi SK, Connolly HM, Freeman WK, Click RL. Impact of intraoperative transesophageal echocardiography among patients undergoing aortic valve replacement for aortic stenosis. *J Am Soc Echocardiogr* 2001; **14**: 863–6.

3. Ionescu AA, West RR, Proudman C, Butchart EG, Fraser AG. Prospective study of routine perioperative transesophageal echocardiography for elective valve replacement: clinical impact and cost-saving implications. *J Am Soc Echocardiogr* 2001; **14**: 659–67.

4. Shapira Y, Vaturi M, Weisenberg DE, *et al.* Impact of intraoperative transesophageal echocardiography in patients undergoing valve replacement. *Ann Thorac Surg* 2004; **78**: 579–84.

5. Eltzschig HK, Rosenberger P, Löffler M, *et al.* Impact of intraoperative transesophageal echocardiography on surgical decisions in 12,566 patients undergoing cardiac surgery. *Ann Thor Surg* 2008; **85**: 845–52.

6. Pouleur AC, le Polain de Waroux JB, Pasquet A, *et al.* Planimetric and continuity equation assessment of aortic valve area: head to head comparison between cardiac magnetic resonance and echocardiography. *J Magn Reson Imaging* 2007; **26**: 1436–43.

7. Donal E, Novaro GM, Deserrano D, *et al.* Planimetric assessment of anatomic valve area overestimates effective orifice area in bicuspid aortic stenosis. *J Am Soc Echocardiogr* 2005; **18**: 1392–8.

8. Oxorn D. The intraoperative quantification of aortic stenosis. *Anesth Analg* 2009; **108**: 10–12.

9. Kadem L, Dumesnil JG, Rieu R, *et al.* Impact of systemic hypertension on the assessment of aortic stenosis. *Heart* 2005; **91**: 354–61.

10. Chambers J. Can high blood pressure mask severe aortic stenosis? *J Heart Valve Dis* 1998; **7**: 277–8.

11. Bermejo J. The effects of hypertension on aortic valve stenosis. *Heart* 2005; **91**: 280–2.

12. Little SH, Chan KL, Burwash IG. Impact of blood pressure on the Doppler echocardiographic assessment of severity of aortic stenosis. *Heart* 2007; **93**: 848–55.

13. Pibarot P, Dumesnil JG. Assessment of aortic valve severity: check the valve but don't forget the arteries! *Heart* 2007; **93**: 780–2.

14. Baumgartner H, Hung J, Bermejo J, *et al.* Echocardiographic assessment of valve stenosis: EAE/ASE recommendations for clinical practice. *Eur J Echocardiogr* 2009; **10**: 1–25.

15. Oh JK, Taliercio CP, Holmes DR, *et al.* Prediction of the severity of aortic stenosis by Doppler aortic valve area determination: prospective Doppler-catheterization correlation in 100 patients. *J Am Coll Cardiol* 1988; **11**: 1227–34.

16. Maslow AD, Haering JM, Heindel S, *et al.* An evaluation of prosthetic aortic valves using transesophageal echocardiography: the double-envelope technique. *Anesth Analg* 2000; **91**: 509–16.

17. Hilberath JN, Shernan SK, Segal S, Smith B, Eltzschig HK. The feasibility of epicardial echocardiography for measuring aortic valve area by the continuity equation. *Anesth Analg* 2009; **108**: 17–22.

18. Vida VL, Hoehn R, Larrazabal LA, *et al.* Usefulness of intra-operative epicardial three-dimensional echocardiography to guide aortic valve repair in children. *Am J Cardiol* 2009; **103**: 852–6.

19. Tribouilloy CM, Enriquez-Sarano M, Fett SL, *et al.* Application of the proximal flow convergence method to calculate the effective orifice area in aortic regurgitation. *J Am Coll Cardiol* 1998; **32**: 1032–9.

20. Pirat B, Little SH, Igo SR, *et al.* Direct measurement of proximal isovelocity surface area by real-time three-dimensional colour Doppler for quantitation of aortic regurgitant volume: an in vitro validation. *J Am Soc Echocardiogr* 2009; **22**: 306–13.

21. Zoghbi WA, Enriquez-Sarano M, Foster E, *et al.* Recommendations for evaluation of the severity of native valvular regurgitation with two-dimensional and Doppler echocardiography. *J Am Soc Echocardiogr* 2003; **16**: 777–802.

22. Tribouilloy CM, Enriquez-Sarano M, Bailey KR, Seward JB, Tajik AJ. Assessment of severity of aortic regurgitation using the width of the vena contracta: a clinical Doppler imaging study. *Circulation* 2000; **102**: 558–64.

23. Enriquez-Sarano M, Seward JB, Bailey KR, Tajik AJ. Effective regurgitant orifice area: a noninvasive Doppler development of an old hemodynamic concept. *J Am Coll Cardiol* 1994; **23**: 443–51.

24. Sutton DC, Kluger R, Ahmed SU, Reimold SC, Mark JB. Flow reversal in the descending aorta: a guide to intraoperative assessment of aortic regurgitation with transesophageal echocardiography. *J Thorac Cardiovasc Surg* 1994; **108**: 576–82.

25. Maslow AD, Mahmood F, Poppas A, Singh A. Intraoperative dobutamine stress echocardiography to assess aortic valve stenosis. *J Cardiothorac Vasc Anesth* 2006; **20**: 862–6.

26. Seeberger MD, Skarvan K, Buser P, *et al*. Dobutamine stress echocardiography to detect inducible demand ischemia in anesthetized patients with coronary artery disease. *Anesthesiology* 1998; **88**: 1233–9.

27. Tornos P, Sambola A, Permanyer-Miralda G, *et al*. Long-term outcome of surgically treated aortic regurgitation. *J Am Coll Cardiol* 2006; **47**: 1012–17.

28. Bonow RO, Carabello BA, Chatterjee K, *et al*. 2008 Focused update incorporated into the ACC/AHA 2006 guidelines for the management of patients with valvular heart disease. A Report of the ACC/AHA Task Force on Practice Guidelines. *Circulation* 2008; **118**: e523–661.

29. Odell JA, Mullany CJ, Schaff HV, *et al*. Aortic valve replacement after previous coronary artery bypass grafting. *Ann Thorac Surg* 1996; **62**: 1424–30.

30. Vahanian A, Baumgartner H, Bax J, *et al*. Guidelines on the management of valvular heart disease: the Task Force on the Management of Valvular Heart Disease of the European Society of Cardiology. *Eur Heart J* 2007; **28**: 230–68.

31. Ruel M, Kapila V, Price J, *et al*. Natural history and predictors of outcome in patients with concomitant functional mitral regurgitation at the time of aortic valve replacement. *Circulation* 2006; **114**: I541–46.

32. Goland S, Trento A, Czer LS, *et al*. Thoracic aortic arteriosclerosis in patients with degenerative aortic stenosis with and without coexisting coronary artery disease. *Ann Thorac Surg* 2008; **85**: 113–19.

33. Jutley RS, Masala N, Sosnowski AW. Transapical aortic cannulation: the technique of choice for type A dissection. *J Thorac Cardiovasc Surg* 2007; **133**: 1393–4.

34. Tingleff J, Joyce FS, Petterson G. Intraoperative echocardiographic study of air embolism during cardiac operations. *Ann Thorac Surg* 1995; **60**: 673–7.

35. Luckie M, Khattar RS. Systolic anterior motion of the mitral valve: beyond hypertrophic cardiomyopathy. *Heart* 2008; **94**: 1383–5.

36. Rahimtoola SH. The problem of valve prosthesis–patient mismatch. *Circulation* 1978; **58**: 20–4.

37. Baumgartner H. The challenge of assessing heart valve prostheses by Doppler echocardiography. *J Am Soc Echocardiogr* 2009; **22**: 394–5.

38. Rosenhek R, Binder T, Maurer G, Baumgartner H. Normal values for Doppler echocardiographic assessment of heart valve prostheses. *J Am Soc Echocardiogr* 2003; **16**: 1116–27.

39. Shernan SK. Intraoperative three-dimensional echocardiography: ready for primetime? *J Am Soc Echocardiogr* 2009; **22**: 27A–28A.

40. Sugeng L, Shernan SK, Salgo IS, *et al*. Live three-dimensional transesophageal echocardiography: initial experience using the fully-sampled matrix array probe. *J Am Coll Cardiol* 2008; **52**: 446–9.

41. Schroeder RA, Mark JB. Is the valve OK or not? Immediate evaluation of a replaced aortic valve. *Anesth Analg* 2005; **101**: 1288–91.

42. Morocutti G, Gelsomino S, Spedicato L, *et al*. Intraoperative transesophageal echo-Doppler evaluation of stentless aortic xenografts. Incidence and significance of moderate gradients. *Cardiovasc Surg* 2002; **10**: 328–32.

43. Popescu WM, Prokop E, Elefteriades JA, Kett K, Barash PG. Phantom aortic valve pressure gradient: discrepancies between cardiac catheterization and Doppler echocardiography. *Anesth Analg* 2005; **100**: 1259–62.

44. Chambers J. Is pressure recovery an important cause of "Doppler aortic stenosis" with no gradient at catheterisation? *Heart* 1996; **76**: 381–3.

45. Niederberger J, Schima H, Maurer G, Baumgartner H. Importance of pressure recovery for the assessment of aortic stenosis by Doppler ultrasound: role of aortic size, aortic valve area, and direction of the stenotic jet in vitro. *Circulation* 1996; **94**: 1934–40.

46. Bach DS. Echocardiographic assessment of stentless aortic bioprosthetic valves. *J Am Soc Echocardiogr* 2000; **13**: 941–8.

47. Jeanmart H, de Kerchove L, Glineur D, *et al*. Aortic valve repair: the functional approach to leaflet prolapse and valve-sparing surgery. *Ann Thor Surg* 2007; **83**: S746–51.

48. le Polain de Waroux JB, Pouleur AC, Goffinet C, *et al*. Functional anatomy of aortic regurgitation: accuracy, prediction of surgical reparability and outcome implications of transesophageal echocardiography. *Circulation* 2007; **116**: I264–9.

49. El Khoury G, Glineur D, Rubay J, *et al*. Functional classification of aortic root/valve abnormalities and their correlation with etiologies and surgical procedures. *Curr Opinion Cardiol* 2005; **20**: 115–21.

50. Cosgrove DM, Frazier CD. Aortic valve repair. In: Cox JL, Sundt TM, eds. *Operative Techniques in Cardiac and Thoracic Surgery*. Philadelphia, PA: Saunders, 1996: Vol. 1, 30–7.

51. Hopkins RA. Aortic valve leaflet sparing and salvage surgery: evolution of techniques for aortic root reconstruction. *Eur J Cardiothoracic Surg* 2003; **24**: 886–97.

52. Yacoub MH, Cohn LH. Novel approaches to cardiac valve repair: from structure to function. *Part II. Circulation* 2004; **109**: 1064–72.

53. Movsowitz HD, Levine RA, Hilgenberg AD, Isselbacher EM. Transesophageal echocardiographic description of the mechanisms of aortic regurgitation in acute type A aortic dissection: implications for aortic valve repair. *J Am Coll Cardiol* 2000; **36**: 884–90.

54. Kouchoukos NT, Dávila-Román VG, Spray TL, Murphy SF, Perrillo JB. Replacement of the aortic root with a pulmonary autograft in children and young adults with aortic valve disease. *N Engl J Med* 1994; **330**: 1–6.

55. Elkins RC, Knott-Craig CJ, Ward KE, McCue C, Lane MM. Pulmonary autograft in children: realized growth potential. *Ann Thorac Surg* 1994; **57**: 1387–94.

56. Rubay JE, Buche M, El Khoury GA, *et al.* The Ross operation: mid-term results. *Ann Thorac Surg* 1999; **67**: 1355–8.

57. David TE, Omran A, Webb G, *et al.* Geometric mismatch of the aortic and pulmonary root causes aortic insufficiency after the Ross procedure. *J Thorac Cardiovasc Surg* 1996; **112**: 1231–9.

58. Practice guidelines for perioperative transesophageal echocardiography. A report by the American Society of Anesthesiologists and the Society of Cardiovascular Anesthesiologists Task Force on Transesophageal Echocardiography. *Anesthesiology* 1996; **84**: 986–1006.

59. Cheitlin MD, Armstrong WF, Aurigemma GP, *et al.* ACC/AHA/ASE 2003 guideline update for the clinical application of echocardiography – summary article: a report of the American College of Cardiology/ American Heart Association Task Force on practice guidelines. *J Am Soc Echocardiogr* 2003; **2**: 954–70.

60. Bonow RO, Carabello BA, Kanu C, *et al.* ACC/AHA 2006 guidelines for the management of patients with valvular heart disease: a report of the American College of Cardiology/American Heart Association

task force on practice guidelines. *Circulation* 2006; **114**: e84–231.

61. Walther T, Falk V, Borger MA, *et al.* Minimally invasive transapical beating heart aortic valve implantation: proof of concept. *Eur J Cardiothorac Surg* 2007; **31**: 9–15.

62. Walther T, Simon P, Dewey T, *et al.* Transapical minimally invasive aortic valve implantation: multicenter experience. *Circulation* 2007; **116** (11 Suppl): I240–5.

63. Ender J, Borger MA, Scholz M, *et al.* Cardiac surgery fast-track treatment in a postanesthetic care unit: six-month results of the Leipzig fast-track concept. *Anesthesiology* 2008; **109**: 61–6.

64. Walther T, Falk V, Kempfert J, *et al.* Transapical minimally invasive aortic valve implantation: the initial 50 patients. *Eur J Cardiothorac Surg* 2008; **33**: 983–8.

65. Grube E, Schuler G, Buellesfeld L, *et al.* Percutaneous aortic valve replacement for severe aortic stenosis in high-risk patients using the second- and current third-generation self-expanding CoreValve prosthesis: device success and 30-day clinical outcome. *J Am Coll Cardiol* 2007; **50**: 69–76.

66. Walther T, Chu MW, Mohr FW. Transcatheter aortic valve implantation: time to expand? *Curr Opin Cardiol* 2008; **23**: 111–16.

67. Shanewise JS, Cheung AT, Aronson S, *et al.* ASE/SCA guidelines for performing a comprehensive intraoperative multiplane transesophageal echocardiography examination: recommendations of the ASE Council for intraoperative echocardiography and the SCA Task Force for certification in perioperative transesophageal echocardiography. *Anesth Analg* 1999; **89**: 870–84.

68. Walther T, Mohr FW. Aortic valve surgery: time to be open-minded and to rethink. *Eur J Cardiothorac Surg* 2007; **31**: 4–6.

Infective endocarditis

John Kneeshaw, Robert Feneck

Introduction

Infective endocarditis is an infection involving the cardiac endothelial surfaces. Although it is commonly associated with infection of the heart valves, other cardiac structures can be primarily or secondarily involved, including the chordae tendineae, mural endocardium, myocardium, and pericardium. Endovascular infection may also occur in association with patent ductus arteriosus, aortic coarctation, or surgically constructed vascular shunts.

The incidence of infective endocarditis has increased in recent years, particularly in patients over 65 years of age [1]. Rates of between 2 and 10 cases per 100 000 person-years have been reported [2–5].

Increased age, an increase in the prevalence of degenerative valvular heart disease, and the more widespread use of implanted heart valves and other intracardiac devices have all been implicated. Furthermore, predisposing medical conditions, such as dialysis-dependent renal disease, diabetes, HIV, and nosocomial infections particularly of central venous catheters may be contributory factors. The recent development of antibiotic resistance may also be a factor. Table 18.1 shows those patients considered to be at risk of endocarditis.

Classification

Four categories have been recently recognized, as described below [1].

Native-valve infective endocarditis

This is classically associated with congenital heart disease and chronic rheumatic heart disease, and more controversially with mitral valve prolapse. The inheritable form of mitral valve prolapse is linked to a dominant marker on chromosome 16 [6]. Only patients with valve regurgitation have an increased risk of infective endocarditis [7,8]. Degenerative valve lesions are a primary cause of age-onset aortic stenosis or mitral regurgitation, which are also risk factors for infective endocarditis. Degenerative valve lesions are present in up to 50% of patients with infective endocarditis who are older than 60 years [9].

Prosthetic-valve infective endocarditis

Prosthetic-valve endocarditis accounts for 1–5% of individuals with infective endocarditis, or 0.3 – 0.6% per patient-year [10,11]. It is not clear whether mechanical or biological valves are more prone to infection [10].

Prosthetic-valve endocarditis may be defined as early (within 60 days of surgery) or late (after 60 days). Progressive endothelialization of the prosthetic material over 2–6 months following implantation reduces the susceptibility of the valve to infection. Both the incidence and the nature of the infecting organisms

Table 18.1. Patients at risk of endocarditis

High risk	Previous episodes of endocarditis
	Prosthetic cardiac valve
	Complex congenital cardiac defect
	Surgically constructed systemic-pulmonary shunts or conduits
Moderate risk	Persistent ductus arteriosus
	Ventricular septal defect, primum atrial septal defect
	Coarctation of the aorta
	Bicuspid aortic valve
	Hypertrophic cardiomyopathy
	Acquired valvular dysfunction
Low risk	Isolated secundum atrial septal defect
	Atrial septal defect, ventricular septal defect, or persistent ductus arteriosus > 6 months post repair
	"Innocent" heart murmur by auscultation in the pediatric population
	"Innocent" heart murmur by echocardiography in adult patients

Core Topics in Transesophageal Echocardiography, ed. Robert Feneck, John Kneeshaw, and Marco Ranucci.
Published by Cambridge University Press. © Cambridge University Press 2010.

Table 18.2. Microbiology of infective endocarditis (IE) in the general population and in specific at-risk groups

| Pathogen | Native-valve IE ($n = 280$) | IE in intravenous drug users ($n = 87$) | Prosthetic-valve IE | |
			Early ($n = 15$)	Late ($n = 72$)
Staphylococci	124 (44%)	60 (69%)	10 (67%)	33 (46%)
Staphylococcus aureus	106 (38%)	60 (69%)	3 (20%)	15 (21%)
Coagulase negative	18 (6%)	0	7 (47%)	18 (25%)
Streptococci	86 (31%)	7 (8%)	0 (0%)	25 (35%)
Oral streptococci	59 (21%)	3 (3%)	0	19 (26%)
Others (non-enterococcal)	27 (10%)	4 (5%)	0	6 (8%)
Enterococcus spp. [a]	21 (8%)	2 (2%)	1 (7%)	5 (7%)
Hacek group	12 (4%) [b]	0	0	1 (1%)
Polymicrobial	6 (2%)	8 (9%)	0	1 (1%)
Other bacteria	12 (4%) [c]	4 (5%)	0	2 (3%)
Fungi	3 (1%)	2 (2%)	0	0
Negative blood culture	16 (6%)	4 (5%)	4 (27%)	5 (7%)

Data from studies providing comparable microbiological details.

[a] > 80% *Enterococcus faecalis*.

[b] Includes *Haemophilus* spp., *Actinobacillus actinomycetemcomitans*, *Cardiobacterium hominis*, *Eikenella corrodens*, and *Kingella kingae*.

[c] Includes four *Escherichia coli*, two *Corynebacterium* spp., two *Proteus mirabilis*, one *Mycobacterium tuberculosis*, and one *Bacteroides fragilis*.

are therefore variable, dependent on the onset of the disease. These are shown in Table 18.2.

Infective endocarditis in intravenous drug users

Patients in this group are usually younger, and 60–80% of patients have no known pre-existing valve lesions. Right-sided endocarditis is more common, with infection of the tricuspid valve accounting for more than 50% of cases. Left-sided valve disease is approximately half as prevalent (aortic valve, 25%; mitral valve, 20%), with mixed right-sided and left-sided infective endocarditis in a few instances [12].

The causative organism usually originates from the skin (Table 18.2); although in HIV-positive patients other agents including *Salmonella*, *Listeria*, and *Bartonella* may be responsible. Mortality from infective endocarditis in HIV-positive patients is inversely related to the CD4 count.

Nosocomial infective endocarditis

This is a growing category, and has been shown to be responsible for up to 22% of patients; with a mortality of greater than 50%. Patients often have no cardiac predisposing factors, and pathogens are frequently associated with catheters or medicosurgical procedures, including central venous catheters in bone marrow recipients (Fig. 18.1; Video 18.1) [13–15].

Hemodialysis may be associated with a disease rate two to three times higher than in peritoneal dialysis patients or in the general population. More than 50% of cases are due to *Staphylococcus aureus* [16,17].

Pathology and microbiology

The processes involved in bacterial colonization of damaged valves have been described in detail [18]. The colonization process may involve damaged epithelium and/or inflamed valve tissue, and it results in the production of numerous factors including tissue-factor activity (TFA) and cytokines. These mediators activate the coagulation cascade, attract and activate platelets, and induce further cytokine, integrin, and TFA production from neighboring endothelial cells, thereby encouraging vegetation growth.

In response to local inflammation, endothelial cells express integrins resulting in endothelial internalization

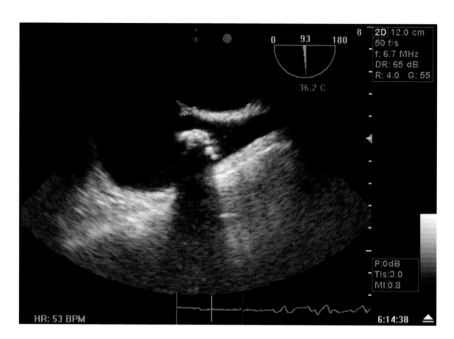

Figure 18.1. Large vegetation on a pacing wire traversing the right atrium.

of bacteria, and the further production of TFA and cytokines. Mechanical damage will trigger blood coagulation, and the coagulum on the damaged endothelia contains large quantities of fibrinogen – fibrin, fibronectin, plasma proteins, and platelet proteins. Pathogens associated with infective endocarditis avidly bind to these structures and colonize them during transient bacteremia.

After valve colonization, the infecting microorganisms become enveloped within the maturing vegetation and persist. Staphylococci and streptococci can trigger tissue-factor production and induce platelet aggregation [19,20], and although activated platelets release platelet microbicidal proteins, microorganisms recovered from patients with infective endocarditis have been shown to be able to resist this effect whilst being able to take advantage of the platelet procoagulant effect.

Tissue invasion and abscess formation are promoted by the production of exoenzymes that convert local host tissues into nutrients for bacterial growth, and exotoxins that are also detrimental. This is particularly a feature of *Staphyloccocus aureus* endocarditis. The risk of mortality from endocarditis is in the range of 5–15% when the infecting organism is *Streptococcus* viridans, 25–45% with *Staphylococcus aureus*, and greater than 50% for fungal endocarditis. Right-sided endocarditis has a mortality of around 10% in intravenous drug abusers. The mortality from endocarditis is increased if there is congestive cardiac failure, abscess formation, or a related neurological event.

Clinical diagnosis

In 1994, the Duke diagnostic criteria were published (Table 18.3) [21]. These are based on both microbiological data and echocardiographic imaging, and have since been extensively validated [22–28]. They have been further refined to more accurately detect infective endocarditis in the case of negative blood cultures and *Staph. aureus*-associated bacteremia [29].

Although patients suspected of having infective endocarditis should undergo at least one echocardiographic assessment, a negative echo does not rule out the disease if other criteria are positive. The importance of blood culture cannot be overemphasized. It remains the best identification method and provides live bacteria for susceptibility testing. For the main causative agents, the first two blood cultures will be positive in more than 90% of cases. Culture-negative disease is often associated with antibiotic consumption within the previous two weeks, and a complex series of procedures may be required to achieve a microbial diagnosis [30,31].

Prophylaxis

Infective endocarditis is a potentially lethal disease and should be prevented whenever possible. Adequate prophylaxis requires establishing those patients at risk, the procedures that might provoke bacteremia, the most effective prophylactic regimen, and a balance

Table 18.3. Modified Duke criteria for diagnosis of infective endocarditis (IE)

Major criteria

Blood culture

- Positive blood cultures (≥ 2/2) with typical IE microorganisms (viridans *Streptococci*, *Strep. bovis*, HACEK group, *Staph. aureus*, or community-acquired enterococci in the absence of primary focus) [a]

- Persistently positive blood cultures, defined as two culture sets drawn > 12 h apart, or three or most of four culture sets with the first and last separated by ≥ 1 h. Single positive culture for *C. burnetti* or antibody titer against phase I > 1 in 800

Endocardial involvement

- Positive echocardiogram for IE (transesophageal echo recommended in patients with prosthetic valves, in patients rated as possible IE by clinical criteria, or in complicated IE (paravalvular abscess); transthoracic echo as first option in other patients)

  (i) oscillating intracardiac mass on valve or supporting structure, or in the path of regurgitant jets, or on implanted material, in the absence of an alternative anatomical explanation, *or*

  (ii) abscess, *or*

  (iii) new partial dehiscence of prosthetic valve

- New valvular regurgitation (worsening of changing or preexisting murmur not sufficient)

Minor criteria

- Predisposing cardiac condition or intravenous drug use, and fever (temperature ≥ 38 °C)

- Vascular factors: major arterial emboli, septic pulmonary infarct, mycotic aneurysms, intracranial hemorrhage, conjunctival hemorrhage, Janeway's lesions

- Immunological factors: glomerulonephritis, Osler nodes, Roth spots, rheumatoid factor

- Microbiology: positive blood cultures, but not meeting major criteria, serological evidence of active infection with plausible microorganisms [b]

- Echocardiogram consistent with disease but not meeting major criteria [c]

Diagnosis

Definite

- Pathology or bacteriology of vegetations, major emboli, or intracardiac abscess specimen, *or*

- Two major criteria, or one major and three minor criteria, or five minor criteria

Possible [d]

- One major and one minor criterion, *or*

- Three minor criteria

Rejected

- Firm alternative diagnosis, *or*

- Resolution of syndrome after ≤ 4 days of antibiotherapy, *or*

- No pathological evidence at surgery or autopsy after ≤ 4 days of antibiotherapy, *or*

- Does not meet criteria mentioned above

[a] Original Duke criteria state: "or community-acquired *S. aureus* or enterococci in the absence of primary focus" [21].

[b] Excludes single positive cultures of coagulase-negative staphylococci and organisms that do not cause endocarditis.

[c] In original Duke criteria [21], but abandoned in revised criteria [29].

[d] Original Duke criteria state: "findings consistent with IE that fall short of *Definite*, but not *Rejected*."

between the risks of side-effects of prophylaxis and of developing the disease.

A number of recommendations have been made, including authoritative recommendations by the European Society of Cardiology (ESC) [32] and the American Heart Association (AHA) [33]. The indications for prophylactic antibiotic therapy for prevention of endocarditis have recently been updated, and these changes are radical and in some opinions controversial. Currently there does not appear to be complete agreement, and the reader is recommended to consult the literature directly for greater detail [34]. However, it should be recognized that the evidence of efficacy of prophylactic antibiotics is largely based on experimental studies. Randomized, placebo-controlled trials raise ethical issues because of the severity of the disease [35], and whilst case–control studies indicate that prophylaxis is effective, most instances of infective endocarditis are not preceded by medicosurgical procedures [36–38]. Therefore, the primary prevention of disease should target infected foci responsible for spontaneous bacteremia – e.g. poor dental hygiene [39,40].

Use of transesophageal echocardiography

In suspected endocarditis, transesophageal echocardiography (TEE) will usually follow a transthoracic (TTE) examination. TEE may be requested to make or refute the diagnosis of endocarditis. In such cases TEE should aim to identify valvular vegetations and other cardiac effects of endocarditis, and to assess cardiac anatomy with regard to factors that might predispose to endocarditis. Figure 18.2 shows an algorithm for the application of TTE and TEE in patients with suspected endocarditis [41].

Where the diagnosis is already made, TEE should:

- seek valvular vegetations and assess their number, size, and location
- assess associated valve abnormalities, particularly regurgitant lesions

- assess the effect of the disease on chamber dimensions and function, in particular ventricular function.
- seek evidence of the complications of endocarditis, i.e. abscesses, fistulae
- provide prognostic information, and assess the risk of embolization and the need for surgical interventions

Vegetations

Vegetations are seen as abnormal echogenic masses attached to the upstream surface of affected valves. They often display exaggerated motion when compared to the motion of the valve leaflets. Aortic valve vegetations are attached to the ventricular surface of the valve leaflets, and may be seen in the aortic root in systole and in the left ventricular outflow tract (LVOT) in diastole. Mitral vegetations are attached to the atrial surface of the leaflets and may be seen in the left atrium in systole and in the left ventricle in diastole. Vegetations vary in size, from up to 3.5 cm in diameter to small lesions that are undetectable with 2D echocardiography. Careful scanning through multiple planes is required to identify vegetations. TEE is superior to TTE in the identification of vegetations, with a sensitivity of 94% and a specificity of 100% reported in some studies [42,43] (Figs. 18.3–18.5; Videos 18.2–18.4).

Aortic valve vegetations may be difficult to distinguish in the presence of aortic stenosis with valvular thickening or calcification, and other non-pathological findings such as the nodules of Arantius (nodular

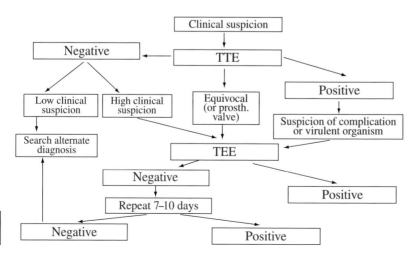

Clinical suspicion

TTE

Negative

Low clinical suspicion | High clinical suspicion

Equivocal (or prosth. valve)

Positive

Search alternate diagnosis

Suspicion of complication or virulent organism

TEE

Negative

Positive

Repeat 7–10 days

Negative

Positive

Figure 18.2. An algorithm for the use of transesophageal echocardiography in suspected infective endocarditis. Adapted from Evangelista & Gonzalez-Alujas, *Heart* 2004; **90**: 614–17 [41].

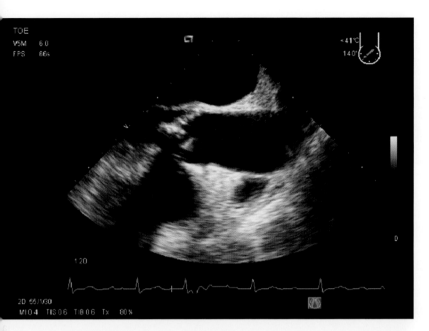

Figure 18.3. Aortic valve ME LAX view showing aortic valve vegetations prolapsing into the LVOT.

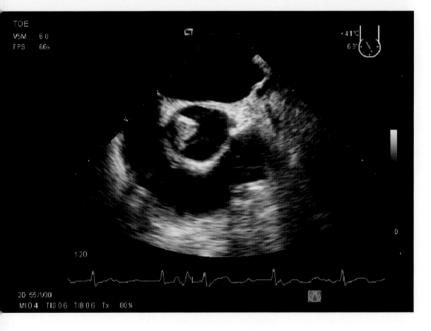

Figure 18.4. Aortic valve ME SAX view showing a vegetation on the non-coronary cusp.

hickenings in the normal cusp apposition regions) or Lambl's excrescences (linear, fibrinous strands attached to the cusp edges). In addition to the mid-esophageal short-axis and long-axis views, the deep transgastric view may be useful in demonstrating vegetations which move into the LVOT in diastole. In patients with aortic valve vegetations there will usually be evidence of valvular dysfunction caused by tissue damage. Mitral valve vegetations are often seen

as rapidly moving or flickering echogenic features which appear in the left atrium. Other pathology which may mimic mitral vegetations includes myxomatous leaflet degeneration and mitral leaflet papillomata. Mitral vegetations should be sought in the full range of views described in Chapter 5 (Fig. 18.6; Video 18.5).

Patients with one left-sided valve affected may have disease of the other valve, and it is important to

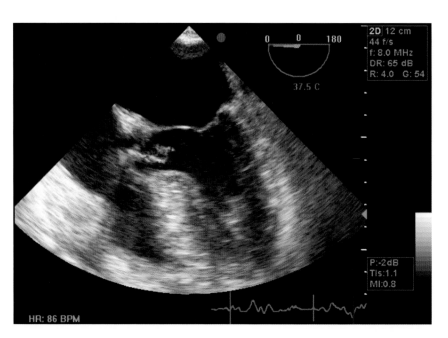

Figure 18.5. Five-chamber view showing aortic valve vegetation prolapsing into the LVOT.

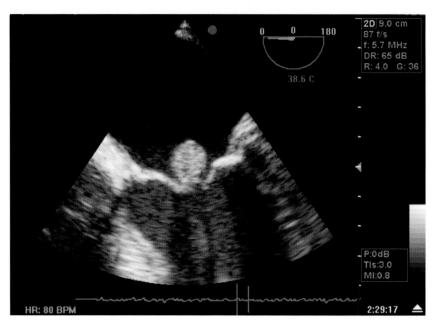

Figure 18.6. Four-chamber view of a large mitral valve vegetation.

thoroughly interrogate both valves if vegetations are seen on one.

Tricuspid valve vegetations, often in patients with a history of intravenous drug abuse, should be sought in the four-chamber view and the mid-esophageal inflow–outflow view. These are often associated with tricuspid regurgitation, which should be assessed, as should any degree of right-heart dilation (Fig. 18.7; Video 18.6).

Vegetations may occur on pacing wire, central venous catheters, and other devices placed on the heart. Any such devices should be imaged thoroughly in a patient with suspected endocarditis.

The risk of embolization of a vegetation increases with the size of vegetations [44]. There is also a greater risk of embolization from the mitral than from the aortic valve. In one study, vegetations greater than 20 mm in diameter presented a 20.8% risk of embolization [45].

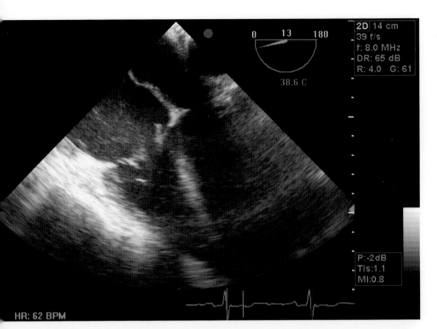

Figure 18.7. Tricuspid valve vegetations.

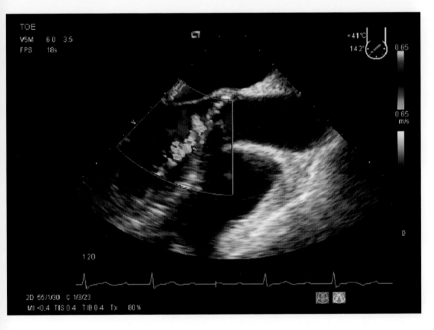

Figure 18.8. Aortic regurgitation produced by endocarditis (same patient as Figure 18.3).

In patients undergoing medical therapy for endocarditis, serial echocardiography may be used to monitor the reduction in size and the healing of vegetations.

Valve dysfunction caused by endocarditis

Regurgitant lesions in valves affected by endocarditis occur because of tissue destruction by the disease process itself, and because of distortion of structures by vegetations (Fig. 18.8; Video 18.7). The severity of regurgitation should be assessed by the Doppler methods (qualitative and quantitative) described in the relevant chapters. Serial echocardiographic examination may be needed to follow the course of the disease and its treatment, and the worsening of valvular regurgitation may be a valuable indicator for the timing of surgical

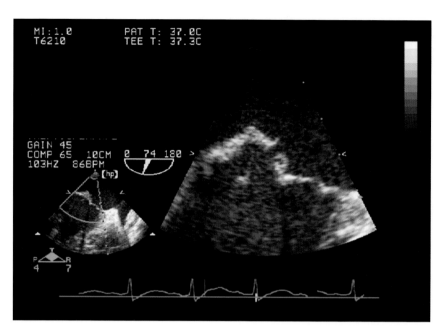

Figure 18.9. Endocarditic leaflet perforation causing mitral regurgitation.

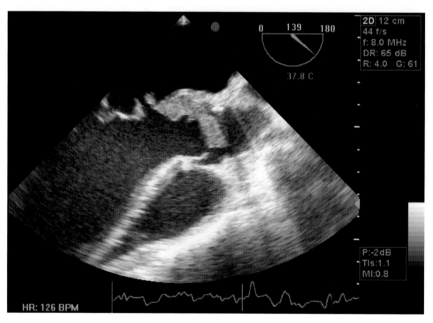

Figure 18.10. Severe aortic endocarditis with extension of the disease into the anterior mitral leaflet causing leaflet perforation.

intervention. Endocarditis usually occurs in previously abnormal valves, and patients with a previously stenotic lesion may re-present with valvular regurgitation. The severity of regurgitant lesions caused by endocarditis can usually be assessed by the methods described for the aortic and mitral valves in Chapters 6 and 7. Where there are destructive lesions which produce leaflet perforation, the perforation itself may sometimes be difficult to visualize. It is, however, usually possible to identify such lesions with color-flow Doppler. Often this will require scanning through multiple planes, and the lesions may be best seen in off-axis or non-standard views (Figs. 18.9–18.12; Videos 18.8–18.10). Valvular stenosis is a rare complication of infective endocarditis, but it may occur if a large mass of vegetative material prolapses into the mitral orifice in diastole.

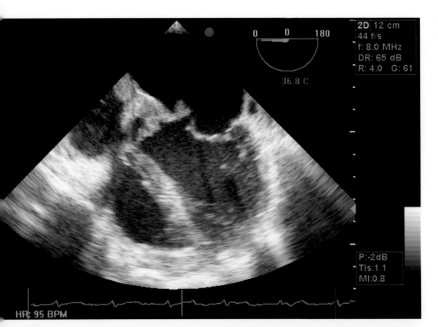

Figure 18.11. Five-chamber view of the same patient as in Figure 18.10.

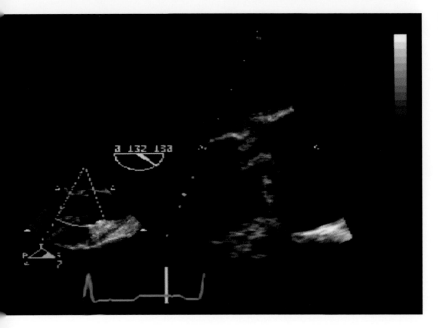

Figure 18.12. Zoomed ME LAX view of the aortic valve showing leaflet perforation by endocarditis.

Perivalvular complications of endocarditis

Endocarditis may be complicated by the formation of perivalvular abscesses and intracardiac fistulae. These are more common around the aortic valve than the mitral. Abscesses appear initially as areas of altered echogenicity in the region of the annulus. This area expands, transgresses the annulus, and then an echo-

free space may form. In aortic valve endocarditis these root abscesses may extend into any adjacent tissues, and may involve the anterior leaflet of the mitral valve, which may itself develop vegetations or become perforated. An abscess cavity may rupture into any adjacent chamber to form an intracardiac fistula (Figs. 18.13–18.15; Videos 18.11–18.14). Because of the anatomical location of the aortic valve, fistulae may form

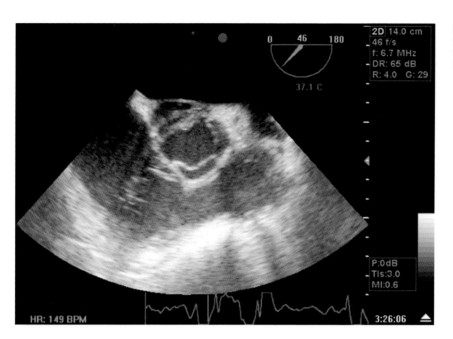

Figure 18.13. ME SAX view of the aortic valve showing perivalvular abscess formation in the area of the non-coronary cusp.

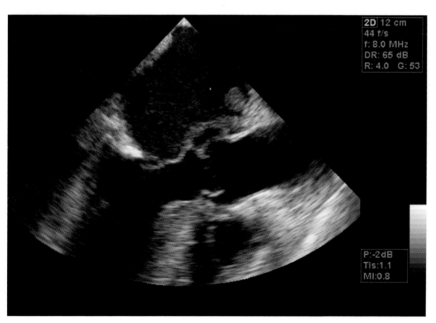

Figure 18.14. ME LAX view of aortic endocarditis with a posterior aortic root abscess and the development of an atrial vegetation.

which communicate with the right ventricular outflow tract, the right atrium, or the left atrium, or through the aortomitral continuity into the LVOT. These fistulae are often identified from the abnormal high-velocity jets that are generated. In mitral endocarditis an abscess may form in the posterior annulus and extend into adjacent segments of ventricular muscle. Similarly tricuspid disease may produce abscesses around the annulus. TEE is a much better modality

for identifying endocarditic abscesses and fistulae than TTE because of the higher ultrasound frequency and hence superior spatial resolution [46,47]. Perivalvular complications of endocarditis should be sought in all patients with endocarditis. Areas of abnormal echo density should be identified with 2D echo and then further interrogated by color-flow Doppler to identify flow through fistulae. This often requires the use of non-standard views. TTE may also be required

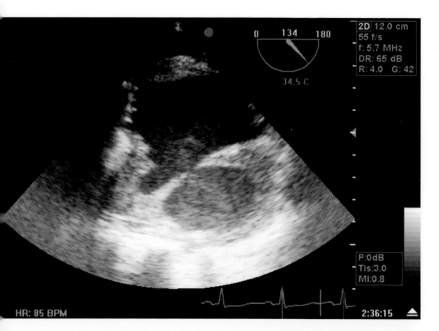

Figure 18.15. ME LAX view of aortic endocarditis with an anterior aortic root abscess in communication with the ascending aorta.

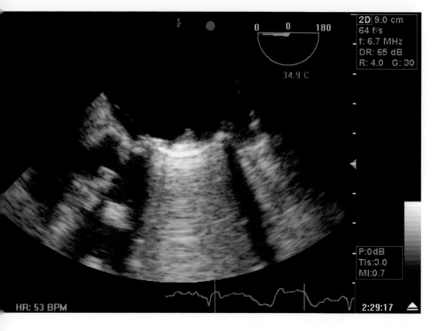

Figure 18.16. Endocarditis affecting a bileaflet prosthetic valve in the mitral position. There are vegetations, and the valve was seen to "rock" in the annulus.

o fully determine the nature of a fistula, because it is easier to align continuous-wave Doppler with abnormal high-velocity flows in TTE than in TEE. The identification of extravalvular phenomena is particularly important in the intraoperative guidance of surgical therapy.

Prosthetic-valve endocarditis

Perivalvular abscess formation is more common with prosthetic than with native-valve endocarditis, because the infection typically involves the interface between the sewing ring and the surrounding tissue. Typically, infection in the area around the sewing ring of a valve

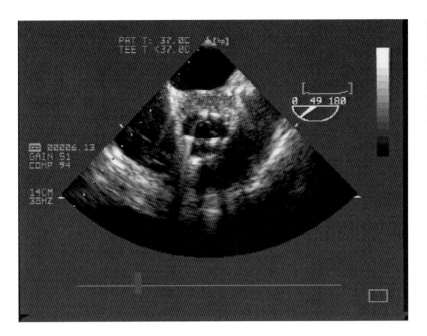

Figure 18.17. Endocarditis affecting a bioprosthetic valve in the aortic position. There is perivalvular extension of the disease with early posterior abscess formation. This is shown by increased distance between the valve and the left atrium, and by a crescent of reduced echogenicity in that area posterior to the annulus.

will produce loosening of the seating of the valve in the annulus, and this will be seen as paraprosthetic regurgitation and a rocking movement of the valve. Perivalvular complications, abscess, and fistula formation are also seen in prosthetic-valve endocarditis, and appear as described for native valves above.

Echocardiographic examination of prosthetic valves is more difficult than that of native valves because of the imaging artifacts (reverberations and echo shadowing) produced by the prosthetic valve. TEE provides better images of prosthetic mitral valves than TTE, but TTE may provide better images of aortic prostheses than TEE. Because of the difficulty in imaging prosthetic valves it is not easy to quantify regurgitation caused by endocarditis. Even without direct measurement of regurgitant flows it is possible to infer that significant regurgitation is present if there is an increase in the velocity of forward flow across the prosthesis. This increase in forward flow velocity occurs because of an increase in the volume of forward flow caused by the regurgitation. There may also be an increase in the velocity of a tricuspid regurgitant jet, reflecting an increase in pulmonary artery pressure caused by a worsening left-sided valvular regurgitation (Figs. 18.16, 18.17; Videos 18.15, 18.16).

In the diagnosis of prosthetic endocarditis a combined approach of TTE followed by TEE is probably sensible (see also Chapter 19).

Indications for surgery

For patients with native-valve endocarditis, the following may constitute acute indications for surgery [48]:

- the development of heart failure from either valve regurgitation or stenosis
- evidence of significantly increased left ventricular end-diastolic or left atrial pressure
- treatment of fungal or other highly resistant organisms
- treatment of intracardiac abscess, perforation, fistulous tracts, and false aneurysms

Surgery may also be indicated for patients with recurrent emboli and persistent vegetations, and for patients with persistent bacteremia despite up to seven days of appropriate antibiotic therapy and in the absence of a metastatic focus of infection.

Large mobile vegetations (> 1.5 cm) may also be considered an indication for surgery in order to prevent embolization. Although valve replacement is historically considered the treatment of choice, valve repair is increasingly considered appropriate in experienced centers.

Such a repair may involve vegetectomy, debridement, the eradication of abscess cavities, and pericardial patch repair of the underlying defect. Leaflet resection and/or placement of an annular ring may be required, according to the intraoperative findings. Valve replacement is necessary when there has been extensive destruction of intracardiac structures, but the increased perioperative and long-term risks associated with valve replacement, compared with valve repair, should be borne in mind, especially when surgery is being considered for prevention of embolization rather than for treatment of heart failure or intracardiac abscess.

The relationship between vegetation size and the risk of embolization has been confirmed, particularly for lesions affecting the anterior leaflet of the mitral valve [44]. The risk of embolization increases significantly if the size of the vegetation exceeds 1.0 cm, and it may also be dependent on patient-specific and bacteriological factors [49]. Thuny *et al.* showed that very large vegetations (> 1.5 cm) may be a reason to consider surgery independent of the severity of the valve dysfunction, the presence or absence of heart failure, or the imputed risk of embolization [50].

The value of surgery in endocarditis has been shown by Vikram *et al.*, who showed that valve surgery was associated with a significant reduction in six-month mortality (16% vs. 33%, $p < 0.001$) compared to medical therapy alone [51], although this benefit was restricted to those patients with moderate or severe heart failure.

Prosthetic-valve endocarditis that relapses after appropriate antibiotic therapy should lead to a careful search for perivalvular extension and metastatic foci of infection. Some patients with relapsed prosthetic-valve endocarditis may respond to a second course of medical treatment, but the majority will require surgery. However, medical therapy should be attempted initially for uncomplicated prosthetic-valve endocarditis caused by first infection with a sensitive organism.

The timing of surgery following CNS embolization is problematic. It is generally advisable to wait up to one week after simple CNS infarction and up to four weeks before undertaking surgery after primary CNS hemorrhage, for example from a ruptured mycotic aneurysm [52].

A number of factors have been implicated in the mortality from surgery for endocarditis, although the trend appears to be improving. Older surgical series have reported mortality rates of 5–25%, but more recent series in selected patients have been more optimistic. A perioperative mortality rate of 3% in a small series of patients following mitral valve repair for endocarditis has been reported [53]. Ten-year survival

in this series was 80%, and freedom from mitral re-operation was 91%. Others have reported perioperative mortality rates of between 9% and 14%, in patients requiring elective/urgent and emergency aortic root homograft reconstruction for complex endocarditis [54].

Although the indications for surgery in the acute phase will be based largely on a collaborative case review, the urgency of surgery is predicated on the patient's hemodynamic status. Acute severe aortic regurgitation is poorly tolerated and usually requires surgery within 24 hours. Patients with acute severe mitral regurgitation can often be stabilized with intensive medical therapy, with surgery delayed for up to several days. Once heart failure intervenes, however, surgery should not be inordinately delayed to provide time for preoperative antibiotic therapy.

Similar considerations apply to considerations for surgery in patients with prosthetic-valve endocarditis. Heart failure, a poorly responsive microorganism, perivalvular extension or an unstable prosthesis are recognized indications. Prosthetic valve dehiscence is defined as a rocking motion of the valve with excursion of 15° or more in at least one plane.

In patients with *Staphylococcus aureus* endocarditis, prosthetic-valve endocarditis is rarely eradicated with antibiotics alone, and retrospective analyses suggest that combined medical and surgical therapy is necessary even in the absence of perivalvular extension or an unstable prosthesis [55].

References

1. Moreillon P, Que YA. Infective endocarditis. *Lancet* 2004; **363**: 139–49.

2. Hogevik H, Olaison L, Andersson R, Lindberg J, Alestig K. Epidemiologic aspects of infective endocarditis in an urban population: a 5-year prospective study. *Medicine (Baltimore)* 1995; **74**: 324–39.

3. Berlin JA, Abrutyn E, Strom BL, *et al.* Incidence of infective endocarditis in the Delaware Valley, 1988–1990. *Am J Cardiol* 1995; **76**: 933–6.

4. Delahaye F, Goulet V, Lacassin F, *et al.* Characteristics of infective endocarditis in France in 1991: a 1-year survey. *Eur Heart J* 1995; **16**: 394–401.

5. Tleyjeh IM, Steckelberg JM, Murad HS, *et al.* Temporal trends in infective endocarditis: a population-based study in Olmsted County, Minnesota. *JAMA* 2005; **293**: 3022–8.

6. Disse S, Abergel E, Berrebi A, *et al.* Mapping of a first locus for autosomal dominant myxomatous

mitral-valve prolapse to chromosome 16p11.2-p12.1. *Am J Hum Genet* 1999; **65**: 1242–51.

7. Zuppiroli A, Rinaldi M, Kramer-Fox R, *et al.* Natural history of mitral valve prolapse. *Am J Cardiol* 1995; **75**: 1028–32.

8. Kim S, Kuroda T, Nishinaga M, *et al.* Relationship between severity of mitral regurgitation and prognosis of mitral valve prolapse: echocardiographic follow-up study. *Am Heart J* 1996; **132**: 348–55.

9. McKinsey DS, Ratts TE, Bisno AL. Underlying cardiac lesions in adults with infective endocarditis: the changing spectrum. *Am J Med* 1987; **82**: 681–8.

10. Sidhu P, O'Kane H, Ali N, *et al.* Mechanical or bioprosthetic valves in the elderly: a 20-year comparison. *Ann Thorac Surg* 2001; **71** (5 Suppl): S257–60.

11. Varstela E. Personal follow-up of 100 aortic valve replacement patients for 1081 patient years. *Ann Chir Gynaecol* 1998; **87**: 205–12.

12. Mathew J, Addai T, Anand A, *et al.* Clinical features, site of involvement, bacteriologic findings, and outcome of infective endocarditis in intravenous drug users. *Arch Intern Med* 1995; **155**: 1641–8.

13. Bouza E, Menasalvas A, Muñoz P, *et al.* Infective endocarditis: a prospective study at the end of the twentieth century – new predisposing conditions, new etiologic agents, and still a high mortality. *Medicine (Baltimore)* 2001; **80**: 298–307.

14. Gouëllo JP, Asfar P, Brenet O, *et al.* Nosocomial endocarditis in the intensive care unit: an analysis of 22 cases. *Crit Care Med* 2000; **28**: 377–82.

15. Martino P, Micozzi A, Venditti M, *et al.* Catheter-related right-sided endocarditis in bone marrow transplant recipients. *Rev Infect Dis* 1990; **12**: 250–7.

16. Abbott KC, Agodoa LY. Hospitalizations for bacterial endocarditis after initiation of chronic dialysis in the United States. *Nephron* 2002; **91**: 203–9.

17. Cabell CH, Jollis JG, Peterson GE, *et al.* Changing patient characteristics and the effect on mortality in endocarditis. *Arch Intern Med* 2002; **162**: 90–4.

18. Moreillon P, Que YA, Bayer AS. Pathogenesis of streptococcal and staphylococcal endocarditis. *Infect Dis Clin North Am* 2002; **16**: 297–318.

19. Bayer AS, Sullam PM, Ramos M, *et al. Staphylococcus aureus* induces platelet aggregation via a fibrinogen-dependent mechanism which is independent of principal platelet glycoprotein IIb/IIIa fibrinogen-binding domains. *Infect Immun* 1995; **63**: 3634–41.

20. Herzberg MC, MacFarlane GD, Gong K, *et al.* The platelet interactivity phenotype of *Streptococcus sanguis* influences the course of experimental endocarditis. *Infect Immun* 1992; **60**: 4809–18.

21. Durack DT, Lukes AS, Bright DK. New criteria for diagnosis of infective endocarditis: utilization of specific echocardiographic findings. *Am J Med* 1994; **96**: 200–9.

22. Bayer AS, Ward JI, Ginzton LE, Shapiro SM. Evaluation of new clinical criteria for the diagnosis of infective endocarditis. *Am J Med* 1994; **96**: 211–19.

23. Gagliardi JP, Nettles RE, McCarty DE, *et al.* Native valve infective endocarditis in elderly and younger adult patients: comparison of clinical features and outcomes with use of the Duke criteria and the Duke Endocarditis Database. *Clin Infect Dis* 1998; **26**: 1165–8.

24. Nettles RE, McCarty DE, Corey GR, Li J, Sexton DJ. An evaluation of the Duke criteria in 25 pathologically confirmed cases of prosthetic valve endocarditis. *Clin Infect Dis* 1997; **25**: 1401–3.

25. Pérez-Vázquez A, Fariñas MC, Garcia-Palomo JD, *et al.* Evaluation of the Duke criteria in 93 episodes of prosthetic valve endocarditis: could sensitivity be improved? *Arch Intern Med* 2000; **160**: 1185–91.

26. Dodds GA, Sexton DJ, Durack DT, *et al.* Negative predictive value of the Duke criteria for infective endocarditis. *Am J Cardiol* 1996; **77**: 403–7.

27. Habib G, Derumeaux G, Avierinos JF, *et al.* Value and limitations of the Duke criteria for the diagnosis of infective endocarditis. *J Am Coll Cardiol* 1999; **33**: 2023–9.

28. Sekeres MA, Abrutyn E, Berlin JA, *et al.* An assessment of the usefulness of the Duke criteria for diagnosing active infective endocarditis. *Clin Infect Dis* 1997; **24**: 1185–90.

29. Li JS, Sexton DJ, Mick N, *et al.* Proposed modifications to the Duke criteria for the diagnosis of infective endocarditis. *Clin Infect Dis* 2000; **30**: 633–8.

30. Brouqui P, Raoult D. Endocarditis due to rare and fastidious bacteria. *Clin Microbiol Rev* 2001; **14**: 177–207.

31. Houpikian P, Raoult D. Diagnostic methods current best practices and guidelines for identification of difficult-to-culture pathogens in infective endocarditis. *Infect Dis Clin North Am* 2002; **16**: 377–92.

32. Horstkotte D, Follath F, Gutschik E, *et al.* Guidelines on prevention, diagnosis and treatment of infective endocarditis executive summary: the task force on infective endocarditis of the European Society of Cardiology. *Eur Heart J* 2004; **25**: 267–76.

33. Baddour LM, Wilson WR, Bayer AS, *et al.* Infective endocarditis: diagnosis, antimicrobial therapy, and management of complications: a statement for healthcare professionals from the Committee on Rheumatic Fever, Endocarditis, and Kawasaki Disease

Council on Cardiovascular Disease in the Young, and the Councils on Clinical Cardiology, Stroke, and Cardiovascular Surgery and Anesthesia, American Heart Association: endorsed by the Infectious Diseases Society of America. *Circulation* 2005; **111**: e394–434.

34. Nishimura RA, Carabello BA, Faxon DP, *et al.* ACC/ AHA 2008 guideline update on valvular heart disease: focused update on infective endocarditis: a report of the American College of Cardiology/American Heart Association Task Force on Practice Guidelines: endorsed by the Society of Cardiovascular Anesthesiologists, Society for Cardiovascular Angiography and Interventions, and Society of Thoracic Surgeons. *Circulation* 2008; **118**: 887–96.

35. Durack DT. Prevention of infective endocarditis. *N Engl J Med* 1995; **332**: 38–44.

36. Strom BL, Abrutyn E, Berlin JA, *et al.* Dental and cardiac risk factors for infective endocarditis: a population-based, case-control study. *Ann Intern Med* 1998; **129**: 761–9.

37. van der Meer JT, Thompson J, Valkenburg HA, Michel MF. Epidemiology of bacterial endocarditis in the Netherlands, 1. Patient characteristics. *Arch Intern Med* 1992; **152**: 1863–8.

38. van der Meer JT, Thompson J, Valkenburg HA, Michel MF. Epidemiology of bacterial endocarditis in the Netherlands, II. Antecedent procedures and use of prophylaxis. *Arch Intern Med* 1992; **152**: 1869–73.

39. Leport C, Horstkotte D, Burckhardt D. Antibiotic prophylaxis for infective endocarditis from an international group of experts towards a European consensus. *Eur Heart J* 1995; **16** (Suppl B): 126–31.

40. Dajani AS, Taubert KA, Wilson W, *et al.* Prevention of bacterial endocarditis: recommendations by the American Heart Association. *JAMA* 1997; **277**: 1794–801.

41. Evangelista A, Gonzalez-Alujas MT. Echocardiography in infective endocarditis. *Heart* 2004; **90**: 614–17.

42. Shapiro SM, Young E, De Guzman S, *et al.* Transesophageal echocardiography in the diagnosis of infective endocarditis. *Chest* 1994; **105**: 377–82.

43. Shively BK, Gurule FT, Roldan CA, Leggett JH, Schiller NB. Diagnostic value of transesophageal compared with transthoracic echocardiography in infective endocarditis. *J Am Coll Cardiol* 1991; **18**: 391–7.

44. Vilacosta I, Graupner C, San Román J, *et al.* Risk of embolization after institution of antibiotic therapy for infective endocarditis. *Am Coll Cardiol* 2002; **39**: 1489–95.

45. Di Salvo G, Habib G, Pergola V, *et al.* Echocardiography predicts embolic events in infective endocarditis. *J Am Coll Cardiol* 2001; **37**: 1069–76.

46. Daniel WG, Mügge A, Martin RP, *et al.* Improvement in the diagnosis of abscesses associated with endocarditis by transesophageal echocardiography. *N Eng J Med* 1991; **324**: 795–800.

47. Graupner C, Vilacosta I, San Román JA, *et al.* Periannular extension of infective endocarditis. *J Am Coll Cardiol* 2002; **39**: 1204–11.

48. O'Gara PT. Infective endocarditis 2006: indications for surgery. *Trans Am Clin Climatol Assoc* 2007; **118**: 187–98.

49. Kupferwasser LI, Hafner G, Mohr-Kahaly S, *et al.* The presence of infection-related antiphospholipid antibodies in infective endocarditis determines a major risk factor for embolic events. *J Am Coll Cardiol* 1999; **33**: 1365–71.

50. Thuny F, Di Salvo G, Belliard O, *et al.* Risk of embolism and death in infective endocarditis: prognostic value of echocardiography: a prospective multicenter study. *Circulation* 2005; **112**: 69–75.

51. Vikram HR, Buenconsejo J, Hasbun R, Quagliarello VJ. Impact of valve surgery on 6-month mortality in adults with complicated, left-sided native valve endocarditis: a propensity analysis. *JAMA* 2003; **290**: 3207–14.

52. Gillinov AM, Shah RV, Curtis WE, *et al.* Valve replacement in patients with endocarditis and acute neurologic deficit. *Ann Thorac Surg* 1996; **61**: 1125–9.

53. Zegdi R, Debieche M, Latrémouille C, *et al.* Long-term results of mitral valve repair in active infective endocarditis. *Circulation* 2005; **111**: 2532–6.

54. Yankah AC, Pasic M, Klose H, *et al.* Homograft reconstruction of the aortic root for endocarditis with periannular abscess: a 17-year study. *Eur J Cardiothorac Surg* 2005; **28**: 69–75.

55. John MD, Hibberd PL, Karchmer AW, Sleeper LA, Calderwood SB. *Staphylococcus aureus* prosthetic valve endocarditis. Optimal management, and risk factors for death. *Clin Infect Dis* 1998; **26**: 1302–9.

Prosthetic valves

John B. Chambers

Introduction

The echocardiography of replacement heart valves is more demanding than for native valves, for the following reasons:

- **Obstruction**. Almost all replacement valves are obstructive compared to normal native valves. The differentiation between normal and pathological obstruction may be difficult.
- **Regurgitation**. Transprosthetic regurgitation is normal for almost all mechanical valves and for many biological valves. This can be mistaken for pathological regurgitation.
- **Normal variability**. The appearance, forward flow, and patterns of regurgitation differ between valve designs. Experience gained from one valve type may lead to confusion if extrapolated to another.
- **Technical difficulties**. Shielding from the ultrasound beam by mechanical parts can obscure vegetations or a regurgitant jet. Blooming or reverberation artifacts can cause overdiagnosis of abnormal masses or of calcification.

Because of the need for multiple views, the echocardiography of replacement heart valves is rarely complete with transesophageal echocardiography (TEE) alone. Furthermore, quantitative Doppler of the aortic valve is more easily performed transthoracically. Left ventricular (LV) function is usually better analyzed transthoracically, and the anterior aortic root may be better visualized transthoracically, while the posterior root is better seen on TEE.

Commonly seen replacement valves are classified in Table 19.1 [1]. There are comprehensive international guidelines for the echocardiographic assessment of prosthetic valves [2] and the management of clinical problems [3,4]. Stented valves placed using transcatheter techniques are rapidly becoming established [5], but these are beyond the scope of this chapter (see

Chapter 17). The aim of this chapter is to summarize the normal appearance of replacement valves by position, and also to describe the diagnosis of pathology.

Echocardiography of the replacement aortic valve

Imaging

The reference view is at the mid-esophageal level, usually with rotation to about 30° to obtain a horizontal section through the valve. It requires more careful and time-consuming positioning of the probe than for a native aortic valve, using multiple positions together with rotation and flexion to insonate the plane of the sewing ring and just below this level in order to localize regurgitant jets. The longitudinal view rotated approximately 90° further shows movement of the cusp or occluder and allows the detection of jets through the valve. The left ventricular outflow tract (LVOT) diameter can be measured in this view for the calculation of effective orifice area using the continuity equation. The deep transgastric five-chamber view is then used to record subaortic velocity on pulsed-wave Doppler, and to obtain transaortic recording on continuous wave. However, quantitative Doppler is more easily and accurately performed transthoracically since more probe and patient positions can be used.

The sutures may be visible on TEE, and should not be mistaken for vegetations. Small fibrin strands are also normal (Fig. 19.1). Early after implantation, a stentless valve inserted as an inclusion will be surrounded by hematoma and edema. This is indistinguishable from an abscess and underlines the fact that an echocardiogram cannot ever be interpreted outside the clinical context. Rocking of the valve suggests dehiscence, which is proved by overlaying color Doppler and demonstrating a paraprosthetic regurgitant jet. Usually rocking in the aortic position implies a large dehiscence, about 40% of the sewing ring.

Core Topics in Transesophageal Echocardiography, ed. Robert Feneck, John Kneeshaw, and Marco Ranucci.
Published by Cambridge University Press. © Cambridge University Press 2010.

Table 19.1. Designs of replacement heart valve

Biological	Autograft (Ross operation)
	Homograft – usually aortic, occasionally pulmonary
	Stented heterograft – e.g. Hancock (porcine), Mosaic (porcine), Baxter Perimount (pericardial), Carpentier–Edwards (standard and supra-annular porcine), Intact (porcine), Labcor (porcine tricomposite), Biocor (porcine tricomposite), Mitroflow (bovine pericardial)
	Stentless heterograft – e.g. Toronto (St. Jude Medical), Cryolife O'Brien, Freestyle (Medtronic), Baxter Prima, Biocor PSB tricomposite, Sorin Pericarbon (pericardial)
Mechanical	Ball-cage – e.g. Starr–Edwards
	Single tilting disk – e.g. Bjork–Shiley, Medtronic Hall, Monostrut, Omniscience, Ultracor
	Bileaflet – e.g. St. Jude Medical, Carbomedics, MCRI On-X, ATS, Sorin Bicarbon, Edwards Tekna, Edwards Mira

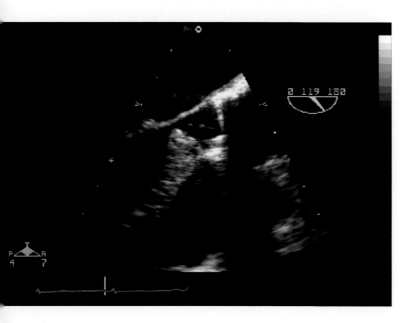

Figure 19.1. Fibrin strand attached to a bileaflet mechanical aortic valve: transesophageal study.

Quantitative Doppler

The minimum dataset is peak velocity, mean pressure difference, and effective orifice area (EOA). It is important to derive the mean pressure difference, because it is calculated using the whole wave-form and reflects function better than using the peak velocity alone. In a normal valve, the subaortic velocity may not be negligible compared with the transaortic velocity, so the long form of the modified Bernoulli equation should be used.

Peak pressure drop across the aortic valve is calculated from the formula

$$\text{Peak } \Delta P = 4 \, (v_2^2 - v_1^2) \qquad (19.1)$$

where V_1 and V_2 are peak velocities in the subaortic and transaortic signal respectively.

Mean pressure difference cannot be derived from the respective mean velocities, but can be calculated from the online software as aortic mean ΔP – subaortic mean ΔP.

Because of the flow dependency of velocity and pressure difference, effective area by the continuity equation (EOA) should be calculated using the formula

$$\text{EOA} = \text{CSA} \times \text{VTI}_1 \, / \, \text{VTI}_2 \qquad (19.2)$$

where

CSA is LV outflow cross-sectional area in cm² calculated from the diameter, assuming circular cross-section

VTI_1 is subaortic velocity integral in cm and VTI_2 is aortic velocity integral in cm

Errors arise if the peak velocity is used in place of the velocity integral [6]. It is almost never appropriate to substitute the labeled size of the replacement valve for the LVOT diameter, because this may differ widely from its true size [7]. For serial studies it is reasonable to use the ratio of the velocity integrals, since this avoids measuring the LVOT diameter [8].

High velocities are common, especially in size 19 or 21 prostheses. The challenge is to differentiate a small but normally functioning valve from a pathologically obstructive valve. The first step is to calculate the EOA using the continuity equation. If this is within the normal range for a valve of that size and design (Appendix 19.1) [9,10], the valve is likely to be normally functioning but small. Patient–prosthesis mismatch is diagnosed if the EOA indexed to body surface area is < 0.85 cm^2/m^2, and severe patient–prosthesis mismatch if the indexed orifice area is < 0.65 cm^2/m^2 [11]. Patient–prosthesis mismatch may reduce the degree of LV mass regression after aortic valve replacement and has been linked with a poorer outcome, particularly if LV systolic function is poor [12–14]. If the EOA is lower than the normal range, pathological obstruction is likely. However, obstruction is most reliably detected by comparing EOA with the baseline study. Allowing for experimental error, a fall of more than 30% is likely to be significant. Finally, and importantly, pathological obstruction is associated with abnormal cusps or occluder on imaging.

Regurgitation

Minor regurgitation is normal in virtually all mechanical valves. Early valves had a closing volume as the leaflet closed, followed by true regurgitation around the occluder. For the Starr–Edwards, there is a small closing volume and usually little or no true regurgitation. The single tilting disk valves have both types of regurgitation, but the pattern may vary. The Bjork–Shiley valve has a minor and major jet from the two orifices, while the Medtronic Hall valve has a single large jet through a central hole in the disk (Fig. 19.2).

The bileaflet valves have continuous leakage through the pivotal points where the lugs of the leaflets are held in the housing (Fig. 19.3). These are thought to prevent the formation of thrombus at sites of stasis and are called "washing jets." They are usually found in formation, two from each pivotal point, giving a characteristic appearance on imaging in a plane just below the valve. Sometimes these single pivotal washing jets divide into two or three separate "plumes," and in some valve designs such as the St. Jude Medical there may be a jet around the edge of one or other leaflet. The jets are invariably low in momentum, so they are homogeneous in color with aliasing confined to the base of the jet.

Regurgitation through the valve is also increasingly reported in normal biological valves. This is mainly because echocardiography machines are increasingly sensitive. Stentless valves, including homografts and autografts, are more likely than the stented valves to have minor regurgitant jets, usually at the point of apposition of all three cusps or at one or more commissure. In stented valves, the regurgitation is usually at the point of apposition of the cusps.

The same methods of quantifying regurgitation can be used as for native regurgitation [15]. However, assessing the height of an aortic jet relative to the LVOT diameter may be difficult if it is eccentric, and care must be taken to measure the diameter of the jet perpendicular to its axis. Multiple small normal transprosthetic jets cannot be quantified accurately, but this is not necessary in clinical practice. For paraprosthetic jets, the proportion of the circumference of the sewing ring occupied by the jet gives an approximate guide to severity: mild ($< 10\%$), moderate (10–25%), severe ($> 25\%$).

Echocardiography of the replacement mitral valve

Imaging

The low esophageal four-chamber view is the reference view, and from here rotation of the probe to two- and three-chamber planes together with anteflexion and retroflexion allows interrogation of the whole of the sewing ring. The transverse short-axis transgastric view is useful for imaging the whole sewing ring, and the location of paraprosthetic jets can be described using a clock-face system. On transthoracic echocardiography, parasternal long- and short-axis views, all apical views, and the subcostal view should be used. Multiple angulation and off-axis views are needed to insonate the whole sewing ring.

The occluder in mechanical valves should open quickly and fully, and reduced opening is a reliable sign of obstruction provided that LV function is good. Severe impairment of LV function may also cause reduced valve opening, but this will be associated with a thin,

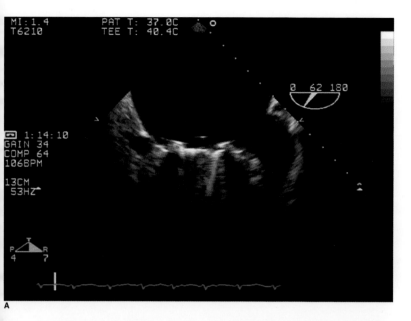

A

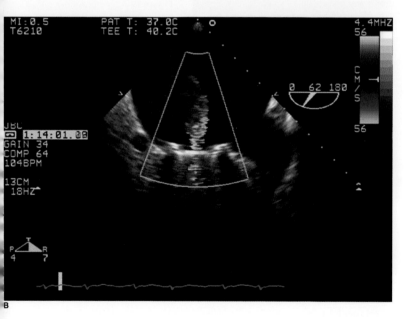

B

Figure 19.2. Medtronic Hall single tilting disk valve in the mitral position. (A) The transesophageal study shows the strut of the Medtronic Hall valve. (B) There is a hole through the leaflet, and a relatively large jet through this is normal.

low-velocity inflow signal on color mapping. In normal bileaflet valves there may be slight oscillation of the leaflets during diastole and slight temporal asymmetry of closure. Off-axis insonation in these valves can show one leaflet better than the other and give the spurious suggestion of obstruction. In biological valves, the cusps should be thin (1–2 mm) and fully mobile with no prolapse behind the plane of the annulus. The color map should entirely fill the orifice in all views. In an obstructed biological valve, it is possible for the color map to be restricted at the orifice but to expand before the tips of the stents, and it is possible to miss this sign. Unlike in the aortic position, rocking of the sewing ring may occur as a result of retention of the native posterior leaflet, but a true dehiscence is obvious from the gap opening between annulus and sewing ring and by the presence of a jet on color mapping.

As for the aortic position, it is normal to see stitches and fibrin strands. It is also normal to see echoes resembling bubbles in the LV (Fig. 19.4). These occur with all

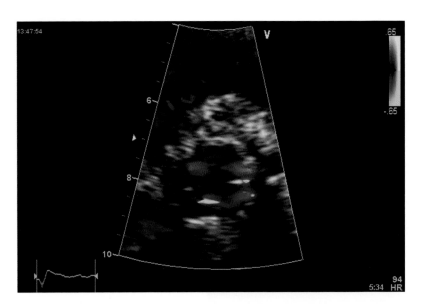

Figure 19.3. Bileaflet mechanical valve in the aortic position. This is a parasternal long-axis transthoracic view. There are two thin washing jets from each pivotal point.

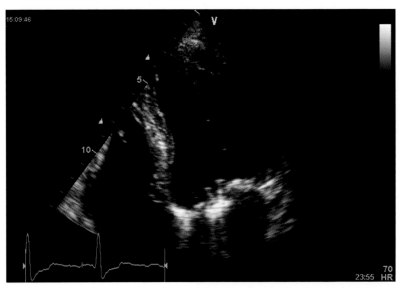

Figure 19.4. Microcavitations associated with a bileaflet mechanical mitral valve: transthoracic study, apical four-chamber view.

designs but are most frequent with bileaflet mechanical valves. Their origin is not firmly established. They are probably benign, although occasional reports link them to abnormalities of higher cognitive function.

Obstruction is diagnosed from thickening and reduced opening of the cusps or occluder with narrowing of the color map through the orifice. TEE is essential for determining the cause of obstruction in mechanical valves [16]: thrombosis, pannus, mechanical obstruction by septal hypertrophy or retained chordae, or vegetations as a result of endocarditis. Thrombus and vegetations (Fig. 19.5) are both associated with low-density echoes, while pannus is typically highly echogenic (Fig. 19.6). A thrombus is usually larger than pannus and more likely to extend into the left atrium and the appendage. However, minor pannus may be overlain by thrombus, so conclusive differentiation may not be possible. The clinical history may also be useful. A shorter duration of symptoms and inadequate anticoagulation suggests thrombus rather than pannus. Onset of symptoms less than a month from surgery predicts thrombus, as a period of six months or more is usually necessary for pannus formation.

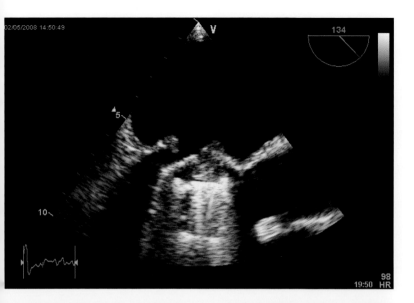

Figure 19.5. Thrombus: transesophageal long-axis view showing a bileaflet mechanical mitral valve with leaflets partially obstructed by thrombus. New thrombus is usually of low echo density and may extend from the left atrial appendage.

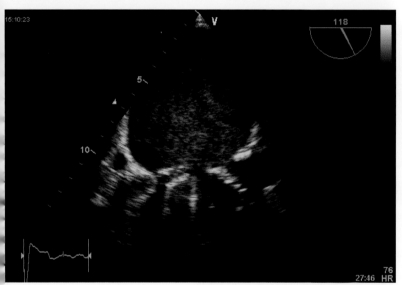

Figure 19.6. Pannus: transesophageal long-axis view showing obstruction of one leaflet of a bileaflet mechanical mitral valve by a layer of highly echogenic pannus.

Quantitative Doppler

The minimum dataset is peak velocity, mean pressure difference, and pressure half-time. The pressure half-time is dependent on LV and left atrial function as well as mitral valve function. In moderate or severe native or prosthetic stenosis, the mitral orifice dominates the pressure half-time, but in a normal prosthetic valve or mild native stenosis, the pressure half-time mainly reflects LV diastolic function. Thus small changes in pressure half-time reflect loading conditions, heart rate, or drugs rather than a change in mitral valve function. The Hatle formula (220/pressure half-time) is not valid in normally functioning mitral prostheses. The mean pressure difference provides a reasonable description of valve function.

In the diagnosis of obstruction, quantitative Doppler is relatively less important in the mitral position than imaging and color mapping. On transthoracic echocardiography, image quality may be poor in a severely breathless patient, and then it is reassuring to have corroboration from a greatly prolonged pressure half-time, usually in excess of 200 ms, associated with a peak transmitral velocity > 2.5 m/s even in the presence of low flow. In less severe obstruction, particularly with restriction of only one leaflet in a bileaflet mechanical valve, the pressure half-time may be only mildly prolonged, to

315

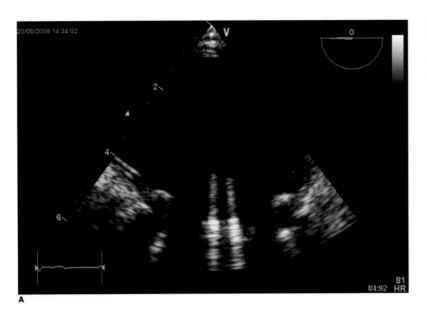

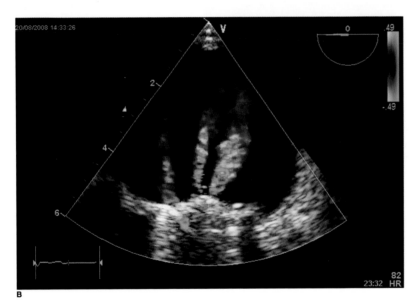

Figure 19.7. Transprosthetic mitral regurgitation on transesophageal imaging. (A) The bileaflet mechanical valve fully open, with (B) two plumes of regurgitation from the pivotal point and one around the leaflet.

around 150 ms. A change from immediate postoperative values may be obvious. Normal ranges are less variable than for the aortic position (Appendix 19.1) [10].

Regurgitation

Normal transprosthetic jets are particularly well seen in the mitral position (Fig. 19.7) and may easily be misdiagnosed as pathological. Although the regurgitant fraction is usually no larger than 10–15%, the associated color jet can look large, up to 5 cm long and 1 cm wide. The regurgitant fraction is directly related to the size of the valve and is also larger at low cardiac output. A

recognized clinical catch is the patient with a low cardiac output as a result of a non-prosthetic cause such as LV failure who is found to have apparently large transprosthetic jets on TEE. It is important not to "treat the echocardiogram" and reoperate in this situation. Abnormal regurgitation through the valve occurs if the leaflet is prevented from closing as a result of thrombus, septal hypertrophy, or a chord (Fig. 19.8).

Paraprosthetic regurgitation is differentiated from transprosthetic regurgitation by the jet having its origin outside the sewing ring (Fig. 19.9). However, it may sometimes be difficult to locate the "neck" of the

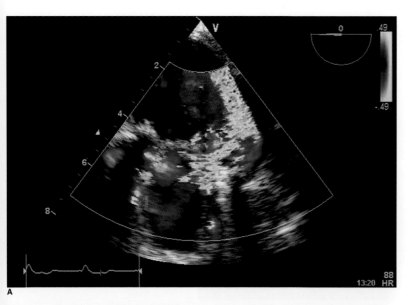

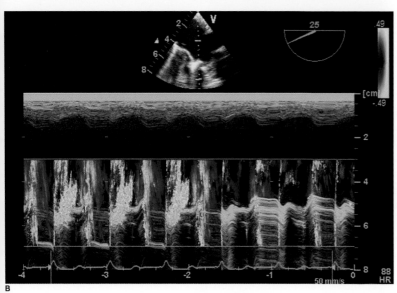

Figure 19.8. Pathological transprosthetic mitral regurgitation. The patient was unstable after implantation of a bileaflet mechanical mitral valve. (A) There was a broad jet of regurgitation, originating inside the sewing ring, which was intermittent, as shown by (B) color M-mode recording. It was caused by intermittent obstruction against the subvalvular apparatus and was cured by rotating the valve within its housing.

jet, and the distal parts of jets detected within the left atrium need to be followed carefully back to their origin. This is easier using 3D TEE. Although paraprosthetic leaks are pathological by definition, they may be small and of no clinical significance. They are particularly frequent immediately after surgery and may resolve as endothelium covers the edge of the sewing ring. Small paraprosthetic jets of no hemodynamic significance may cause hemolysis, and hemolytic anemia is an indication for TEE.

Quantifying regurgitation uses the same methods as for native regurgitation [15], although, as in the aortic position, the proportion of the circumference of

the sewing ring occupied by a paraprosthetic jet gives an additional guide to severity: mild (< 10%), moderate (10–25%), severe (> 25%). The width of the jet is better determined by 3D echocardiography.

Echocardiography of the replacement tricuspid valve

The tricuspid valve is imaged from the bicaval view obtained in the low esophageal four-chamber view, with further 90° rotation and the probe turned counterclockwise. It is also shown from a transgastric view with 90° rotation. It is imaged transthoracically from

317

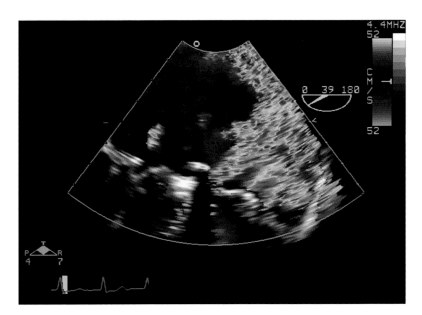

Figure 19.9. Paraprosthetic mitral regurgitation. There is a broad jet originating outside the sewing ring. The small, normal transprosthetic jets are also visible.

the parasternal long-axis view rotated towards the right ventricle, the parasternal short-axis view, the apical four-chamber view, and the subcostal view. The minimum dataset is peak velocity, mean pressure difference, and pressure half-time.

Obstruction is shown by reduced cusp or occluder motion with a narrowed color signal. On transthoracic imaging, an engorged, unreactive inferior vena cava with a dilated right atrium and small right ventricle are useful indirect signs. A transtricuspid peak velocity > 1.5 m/s and mean pressure difference > 5 mmHg are also suggestive [17,18]. The pressure half-time is variable and not helpful unless markedly prolonged to > 240 ms. As for the mitral position, TEE is essential for determining the cause of obstruction in mechanical valves: thrombosis, pannus, mechanical obstruction by septal hypertrophy or retained chordae, or vegetations as a result of endocarditis.

As for the mitral position, minor transprosthetic tricuspid regurgitation is normal. A paraprosthetic jet should be assessed by its width, which is most easily measured using 3D. Other methods of quantification are as for native tricuspid regurgitation [15]: jet shape and density, right ventricular volume load, hepatic vein systolic flow reversal.

Echocardiography of the replacement pulmonary valve

The pulmonary valve is imaged from the low esophageal view by rotating clockwise from the long-axis view of the aorta. It can also be imaged from a deep transgastric view in a 120° imaging plane. However, it is better assessed transthoracically using parasternal long-axis and short-axis views as well as from the substernal view. The minimum dataset is peak velocity and mean pressure difference. Obstruction is suggested by cusp thickening or immobility with narrowing of the color-flow signal. A single peak velocity > 3m/s is suspicious, although a progressive rise in serial estimates is more reliable. New impairment of right ventricular function may also result from pulmonary valve obstruction [19].

Pulmonary regurgitation can be quantified by comparing the jet width to the annulus diameter as mild (< 25%), moderate (26–50%) and severe (> 50%). In severe pulmonary regurgitation, the pressure half-time is short, often < 100 ms [20], the jet is dense, and the right ventricle is dilated and hyperdynamic.

Conclusions

- Quantitative Doppler should always be interpreted in the clinical context; normal ranges vary with design, position, and size.
- Velocities are flow-dependent; always calculate effective orifice area for valves in the aortic position.
- Do not use valve size in place of left ventricular outflow tract diameter in calculating the effective orifice area.

- The pressure half-time method for calculating effective orifice area is not valid in normal replacement mitral valves.
- Transvalvular regurgitation is normal in almost all mechanical valves and many biological valves.
- Tranthoracic and transesophageal echocardiography are complementary and should not be considered in isolation.

References

1. Jamieson WRE. Advanced technologies for cardiac valvular replacement, transcatheter innovations and reconstructive surgery. Surgical Technology International XV Cardiovascular Surgery. *Surgical Technology International Online*. www.ump.com/15-149-CS-Page1-.html (accessed September 2009).

2. Zoghbi WA, Chambers JB, Dumesnil JG, *et al.* Recommendations for evaluation of prosthetic valves with echocardiography and doppler ultrasound: a report from the American Society of Echocardiography's Guidelines and Standards Committee and the Task Force on Prosthetic Valves. *J Am Soc Echocardiog* 2009; **22**: 975–1014.

3. Bonow RO, Carabello BA, Kanu C, *et al.* ACC/AHA 2006 guidelines for the management of patients with valvular heart disease: a report of the American College of Cardiology/American Heart Association task force on practice guidelines. *Circulation* 2006; **114**: e84–231.

4. Vahanian A, Baumgartner H, Bax J, *et al.* Guidelines on the management of valvular heart disease: the Task Force on the Management of Valvular Heart Disease of the European Society of Cardiology. *Eur Heart J* 2007; **28**: 230–68.

5. Descoutures F, Himbert D, Lepage L, *et al.* Contemporary surgical or percutaneous management of severe aortic stenosis in the elderly. *Eur Heart J* 2008; **29**: 1410–17.

6. Chambers JB, Spiropoulos G. Estimation of the aortic orifice area: comparison of the classical and modified forms of the continuity equation. *Am J Noninvasive Cardiol* 1993; **7**: 259–62.

7. Chambers J, Oo L, Naracott A, Lawford P, Blauth C. Nominal size in six bileaflet mechanical aortic valves: a comparison with orifice size and a biological equivalent. *J Thorac Cardiovasc Surg* 2003; **125**: 1388–93.

8. Dumesnil JG, Honos GN, Lemieux M, Beauchemin J. Validation and applications of indexed aortic prosthetic valve areas calculated by Doppler echocardiography. *J Am Coll Cardiol* 1990; **16**: 637–43.

9. Rajani R, Mukherjee D, Chambers J. Doppler echocardiography in normally functioning replacement aortic valves: a review of 129 studies. *J Heart Valve Dis* 2007; **16**: 519–35.

10. Rosenhek R, Binder T, Maurer G, Baumgartner H. Normal values for Doppler echocardiographic assessment of heart valve prostheses. *J Am Soc Echocardiogr* 2003; **16**: 1116–27.

11. Pibarot P, Dumesnil JG. Prosthesis–patient mismatch: definition, clinical impact, and prevention. *Heart* 2006; **92**: 1022–9.

12. Blais C, Dumesnil JG, Baillot R, *et al.* Impact of prosthesis–patient mismatch on short-term mortality after aortic valve replacement. *Circulation* 2003; **108**: 983–8.

13. Tasca G, Mhagna Z, Perotti S, *et al.* Impact of prosthesis–patient mismatch on cardiac events and midterm mortality after aortic valve replacement in patients with pure aortic stenosis. *Circulation* 2006; **113**: 570–6.

14. Mohty D, Malouf JF, Girard SE, *et al.* Impact of prosthesis–patient mismatch on long-term survival in patients with small St. Jude medical mechanical prostheses in the aortic position. *Circulation* 2006; **113**: 420–6.

15. Zoghbi WA, Enriquez-Sarano M, Foster E, *et al.* Recommendations for evaluation of the severity of native valvular regurgitation with two-dimensional and Doppler echocardiography. *J Am Soc Echocardiogr* 2003; **16**: 777–802.

16. Grunkemeier GL, Li HH, Naftel DC, Starr A, Rahimtoola SH. Long-term performance of heart valve prostheses. *Curr Probl Cardiol* 2000; **25**: 73–154.

17. Connolly HM, Miller FA, Taylor CL, *et al.* Doppler hemodynamic profiles of 82 clinically and echocardiographically normal tricuspid valve prostheses. *Circulation* 1993; **88**: 2722–7.

18. Kobayashi Y, Nagata S, Ohmori F, *et al.* Serial Doppler echocardiographic evaluation of bioprosthetic valves in the tricuspid position. *J Am Coll Cardiol* 1996; **27**: 1693–7.

19. Novaro GM, Connolly HM, Miller FA. Doppler hemodynamics of 51 clinically and echocardiographically normal pulmonary valve prostheses. *Mayo Clin Proc* 2001; **76**: 155–60.

20. Rodriguez RJ, Riggs TW. Physiologic peripheral pulmonary stenosis in infancy. *Am J Cardiol* 1990; **66**: 1478–81.

Appendix 19.1: Normal ranges for replacement heart valves

Values are expressed as mean (standard deviation).

Aortic position

Homograft

	V$_{max}$ (m/s)	Mean ΔP (mmHg)	EOA (cm²)
22 mm	1.7 (0.3)	5.8 (3.2)	2.0 (0.6)
26 mm	1.4 (0.6)	6.8 (2.9)	2.4 (0.7)

Porcine

	V$_{max}$ (m/s)	Mean ΔP (mmHg)	EOA (cm²)
Carpentier–Edwards			
21 mm	2.8 (0.5)		1.2 (0.2)
23 mm	2.8 (0.7)		1.1 (0.2)
25 mm	2.6 (0.6)		1.2 (0.3)
27 mm	2.5 (0.5)		1.3 (0.3)
29 mm	2.4 (0.4)		1.4 (0.1)
Intact			
21 mm	1.0 (0.1)	19.3 (7.4)	1.5 (0.3)
23 mm	1.3 (0.1)	18.8 (6.1)	1.6 (0.3)
25 mm	1.4 (0.2)	18.8 (8.0)	1.9 (0.3)
27 mm		15.0 (3.7)	
Hancock			
23 mm		12.0 (2.0)	
25 mm	2.4 (0.4)	11.0 (2.0)	
27 mm	2.4 (0.4)	10.0 (3.0)	

Bovine pericardial

	V$_{max}$ (m/s)	Mean ΔP (mmHg)	EOA (cm²)
Labcor–Santiago			
19 mm		10.1 (3.1)	1.3 (0.1)
21 mm		8.2 (4.5)	1.3 (0.1)
23 mm		7.8 (2.9)	1.8 (0.2)
25 mm		6.8 (2.0)	2.1 (0.3)

Single tilting disk

	V$_{max}$ (m/s)	Mean ΔP (mmHg)	EOA (cm²)
Bjork–Shiley			
21 mm	3.0 (0.9)		1.1 (0.3)
23 mm	2.4 (0.5)	14.0 (7.0)	1.3 (0.3)
25 mm	2.1 (0.5)	13.0 (5.0)	1.4 (0.4)
27 mm	2.0 (0.3)	10.0 (2.0)	1.6 (0.3)
Medtronic Hall			
21 mm		13.0 (4.0)	1.4 (0.1)
23 mm	2.3 (0.9)		
25 mm	2.1 (0.3)		
Omnicarbon			
21 mm	3.0 (0.3)	20.0 (5.0)	
23 mm	2.7 (0.3)	18.0 (5.0)	
25 mm	2.5 (0.3)	15.0 (4.0)	
27 mm	2.1 (0.2)	12.0 (2.0)	

Bileaflet mechanical

	V$_{max}$ (m/s)	Mean ΔP (mmHg)	EOA (cm²)
St Jude			
19 mm	3.0 (0.6)	19.4 (7.2)	1.0 (0.3)
21 mm	2.6 (0.3)	14.8 (4.3)	1.3 (0.2)
23 mm	2.5 (0.5)	13.5 (5.9)	1.3 (0.3)
25 mm	2.4 (0.5)	12.2 (5.9)	1.8 (0.4)
27 mm	2.2 (0.5)	11.0 (5.0)	2.4 (0.6)
29 mm	2.0 (0.1)	7.0 (1.0)	2.7 (0.3)
Carbomedics			
19 mm	3.2 (0.4)	19.3 (8.5)	0.9 (0.3)
21 mm	2.5 (0.5)	13.7 (5.5)	1.3 (0.4)
23 mm	2.4 (0.4)	11.0 (4.6)	1.6 (0.4)
25 mm	2.3 (0.3)	9.1 (3.5)	1.8 (0.4)
27 mm	2.1 (0.4)	7.9 (3.4)	2.2 (0.6)
29 mm	1.8 (0.4)	5.6 (3.0)	3.2 (1.6)

321

Ball and cage

	V$_{max}$ (m/s)	Mean ΔP (mmHg)	EOA (cm²)
Starr–Edwards			
23 mm	3.4 (0.6)		1.1 (0.2)
24 mm	3.6 (0.5)		1.1 (0.3)
26 mm	3.0 (0.2)		

Mitral position

Porcine

	V$_{max}$ (m/s)	Mean ΔP (mmHg)	PHT (ms)
Carpentier–Edwards			
27mm		6.0 (2.0)	95 (12)
29mm	1.5 (0.3)	4.7 (2.0)	110 (30)
31mm	1.5 (0.3)	4.5 (2.0)	102 (34)
33mm	1.4 (0.2)	5.4 (4.0)	94 (26)
Intact			
25mm		7.8 (2.4)	
27mm		5.4 (1.5)	
Hancock			
29mm		2.0 (0.7)	
31mm		4.9 (1.7)	
33mm	5.0 (2.0)		

Bovine pericardial

	V$_{max}$ (m/s)	Mean ΔP (mmHg)	PHT (ms)
Labcor–Santiago			
27 mm		2.8 (1.5)	85 (18)
29 mm		3.0 (1.3)	80 (34)

Single tilting disk

	V$_{max}$ (m/s)	Mean ΔP (mmHg)	PHT (ms)
Bjork–Shiley			
25 mm	1.6 (0.3)		
27 mm	1.5 (0.2)	2.7 (0.8)	94 (31)
29 mm	1.4 (0.4)	2.0 (0.1)	85 (22)
31 mm	1.5 (0.3)	3.4 (2.2)	81 (20)
33 mm	1.3 (0.6)		75 (25)

Single tilting disk (*cont.*)

	V$_{max}$ (m/s)	Mean ΔP (mmHg)	PHT (ms)
Medtronic Hall			
29 mm	1.6 (0.1)		69 (15)
31 mm	1.5 (0.1)		77 (17)
Omnicarbon			
25 mm		6.0 (2.0)	
27 mm		6.0 (2.0)	
29 mm		5.0 (2.0)	
31 mm		6.0 (2.0)	

Bileaflet mechanical

	V$_{max}$ (m/s)	Mean ΔP (mmHg)	PHT (ms)
St Jude			
27 mm	1.6 (0.3)	5.0 (2.0)	
29 mm	1.6 (0.3)	4.5 (2.4)	81 (9)
31 mm	1.7 (0.4)	5.2 (3.0)	84 (12)
Carbomedics			
25 mm	1.6 (0.2)	4.3 (0.7)	92 (20)
27 mm	1.6 (0.3)	3.7 (1.5)	91 (24)
29 mm	1.8 (0.3)	3.7 (1.3)	79 (11)
31 mm	1.6 (0.4)	3.3 (1.1)	92 (20)
33 mm	1.4 (0.3)	3.4 (1.5)	79 (18)
Edwards–Duromedics			
27 mm	1.9 (0.3)		105 (14)
29 mm	1.8 (0.2)		89 (18)
31 mm	1.7 (0.3)		99 (18)

Caged ball

	V$_{max}$ (m/s)	Mean ΔP (mmHg)	PHT (ms)
Starr–Edwards			
28 mm	1.8 (0.2)		130 (25)
30 mm	1.8 (0.2)		100 (40)
32 mm	1.9 (0.4)		125 (60)

References

Wang Z, Grainger N, Chambers J. Doppler echocardiography in normally functioning replacement heart valves: a literature review. *J Heart Valve Dis* 1995; **4**: 591–614.

Rimington H, Chambers J. *Echocardiography: Guidelines for Reporting*, 2nd edn. London: Informa Healthcare, 2007.

20

Adult congenital heart disease
TEE guidance of interventional catheter-delivered devices

Mario Carminati, Diana Negura, Luciane Piazza, Massimo Chessa, Gianfranco Butera, Robert Feneck

Introduction

Congenital heart disease (CHD) represents a series of complex lesions, many of which present at or soon after birth. The echocardiography of CHD is therefore highly specialised. A detailed review of pediatric cardiology and echocardiography for CHD is outside the scope of this book. Furthermore, the syllabus and accreditation for the echocardiography of congenital heart disease in Europe is provided for by a separate accreditation process [1].

The diagnosis and management of patients with adult CHD has been the focus of much interest, and recently guidelines have been published which are both timely and comprehensive [2]. This and the associated publications are highly recommended to those who wish to gain a greater understanding of the recommendations for the management of adults with CHD.

Adult patients with either corrected or uncorrected CHD may present in a variety of circumstances. Although transthoracic echocardiography (TTE) remains the mainstay of the echocardiographic investigation of CHD, transesophageal echocardiography (TEE) may be of value either to aid in the initial diagnosis, or to guide therapy.

It is not proposed to discuss those congenital diseases that have been identified as being of great or moderate complexity, since these are specialized conditions that should be managed specifically within adult congenital heart centers [2]. Some have already been mentioned elsewhere in this book (Tables 20.1, 20.2).

The conditions described in this chapter are those that are regarded as being manageable outside of specialist centers (Table 20.3).

The non-surgical treatment of a variety of congenital heart malformations by interventional cardiac catheterization is well established, and up to 40% of cases can be treated in this way.

While most procedures are carried out under radiographic screening, in some circumstances TEE

Table 20.1. Types of adult congenital heart disease of great complexity [2]

- Conduits, valved or non-valved
- Cyanotic congenital heart (all forms)
- Double-outlet ventricle
- Eisenmenger syndrome
- Fontan procedure
- Mitral atresia
- Single ventricle (also called double inlet or outlet, common, or primitive)
- Pulmonary atresia (all forms)
- Pulmonary vascular obstructive disease
- Transposition of the great arteries
- Tricuspid atresia
- Truncus arteriosus/hemitruncus
- Other abnormalities of atrioventricular or ventriculoarterial connection not included above (e.g. crisscross heart, isomerism, heterotaxy syndromes, ventricular inversion)

improves their success and safety. TEE may be an important imaging modality for the following procedures:

- closure of atrial septal defects (ASDs)
- occlusion of baffle fenestrations following the total cavopulmonary connection
- closure of ventricular septal defects (VSDs) (muscular, perimembranous, and post-infarction)

Development of the atrial septum and atrial septal defects

Figure 20.1 shows the heart at four weeks gestation. The endocardial tubes have fused together, and a common atrium is linked to a common ventricle by a single atrioventricular canal. Blood then passes from the common ventricle into the truncus arteriosus and thence to the primitive circulation.

Core Topics in Transesophageal Echocardiography, ed. Robert Feneck, John Kneeshaw, and Marco Ranucci.
Published by Cambridge University Press. © Cambridge University Press 2010.

Table 20.2. Diagnoses in adult patients with congenital heart disease of moderate complexity [2]

- Aorto-left ventricular fistulas
- Anomalous pulmonary venous drainage, partial or total
- Atrioventricular septal defects (partial or complete)
- Coarctation of the aorta
- Ebstein's anomaly
- Infundibular right ventricular outflow obstruction of significance
- Ostium primum atrial septal defect
- Patent ductus arteriosus (not closed)
- Pulmonary valve regurgitation (moderate to severe)
- Pulmonary valve stenosis (moderate to severe)
- Sinus of Valsalva fistula/aneurysm
- Sinus venosus atrial septal defect
- Subvalvular aortic stenosis or supravalvular aortic stenosis (except hypertrophic obstructive cardiomyopathy)
- Tetralogy of Fallot
- Complicated ventricular septal defect

Table 20.3. Diagnoses in adult patients with simple congenital heart disease [2]

Native disease	Isolated congenital aortic valve disease
	Isolated congenital mitral valve disease (e.g. except parachute valve, cleft leaflet)
	Small atrial septal defect
	Isolated small ventricular septal defect (no associated lesions)
	Mild pulmonary stenosis
	Small patent ductus arteriosus
Repaired conditions	Previously ligated or occluded ductus arteriosus
	Repaired ventricular septal defect without residua
	Repaired secundum or sinus venosus atrial septal defect without residua

At the end of the fourth gestational week, the crescent-shaped septum primum grows from the roof of the primitive atrium towards the endocardial cushion. The diminishing opening between the septum primum and the endocardial cushion is called the ostium primum. This opening allows blood to pass from the right atrium to the left. The septum primum gradually becomes complete, but before the ostium primum finally closes a number of fenestrations appear higher up, and these enlarge to form a single opening, the foramen secundum.

A second crescent-shaped ridge of tissue – the septum secundum – grows towards the endocardial cushion. This tissue is thick and muscular, in contrast to the septum primum, which is thin and membraneous.

At the end of six weeks gestation the septum secundum finishes growing. It contains a permanent opening on its posteroinferior surface, the foraman ovale. The septum primum degenerates and its remnant acts as a flap valve covering the foramen ovale. This flap valve allows blood flow from right to left. After birth, as the left atrial pressure exceeds the right, the flap valve closes, and over the next three months the septum secundum and the valve of the foramen ovale fuse. This area becomes the fossa ovalis.

The development of the superior and inferior venae cavae is also important embryologically. The right horn of the sinus venosus encompasses the right superior and inferior venae cavae. Normally the sinus venosus shifts to the right and becomes incorporated into the right atrium and interatrial septum. The sinus venosus may be incompletely incorporated, or else may not shift to the right enough to be fully incorporated into the septum.

The coronary sinus develops as a venous drainage structure receiving the small, middle, and great cardiac veins. It normally drains into the right atrium, but developmental failure of the left atrial roof may occur, leading to the development of a permanent shunt at atrial level.

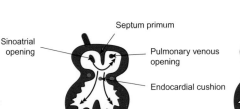
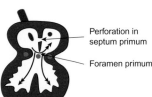

Sinoatrial opening

Septum primum

Pulmonary venous opening

Endocardial cushion

Perforation in septum primum

Foramen primum

Early week 4

Mid week 4

Figure 20.1. The heart at early and mid four weeks gestation, showing atrial septal development.

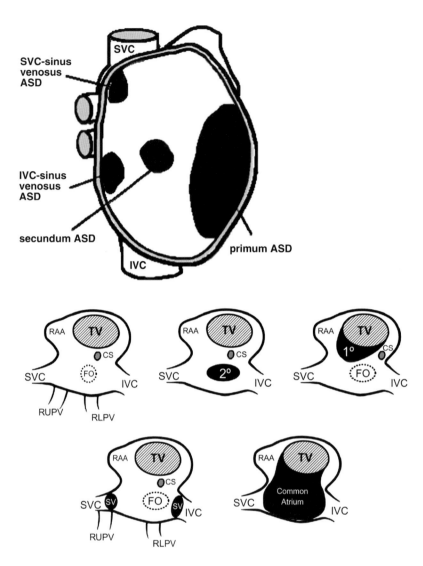

Figure 20.2. Common types of atrial septal defect. CS, coronary sinus; FO, foramen ovale; IVC, inferior vena cava; RAA, right atrial appendage; RLPV, right lower pulmonary vein; RUPV, right upper pulmonary vein; SV, sinus venosus; SVC, superior vena cava; TV, tricuspid valve; 1°, primum atrial septal defect; 2°, secundum atrial septal defect.

Atrial septal defects

The morphology of the various types of ASD has been known since the early description by Rokitansky [3], and they are classified as follows:

- ostium secundum (fossa ovalis) (70%)
- ostium primum (partial atrioventricular septal defect) (15–20%)
- superior and inferior sinus venosus (combined incidence 10%, but superior more common than inferior)
- coronary sinus type, or common atrium (1%) (Fig. 20.2).

The most common type of ASD is the ostium secundum (or fossa ovalis) defect (Videos 20.1, 20.2).

These defects may extend outside the true limits of the fossa ovalis when there is a deficiency of the infolding tissue. They may therefore extend posteriorly to the mouth of the coronary sinus, inferiorly to the atrioventricular junction, posteroinferiorly to the mouth of the inferior caval vein, or superiorly to the mouth of the superior caval vein. With posterosuperior extension, the defect may extend to the orifice of the pulmonary veins, particularly to the right upper pulmonary vein, while anterior encroachment is near to the aorta. These extensions of the secundum ASD are commonly called "rims of the defect."

In contrast, a superior sinus venosus interatrial communication is found within the mouth of the superior caval vein. There is a biatrial connection, overriding the rim of the fossa ovalis, which produces "extracardiac" interatrial communication [4].

Coronary sinus atrial septal defects are extremely rare. They occur as a result of a partial defect in the wall between the coronary sinus and the left atrium and produce an interatrial communication through the orifice of the coronary sinus.

A primum ASD is part of an atrioventricular septal defect. Its superior boundary is the inferior border of the fossa ovalis and its inferior boundary is the superior and inferior bridging leaflets of the common atrioventricular valve [5].

Lesions associated with different ASDs are shown in Table 20.4.

TEE imaging of the atrial septum

The standard views for imaging the atrial septum are as follows:

- Four-chamber mid-esophageal view. This is useful for demonstrating ostium secundum and ostium primum defects.
- Bicaval mid-esophageal view. This is useful for demonstrating a sinus venosus defect and for identifying anomalous pulmonary veins.
- Mid-esophageal AV short-axis view. This may need to be rotated slightly to bring the atrial septum into the center of the image.

It is particularly important to identify other features which may be present, including atrioventricular valve abnormalities, chamber enlargement suggesting shunting and volume overload, and ventricular dysfunction. The optimum TEE windows for these assessments are described in the relevant sections of this book.

Transcatheter device closure of ASDs

It is important to be aware that only secundum ASDs are suitable for transcatheter device closure, provided that there is at least a 4–5 mm rim between the defect and the atrioventricular valves, the superior and inferior caval veins, and the entry of the pulmonary veins into the left atrium. The shape and borders of a fossa ovalis defect can be well demonstrated by three-dimensional echocardiography [6]. Depending on the location, any attempt to close one of the other types of interatrial communications is likely to result in obstruction to the systemic or pulmonary venous pathways or of the coronary sinus, or may interfere with atrioventricular valve function. Anomalous pul-

Table 20.4. Types of lesion associated with atrial septal defect

ASD	Lesions
Secundum	Pulmonic stenosis
	Mitral valve prolapse
	Partial anomalous pulmonary venous connection`
Primum	Cleft mitral valve
	Discrete subaortic stenosis
	Sinus venosus
	Partial anomalous pulmonary venous return
Coronary sinus	Partial anomalous pulmonary venous return
	Persistent left superior vena cava

monary venous drainage is also a contraindication for device closure of the defect [7].

In addition, the presence of an atrial septal aneurysm (ASA) may complicate the use of transcatheter devices for closure of an ASD. One estimate of the incidence of ASA suggests it may be as high as 2.2% [8]. Ewert et al. classified ASAs on the basis of the findings at TEE as follows [9]:

- ASA with patent foramen ovale (type A)
- ASA with single atrial septal defect (type B)
- ASA with two perforations or few perforations located in no more than two clusters requiring placement of more than one device (type C)
- ASA with multiple perforations located in more than two areas of atrial septal (type D) (Fig. 20.3).

In their series, all patients with type A and approximately 50% of patients with type B aneurysms were suitable for device closure. Although device closure was attempted in patients with type C lesions, 50% had a residual shunt. All patients with type D lesions required surgery.

The initial selection of patients for transcatheter closure of ASDs is made by TTE, which allows the various types to be distinguished. The final arbiter of suitability is TEE, usually performed immediately before the procedure.

Biplane or omniplane echocardiography allows the exact morphology and diameter of the defect to be determined, as well as the dimensions of the rim and the diameter of the septum itself. It is important to exclude a sinus venosus, coronary sinus, or ostium primum defect, which will be unsuitable for the device closure. Before starting, it is necessary to identify

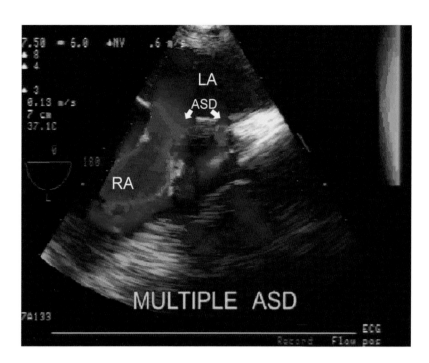

Figure 20.3. Short-axis section of the atria showing multiple atrial septal defect, o.s. type with left-to-right shunt.

additional fenestrations within the fossa ovalis, or alternatively multiple fenestrations within the fossa ovalis, often associated with an aneurysm.

The role of TEE during the percutaneous procedure is to identify the number of defects and monitor the implantation of the device. This must be done without obstructing fluoroscopy. During implantation the location of catheters, balloon sizing, and the position of the device both before and after release should be assessed [6].

It is important to interrogate the entire atrial septum to ensure that small defects at the margins of the septum are not missed. Utilizing the mid-esophageal four-chamber view in the horizontal plane (0°), the entire septum is interrogated from the superior vena cava–right atrium superiorly to the coronary sinus–right atrium junction inferiorly. Rotation of the image plane to the bicaval view (90°) as described in Chapter 4 displays the septum in an orthogonal plane, from the inferior vena cava to the superior vena cava. The tip of the catheter or sheath can be visualized only if the catheter can be depicted in its long axis. This almost always requires imaging in oblique planes, and is sometimes difficult.

Prior to the delivery of the device, the tip of the sheath should be in the left atrium, well away from the mitral valve, pulmonary veins, and left atrial appendage.

It is important to confirm that the catheter or the guidewire passes through the main or largest ASD, or in the case of multiple fenestrations that it passes through one of the more central defects. A sizing balloon is then passed over the guide wire into the left atrium. The defect is completely occluded with an inflated balloon, and color-flow Doppler is used to identify any residual shunting (Fig. 20.4); this requires the rapid acquisition of multiple views using color-flow mapping of the entire area around the balloon. The balloon is measured by taking the distance between the rims of the septal defect with the balloon occluding the septal deficiency, checking the remainder of the atrial septum for other secondary defects. Occasionally, if there are two large defects, it is important to balloon-size both of them, because two closure devices may be required. In the presence of multiple fenestrations, sizing is not required and only one device is usually needed. When there is an aneurysm of the fossa ovalis, multiple fenestrations may occur. Closure using two devices has been described [9,10].

During sizing, the balloon should be preferably perpendicular to the interatrial septum.

The catheter or sheath used for delivery of the device crosses the defect at an angle of between 45° and 90°, and frequently pushes the septal remnant in a posterosuperior direction. It is advisable to adjust the

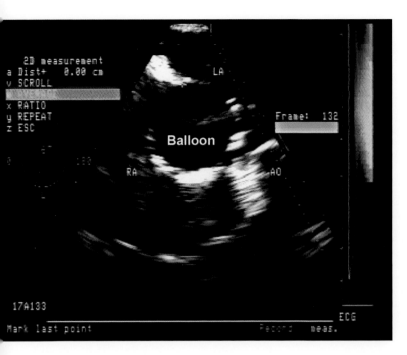

Figure 20.4. Short-axis section of the atria during balloon sizing of atrial septal defect. AO, aorta; LA, left atrium; RA, right atrium.

imaging plane to that which shows the largest part of the left atrium. The tip of the sheath should be positioned in the body of the left atrium before the atrial disk of the device is opened. If the sheath with the device is then pulled towards the rims of the septal defect, the septum shifts back in an anteroinferior direction, increasing the dimensions of the left atrium. The device can then be visualized relative to the atrial septum, the right pulmonary veins, and the mitral valve. During the opening of the left atrial component, the device is mostly at an angle with the atrial septum, with the anterosuperior part of the device usually close to it. Echocardiography at this point serves to confirm that all parts of the left atrial disk remain within the left atrium, and do not become attached to the mitral valve or the pulmonary veins.

Once the right atrial disk is opened, the rims of the fossa ovalis and the septal remnant should be sandwiched between the two sides of the atrial septum (Fig. 20.5). Then the device is released. Before this release, the device can easily be retrieved by withdrawing it into the sheath by traction on the delivery wire. A final assessment of the position of the device is performed by TEE following its release [11]. Once the device has been released, a complete assessment is mandatory. This includes careful checking for residual leaks. The best views can be obtained using the mid-esophageal AV short-axis view at 50–55° and the bicaval view at 90° (Fig. 20.6).

Video 20.3 shows some of the key stages in transcatheter closure of an ASD. Video 20.4 shows aspects of the transcatheter closure of multiple ASDs.

Patent foramen ovale (PFO)

Methodologies for diagnosis and anatomic and functional sizing of a PFO include TTE, TEE, and transcranial Doppler, with saline contrast [12].

TEE is currently considered the reference standard for PFO diagnosis, allowing direct imaging of the interatrial septum (Fig. 20.7) and saline contrast shunting through a PFO. If color-flow Doppler or peripheral saline contrast injection are able to detect right-to-left flow during normal respiration, this is termed a resting PFO. Enhanced right-to-left flow may be noted upon release of the Valsalva maneuver. The TEE can help show the morphology of the PFO and direct the catheter through the communication. PFO closure can be carried out using either a STARflex device (Figs. 20.8, 20.9; Video 20.5) or an Amplatzer device (Video 20.6).

The closure should be followed by a TEE examination as described for other ASDs (Fig. 20.10).

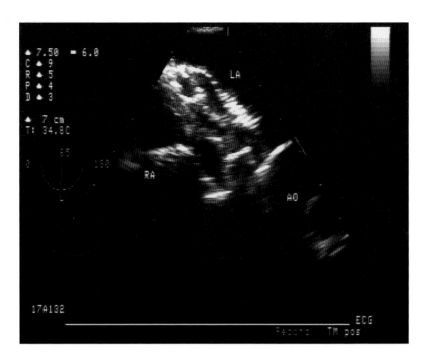

Figure 20.5. Short-axis section of the atria during Amplatzer atrial septal occluder (ASO) device positioning, showing the left disk opened in the left atrium and the right disk opened in the right atrium. The device is still anchored to the delivery system. AO, aorta; LA, left atrium; RA, right atrium.

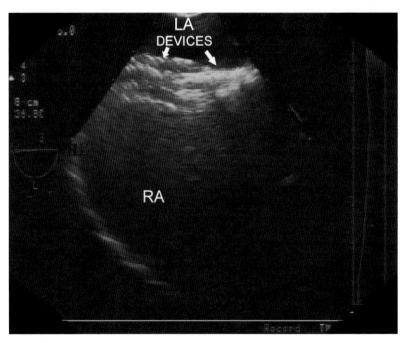

Figure 20.6. Short-axis section of the atria after two Amplatzer ASO device deployments. LA, left atrium; RA, right atrium.

Development of the ventricular septum and ventricular septal defects

At the end of the fourth gestational week, a muscular ventricular septum starts to grow superiorly from the floor of the ventricle (Fig. 20.1). Thus the common ventricle becomes partially divided into the left and right ventricles, with an interventricular foramen located between the fused endocardial cushions and the muscular septum, connecting the two ventricles.

At the end of the fifth week two ridges of tissue (conotruncal ridges) appear in the truncus arteriosus

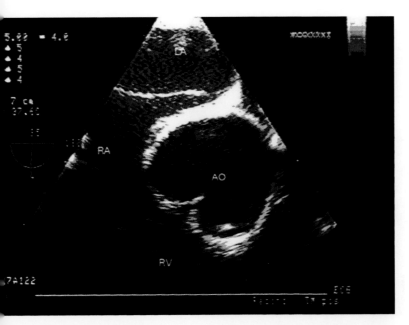

Figure 20.7. Short-axis view of patent foramen ovale (PFO).

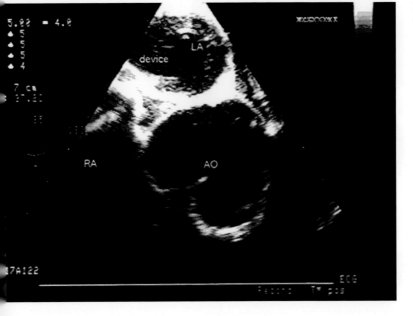

Figure 20.8. Implantation of a STAR-flex device (still attached to the delivery cable).

These ridges grow towards each other and form a spiral septum called the aorticopulmonary septum. This divides the truncus arteriosus into the aorta and pulmonary trunk.

The aorticopulmonary septum grows into the ventricles and fuses with the already fused endocardial cushions and muscular ventricular septum. Once this has occurred, by the end of week 8, these three components form the membraneous ventricular septum, which closes off the interventricular foramen.

In the left ventricle, a prominent horseshoe-shaped myocardial ridge runs from the anterior wall through the apex to the posterior wall of the left ventricle. In the atrioventricular region this ridge is continuous with atrial myocardium and covered with cushion tissue.

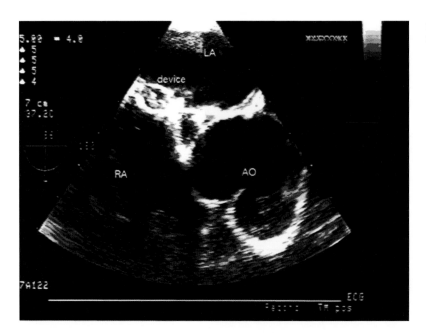

Figure 20.9. STAR-flex device delivered from the delivery cable.

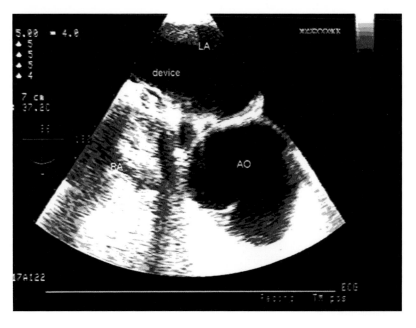

Figure 20.10. Contrast echo after device implantation showing no evidence of residual right-to-left shunt.

The anterior and posterior parts of the ridge enlarge, loosening their connections with the atrial myocardium, and the lateral sides gradually delaminate from the left ventricular wall. The continuity between the two parts is incorporated into the apical trabecular network. In this way the anterior and posterior parts of the ridge transform into the anterolateral and the posteromedial papillary muscles, respectively [13].

Ventricular septal defects

The first description of transcatheter closure of a ventricular septal defect was that of Lock and colleagues in 1988 [14]. The paucity of information available may be a reflection of the technical difficulties that can be encountered. Suitable candidates are those with a congenital muscular or perimembranous VSD, a residual defect at the patch margins following cardiac

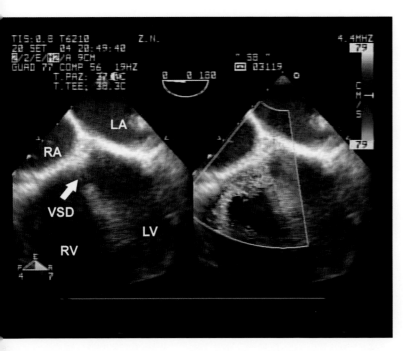

Figure 20.11. Four-chamber view showing a perimembranous ventricular septal defect (VSD) (left) with left-to-right shunt demonstrated by colour flow. LA, left atrium; LV, left ventricle; RA, right atrium; RV, right ventricle.

surgery, and ischemic defects following myocardial infarction [15]. Defects unsuitable for device closure include those which are doubly committed or associated with aortic valve prolapse (Fig. 20.11).

The majority of muscular VSDs, located in the mid portion or apical part of the septum, are closed with a device delivered through a long transseptal sheath introduced through the right internal jugular vein. For defects located in the high muscular portion of the septum, or for perimembranous defects, the sheath is inserted into a femoral vein. Whichever route is used, the guidewire must be identified traversing the main defect, and in the case of multiple defects crossing one that is situated centrally in the ventricular septum. In a similar fashion to atrial septal defects, a combination of fluoroscopy and TEE is required.

Balloon sizing of the defect is not essential, but the type of closure device selected will depend on many factors, including the preference and experience of the operator, the thickness of the ventricular septum, and the exact morphology of the defect.

The ventricular septum is a complex structure that requires careful interrogation in multiple planes. From the mid-esophageal window (0°), flexion displays the left ventricular outflow tract (LVOT) and thin membranous part of the septum. Advancing the probe reveals the muscular/trabecular part of the septum. Image plane rotation to 30–45° produces a short-axis view of the heart analogous to an inverted parasternal short-axis view. By rotating the probe to obtain an image in a plane passing below the level of the aortic valve, perimembranous and doubly committed VSDs can be seen. Further rotation of the image plane to 130° produces an approximation of the TTE apical long-axis view, providing further imaging of the perimembranous septum. Although it may be difficult to align the Doppler beam parallel to VSD flow, it is important to look out for turbulence within the right ventricular cavity and a flow convergence zone within the left ventricular cavity. In patients with a perimembranous VSD, TEE is valuable in identifying the mechanism of spontaneous closure and associated findings – for example, suction of the right aortic cusp into the defect resulting in aortic regurgitation, or involvement of tricuspid subvalvular tissue [16].

The principles of echocardiographic guidance of device closure of VSDs are similar to those for ASDs, but several factors make this procedure more complicated. The technique of transcatheter closure of perimembranous VSDs is similar to that developed for muscular VSDs. Echocardiography both before and during the implantation of the device is the most

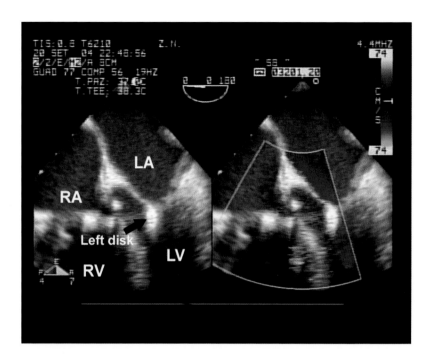

Figure 20.12. VSD closure. Four-chamber view showing Amplatzer VSD Occluder device with left disk (black arrow) opened in left ventricle (left). LA, left atrium; LV, left ventricle; RA, right atrium; RV, right ventricle.

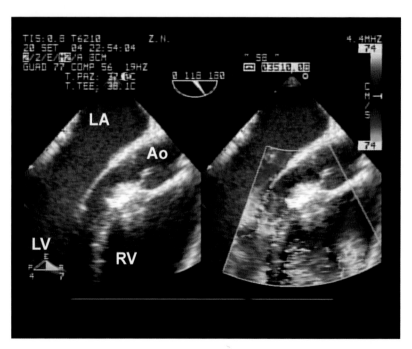

Figure 20.13. VSD closure. Long-axis view after Amplatzer VSD Membranous Occluder device deployment (left) and with colour flow (right): no evidence of residual shunt. AO, aorta; LA, left atrium; LV, left ventricle; RV, right ventricle.

important imaging modality (Figs. 20.12–20.14). TEE is used to determine the morphology and diameter of the defect, and the relation to the semilunar and atrioventricular valves and their tensor apparatus. There is frequently a need for the transgastric views, which

are particularly useful for delineating the defect. Important information is provided about the position of the wire, the tip of the sheath, and the opened distal disk when pulled into the VSD. Once the device is at the tip of the sheath, the echo is checked to ensure

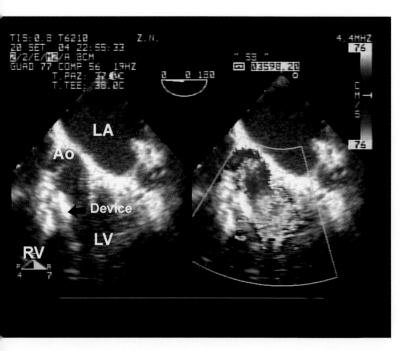

Figure 20.14. VSD closure. Five-chamber view after Amplatzer VSD Membranous Occluder device (black arrow) deployment (left) and with colour flow (right), demonstrating a complete closure. AO, aorta; LA, left atrium; LV, left ventricle; RV, right ventricle.

hat the device does not open inside the mitral tensor apparatus. The deployment of the device is monitored mainly by echo. The right ventricular disk may need time to fully configure. If the lips of the device are tilted in to the defect then the sheath can be advanced back over the device to recapture it and redeploy it. TEE and angiography may then be used to check its final position prior to release of the device [15,16]. After the release of the occluder, color Doppler is performed to detect aortic or tricuspid valve regurgitation and residual shunts. Some flow through the device may be detected at the end of the procedure. It is important to determine whether it is occuring during diastolic filling of the right ventricle or during systolic left ventricular contraction.

Video 20.7 shows some of the key stages in transcatheter closure of a perimembranous VSD.

Development of the tricuspid and mitral valves and residual atrioventricular canal

By the end of the fifth week, the developing left ventricle supports the larger part of the circumference of the atrioventricular canal, while the developing right ventricle provides most of the muscular support for the developing ventricular outflow tract. The lumen of the atrioventricular canal is largely occupied by the superior and inferior atrioventricular endocardial cushions [17].

Fusion of the atrioventricular endocardial cushions during the sixth week of development divides the atrioventricular canal into right and left atrioventricular junctions, to which the developing leaflets of the mitral and tricuspid valves will eventually be anchored. Septation of the AV canal, the atrium, and the ventricle occurs at a similar time. The endocardial cushions remodel into valve leaflets and chordae, with the chordal part of the cushions remaining attached to the developing papillary muscles (Fig. 20.15).

On the right side, following similar delamination of the tension apparatus within the myocardium, the leaflets of the tricuspid valve become freely movable.

Failure of fusion of the superior and inferior cushions is the process usually held responsible for producing atrioventricular septal, or canal, defects [18], previously termed endocardial cushion defects.

In a partial atrioventricular septal defect (AVSD) the atrioventricular valve rings are normal, but there is a cleft in one of the mitral valve leaflets. This results when the endocardial cushion fails to obliterate the

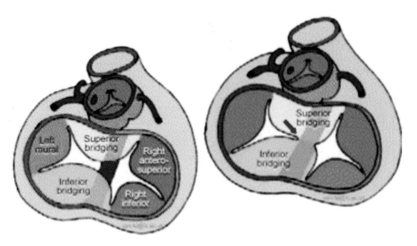

Figure 20.15. Septation and division of endocardial cushion.

Box 20.1 Case report

A 53-year-old male patient presented as an emergency admission for breathlessness and right-sided pleuritic pain. The patient was hypertensive (230/130) but renal function was within normal limits. He was found to have severe mitral regurgitation, and was acutely stabilized, but worsened over three weeks, with reducing exercise tolerance. Coronary angiography suggested the need for myocardial revascularization, and the patient was scheduled for CABG surgery and mitral valve repair.

Intraoperative TEE showed a complex series of anterior, central, and posterior directed jets of mitral regurgitation, in addition to tricuspid regurgitation and a low atrial septal defect.

Surgical exploration revealed a partial atrioventricular septal defect (Videos 20.8–20.11).

---

ostium primum. Normally the leaflets are free to move, but in a partial AVSD, two of the five leaflets (superior and inferior bridging leaflets) become tethered to the ventricle, and only atrial communication may be left. The left and right sides of the heart are still separate. However, recent evidence suggests that AVSDs can exist without interatrial or interventricular communications [19].

A complete AVSD occurs when the atrioventricular valve is complete but the atrioventricular valve rings are incomplete, resulting in a common atrioventricular orifice. The superior and inferior bridging leaflets of the mitral valve are free-floating and incapable of functionally separating the left and right sides of the heart. There is subsequent interatrial and interventricular communication.

Formation of the normal mitral valve not only requires division of the atrioventricular canal, but also cannot proceed until the developing aorta becomes committed to the left ventricle. In the definitive heart, almost always there is fibrous continuity between two

of the leaflets of the aortic valve and one of the leaflets of the mitral valve.

Although AVSDs usually present early in childhood, a partial AVSD may present in adulthood (Box 20.1).

Another defect that usually presents in childhood but may present in adult life is a parachute mitral valve [20]. In contrast to an AVSD, this results from an abnormality of the papillary muscles, such that all the chordae to the mitral valve are attached to one papillary muscle only. These are usually short and restricted, resulting in severe mitral stenosis. Associated lesions include a supravalvular ring of the left atrium, subaortic stenosis, and coarctation of the aorta.

TEE of atrioventricular septal defects

Possible partial AVSD should be considered in patients who have complex patterns of mitral regurgitation (MR). Centrally, anteriorly, or posteriorly directed jets of MR may be apparent, and the degree of regurgitation is usually severe.

Optimum TEE windows for examining the mitral valve are the non-standard five-chamber mid-esophageal view, the mid-esophageal four-chamber, two-chamber, mitral commissural, and long-axis views, and the transgastric basal short-axis and long-axis two-chamber views (see Chapter 7).

Conclusion

The medical care of both corrected and uncorrected adult congenital heart disease has improved substantially in recent years, and those performing adult TEE should be familiar with the basic echocardiography of the simpler lesions.

TEE guidance during transcatheter closure of ASD, PFO, and VSD is now standard practice. Echocardiography is used to determine the size and location of the defect and its relationship with the surrounding structures. TEE provides an accurate assessment of the atrial and ventricular septum, the position and the size of the defects, and the adequacy of the rims of the defect. It also allows control of the position of the device, and can check for the presence of residual shunts. Finally, TEE gives the interventional cardiologist the potential to obtain an excellent anatomical definition during the catheterization procedure.

References

1. European Association of Echocardiography. Accreditation in echocardiography. www.escardio.org/communities/EAE/accreditation/Pages/welcome.aspx (accessed September 2009).

2. Warnes CA, Williams RG, Bashore TM, et al. ACC/AHA 2008 guidelines for the management of adults with congenital heart disease: executive summary. Circulation 2008; 118: 2395–451.

3. Rigby ML. Transoesophageal echocardiography during interventional cardiac catheterisation in congenital heart disease. Heart 2001; 86 (Suppl 2): II23–9.

4. Houston A, Hillis S, Lilley S, Richens T, Swan L. Echocardiography in adult congenital heart disease. Heart 1998; 80 (Suppl 1): S12–26.

5. Ho S, McCarthy K, Rigby M. Anatomy of atrial and ventricular septal defects. J Interven Cardiol 2000; 13: 475–85.

6. Chessa M, Carminati M, Butera G, et al. Early and late complications associated with transcatheter occlusion of secundum atrial septal defect. J Am Cardiol 2002; 39: 1061–5.

7. Műgge A, Daniel WG, Angermann C, et al. Atrial aneurysm in adult patients: a multicenter study using transthoracic and transesophageal echocardiography. Circulation 1995; 91: 2785–92.

8. Agmon Y, Khandheria BK, Meissner I, et al. Frequency of atrial septal aneurysms in patients with cerebral ischemic events. Circulation 1999; 99: 1942–4.

9. Ewert P, Berger F, Vogel M, et al. Morphology of perforated atrial septal aneurysm suitable for closure by transcatheter device placement. Heart 2000; 84: 327–31.

10. Butera G, Carminati M, Chessa M, et al. CardioSEAL/STARflex versus Amplatzer devices for percutaneous closure of small to moderate (up to 18 mm) atrial septal defects. Am Heart J 2004; 148: 507–10.

11. Kerut EK, Norfleet WT, Plotnick GD, Giles TD. Patent foramen ovale: a review of associated conditions and the impact of physioloical size. J Am Coll Cardiol 2001; 38: 613–23.

12. Masani ND. Transoesophageal echocardiography in adult congenital heart disease. Heart 2001; 86 (Suppl 2): II30–40.

13. Oosthoek PW, Wenink AC, Wisse LJ, Gittenberger-de Groot AC. Development of the papillary muscles of the mitral valve: morphogenetic background of parachute-like asymmetric mitral valves and other mitral valve anomalies. J Thor Cardiovasc Surg 1998; 116: 36–46.

14. Lock JE, Block PC, McKay RG, Baim DS, Keane JF. Transcatheter closure of ventricular septal defects. Circulation 1988; 78: 361–8.

15. Thanopoulos BD, Tsaousis GS, Karanasios E, Eleftherakis NG, Paphitis C. Transcatheter closure of perimembranous ventricular septal defects with the Amplatzer asymmetric ventricular septal defect occluder: preliminary experience in children. Heart 2003; 89: 918–22.

16. Rosenhek R, Binder T. Monitoring of invasive procedures: the role of echocardiography in cathlab and operating room. J Clin Basic Cardiol 2002; 5: 139–43.

17. Kanani M, Moorman AF, Cook AC, et al. Development of the atrioventricular valves: clinicomorphological correlations. Ann Thorac Surg 2005; 79: 1797–804.

18. Lamers WH, Virágh S, Wessels A, Moorman AF, Anderson RH. Formation of the tricuspid valve in the human heart. *Circulation* 1995; **91**: 111–21.

19. Kaski JP, Wolfenden J, Josen M, Daubeney PE, Shinebourne EA. Can atrioventricular septal defects exist with intact septal structures? *Heart* 2006; **92**: 832–5.

20. Fitzsimons B, Koch CG. Parachute mitral valve. *Anesth Analg* 2005; **101**: 1613–14.

Critical and emergency care

Luca Lorini, Erik Sloth

Introduction

The value of echocardiography in the critically ill has been recognized for many years. Although initially utilized in patients following cardiac surgery [1–3], the technique has expanded to include diagnosis and monitoring on the general intensive care unit (ICU) [4–6]. It is able to provide additional data to those available from standard invasive hemodynamic monitoring [5–8], and these data may be more useful than some available through conventional techniques, specifically pulmonary artery catheterization (PAC) [9–11].

Although there are few data to demonstrate the benefit of echocardiography in intensive care, some studies have indicated its potential usefulness in changing the diagnosis and management of the critically ill [12–15], by providing an effective means of assessing ventricular function [16–17], fluid responsiveness [18], and the hemodynamics of shock states [5,6,8,19].

A recent comprehensive document has indicated the requirements for echocardiography practice, training, and accreditation in intensive care. These include the need to interpret findings from both transthoracic and transesophageal studies, to expeditiously answer specific questions in the context of the rapidly changing pathophysiological status of the critically ill patient, and to be accessible for continued echocardiographic monitoring [20]. To that end, different levels of training and expertise have been suggested. These differ from conventional routes in transthoracic and transesophageal accreditation by being more problem-focused than image-modality focused, and in particular by an entry-level practice of emergency, or resuscitation echocardiography, which is based on transthoracic imaging (Fig. 21.1).

Transthoracic echocardiography in intensive care

Since transthoracic echocardiography (TTE) forms the basis of the proposed entry-level practice, it is useful to briefly identify the role of TTE in the ICU. TTE

is less invasive and is attainable within minutes. The quality of images in intensive care is often inferior to images obtained by transesophageal echo (TEE). However, technical refinements, including second harmonic imaging and contrast echocardiography, have improved its capabilities [21,22]. Edema, mechanical ventilation with high levels of end-expiratory pressure, subcostal drainage, dressings, and an unfavorable supine position with restricted patient positioning are the main reasons for the limited acoustic windows seen with TTE in the critically ill [23,24]. The examination is estimated to be inadequate in approximately 50% of patients on mechanical ventilation [23,25].

In some situations transthoracic imaging provides better image quality and diagnostic Doppler data. Anterior structures, for example, such as a prosthetic aortic valve, may be better imaged from the transthoracic view. In many situations, a limited view may still be of value. Evaluation of the hypotensive patient with respect to load and contractility, and assessing the response to intervention, is often possible without the high-quality acoustic windows that are necessary for a comprehensive diagnostic examination. The feasibility of an abbreviated, focus assessed transthoracic echo (FATE) protocol as a means of visualizing the hemodynamic determinants for assessment and optimization has been demonstrated [13]. The quick and readily obtainable scanning of the pleura on both sides is an additional strength of the TTE approach.

Recent technical advances have made the use of portable echocardiographic equipment a viable alternative in selected situations. These devices offer the opportunity for rapid, repeated evaluation and treatment control regardless of patient location, and reach a sensitivity of 70–90% when compared with conventional echocardiography [26].

Focus assessed transthoracic echocardiography (FATE)

FATE has been created for use in the hemodynamically unstable patient in ICU. The importance of rapid

Core Topics in Transesophageal Echocardiography, ed. Robert Feneck, John Kneeshaw, and Marco Ranucci.
Published by Cambridge University Press. © Cambridge University Press 2010.

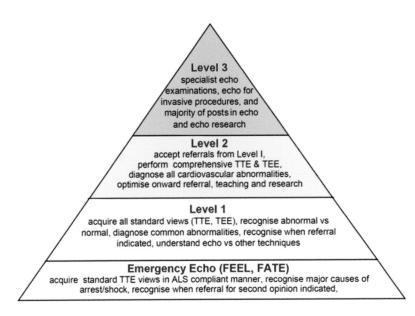

Figure 21.1. Proposed levels of competence for echocardiography in ICU Note that "emergency echo" represents an entry level, a first basic step in competence, and does not equate to level 1. ALS, advanced life support; FATE focus assessed transthoracic echocardiography; FEEL, focused echocardiographic evaluation in life support; TEE, transesophageal echocardiography; TTE, transthoracic echocardiography. Reprinted with permission from Price *et al. Cardiovasc Ultrasound* 2008; 6: 49 [20].

access to images of the heart and great vessels, even via acoustic windows of inferior quality, has been recognized. One or more useful images are obtainable in 97% of critically ill patients [13]. FATE implies a rapid examination of the heart via the apical, subcostal, and parasternal windows (Figs. 21.2, 21.3). Pleurae are visualized via scanning laterally on both sides.

FATE is performed from the four positions shown in Figure 21.2 in a rapid sequence with the following goals:

- exclude obvious pathology
- assess wall thickness and dimensions of chambers
- assess contractility
- visualize pleura on both sides
- relate the information to the clinical context

In many circumstances FATE may be sufficient. Case series describe limited-scope goal-directed echo examination as a rapid, safe, and reliable means of obtaining selected information in the critically ill patient [13,27].

Transesophageal echocardiography in the ICU

The importance of TEE in the general intensive care setting has gradually increased, even in non-cardiac critically ill patients. The image quality in ventilated patients is usually much better with TEE than with TTE [24,28]. There is substantial evidence that TEE complements the usual hemodynamic monitoring, in particular in the monitoring of global and regional systolic function and the guidance of fluid administration in critically ill patients [29,30]. TEE may help to define pathophysiological abnormalities even in patients with established continuous invasive monitoring of pulmonary artery pressures. In patients monitored with pulmonary artery catheters, poor concordance has been demonstrated between the hemodynamic and the echocardiographic diagnosis [29–32]. Unexpected clinical findings are discovered by TEE in 25–59% of patients, and may lead to a change in treatment in 32–64% of patients [28,30–33]. Case series have demonstrated that monitoring in intensive care with TEE is associated with higher inter-observer agreement in diagnosing and excluding significant causes of hemodynamic instability for postoperative cardiac surgical patients than hemodynamic data alone [14].

The major drawback of TEE is the difficulty of continuously monitoring the conscious patient. This is particularly important for patients with unexplained hypotension, in which the relative contributions of volume and contractility may change over time. Pediatric probes left for prolonged imaging have been shown to provide useful data in intensive care [34] and transnasal TEE probes in the awake patient have been evaluated [35].

Safety and probe insertion

General safety considerations and techniques of probe insertion are as described in Chapter 3. Intensive care

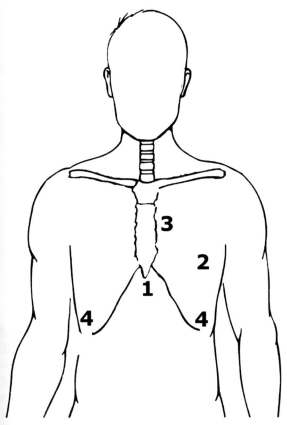

Figure 21.2. Examination of the heart via (1) subcostal, (2) apical, (3) parasternal, and (4) pleural windows.

patients frequently have an endotracheal tube *in situ*, and may be undergoing sophisticated forms of controlled ventilation. If patients are receiving enteral feeding, this may need to be stopped and the stomach aspirated. This may also be necessary if there is significant abdominal distension and gastric air present.

Probe insertion may be a noxious stimulus and may produce tachycardia and a significant hypertensive response. Intensive care patients are frequently sedated, but not anesthetized, and appropriate sedation may be required for the procedure. This may include muscular relaxation if necessary. The use of a bite block is strongly recommended, to reduce the damage inflicted on the probe by dental trauma.

Probe insertion in intensive care may be done blindly or under direct vision. There are drawbacks to both techniques, and a judgment should be made on each case. Blind insertion may be facilitated by inserting the thumb into the mouth behind the teeth and thrusting the mandible upward, inserting the probe with the rotating transducer element facing anteriorly and the probe tip gently anteflexed. In some situations it may help to slightly anteflex the neck. Alternatively the transducer can be inserted under direct vision using a laryngoscope as described in Chapter 3. Whichever technique is used, a gentle approach is essential. ICU patients have especially fragile tissues and the risk of traumatic damage is increased.

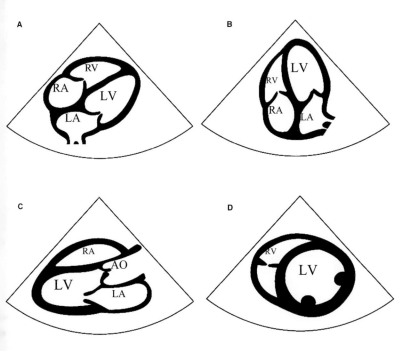

Figure 21.3. Views obtained using the FATE protocol. Schematic drawing of the four most important image planes as they appear on the monitor during TTE. (A) Subcostal four-chamber view (position 1, Fig. 21.2). The right ventricular free wall, the mid-section of the interventricular septum, and the posterolateral left ventricular wall are seen. (B) Apical four-chamber view (position 2, Fig. 21.2). The left-sided chambers are seen to the right, the right-sided to the left of the screen. (C) Parasternal long-axis view (position 3, Fig. 21.2). The right ventricular outflow tract is seen anteriorly. The aortic root and valve, the mitral valve, the interventricular septum, and the left ventricular posterior wall are further displayed. The left atrium is seen posterior to the aortic root, with a similar anteroposterior dimension to the aortic root. (D) Parasternal short-axis view (position 3, Fig. 21.3). Left and right ventricles and papillary muscles. AO, aorta; LA, left atrium; LV, left ventricle; RA, right atrium; RV, right ventricle. Reproduced with permission from Jensen *et al.*, *Eur J Anaesthesiol* 2004; **21**: 700–7 [13].

341

Table 21.1. Indications for transesophageal echocardiography in intensive care

- Monitoring and evaluation of hemodynamic instability
- Suspected endocarditis
- Pericardial effusion
- Assessment of valvular function
- Evaluation of aortic dissection
- Complications of myocardial infarction
- Hypoxemia and pulmonary emboli
- Source of systemic embolism
- Evaluation of chest trauma
- Evaluation of heart transplant donors

Table 21.2. Echocardiographic assessment of three hemodynamic determinants

Parameter	Assessed by
Preload	LV dimensions (long and short axis)
Afterload	LV dimensions and pressure (LVEDP)
Contractility	LV dimensions (dynamic: long and especially short axis)

Despite the precarious status of many intensive care patients, the complication rate with TEE in this population is only slightly greater than in other groups of patients [30,36,37].

The contraindications to TEE are the same as in other settings and include significant disease of the pharynx and esophagus. Anticoagulation within therapeutic levels is not considered a contraindication.

Indications

The most frequent indications for TEE in ICU are listed in Table 21.1. Hemodynamic instability, suspected endocarditis, aortic dissection, and source of embolus are common indications, but the case distribution in different studies is due to differences in patient population and in the trends for performing TEE [31,32,36,37].

Hemodynamic assessment and the monitoring of cardiac function

The threshold for the use of echocardiography in intensive care has decreased. Echocardiography is a fast and accurate method in the diagnosis of the cause of hemodynamic instability. In the critically ill patient, however, there are significant differences in the relative value of TEE versus TTE [24,32]. In the hypotensive patient, the relative contributions of left ventricular (LV) systolic dysfunction, excessive afterload, and inadequate preload are often unclear, even when invasive hemodynamic monitoring is utilized. Table 21.2 illustrates the simplified basic concept of echocardiographic assessment of the three hemodynamic determinants preload, afterload, and contractility.

The methodology and value of TEE in assessing these parameters are discussed extensively in Chapters 9 and 13. Only those aspects that pertain specifically to intensive care will be discussed here.

Preload

Accurate determination of preload is essential for the optimization of hemodynamic performance in ICU patients. Preload is more accurately estimated by left ventricular end-diastolic volume (LVEDV) than by pressure measurements. Estimates of preload by pulmonary wedge pressure measurements may be inaccurate, frequently masking relative hypovolemia which becomes more evident on TEE imaging. In patients receiving intermittent positive pressure ventilation (IPPV), pulmonary capillary wedge pressure (PCWP) may be influenced by both ventricular compliance and the mode of ventilation, and it therefore may not reflect accurately the volume status of the patient.

Two-dimensional (2D) imaging is able to provide measurements of area and cavity dimensions, and Doppler studies at the level of the mitral valve and the pulmonary veins offer additional preload information. A reliable appraisal of preload requires a direct estimate of LV volume, preferably obtained from a transgastric mid-cavity short-axis view. This view is used because of its reproducibility and because acute changes in LV volume affect the short axis to a much greater degree than the long axis [38].

LV short-axis area and dimension may be valuable estimates of preload, and end-diastolic area (EDA) measured with TEE has been shown to correlate well with LV volumes determined by radionuclide studies [39]. The simple dimension may be measured with M-mode echo, and EDA may be calculated by planimetry of the endocardial border. Less formally, inadequate preload may be estimated by visual assessment of the LV end-diastolic cavity dimension, and "kissing" or touching of the papillary muscles in systole may indicate significant hypovolemia. Larger volume losses will result in systolic obliteration of the LV cavity.

A reduction in EDA may occur in other settings in ICU patients, for example in septic shock, where a profound decrease of systemic vascular resistance results in complete emptying of the LV during systole [40,41].

Doppler analysis of the pulmonary vein flows may also give valuable information on preload. The ratio between systolic flow wave (S) and diastolic flow velocity (D) of pulmonary veins, however, has shown excellent inverse correlation with PCWP [42]. It is not appropriate to use this sign in patients with mitral regurgitation.

Patients with a chronically dilated left ventricle may demonstrate inadequate preload at a higher LV filling status than patients with normal LV function. Therefore, the evaluation of optimal LV size becomes challenging (Video 21.1).

Cardiac tamponade is a specialized example of inadequate preload, in which external cardiac compression from blood or clots restricts cardiac filling, leading to a low output state.

Systolic and diastolic function

Left ventricular systolic and diastolic function is extensively covered in Chapter 9.

The normal 2D indices of systolic function (fractional shortening, fractional area of change, ejection fraction) and Doppler-based indices may be used. As in other situations, a visual assessment by an experienced echocardiographer may be adequate. Both 2D and Doppler measurements may be used to calculate stroke volume and cardiac output. Several studies have compared TEE Doppler estimates of cardiac output with hemodilution estimates using PAC. Irrespective of the Doppler-derived method used, good correlations between TEE and thermodilution have been noted.

Diastolic function is more difficult to assess visually, and formal measurements may be made. Transmitral flow and propagation velocity, pulmonary vein flow velocity, and tissue Doppler velocity may all be valuable in assessing diastolic dysfunction. The importance of diastolic function is demonstrated by the observation that up to 50% of patients with acute pulmonary edema have been shown to have normal systolic function, and in most of these cases the underlying cause was thought to be diastolic dysfunction

[42]. Diastolic function is an important determinant of LV filling. Ventricular compliance and the rate of LV relaxation influence the transmitral pressure gradient, which is the actual physical determinant of LV filling [38,42].

In the hypotensive patient, the relative contributions of LV systolic dysfunction, excessive afterload, and inadequate preload are often unclear, even when invasive hemodynamic monitoring is utilized.

Chest trauma

Either TTE or TEE may be performed in the emergency room to assess the effects of blunt and penetrating chest trauma. Indications for emergency assessment are well recognized [13,43], and the use of echocardiography in this setting is undisputed. There are several considerations in the echocardiography of patients with chest trauma that are admitted to the ICU. TTE has a relatively low diagnostic yield compared with TEE [44], but where tamponade is suspected TTE may provide the diagnosis rapidly. It is also particularly useful in the diagnosis of aortic disruption [45].

Delayed tamponade is not uncommon, but in addition a large range of abnormalities have been described following chest trauma, and therefore, where time permits, a comprehensive study should be performed (Table 21.3).

Where concomitant pneumothorax exists, TTE may be unhelpful and TEE may be required. TEE may be contraindicated if there is esophageal, maxillofacial, or cervical spine injury. Both computed tomography (CT) and magnetic resonance imaging (MRI) are less invasive alternatives, although both procedures are time-consuming and involve moving the patient to a scanner. In contrast, TEE can be performed safely and rapidly at the bedside, in the operating room, emergency room, or ICU.

Table 21.3. Conditions associated with chest trauma

- Hemopericardium
- Pleural collections
- Aortic valve disruption
- Aortic disruption
- Ventricular septal defect
- Coronary artery disruption
- Mitral valve disruption
- Myocardial contusion

Injuries due to acute deceleration may result in lesions in the ascending aorta, or more commonly in the descending aorta 2–3 cm distal to the origin of the left subclavian artery. The aortic arch is rarely involved. TEE is capable of imaging the proximal ascending aorta, the distal arch, and the descending thoracic aorta. The distal ascending aorta and the proximal arch are usually poorly visualized.

Recent studies have demonstrated that TEE has a 75% specificity and a 100% sensitivity in the diagnosis of mediastinal hematomas [46–48]. The diagnosis is based upon imaging of signs such as an increased distance, of more than 3 mm, between the TEE probe and the descending aorta, a double contour aspect of the aortic wall, and ultrasound signals between the aorta and the visceral pleura.

A mediastinal hematoma does not always signify the presence of an aortic injury, but may be due to injuries to bony structures or other vessels. Traumatic aortic injury may cause intimal tears with or without dissection, as well as aortic lesions with false aneurysm formation or transection [49].

Placement of assist devices

TEE plays an important role in evaluating both the type of ventricular assist device (VAD) to be used and also its efficacy. The assessment of ventricular function is important in choosing the most suitable type of mechanical ventricular support (e.g. left ventricular assist device, LVAD; biventricular assist device, BIVAD) [50].

TEE may also diagnose intracardiac defects that complicate LVAD implantation, including the presence of a patent foramen ovale (PFO), stenosis of the atrioventricular valves, or incompetence of the semilunar valves. An atrial septal defect and significant mitral or tricuspid stenosis may prevent adequate VAD performance. Retrograde flow from the VAD cannula through a regurgitant semilunar valve may lead to ventricular distension and failure.

TEE may also be useful in the following:

- guiding placement of a VAD cannula
- assessing blood flow through it
- detecting the presence of intracavity air
- evaluating VAD function
- imaging the descending aorta and the pulmonary artery to detect air (e.g. from a BIVAD)
- identifying intracavity tumors or thrombi

Adequate function of an LVAD is monitored by assessing emptying of both the left atrium and ventricle.

Because LVAD flow is volume-dependent, appropriate preload must be maintained, to allow normal function and prevent thrombosis and occlusion of the inflow cannula. LV collapse, with resultant occlusion of the LVAD inlet cannula, generates a subatmospheric pressure and may cause air embolism through the suture lines.

TEE is also important in the evaluation of both the position and the direction of the VAD inflow cannula. This is typically implanted at the ventricular apex and positioned away from the interventricular septum (toward the ventricular inflow valve), maximizing VAD filling and ventricular empting. Two-dimensional imaging evaluates both the patency of the orifice and the correct alignment of the inflow cannula in the ventricle.

When an LVAD is used, the presence of air is more readily seen in the descending aorta, because the proximal aorta and arch may be visualized poorly. Following cardiopulmonary bypass and after LVAD placement, the use of TEE becomes important for monitoring right ventricular function, by evaluating both the size and contractility of the ventricle and the extent of tricuspid regurgitation.

Evaluation of the potential cardiac donor

Echocardiography may be useful in the selection of suitable donors for heart transplantation. In some cases it is important to exclude cardiac lesions resulting from chest trauma, which may easily and safely be diagnosed by TEE in the hands of an experienced operator. Right ventricular contusions are approximately twice as common as left ventricular contusions. Traumatic lesions may include tricuspid valve disruption resulting in tricuspid regurgitation, aortic rupture, and pericardial effusion.

TEE provides images of excellent quality, whereas transthoracic examination may be inadequate in this setting. Brainstem death causes severe left ventricular dysfunction in almost 20% of cases. In a direct comparison of TTE and TEE in a small series of brain-dead patients being considered as cardiac transplant donors, TEE revealed significant abnormalities of valve morphology and left ventricular function which were not identified by a TTE examination [51]. However, the use of a single echocardiogram to determine the physiological suitability of a donor is not supported by evidence. The value of TEE in the management of potential donors may however be limited by the short time in which the examination must be accurately performed, and by the knowledge and experience of the person performing the TEE in some donor hospitals. Under such circumstances the accuracy of echocardiography interpretation may be suboptimal [52], and some usable donor organs may be excluded because of over-reporting of trivial abnormalities of morphology or function.

Conclusion

The critical care and emergency room setting provides an opportunity to utilize basic echo screening protocols, as well as formal transthoracic and transesophageal echocardiography. It is therefore important to recognize both the potential benefits and the limitations of each technique. Screening protocols are highly valuable for a rapid assessment of cardiac function, but more definitive diagnosis may need more sophisticated imaging. TEE is indicated particularly where this imaging modality is primarily indicated (see Chapter 1) or where surface imaging is unable to produce images of sufficient quality.

References

1. Shanewise JS, Cheung, AT, Aronson S, et al. ASE/SCA guidelines for performing a comprehensive intraoperative multiplane transesophageal echocardiography examination. *J Am Soc Echocardiogr* 1999; **12**: 884–900.

2. Cahalan MK, Abel M, Goldman M, et al. American Society of Echocardiography and Society of Cardiovascular Anesthesiologists task force guidelines for training in perioperative echocardiography. *Anesth Analg* 2002; **94**: 1384–8.

3. Cheitlin MD, Armstrong WF, Aurigemma GP, et al. ACC/AHA/ASE 2003 guideline update for the clinical application of echocardiography: summary article. A report of the American College of Cardiology/ American Heart Association Task Force on Practice Guidelines (ACC/AHA/ASE Committee to Update the 1997 Guidelines for the Clinical Application of Echocardiography). *Circulation* 2003; **108**: 1146–62.

4. Beaulieu Y, Marik PE. Bedside ultrasonography in ICU: part 1. *Chest* 2005; **128**: 881–95.

5. Marik PE, Baram M. Noninvasive hemodynamic monitoring in the intensive care unit. *Crit Care Clin* 2007; **23**: 383–400.

6. Vignon P. Hemodynamic assessment of critically ill patients using echocardiography Doppler. *Curr Opin Crit Care* 2005; **11**: 227–34.

7. Price S, Nicol E, Gibson DG, Evans TW. Echocardiography in the critically ill: current and potential roles. *Intensive Care Med* 2000; **32**: 48–59.

8. Vieillard-Baron A, Prin S, Chergui K, Dubourg O, Jardin F. Hemodynamic instability in sepsis: bedside assessment by Doppler echocardiography. *Am J Resp Crit Care* 2003; **168**: 1270–6.

9. Shah MR, Hasselblad V, Stevenson LW, et al. Impact of the pulmonary artery catheter in critically ill patients: meta-analysis of randomized clinical trials. *JAMA* 2005; **294**: 1664–70.

10. Harvey S, Harrison DA, Singer M, et al. PAC-Man study collaboration. Assessment of the clinical effectiveness of pulmonary artery catheters in management of patients in intensive care (PAC-Man): a randomised controlled trial. *Lancet* 2005; **366**: 472–7.

11. Richard C, Warszawski J, Anguel N, et al. Early use of the pulmonary artery catheter and outcomes in patients with shock and acute respiratory distress syndrome: a randomized controlled trial. *JAMA* 2003; **290**: 2713–20.

12. Hüttemann E, Schelenz C, Kara F, Chatzinikolaou K, Reinhart K. The use and safety of TEE in the general ICU: a minireview. *Acta Aanaesthesiol Scand* 2004; **48**: 827–36.

13. Jensen MB, Sloth E, Larsen KM, Schmidt MB. Transthoracic echocardiography for cardiopulmonary monitoring in intensive care. *Eur J Anaesthesiol* 2004; **21**: 700–7.

14. Costachescu T, Denault A, Guimond JG, et al. The hemodynamically unstable patient in the intensive care unit: hemodynamic vs. transesophageal echocardiographic monitoring. *Crit Care Med* 2002; **30**: 1214–23.

15. Joseph MX, Disney PJ, Da Costa R, Hutchison SJ. Transthoracic echocardiography to identify or exclude cardiac cause of shock. *Chest* 2004; **126**: 1592–7.

16. Poelaert JI, Schüpfer G. Hemodynamic monitoring utilizing TEE: the relationships among pressure, flow and function. *Chest* 2005; **127**: 379–90.

17. Slama M, Maizel J. Echocardiographic measurement of ventricular function. *Curr Opin Crit Care* 2006; **12**: 241–8.

18. Charron C, Caille V, Jardin F, Vieillard-Baron A. Echocardiographic measurement of fluid responsiveness. *Curr Opin Crit Care* 2006; **12**: 249–54.

19. Jones AE, Tayal VS, Sullivan DM, Kline JA. Randomized, controlled trial of immediate versus delayed goal-directed ultrasound to identify the cause of nontraumatic hypotension in emergency department patients. *Crit Care Med* 2004; **32**: 1703–8.

20. Price S, Via G, Sloth E, et al. Echocardiography practice, training and accreditation in the intensive care: document for the World Interactive Network Focused on Critical Ultrasound (WINFOCUS) *Cardiovasc Ultrasound* 2008; **6**: 49.

345

21. Kornbluth M, Liang DH, Paloma A, Schnittger I. Native tissue harmonic imaging improves endocardial border definition and visualization of cardiac structures. *J Am Soc Echocardiogr* 1998; **11**: 693–701.

22. Kornbluth M, Liang DH, Brown P, Gessford E, Schnittger I. Contrast echocardiography is superior to tissue harmonics for assessment of left ventricular function in mechanically ventilated patients. *Am Heart J* 2000; **140**: 291–6.

23. Cook CH, Praba AC, Beery PR, Martin LC. Transthoracic echocardiography is not cost-effective in critically ill surgical patients. *J Trauma* 2002; **52**: 280–4.

24. Vignon P, Mentec H, Terré S, et al. Diagnostic accuracy and therapeutic impact of transthoracic and transesophageal echocardiography in mechanically ventilated patients in the ICU. *Chest* 1994; **106**: 1829–34.

25. Parker MM, Cunnion RE, Parillo JE. Echocardiography and nuclear cardiac imaging in the critical care unit. *JAMA* 1985; **254**: 2935–9.

26. Ashrafian H, Bogle RG, Rosen SD, Henein M, Evans TW. Portable echocardiography. *BMJ* 2004; **328**: 300–1.

27. Benjamin E, Griffin K, Leibowitz AB, et al. Goal-directed transesophageal echocardiography performed by intensivists to assess left ventricular function: Comparison with pulmonary artery catheterization. *J Cardiothorac Vasc Anesth* 1998; **12**: 10–15.

28. Heidenreich PA, Stainback RF, Redberg RF, et al. Transesophageal echocardiography predicts mortality in critically ill patients with unexplained hypotension. *J Am Coll Cardiol* 1995; **26**: 152–8.

29. Fontes M, Bellows W, Ngo L, Mangano D. Assessment of ventricular function in critically ill patients: limitations of pulmonary artery catheterization. *J Cardiothorac Vasc Anesth* 1999; **5**: 521–7.

30. Poelaert JI, Trouerbach J, De Buyzere M, Everaert J, Colardyn FA. Evaluation of transesophageal echocardiography as a diagnostic and therapeutic aid in a critical care setting. *Chest* 1995; **107**: 774–9.

31. Wake PJ, Ali M, Carroll J, Siu SC, Cheng DC. Clinical and echocardiographic diagnoses disagree in patients with unexplained hemodynamic instability after cardiac surgery. *Can J Anaesth* 2001; **48**: 778–83.

32. Colreavy FB, Donovan K, Lee KY, Weekes J. Transesophageal echocardiography in critically ill patients. *Crit Care Med* 2002; **30**: 989–96.

33. Schmidlin D, Schuepbach R, Bernard E, et al. Indications and impact of postoperative transesophageal echocardiography in cardiac surgical patients. *Crit Care Med* 2001; **29**: 2143–8.

34. Voci P, Marino P. Transesophageal echocardiography in critically-ill patients using a miniaturized probe:

feasibility, efficacy and indications. *Cardiologia* 1996; **41**: 855–9.

35. Spencer KT, Krauss D, Thurn J, et al. Transnasal transesophageal echocardiography. *J Am Soc Echocardiogr* 1997; **10**: 728–37.

36. Khoury AF, Afridi I, Quiñones MA, Zoghbi WA. Transesophageal echocardiography in critically ill patients: feasibility, safety and impact on management. *Am Heart J* 1994; **127**: 1363–71.

37. Hwang JJ, Shyu KG, Chen JJ, et al. Usefulness of transesophageal echocardiography in the treatment of critically ill patients. *Chest* 1993; **104**: 861–6.

38. Troianos CA, Porembka DT. Assessment of left ventricular function and hemodynamics with transesophageal echocardiography. *Crit Care Clin* 1996; **12**: 253–72.

39. Clements FM, Harpole DH, Quill T, Jones RH, McCann RL. Estimation of left ventricular volume and ejection fraction by two-dimensional transoesophageal echocardiography: comparison of short axis imaging and simultaneous radionuclide angiography. *Br J Anaesth* 1990; **64**: 331–6.

40. Feinberg MS, Hopkins WE, Davila-Roman VG, Barzilai B. Multiplane transesophageal echocardiographic Doppler imaging accurately determines cardiac output measurements in critically ill patients. *Chest* 1995; **107**: 769–73.

41. Dabaghi SF, Rokey R, Rivera JM, Saliba WI, Majid PA. Comparison of echocardiographic assessment of hemodynamics in the intensive care unit with right-sided cardiac catheterization. *Am J Cardiol* 1995; **6**: 392–5.

42. Appleton CP, Firstenberg MS, Garcia MJ, Thomas JD. The echo-Doppler evaluation of left ventricular diastolic function: a current perspective. *Cardiol Clin* 2000; **18**: 513–46.

43. Breitkreutz R, Walcher F, Seeger F. Focused echocardiographic evaluation in resuscitation management: concept of an advanced life support-conformed algorithm. *Crit Care Med* 2007; **35**: S150–61.

44. Chirillo F, Totis O, Cavarzerani A, et al. Usefulness of transthoracic and transoesophageal echocardiography in recognition and management of cardiovascular injuries after blunt chest trauma. *Heart* 1996; **75**: 301–6.

45. Smith MD, Cassidy JM, Souther S, et al. Transesophageal echocardiography in the diagnosis of traumatic rupture of the aorta. *N Engl J Med* 1995; **332**: 356–62.

46. Catoire P, Orliaguet G, Liu N, et al. Systematic transesophageal echocardiography for detection of mediastinal lesions in patients with multiple injuries. *J Trauma* 1995; **38**: 96–102.

47. Vlahakes GJ, Warren RL. Traumatic rupture of the aorta. *N Engl J Med* 1995; **332**: 389–90.

48. Goldstein SA, Mintz GS, Lindsay J. Aorta: comprehensive evaluation by echocardiography and transesophageal echocardiography. *J Am Soc Echocardiogr* 1993; **6**: 634–59.

49. Fernandez LG, Lain KY, Messersmith RN, *et al.* Transesophageal echocardiography for diagnosing aortic injury: a case report and summary of current imaging techniques. *J Trauma* 1994; **36**: 877–80.

50. Heath MJS, Dickstein ML. Perioperative management of the left ventricular assist device recipient. *Prog Cardiovasc Dis* 2000; **43**: 47–54.

51. Stoddard MF, Longaker RA. The role of transesophageal echocardiography in cardiac donor screening. *Am Heart J* 1993; **125**: 1676–81.

52. Zaroff JG, Rosengard BR, Armstrong WF, *et al.* Consensus conference report: maximizing use of organs recovered from the cadaver donor. *Circulation* 2002; **106**: 836–41.

22

Three-dimensional imaging

Heinz D. Tschernich

Introduction

In 1974 Decker *et al.* first demonstrated cardiac images using 3D echocardiography [1]. Subsequent publications focused on reconstructive 3D echocardiography, reporting of different approaches for image acquisition and 3D reconstruction in adults and children [2–7]. However, image reconstruction took a long time due to low processor power.

In 1986 Martin and colleagues were the first to report 3D-TEE image reconstruction by angulating the probe tip automatically to achieve different levels of cut planes [8]. In 1992 Pandian *et al.* described the use of a "prototype tomographic transesophageal echocardiographic probe" that was computer-automated to record parallel images [9]. The current approach, using rotational scanning for data acquisition, was first published in 1993 by Sapin *et al.* [10], followed by publications reporting in-vivo data in 1994 [11].

The breakthrough in 3D echocardiography technology occurred when matrix transducer technology for real-time 3D echocardiography became available in 2000 [12]. Miniaturization finally led to the development of the first real-time 3D-TEE probe (RT3D-TEE) [13], which became commercially available in 2007.

Currently available techniques follow two principles:

- 3D reconstruction from sequentially recorded 2D planes
- real-time 3D echocardiography, a technology capable of scanning and construction in real time

3D reconstruction

Three-dimensional reconstruction was the first approach used. Initially three different scan and data acquisition techniques were proposed:

- linear scanning
- fan-like scanning
- rotational scanning

With linear scanning, parallel images were sequentially recorded at a predefined rate (1 mm steps) along the long axis of the heart to create a 3D volume of prismatic shape. Using fan scanning, images were obtained by moving the transducer and the imaging plane like a fan in an angular sweep, resulting in an acquired 3D volume with a pyramidal shape.

Rotational scanning is performed by rotation of the transducer around the central axis of the imaging plane (Fig. 22.1). Thus a conical volume is created. Recent commercially available systems use rotational scanning on a conventional multiplane probe.

All three techniques may be used with TEE, but the advantage of the rotational approach is that only a small acoustic window is required through which 2D cut planes can be recorded. Thus one can focus on the area of interest throughout the acquisition time.

With all reconstruction techniques it is extremely important to have exact information on the spatial position of each image plane, the position of the heart relative to the scan plane (translation of the heart and

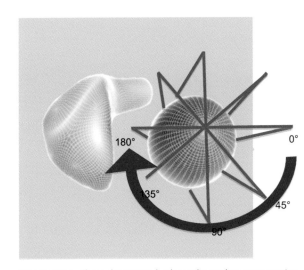

Figure 22.1. Three-dimensional echocardiography reconstruction technique: rotation around a central axis from 0° to 180°, thus creating a conical 3D volume.

Core Topics in Transesophageal Echocardiography, ed. Robert Feneck, John Kneeshaw, and Marco Ranucci.
Published by Cambridge University Press. © Cambridge University Press 2010.

respiration mainly interferes with freeze-positioning the heart), and temporal information. Therefore, respiration and ECG gating was implemented in order to stabilize the position of the heart and localize the transducer relative to the heart. Using the rotational approach, it is necessary to record a full 180° arc to achieve the completed conical volume. Current 3D-reconstruction systems perform rotation automatically in 3–5° steps, recording one heart cycle at each cut plane. Thus a full 180° scan needs at least 36–60 seconds.

Real-time 3D echocardiography

Real-time 3D echocardiography (RT3D) is dependent on fast processor power and the latest generation of matrix transducer technology.

RT3D is based on the phased array and parallel processing principle to enhance line density within the scan volume and to provide rapid image acquisition. A 2D matrix probe uses 64 elements in several rows, but the RT3D matrix transducer consists of about 2800 elements, the RT3D-TEE matrix of about 2500 elements (Fig. 22.2). By parallel processing, the 3D system uses multiple emission lines for any given receiver line to create the 3D volume (up to 16 : 1). Due to the huge computing workload, volume size and temporal resolution are linked to and dependent on each other within narrow confines. Once a 3D volume is built, post-processing is needed to discriminate signal from noise, and complex rendering algorithms are necessary to extract the surface contours.

Resolution in RT3D

In comparison with 2D scanning, physical and technical limitations in 3D imaging are ubiquitous, and the examiner has to handle them in daily practice. Therefore a basic understanding is necessary for good image results.

The most important fact is that spatial and temporal resolution are closely but inversely linked. Once scanning is optimized to either spatial or temporal resolution, the settings will interfere with the quality of the other.

Spatial resolution

The location of every point within a 3D-volume dataset is defined by three determinants: the distance on the x-axis equals the distance from the transducer (the depth within the 3D volume), the y-axis defines the azimuth plane, and the z-axis defines the elevation plane (Fig. 22.3). Spatial resolution is different along the different axes: along the x-axis it is the same as in 2D scanning (1/2 wavelength), but it is two to three times worse in the other two planes.

Once the object plane within the 3D dataset is perpendicular to the ultrasound beam the object will be displayed in axial resolution (Fig. 22.4A). If the object plane is parallel to the ultrasound beam the resolution will be much worse (Fig. 22.4B). Clinically, the difference is easy to observe: while the mitral valve can be imaged in good resolution from an en-face view, it is much more difficult to visualize the aortic valve in good resolution, because the valve plane is close to 40° to the insonation direction.

Temporal resolution

Despite parallel processing, ultrasound transmission remains dependent on the conventional laws of physics when traveling through tissue. At a tissue velocity of

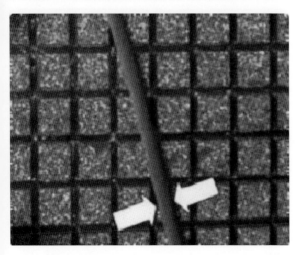

Figure 22.2. Multiple transducer elements arranged in a gridlike fashion in a matrix phased-array transducer. A human hair is shown for size comparison. Reproduced with permission from Hung J *et al.* 3D echocardiography: a review of the current status and future directions. *J Am Soc Echocardiogr* 2007; **20**: 213–33.

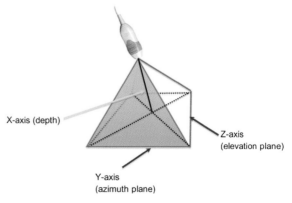

X-axis (depth)

Z-axis (elevation plane)

Y-axis (azimuth plane)

Figure 22.3. 3D coordinate system: *x*-axis (depth), *y*-axis (azimuth plane), *z*-axis (elevation plane)

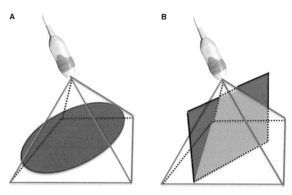

Figure 22.4. In 3D echocardiography the relationship between object plane and ultrasound beam direction determines spatial resolution: (A) axial resolution if perpendicular; (B) lateral resolution if parallel to beam direction.

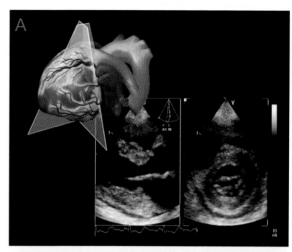

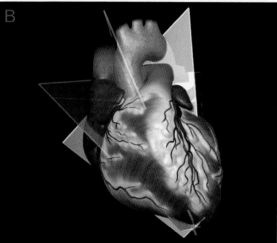

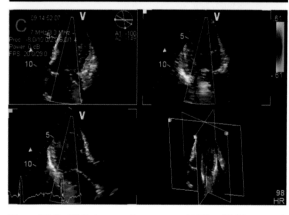

1540 cm/s it takes an ultrasound beam 13 µs to cover a distance of 1 cm to and fro. For a volume sector of 60 × 30°, the whole sector needs 1800 scan lines to generate one volume dataset. Supposing a frame rate of 20 Hz, 36 000 scan lines per second, or a pulse repetition frequency of 36 kHz, is required, and subsequently the maximal interval between two consecutive pulses is only 18 µs. These obstacles can be overcome by the following:

1. Optimize the size of the 3D volume needed, the depth, or the line density – either by reducing the line-density mode or by changing the frame rate, depending on the ultrasound system. Decreased line density will lead either to an increase in the 3D volume, at a given frame rate, or to an increase in frame rate at a fixed volume size.

2. Alternatively, switch from real-time 3D scanning to a multiple volume-gated mode called "full-volume," stitching several single volumes together.

Image acquisition in RT3D

Current 3D probes offer 2D, spectral and CFD, 3D, 3D-CFD in real time (General Electric), and multi-beat acquisition (General Electric, Philips). RT3D technology is available for TTE (General Electric, Philips, Siemens, Toshiba) and TEE (Philips). Technical aspects and modalities as described in the following refer to General Electric (GE) and Philips systems, as systems from other suppliers were not tested.

To optimize workflow and handle current limitations in RT3D the ultrasound companies provide different scanning modes on their systems [14]:

Figure 22.5. (A) Biplane mode: parasternal LAX and SAX are simultaneously obtained and displayed. (B,C) Triplane mode: apical four-chamber, apical two-chamber, and apical LAX are simultaneously obtained and displayed.

1. Multiplane (bi-/triplane) mode (GE) or x-plane (biplane) mode (Philips). Two to three reference

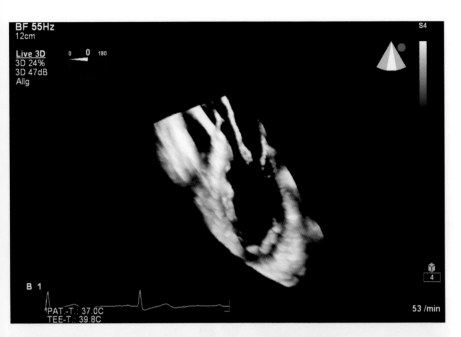

Figure 22.6. Thick slice: a thin 3D volume of 90 × 4°.

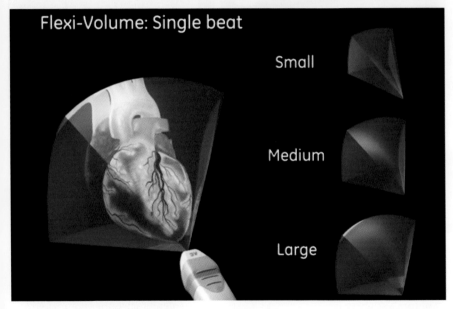

Figure 22.7. Single-beat acquisition at different volume sizes (small, medium, large) adjusted to different requirements of temporal and spatial resolution, volume size. Reproduced with permission of GE Healthcare.

planes are displayed simultaneously in B-mode or CFD (Fig. 22.5).

2. Thick slice mode (Philips) provides a small 3D volume of 90 × 4° size, which adds some 3D impression to a "thick" semi-2D image (Fig. 22.6).

3. Single-beat acquisition (GE) or Live-3D mode (Philips). While Philips Live-3D mode has a fixed volume size of 90 × 30°, the single-beat mode on General Electric's E9 system offers three different volume sizes: 35 × 35°, 50 × 50°, and a large volume of up to 90 × 90°. In addition, the volume shape can be changed from square to rectangle in several steps (Fig. 22.7). CFD is not provided in Live-3D mode on Philips systems. The beam direction is deflected to several angles in the elevation plane in fixed steps (center, front, back).

4. Zoom modes are available on all 3D systems. A further reduction of the region of interest in both the azimuth and the elevation planes leads to an increase in temporal and spatial resolution

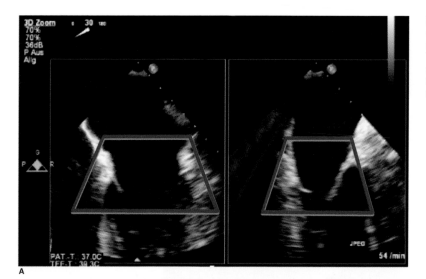

Figure 22.8. Zoom mode: adjustment of volume size to the region of interest optimizes temporal and spatial resolution. This kind of pre-cropping makes navigation through the obtained 3D volume much easier. (A) Pre-crop window; (B) 3D zoom image.

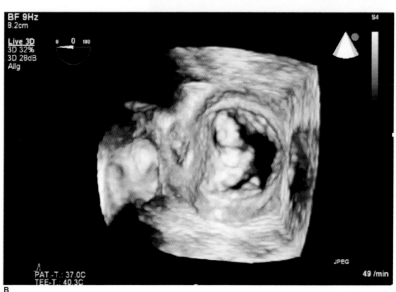

(Fig. 22.8). The zoom mode is a valuable tool for pre-cropping the volume to the structures of interest, making orientation within the 3D dataset after acquisition much easier.

5. Multi-beat acquisition (GE) or Full-volume mode (Philips). Due to technical restrictions, large volumes of realistic depth cannot be scanned in real time, or only at unacceptably low frame rates. To obtain large pyramidal volumes (101 × 104°, Philips; 90 × 90°, GE) single adjacent volumes may be stitched together (Fig. 22.9). To avoid artifacts at the borders ("stitching artifacts"), image acquisition is ECG-triggered. To enhance either volume size or frame rate the number of stitched volumes can be varied from two to seven in B-mode, and seven in CFD. Acquisition is best done on breath-hold, and ECG artifacts due to manipulation or surgical interaction (e.g. diathermy) will interfere and lead to stitching artifacts. To obtain CFD images, single- and multi-beat mode can be used on GE systems, while Philips systems only provide CFD in full-volume mode (Fig. 22.10).

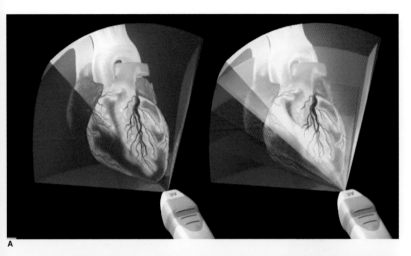

Figure 22.9. Multi-beat acquisition: several adjacent volumes, acquired by elevation steering, are stitched together to one large volume. Volume size and/or temporal resolution can be improved with this type of acquisition. ECG-gating is needed to avoid stitching artifacts. (A) Schematic model of multi-beat acquisition from four volumes (reproduced with permission of GE Healthcare). (B) Full volume from mitral valve and left ventricle.

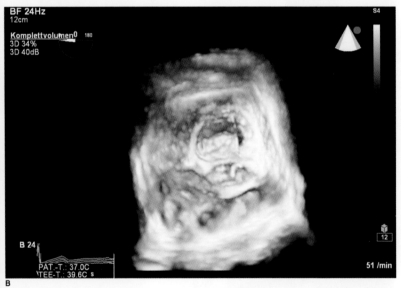

Figure 22.10. Full volume in CFD mode.

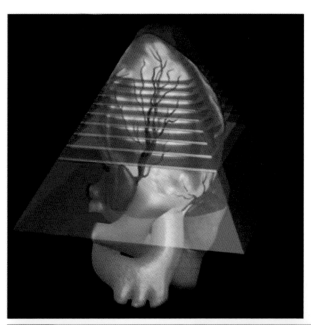

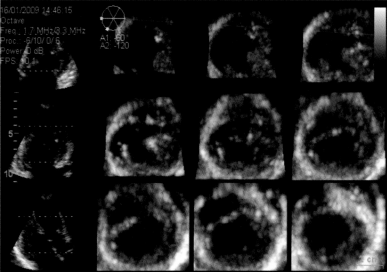

Figure 22.11. Twelve-slice mode (B-mode): schematic model of nine parallel planes through the LV (reproduced with permission of GE Healthcare), together with the three standardized long-axis planes as displayed in 12-slice mode from a patient 12 weeks after repeat heart transplantation.

6. Slice-mode (post-processing). An acquired 3D dataset can be presented in a slice-mode with 9 (Philips) or 9–12 (GE) parallel slices through the dataset in B-mode, and 6 slices in CFD (GE) (Figs. 22.11, 22.12).

Post-processing and navigation in RT3D

Once a dataset is obtained, 3D post-processing tools are required to render an image. Three-dimensional echo tends to display surfaces of cardiac structures, and not cut slices as with 2D echo. Since blood has its own echogenicity it is sometimes difficult to suppress noise and visualize tissue that might have similar reflectivity.

Basic adjustments are made on the settings of 2D gain (overall gain), time gain control, and lateral gain control, and on 4D gain (compression), enhancing the 3D impression and increasing signal-to-noise ratio. Even more complex algorithms such as "UD clarity" (GE) adjust the image in terms of spatial filtering, edge enhancement, smoothness, and crispness.

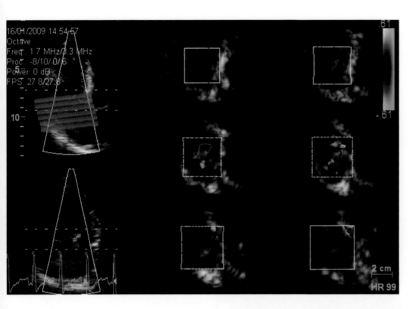

Figure 22.12. Six-slice mode (CFD): the same principle as for B-mode. A valuable feature for planimetry of effective orifice area of the mitral valve, as shown in this example.

Volume optimization (another post-processing tool) provides default sets for adjusting brightness, temporal filtering, and gray-scale correction.

Post-processing algorithms on Philips ultrasound systems are packed into "3D vision controls" (Vision A–H, with the highest resolution in F, G, H), whereas others, such as brightness or smoothing, are very similar to GE ultrasound systems. Substantial attempts have been made to simplify optimizing the 3D image quality of the dataset by providing post-processing setting packages. Adjustments are mainly made by changing several settings together, and although individual changes are possible it may be difficult to understand exactly which image characteristic has been changed.

The impression of depth of a 3D dataset is not well displayed on a 2D monitor. Post-processing can give a more three-dimensional impression, but two-color maps that add color to define depth are more effective. Finally, in stereoscopic vision mode a volume is displayed in two different colors, each from a slightly different viewing angle. Using polarized lenses the stereo effect can be visualized, and information is integrated to a very vivid three-dimensional image.

Structures of primary interest are contained within the 3D volume, but navigation through the 3D dataset can be challenging. Crop tools help to cut into the dataset and reduce tissue information to the volume of interest (VOI). Available crop features are crop boxes, arbitrary crop planes, parallel crop, and flip crop. Using the crop-box tool a virtual box is put around the dataset that helps to define cropping from each side. Arbitrary crop planes may be used to cut

into the dataset from any direction. The parallel-crop feature defines two parallel crop planes that can be manipulated, with an adjustable distance between the planes. Flip crop changes the viewing direction by 180°, for example allowing an easy switch from a ventricular view of a mitral valve to a surgeon's view from the atrial side (Fig. 22.13).

The latest generation of 3D echo systems offer semi-automatic navigation tools based on the adjustment of the 3D LV dataset to standardized orientation. Once this is done, the tool provides easy navigation to standardized 2D cut planes, for example of the mitral valve from the ventricular and atrial side, and of the aortic valve (Fig. 22.14).

Artifacts

In addition to the common ultrasound artifacts, two types of artifact are characteristic of 3D echo. These are stitching artifacts and drop-outs.

Stitching artifacts

All 3D reconstruction modes are at risk of artifacts at the interfaces of the adjacent volumes. These are caused by irregularities in cardiac rhythm, patient motion (breathing), probe movement, or electrical interference (diathermic knife) during image acquisition, and are easy to detect (Fig. 22.15). To avoid stitching artifacts, images should be acquired during breath-holding, the ECG should be optimized (positive

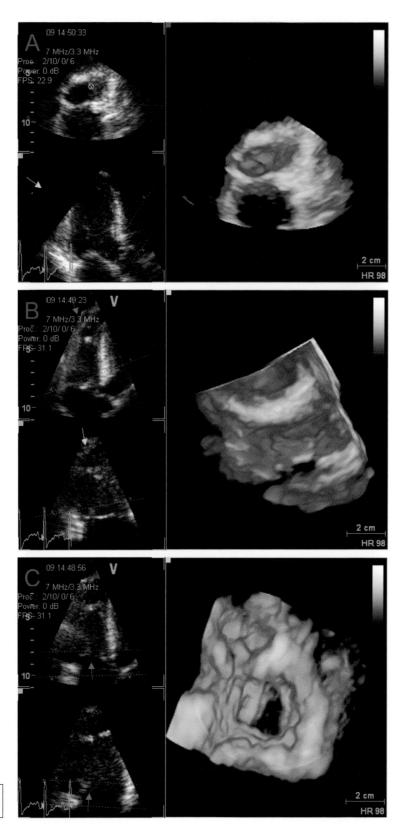

Figure 22.13. Crop tools: (A) parallel-crop tool to obtain a view of the aortic valve; (B,C) flip-crop tool for a fast change of the viewing direction from en-face view of the mitral valve to a surgeon's view from the atrial side.

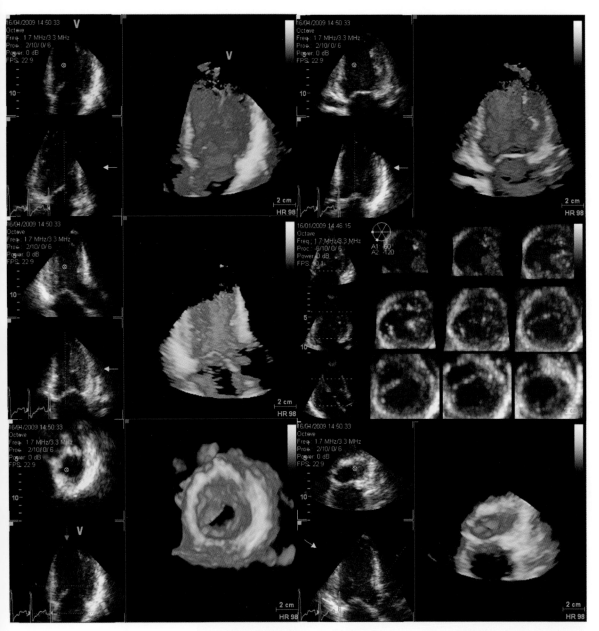

Figure 22.14. Apical alignment tool offers semi-automatic navigation to standardized views after adjustment of the LV volume to standardized orientation.

R-waves), the number of stitch volumes should be decreased, and other intereference should be discontinued for the time of image acquisition.

Dropout artifacts

Since dropout artifacts are very common in 3D echo, it can sometimes be challenging to differentiate between dropout and real defects (e.g. atrial septal defect,

ventricular septal defect, valvular perforation). The artifacts are caused by low gain settings, by the inablility of algorithms to differentiate signal from noise, and by the limitations of lateral spatial resolution (Fig. 22.16). To overcome those artifacts, 2D and 4D gain settings need to be optimized, and the cardiac structure of interest should be imaged from a view that ensures an insonation angle of 90° to the object plane.

357

Clinical applications of RT3D and RT3D-TEE

The great potential of RT3D-TEE lies in improved visualization of cardiac structures, and it is therefore ideally suited for evaluating valve disease, guiding interventional procedures, and evaluating the success of valve repair.

Mitral valve

Recent studies have focused on the feasibility and accuracy of RT3D-TEE for evaluating mitral valve (MV) disease. RT3D-TEE has been shown to be more useful in correctly diagnosing and localizing

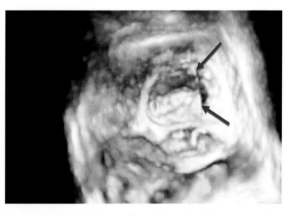

Figure 22.15. Stitching artifact: discontinuation on interface between adjacent volumes (arrow).

MV prolapse and/or chordal rupture [15,16], and 3D image acquisition has been shown to be quick and easy [17]. RT3D-TEE has been shown to improve accuracy in the diagnosis of A2, A3 and posterior leaflet disease [17,18]. The annuloplasty ring size can be determined preoperatively [19], with good visualization of MV prosthesis and annuloplasty and close agreement with surgical findings [20]. The spatial relationship between the anterior MV leaflet and septum in hypertrophic obstructive cardiomyopathy patients undergoing MV repair has also been reported [21].

A comprehensive assessment of the MV with RT3D-TEE involves the acquisition of the so-called en-face view, a full volume, and a 3D color full-volume image (Fig. 22.17). Instead of performing a conventional 2D MV study, x-plane mode (biplane) can be used to obtain standardized 2D cut planes and display them side by side (ME four-chamber/two-chamber, or ME four-chamber/LAX), in either B-mode or CFD. This can be supplemented by offline analysis using a quantitative assessment tool.

The en-face view mirrors the surgical view from the left atrium down to the MV and is therefore probably the most important view for the surgeon. It is usually obtained in 3D zoom mode based on the ME four-chamber view. In a second step the 3D dataset is rotated to display the aortic valve at 12 o'clock, with the anterior leaflet at the top and the posterior leaflet at the bottom of the image. The dataset can then be

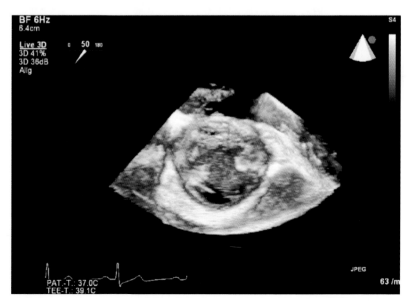

Figure 22.16. Dropout artifact: caused by low gain settings and thin tissue texture with a low signal-to-noise ratio.

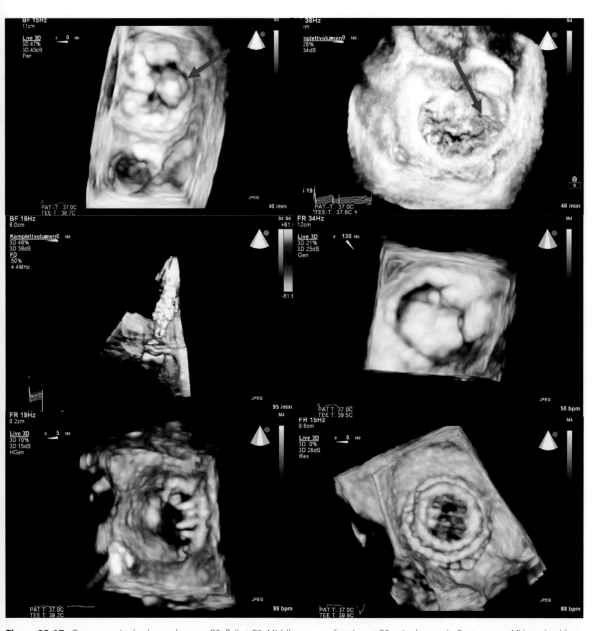

Figure 22.17. Top row: mitral valve prolapse at P2, flail at P3. Middle row: perforation at P2, mitral stenosis. Bottom row: MV repair with an open band, bileaflet mechanical prosthesis.

manipulated by looking from atrial or ventricular perspectives, by focusing on the close relationship of the anterior MV and left ventricular outflow tract (LVOT), or by cutting into the dataset to obtain cut planes through the leaflets where required. Three-dimensional color adds information about the localization and distribution of regurgitation jets and the size of any con-

vergence phenomenon. Using slice mode, the effective regurgitant orifice area can be measured. After MV replacement, 3D-CFD is useful to detect and localize any paravalvular leak.

Mitral valve quantification software packages, developed by Philips (QLAB MVQ) or TomTec (4D MV-Assessment), allow extensive analysis of valve morphology and function. By defining key points at the annulus, coaptation line, atrioventricular valve plane, nadir, and papillary muscles, the software reconstructs a 3D schematic model of the valve and calculates key dimensions and areas (Fig. 22.18). It may also enable quite subtle repairs to be undertaken (Fig. 22.19).

Aortic valve, aorta, minimal invasive cardiac surgery techniques

Imaging the aortic valve (AV) with RT3D-TEE is significantly more difficult than imaging the MV [22]. Whereas the commissures can usually be easily seen, imaging the leaflet body is more difficult, especially

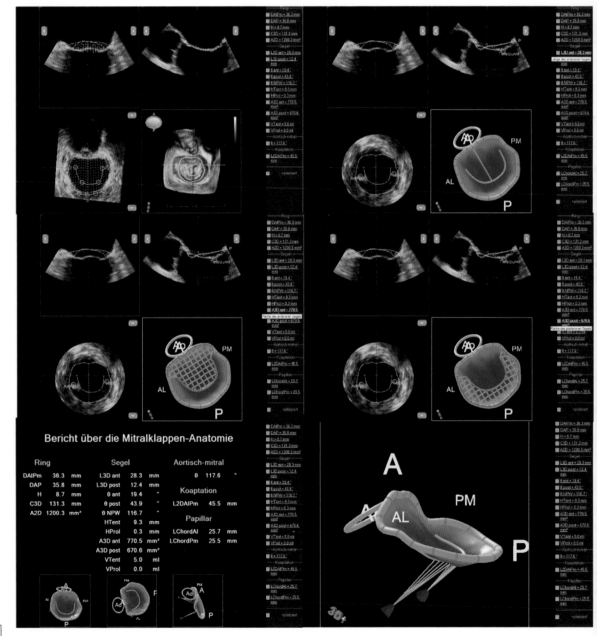

Figure 22.18. MVQ mitral valve quantification tool (Philips). From the definition of key points throughout the ring and coaptation line a schematic model is built and several dimensions and areas are calculated.

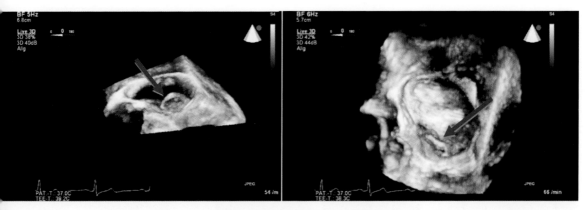

Figure 22.19. Case 3: old MV endocarditis with covered perforation at the anterolateral commissure.

with thin leaflet tissue [23], partly because of the spatial orientation of the valve plane and the direction of the ultrasound beam. Calcification may also cause artifacts, resulting in significant dropout. However, the AV area (AVA) may be calculated from multiplane reconstructive mode (MPR) before and after AV replacement [24], and has been shown to correlate well with conventional methods [25]. Several case reports have suggested that RT3D-TEE may provide additional information in infectious endocarditis [26–28]. Furthermore, initial case reports indicate that transcatheter AV replacement procedures or endoluminal clamp during heart-port procedures will profit from 3D guidance (Fig. 22.20).

Image acquisition of the AV can be achieved using live 3D mode or 3D zoom from the ME LAX view by adjusting the volume borders to include the LVOT or AV root. Using the same modes, the aorta can be assessed in long-axis views. Cropping one-half of the circumference leads to free visual access to the lumen inside. AV failure due to thrombus may easily be identified (Fig. 22.21).

Right heart valves

Because of the same technical limitations as for the aortic valve, right heart valves are extremely difficult to image on RT3D. The tricuspid valve can be optimally visualized in only 11–39% [22,23], and the pulmonary valve only in 13%. Surgical decision making on the basis of visual information is possible in 13% (tricuspid valve) and 0% (pulmonary valve) respectively [23].

The morphology of the tricuspid valve can be assessed using 3D zoom. The ME RV inflow–outflow view is the best approach (Fig. 22.22).

ASD closure and atrial findings

Three-dimensional TEE is valuable for assessing the size and location of atrial septal defects and their relationship to neighboring structures, and for measuring the defect and rim size (Fig. 22.23). 3D-TEE was evaluated against balloon stretched size measurement (BSD) for transcatheter ASD closure, and was found to correlate well with BSD in cases with a single ASD, but poorly in multiple defects. The authors therefore described 3D-TEE and transcatheter methods as complementary techniques [29].

RT3D-TEE may also provide information that helps to differentiate between thrombus and atrial structures (Eustachian valve, pectinate muscles, coumadin ridge). Further reports demonstrate the capacity to evaluate atrial tumors [30], and assess the morphology of the left atrial appendage (Figs. 22.24, 22.25) [31].

Ventricular function

Determination of global and regional ventricular function is an essential part of every TEE examination. Ejection fraction (EF) calculation using Simpson's rule has been the gold standard for many years. However, the method has significant limitations.

With the introduction of RT3D, 3D-based LV volume calculation is possible, and along with semi-automated endocardial detection and automatic tracking this method presents a big step forward for obtaining LV volumes and EF. The 3D-TTE approach has been validated compared to 2D and cardiac magnetic resonance (CMR) techniques [32–35]. Case reports indicate that 3D-TEE is feasible, although further validation is required [30].

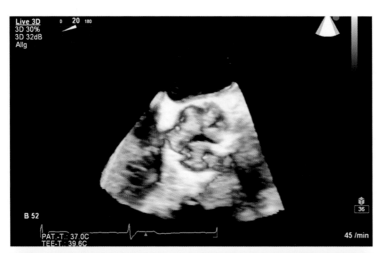

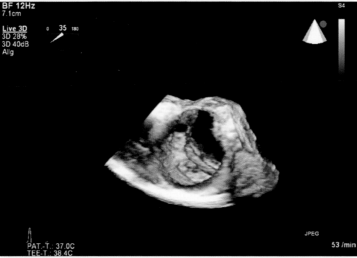

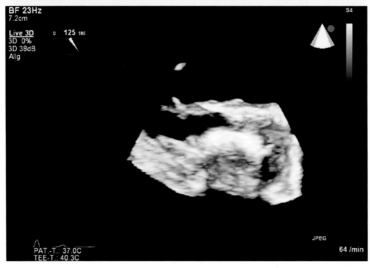

Figure 22.20. From top to bottom: heavily calcified stenotic AV, bicuspid AV, transapical transcatheter AV replacement with the device catheter in place.

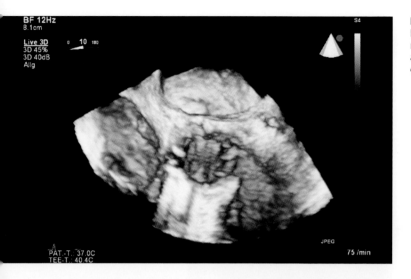

Figure 22.21. Case 4: a patient with history of AV replacement, with a mechanical prosthesis four months ago, and a stuck AV prosthesis due to partial clotting.

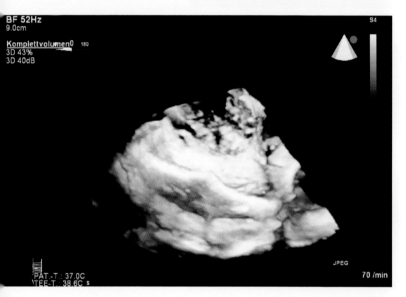

Figure 22.22. Tricuspid valve obtained from RT3D-TEE. Due to the thin leaflets the leaflet body does not appear as continuous tissue but multiply perforated.

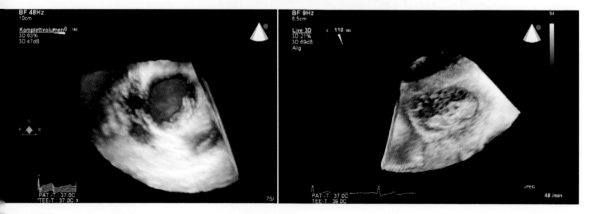

Figure 22.23. Atrial septal defect (left); persistent foramen ovale (right).

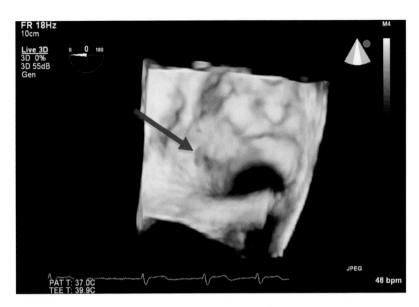

Figure 22.24. Spontaneous contrast ascending from the left atrial appendage.

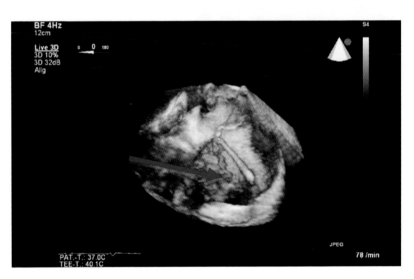

Figure 22.25. A thrombus floating within the cavity of the right atrium, with its origin most likely from a central venous catheter tip.

Three-dimensional volume acquisition for global and regional LV function assessment is achieved in single-beat or multibeat (full volume) mode, based on four-chamber views from either apical windows (TTE) or mid-esophageal level (TEE). Using built-in software, the mitral aspect of the inferoseptal, anterolateral, anterior, and inferior walls and the apex has to be defined in end-diastolic and end-systolic frames, followed by automated border tracking. The system will then calculate LV volume frame by frame throughout the cardiac cycle, finally calculating EF from end-diastolic and end-systolic volumes.

To obtain regional information, the total volume is subdivided into 17 segmental volumes. Each segmental volume is analyzed separately to obtain regional information and timing information (Fig. 22.26).

Because of its complex shape, quantifying RV function remains challenging, and currently it is done by visual assessment. TomTec has a tool that calculates RV volume and RVEF based on 3D data sets. Similar to the LV, RV volume calculation is based on a dynamic surface model and semi-automated tracking in four-chamber, sagittal, and coronal planes. RV volumes and RVEF correlated reasonably well against magnetic resonance quantification (Fig. 22.27) [36].

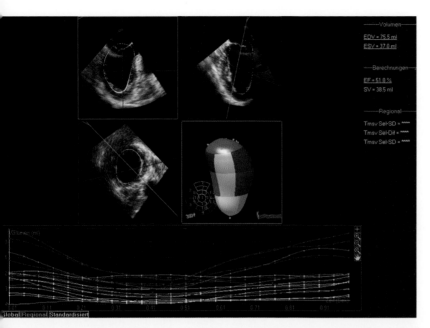

Figure 22.26. LV volume and LVEF calculation from 3D dataset. LV volumes are calculated frame by frame in an semi-automated fashion after key points of MR and apex in both end-diastolic and end-systolic frames have been marked. Besides global information, the tool provides regional information calculated from a 17- segment volume model.

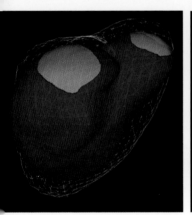
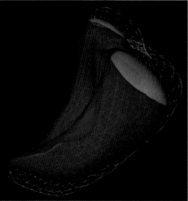
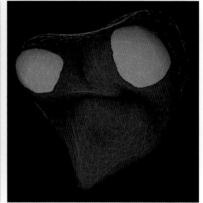

Figure 22.27. RV volumes and RVEF can be calculated using a TomTec software package. Following the same principle as the LV model, it relies on a dynamic surface model and semi-automated tracking. Schematic model reprinted with permission of TomTec.

Future prospects

Despite the recent developments in 3D echocardiography, further progress will depend on resolving the current limitations in RT3D technology, particularly on temporal and spatial resolution. Improvements in spatial resolution in lateral dimensions will enable the evaluation of right heart valves and other cardiac structures of a thin texture. The merger of enhanced 3D technology with myocardial deformation imaging will facilitate rapid, accurate, and powerful functional analysis of the heart.

References

1. Dekker DL, Piziali RL, Dong E. A system for ultrasonically imaging the human heart in three dimensions. *Computers and Biomedical Research* 1974; 7: 544–53.

2. Matsumoto M, Matsuo H, Kitabatake A, *et al.* Three-dimensional echocardiograms and two-dimensional echocardiographic images at desired planes by a computerized system. *Ultrasound Med Biol* 1977; **3**: 163–78.

3. Geiser EA, Lupkiewicz SM, Christie LG, *et al.* A framework for three-dimensional time-varying

reconstruction of the human left ventricle: sources of error and estimation of their magnitude. *Comput Biomed Res* 1980; **13**: 225–41.

4. Ghosh A, Nanda NC, Maurer G. Three-dimensional reconstruction of echo-cardiographic images using the rotation method. *Ultrasound Med Biol* 1982; **8**: 655–61.

5. Nixon JV, Saffer SI, Lipscomb K, Blomqvist CG. Three-dimensional echoventriculography. *Am Heart J* 1983; **106**: 435–43.

6. Snyder JE, Kisslo J, von Ramm O. Real-time orthogonal mode scanning of the heart. I. System design. *J Am Coll Cardiol* 1986; **7**: 1279–85.

7. Fulton DR, Marx GR, Pandian NG, *et al.* Dynamic three-dimensional echocardiographic imaging of congenital heart defects in infants and children by computer-controlled tomographic parallel slicing using a single integrated ultrasound instrument. *Echocardiography* 1994; **11**: 155–64.

8. Martin RW, Bashein G, Zimmer R, Sutherland J. An endoscopic micromanipulator for multiplanar transesophageal imaging. *Ultrasound Med Biol* 1986; **12**: 965–75.

9. Pandian NG, Nanda NC, Schwartz SL, *et al.* Three-dimensional and four-dimensional transesophageal echocardiographic imaging of the heart and aorta in humans using a computed tomographic imaging probe. *Echocardiography* 1992; **9**: 677–87.

10. Sapin PM, Schroeder KD, Smith MD, DeMaria AN, King DL. Three-dimensional echocardiographic measurement of left ventricular volume in vitro: comparison with two-dimensional echocardiography and cineventriculography. *J Am Coll Cardiol* 1993; **22**: 1530–7.

11. Roelandt JR, ten Cate FJ, Vletter WB, Taams MA. Ultrasonic dynamic three-dimensional visualization of the heart with a multiplane transesophageal imaging transducer. *J Am Soc Echocardiogr* 1994; **7**: 217–29.

12. Kisslo J, Firek B, Ota T, *et al.* Real-time volumetric echocardiography: the technology and the possibilities. *Echocardiography* 2000; **17**: 773–9.

13. Pua EC, Idriss SF, Wolf PD, Smith SW. Real-time 3D transesophageal echocardiography. *Ultrason Imaging* 2004; **26**: 217–32.

14. Yang HS, Bansal RC, Mookadam F, *et al.* Practical guide for three-dimensional transthoracic echocardiography using a fully sampled matrix array transducer. *J Am Soc Echocardiogr* 2008; **21**: 979–89.

15. Garcia-Orta R, Moreno E, Vidal M, *et al.* Three-dimensional versus two-dimensional transesophageal echocardiography in mitral valve repair. *J Am Soc Echocardiogr* 2007; **20**: 4–12.

16. Manda J, Kesanolla SK, Hsuing MC, *et al.* Comparison of real time two-dimensional with live/real time three-dimensional transesophageal echocardiography in the evaluation of mitral valve prolapse and chordae rupture. *Echocardiography* 2008; **25**: 1131–7.

17. Grewal J, Mankad S, Freeman WK, *et al.* Real-time three-dimensional transesophageal echocardiography in the intraoperative assessment of mitral valve disease. *J Am Soc Echocardiogr* 2009; **22**: 34–41.

18. Jungwirth B, Mackensen GB. Real-time 3-dimensional echocardiography in the operating room. *Semin Cardiothorac Vasc Anesth* 2008; **12**: 248–64.

19. Ender J, Koncar-Zeh J, Mukherjee C, *et al.* Value of augmented reality-enhanced transesophageal echocardiography (TEE) for determining optimal annuloplasty ring size during mitral valve repair. *Ann Thorac Surg* 2008; **86**: 1473–8.

20. Sugeng L, Shernan SK, Weinert L, *et al.* Real-time three-dimensional transesophageal echocardiography in valve disease: comparison with surgical findings and evaluation of prosthetic valves. *J Am Soc Echocardiogr* 2008; **21**: 1347–54.

21. Jungwirth B, Adams DB, Mathew JP, *et al.* Mitral valve prolapse and systolic anterior motion illustrated by real time three-dimensional transesophageal echocardiography. *Anesth Analg* 2008; **107**: 1822–4.

22. Sugeng L, Shernan SK, Salgo IS, *et al.* Live 3-dimensional transesophageal echocardiography: initial experience using the fully-sampled matrix array probe. *J Am Coll Cardiol* 2008; **52**: 446–9.

23. Tschernich HD, Mora B, Hiesmayr M. Visibility of cardiac valves using real-time 3D-transoesophageal echocardiography (RT3D-TOE) in the OR: a feasibility study. *J Cardiothorac Vasc Anesth* 2008; **22**: S8.

24. Scohy TV, Soliman OI, Lecomte PV, *et al.* Intraoperative real time three-dimensional transesophageal echocardiographic measurement of hemodynamic, anatomic and functional changes after aortic valve replacement. *Echocardiography* 2009; **26**: 96–9.

25. Blot-Souletie N, Hébrard A, Acar P, Carrié D, Puel J. Comparison of accuracy of aortic valve area assessment in aortic stenosis by real time three-dimensional echocardiography in biplane mode versus two-dimensional transthoracic and transesophageal echocardiography. *Echocardiography* 2007; **24**: 1065–72.

26. Armen TA, Vandse R, Bickle K, Nathan N. Three-dimensional echocardiographic evaluation of an incidental quadricuspid aortic valve. *Eur J Echocardiogr* 2008; **9**: 318–20.

27. Medina HM, Vazquez J, Pritchett A, Lakkis N, Dokainish H. Comprehensive imaging including

three-dimensional echocardiography of an infected, ruptured sinus of Valsalva aneurysm. *Echocardiography* 2007; **24**: 1096–8.

28. Malagoli A, Barbieri A, Modena MG. Bicuspid aortic valve regurgitation: quantification of anatomic regurgitant orifice area by 3D transesophageal echocardiography reconstruction. *Echocardiography* 2008; **25**: 797–8.

29. Abdel-Massih T, Dulac Y, Taktak A, *et al.* Assessment of atrial septal defect size with 3D-transesophageal echocardiography: comparison with balloon method. *Echocardiography* 2005; **22**: 121–7.

30. Scohy TV, Lecomte PV, McGhie J, *et al.* Intraoperative real time three-dimensional transesophageal echocardiographic evaluation of right atrial tumor. *Echocardiography* 2008; **25**: 646–9.

31. Shah SJ, Bardo DM, Sugeng L, *et al.* Real-time three-dimensional transesophageal echocardiography of the left atrial appendage: initial experience in the clinical setting. *J Am Soc Echocardiogr* 2008; **21**: 1362–8.

32. Caiani EG, Corsi C, Zamorano J, *et al.* Improved semiautomated quantification of left ventricular volumes and ejection fraction using 3-dimensional echocardiography with a full matrix-array transducer: comparison with magnetic resonance imaging. *J Am Soc Echocardiogr* 2005; **18**: 779–88.

33. Corsi C, Lang RM, Veronesi F, *et al.* Volumetric quantification of global and regional left ventricular function from real-time three-dimensional echocardiographic images. *Circulation* 2005; **112**: 1161–70.

34. Soliman OI, Krenning BJ, Geleijnse ML, *et al.* Quantification of left ventricular volumes and function in patients with cardiomyopathies by real-time three-dimensional echocardiography: a head-to-head comparison between two different semiautomated endocardial border detection algorithms. *J Am Soc Echocardiogr* 2007; **20**: 1042–9.

35. Sugeng L, Mor-Avi V, Weinert L, *et al.* Quantitative assessment of left ventricular size and function: side-by-side comparison of real-time three-dimensional echocardiography and computed tomography with magnetic resonance reference. *Circulation* 2006; **114**: 654–61.

36. Niemann PS, Pinho L, Balbach T, *et al.* Anatomically oriented right ventricular volume measurements with dynamic three-dimensional echocardiography validated by 3-Tesla magnetic resonance imaging. *J Am Coll Cardiol* 2007; **50**: 1668–76.

23

Recent developments in Doppler imaging

Heinz D. Tschernich

Introduction

Recent developments in Doppler imaging have enhanced our capability to quantify myocardial function. Conventional techniques, including two-dimensional (2D) imaging, spectral and color-flow Doppler, have clear limitations. Quantification of ventricular function or detection of ischemia from blood-pool measurements have been shown to be load-dependent, insensitive, and unspecific.

To overcome these limitations, a number of technologies have been introduced, placing special emphasis on myocardial quantification. These include pulsed-wave tissue Doppler imaging (PW-TDI), color Doppler myocardial imaging (CDMI), and speckle-tracking echocardiography (STE).

All of these technologies are available in both transthoracic (TTE) and transesophageal echocardiography (TEE). The aim of this chapter is to introduce these recent developments, outlining their physical background and discussing their main areas of application and their limitations.

Tissue Doppler imaging

Historical background

The technique of using pulsed-wave Doppler (PWD) to measure myocardial velocities was first published in 1989 [1,2]. A technical principle in pulsed Doppler blood-flow studies that was developed to improve signal quality was to filter out the low-frequency Doppler noise generated by the contracting myocardium. In the late 1980s this filtered noise was recognized as a potential source of information for the assessment of myocardial motion, leading to the development of tissue Doppler. Further developments based on PWD technology tended to describe myocardial motion not only in terms of velocity but also by quantifying myocardial deformation. The concept of using color-flow Doppler imaging – a technique also based on PWD – as a means of assessing myocardial motion was first described in 1992 [3]. In 1998, Heimdal et al. [4] introduced cardiac real-time strain and strain rate analysis as a novel extension of tissue Doppler. The research group from the Norwegian University of Science and Technology published basic concepts and showed practical applications of color-coded strain rate displays in echocardiography [5]. Subsequently, Sutherland et al. [6] and Hatle [7] summarized the emerging methods in tissue Doppler analysis of left ventricular (LV) wall motion.

Since traditional Doppler techniques for evaluating myocardial function are limited by angle dependency, recent technical developments have chosen a different approach for assessing myocardial motion. Myocardial tissue motion information has been extracted from the gray scale of the 2D image. The principles of this technique, called speckle tracking, were first published between 2001 and 2004 [8–10].

Technology

Tissue Doppler imaging (PW-TDI) uses Doppler technology to measure velocities at a certain point in the myocardium. The PWD principle not only allows the detection of velocities but is also able to obtain spatial information. In pulsed-wave mode ultrasound pulses are transmitted along an image line at a constant rate (pulsed repetition frequency, PRF). Rather than acquiring the complete wave, backscattered from the object, only one sample of the reflected wave is analyzed, at a fixed time after transmission of the pulse. The time is defined by the distance between the scanner and the object and is called the range gate. For a non-moving object the reflected signal will be identical, whereas for a moving object the backscattered signals will be shifted in phase according to the velocity of the moving object. By analyzing the phase shift of two pulses transmitted at an interval of a quarter of a wavelength, not only the velocity but also the direction of movement of the object can be obtained.

Core Topics in Transesophageal Echocardiography, ed. Robert Feneck, John Kneeshaw, and Marco Ranucci.
Published by Cambridge University Press. © Cambridge University Press 2010.

PWD technique for assessment of myocardial velocities

Signals from blood flow and the moving myocardium can be discriminated by their signal characteristics. Blood will generate signals of high Doppler-shift frequencies (reflecting blood velocities in about the meter/second range) but low amplitude, whereas moving myocardium will generate signals characterized by low Doppler-shift frequencies (centimeter/second range) but high amplitude (up to 40 dB) (Fig. 23.1). While those low-velocity/high-amplitude signals are filtered out for blood-flow measurements, they are used as the primary signals in tissue Doppler imaging (Fig. 23.2).

Data acquisition

PW-TDI is the simplest approach to data acquisition, and is available on all current cardiac ultrasound systems, during both TTE and TEE exams. It measures the instantaneous peak velocities from the myocardium at a distinct area defined by the sample volume. An area and not a point is chosen, since the myocardial wall moves during the cardiac cycle, but the sample volume remains at the same point. For longitudinal motion the sampled area may measure up to 12–16 mm for velocity data collected from basal LV segments, and up to 20–22 mm for data collected from basal right ventricular (RV) segments (Fig. 23.3). Therefore spatial resolution is poor. On the other hand, PW-TDI has an excellent temporal resolution of about 3–4 ms, based on a typical sampling rate of approximately 250 samples per second.

A standard sample volume should be 6 mm in size, as a compromise between maximizing axial resolution and keeping the sample volume within the myocardium during the cardiac cycle. The sample volume should be positioned in the center of the myocardium with ideally no (or insignificant) angle between the insonating ultrasound beam and the direction of the moving myocardial wall. To ensure

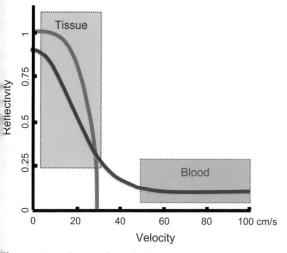

Figure 23.1. Ultrasound signal characteristics: blood (red) versus myocardium (blue).

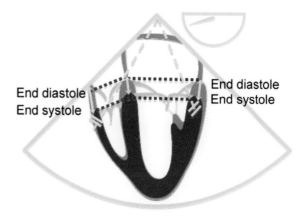

Figure 23.3. Spatial resolution of the PW-TDI signal collected from basal segments of the LV lateral wall and RV free wall. The range gate of the PWD remains at the same point, while the myocardial walls move towards the apex.

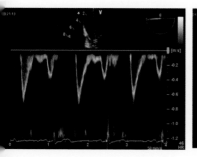
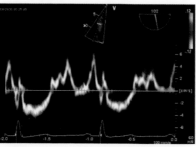

Figure 23.2. Comparison of PWD signals received from blood pool (mitral inflow, left) and tissue (LV inferior wall, right).

369

aliasing is avoided, the Doppler velocity range should be set to values slightly above normal myocardial velocities. These will rarely exceed 20 cm/s, but since increased values may be found in young or hypovolemic patients, and in patients with decreased afterload or receiving inotropic treatment, the velocity range should be adapted to higher values in these cases.

Color Doppler myocardial imaging

PW-TDI suffers from the following limitations:

- the need for manual mapping
- limited spatial resolution
- the inability to simultaneously record different ventricular wall segments

This information may be acquired by defining different range gates along the scan line. Many transmitted pulses would be needed to estimate the regional velocities, which again would result in a poor frame rate.

In contrast, color Doppler myocardial imaging (CDMI) uses the principle of color-flow mapping to measure velocities in different directions at a reasonable frame rate. The underlying principle relies on the measurement of the local phase shift from captured signals of subsequent pulses (at least two) along a scan line. To determine the phase of a sinusoid, two samples transmitted with a maximum delay of a quarter of wavelength are required. To obtain the phase shift between two subsequently received signals, two pairs of samples are required. Finally, the information along all the scan lines is put together to define velocity and direction within the myocardium. The method is called "autocorrelation" and is used in the same way as in conventional color-flow Doppler (CFD). The only difference is the velocity range of their primary signals and the filtering they use to eliminate noise: CFD filters out the slow-moving, strongly reflecting structures of the myocardial walls, which generate the primary signal in CDMI.

PW-TDI, CDMI, and transesophageal echocardiography

Although TDI was primarily developed and evaluated for TTE, its feasibility in TEE has been shown in several studies. Simmons et al. compared TTE with TEE-CDMI data at several stages of cardiac surgery and found similar data from comparable segments [11]. In an animal model, Cheung et al. found TTE and TEE-TDI data to

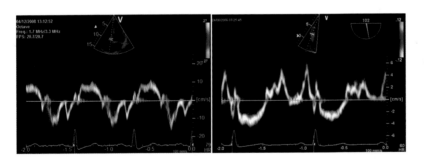

Figure 23.4. Comparison of PW-TDI signals from TTE (left) and TEE (right). Because of the direction of motion of the myocardium and the probe position, the TEE curves appear as a mirror image of the TTE curves from the same segments.

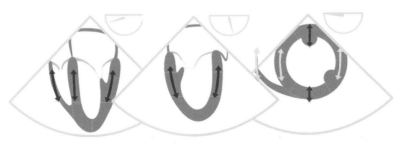

Figure 23.5. Main motion directions of the myocardium that can be assessed by TEE and relevant TEE views.

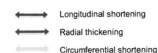

Longitudinal shortening

Radial thickening

Circumferential shortening

be comparable from measurements during the isovolumic (IVA) and ejection phase (S) of systole, and from early diastole (E) [12]. Skarvan and colleagues studied global and regional systolic and diastolic function before and after coronary bypass surgery using PW-TDI. Comparing it to the transmitral filling pattern, they found early changes in myocardial function after mammary artery grafting, indicating an improvement in systolic function accompanied by impairment in diastolic function [13]. Radial function from transgastric short-axis views during cardiac surgery and one hour postoperatively were investigated using CDMI by Sloth *et al.* [14]. At different stages of loading and unloading and during withdrawal from cardiopulmonary bypass they demonstrated the reliability of myocardial velocity data.

Normal data, parameters, and curve interpretation

In interpreting velocity, displacement, and strain rate data, curves acquired from TEE are like a mirror image of the equivalent TTE data. To obtain, for example, longitudinal TEE views, the probe is positioned at mid-esophageal level behind the atria, but it needs to be placed at the apex to receive similar views from TTE. Longitudinal motion of the myocardium is therefore displayed in a different orientation, depending on which approach was used to acquire the image. Thus, TTE-TDI data shows positive systolic and negative diastolic values, whereas TEE-TDI data presents negative in systole and positive in diastole (Fig. 23.4).

For correct interpretation of myocardial velocity and deformation, the main direction of motion of the ventricle needs to be identified. From the TEE view, the following motion can be assessed by Doppler myocardial imaging (PW-TDI and CDMI):

- The longitudinal motion of LV walls can be obtained from mid-esophageal level in the four-chamber view (ME four-chamber) for the inferoseptal and anterolateral walls, in the two-chamber view (ME two-chamber) for the anterior and inferior walls, and in the long-axis view (ME LAX) for the anteroseptal and inferolateral walls. RV longitudinal motion is difficult to obtain from TEE views since there is a significant angle between insonation and the direction of the RV wall motion. The exception is the free posterior wall in the ME RV inflow–outflow view (Fig. 23.5). Radial motion can be recorded from transgastric (TG) short-axis planes (TG mid SAX, TG basal SAX). Since only walls with a radial motion vector that is parallel to insonation can be assessed, radial motion can only be measured from the anterior and inferior wall at basal and mid-papillary level by TDI using TEE (Fig. 23.5).

- The assessment of circumferential motion using TEE has the same limitations as radial motion. It can only be obtained from TG basal SAX and TG mid SAX, but the inferoseptal and anterolateral walls will be in line with the ultrasound beams. Once the probe is turned to the right, the circumferential motion pattern of the RV free wall can be assessed.

Myocardial architecture

The ventricular myocardium in normal hearts is composed of three layers of muscle fibers: a superficial (subepicardial), a middle, and a deep layer (subendocardial) [15]. The three layers can be identified by the different orientation of the muscle fibers. All three layers are present in the LV. The middle layer is missing in the RV.

The superficial layer of the heart (Fig. 23.6) consists of muscle fibers running from the base to the apex in an oblique manner, crossing the anterior and

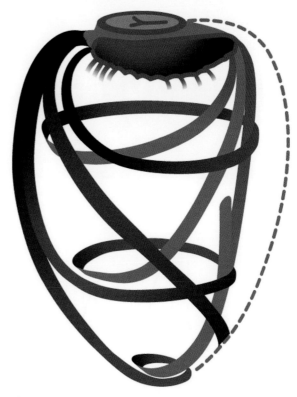

Figure 23.6. Helical fiber orientation of the myocardium, consisting of three layers.

posterior interventricular groove. The fibers in the superficial layer of the RV are arranged more circumferentially than in the LV.

The middle layer in LV myocardium consists of circumferentially orientated myocardial fibers. This layer is thickest at the middle, thinning out towards both the basal and apical regions, with a small apical aperture through which the superficial muscle fibers invaginate to become subendocardial, and a large oval aperture at the base. No proper middle layer can be defined in the normal RV.

Longitudinally arranged fibers form the deep (subendocardial) layer, passing through the vortices toward the papillary muscles, the atrioventricular orifices, and the arterial orifices, and to the ventricular septum.

Myocardial velocity: waveform

Several components define a typical myocardial velocity curve during one cardiac cycle. Whereas systole is characterized by two spikes, isovolumic contraction (IVC) and ejection phase (systolic contraction, S'), in diastole three spikes can be identified: isovolumic relaxation (IVR), early relaxation (E'), and atrial contraction (A') (Fig. 23.7). Since each phase contains essential information, proper timing is essential for interpretation of each specific spike in the curve. The easiest way to achieve accurate timing is by using conventional spectral Doppler flow curves of both mitral inflow and aortic flow (Fig. 23.8).

Comparison of PW-TDI and CDMI velocity data

Curves acquired from PW-TDI and CDMI appear similar in shape. However, on closer inspection there are differences. Although the spikes occur at the same time, velocities measured from PW-TDI will be higher than from CDMI. In addition, the PW-TDI

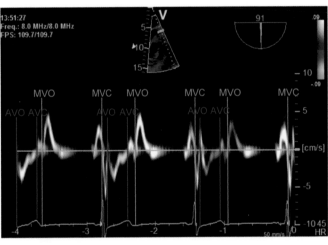

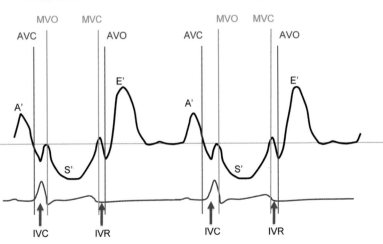

Figure 23.7. Typical waveforms of PW- and CDMI. Systole with isovolumic contraction (IVC) and ejection phase (S') diastole with isovolumic relaxation (IVR) E', A'. Correct allocation of the different phases using timing. AVC, aortic valve closure; AVO, aortic valve opening; MVC mitral valve closure; MVO, mitral valve opening;.

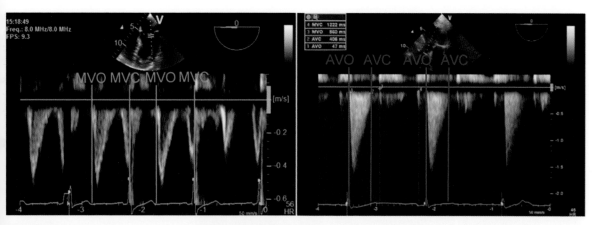

Figure 23.8. Timing performed using mitral inflow (left) and flow across the aortic valve (right).

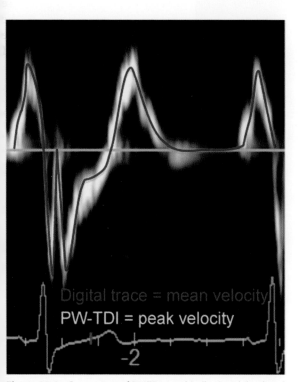

Figure 23.9. Comparison of PW-TDI signal (yellow) and the digital processed signal of the CDMI (red).

signal does not look as sharp as the CDMI curves. The low spatial resolution leads to a range of velocities being measured at the same time, from minimum to maximum velocities. Peak values measured using PW-TDI are therefore higher than the "mean velocities" of the digitally processed CDMI signal (Fig. 23.9).

A complete regional myocardial mapping of all segments using PW-TDI can only be performed sequentially segment by segment (Fig. 23.10), whereas with CDMI there is the possibility of analyzing multiple velocity profiles from anywhere within the acquired scanned sector. The software therefore allows parallel analysis of all six segments of both LV walls in one plane (Fig. 23.11). The advantage of an immediate comparison of the curves from different segments becomes clear in the case of arrhythmias, or for an easy overview of the regional distribution of a functional pathology.

Color Doppler myocardial imaging: from velocity to strain rate

CDMI allows us not only to superimpose myocardial velocity on the 2D image by velocity color coding, but also to track serial changes in ventricular wall motion velocity over time with the use of M-mode CDMI. Two-dimensional CDMI provides a rapid qualitative visual assessment of wall dynamics, allowing us to analyze simultaneously various myocardial regions, and provides a good spatial resolution that even permits differentiation of the velocity profiles between the subendocardial and subepicardial layers (Fig. 23.12).

Two-dimensional CDMI, however, is limited by its temporal resolution. In contrast, M-mode CDMI is characterized by high spatial and temporal resolution, as sampling is performed only on a single line (Fig. 23.12). Since the analysis of CDMI data is done by post-processing digital raw data, M-mode presentation is not limited by the physical lines of the ultrasound beams but can also be modified to follow the shape of the myocardial wall, for instance (curved anatomical M-mode, CAMM) (Fig. 23.13).

373

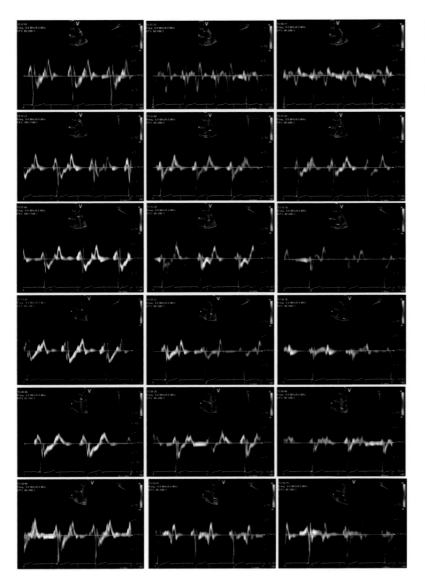

Figure 23.10. PW-TDI curves from anterolateral (1st row), anterior (2nd row), anteroseptal (3th row), inferoseptal (4th row), inferior (5th row), and inferolateral wall (6th row). Samples from basal, mid, and apical segments show base-to-apex gradient in velocities.

Velocity is the basic parameter obtained from myocardial motion analysis. However, the velocity of a myocardial region can be generated either through active contraction or passively through normally contracting segments exerting force on a non-contracting segment. Since myocardial function is expressed by contractility, it is necessary not only to measure velocity but also to quantify myocardial deformation.

Myocardial deformation describes the ability of the muscle fibers to shorten in systole and lengthen in diastole. Deformation can be defined by two parameters: strain and strain rate. In cardiac muscle physiology, strain is directly related to fiber shortening and strain rate to the velocity of shortening, which is a measure of contractility.

Strain (ε)

Strain is defined as the extent of deformation of an object (shortening, lengthening), normalized to its original dimension:

$$\varepsilon = \frac{L_1 - L_0}{L_0} = \frac{\Delta L}{L_0} \qquad (23.1)$$

where L_0 is the initial length of the object and L_1 its length after deformation (Fig. 23.14). Strain is a dimensionless quantity, and the resulting deformation

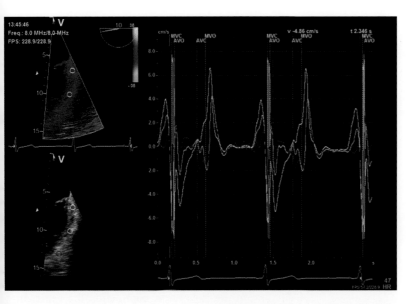

Figure 23.11. CDMI analysis of the LV lateral wall. Simultaneously obtained curves from the basal, mid, and apical segments, showing a typical base-to-apex gradient of myocardial velocities.

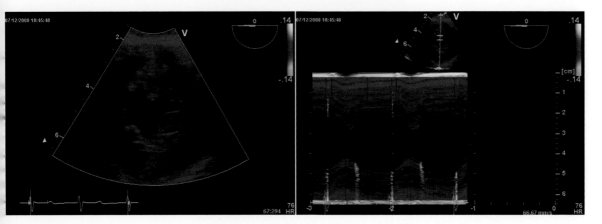

Figure 23.12. Possibilities in acquisition of CDMI images: 2D CDMI (left) and CDMI M-mode (right).

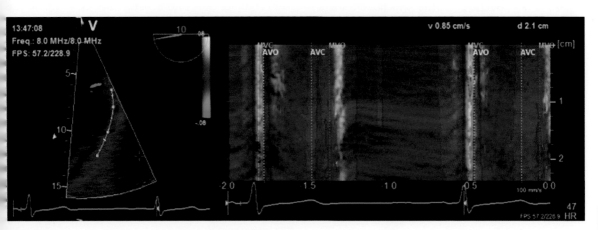

Figure 23.13. Curved anatomical M-mode analysis of a CDMI image.

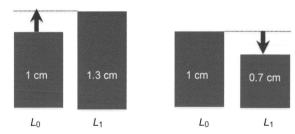

Figure 23.14. Two examples of strain. Lengthening of 30% = 30% strain (left); shortening of 30% = −30% strain (right).

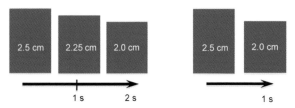

Figure 23.15. Two examples of strain rate. In both cases the object shortens 20% (−20% strain). On the left, deformation occurs in 2 seconds, an average strain rate of 0.2/2 s = 0.1 s^{-1}. On the right, the object needs just 1 second to shorten by the same amount, a strain rate of 0.2/1 s = 0.2 s^{-1}.

of the myocardium is expressed as either a fractional or a percentage change from the original dimension.

Strain rate (SR)

Strain rate (SR) is the change of strain over time (t), in other words the speed of deformation, and it can be derived from

$$SR = \frac{\Delta L}{L_0 t} \qquad (23.2)$$

with ΔL being the change of length, L_0 the original length, and t the time during which deformation occurs. Therefore, although the extent of deformation may be the same, SR may differ according to the time taken for the deformation to occur (Fig. 23.15).

The measurement unit of SR is s^{-1}.

Clinical applications of PW-TDI and CDMI

Myocardial motion and deformation

The determination of contractile force by blood-flow-derived parameters is hampered by major limitations, including load dependency. The assessment of contractility based on myocardial motion and deformation appears much more promising. The following describes the approach to and the clinical value of myocardial motion and deformation analysis for evaluating ventricular function.

Global systolic function

Systole consists of two phases of contraction, the isovolumic contraction time (ICT) and the ejection time (ET). During isovolumic contraction the ventricle is not influenced by load changes, and thus the ventricle applies force to a specific volume (end-diastolic) which does not change within that phase. During the ejection phase the LV volume is ejected until LV pressure drops below aortic pressure and the aortic valve closes. Parameters measured during ICT may indicate systolic function independent of load, while ejection-phase indices will tend to be influenced by load changes.

Isovolumic phase indices: acceleration during isovolumic contraction

Isovolumic contraction can easily be quantified by PW-TDI or CDMI. To measure isovolumic acceleration (IVA) one has to image LV walls (anterior, anterolateral) or RV walls (free, inferior) from the mid-esophageal level. In PW-TDI, sample volumes should be placed at the base immediately below the insertion of the mitral valve leaflets (LV) or the tricuspid valve leaflets (RV) (Fig. 23.16). In CDMI, recordings from the basal wall regions must be made. Analysis can be performed off-line, locating the sample volume as described above.

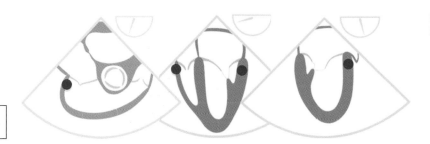

Figure 23.16. Sample regions in TEE for IVA acquisition.

Tissue velocity traces show a characteristic spike representing isovolumic contraction of the myocardium. The slope of the spike equals the acceleration of myocardial velocities and therefore determines contractility (Fig. 23.17) Studies have suggested that IVA is a load-independent measure of contractility [16,17], with a normal range for IVA of 2.86 ± 1.23 m/s^2, decreasing with reduced systolic function. Limitations of IVA are caused by the brief duration of the event (10–40 ms), and therefore high frame rates (150–250 frames per second) are required to display isovolumic contraction. Isovolumic contraction may be determined from myocardial deformation using SR [18].

Ejection-phase indices

During the ejection phase of systole, the mitral ring moves downwards to the apex, the aortic valve opens, and blood is ejected. In contrast to blood-pool-derived parameters (e.g. ejection fraction, stroke volume), myocardial deformation parameters (velocity, strain, and strain rate) can be used in order to primarily define the contractile force causing ejection.

Atrioventricular displacement: mitral ring motion and tricuspid annular plane systolic excursion (TAPSE)

Annular displacement during systole is the result of the longitudinal shortening of both ventricles, and it is therefore a measure of overall systolic function. It can be quantified either by M-mode or by CDMI.

Using CDMI, the velocity of the atrioventricular plane during systole is measured. From these velocity

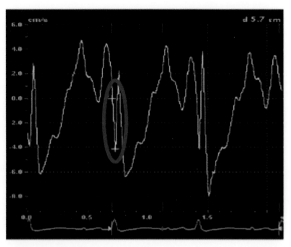

Figure 23.17. Spike during isovolumic contraction. The ascending slope represents contractile force (= IVA).

data, spatial displacement of the atrioventricular level can be calculated in terms of distances. The atrioventricular plane motion is then displayed either by color-coding segments according to the amount of spatial displacement or by individual curves obtained from sample volumes, placed at the region of the septal and/or lateral mitral ring, or the lateral tricuspid ring, respectively (Fig. 23.18). Normal values are shown in Table 23.1.

Myocardial velocities of the mitral and tricuspid ring

While annular displacement obtained from CDMI is derived from velocity data, peak systolic velocity

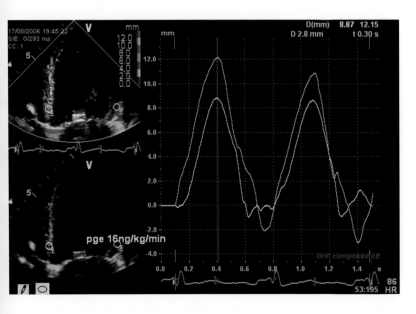

Figure 23.18. Annular displacement: parametric display (left upper) and curve presentation (right).

377

Table 23.1. Normal values for tricuspid ring motion and mitral ring motion

	Systolic ring excursion (mm, mean ± SD)
Tricuspid	20 ± 0.3
Mitral (septal)	12 ± 0.2
Mitral (lateral)	15 ± 0.3

Table 23. 2. Normal values of tricuspid and mitral ring velocities (in cm/s)

Segment	Ring velocity (cm/s)
RV free wall	9.96 ± 1.97
Inferoseptal	6.85 ± 1.34
LV anterolateral wall	8.64 ± 2.13

Table 23. 3. Normal strain and strain rate values of the RV and LV at basal segments

View	Segment	Peak systolic strain (%)	Peak systolic strain rate (s^{-1})
Apical four-chamber	Inferoseptal basal	21 ± 5	1.51 ± 0.35
	Anterolateral basal	13 ± 4	1.19 ± 0.26
	RV anterolateral basal	19 ± 6	1.50 ± 0.41
Apical two-chamber	Anterior basal	17 ± 6	1.50 ± 0.44

Table 23.4. Normal values of diastolic velocities and strain rate

View	Segment	Velocity (cm/s)		Strain rate (s^{-1})	
		E_m	A_m	E_m	A_m
Apical four-chamber	Inferoseptal basal	8.82 ± 2.49	5.01 ± 1.67	2.03 ± 0.48	1.09 ± 0.47
	Anterolateral basal	12.34 ± 2.1	4.35 ± 1.54	1.62 ± 0.65	0.74 ± 0.39
	RV anterolateral basal	10.04 ± 2.2	2.15 ± 7.90	2.10 ± 2.28	1.08 ± 1.16

can also be used to quantify left and right ventricular function.

Studies of left and right ventricular long-axis function have identified normal values [19,20], and have shown longitudinal shortening to be dominant over radial shortening in healthy young subjects, changing with age. Normal values are shown in Table 23.2. Data comparing RV fractional area change (FAC), TAPSE, and peak tricuspid annulus systolic (TA Sa) velocities suggested an excellent correlation between all of them, and have defined normal values for TA Sa velocities as > 10.5 cm/s [21].

Myocardial deformation is directly related to the amount and velocity of fiber shortening. Therefore ε and SR have been demonstrated to be superior over tissue Doppler velocity for tracking local systolic function [22]. This is because ε and SR are less sensitive to segment tethering and cardiac translation. Peak systolic strain and peak systolic strain rate obtained from basal segments of the left ventricle may accurately reflect global ventricular function. Normal values are shown in Table 23.3.

Global diastolic function

Conventional methods, including mitral inflow and pulmonary venous flow, are strongly influenced by loading conditions. Combining TDI information with data from mitral inflow and pulmonary venous flow improves the assessment of diastolic function and yields additional information about diastolic left atrial (LA) and end-diastolic LV pressures.

Interpretation of myocardial velocity data in diastole

There are two waves, corresponding to early filling (E_m = E′) and atrial contraction (A_m = A′). In healthy humans, the peak of E_m precedes the peak of LV-filling E velocity, suggesting that LV filling is initiated by active relaxation of the myocardium generating a negative pressure in the LV cavity. Normal values are shown in Table 23.4 [20].

Myocardial velocities and diastolic grading

Compared to LV filling profiles, myocardial velocities show a decrease in peak velocities in early filling and an increase in atrial contraction, suggesting an inverse E_m/A_m ratio, becoming more pronounced with increasing deterioration of diastolic dysfunction (Fig. 23.19).

Since there is no pseudonormalization in myocardial relaxation, TDI can be used to unmask pseudonormalization in diastolic dysfunction (Fig. 20.20).

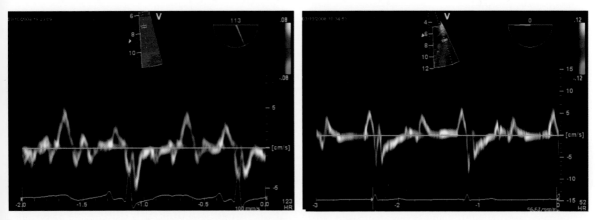

Figure 23.19. Normal diastolic myocardial velocity profile (left) versus diastolic dysfunction with inverse E_m/A_m ratio and decreased absolute velocities (right).

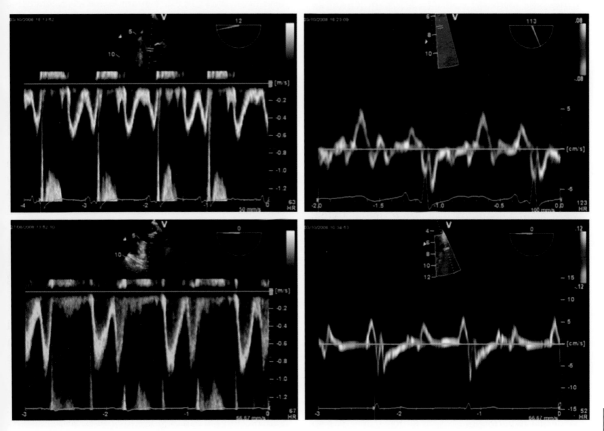

Figure 23.20. Normal diastolic function versus pseudonormalization: mitral inflow profile (left) and myocardial velocity profile (right).

Evaluation of left ventricular filling pressures

Standard Doppler methods (mitral E/A ratio, S/D ratio, isovolumic relaxation time, deceleration time) are limited for estimating LV filling pressures since they cannot separate the effects of LV relaxation from preload as confounding variables. However, when combined with TDI velocities, these confounding effects can be separated. Since mitral E velocity results from an interaction of both LA pressure and LV relaxation, whereas E_m is related primarily to LV relaxation, the E/E_m ratio may be used to predict LA pressure. This theoretical concept has been validated in a relatively heterogeneous population of patients undergoing right heart catheterization [23]. Three stages can be discriminated:

- when LV relaxation is normal and LA pressure is normal, both E and E_m are elevated
- when LV relaxation is impaired but LA pressure remains normal, both E and E_m are decreased
- when LV relaxation is impaired and LA pressure is increased, E is elevated but E_m is decreased.

Thus the E/E_m ratio will increase with deterioration of diastolic function. An E/E_m ratio > 15 is associated with a mean LA pressure > 15 mmHg.

Since the E/E_m ratio is easy to obtain and is closely related to LV filling pressures, its clinical value is proven as a predictor of survival, especially after myocardial infarction [24,25]. It has therefore been incorporated in the European diastolic heart failure guidelines [26]. In "heart failure with normal EF" (HFNEF), an E/E_m > 15 suggests diagnostic evidence of diastolic LV dysfunction from the use of TDI alone. If TDI yields values suggestive of diastolic LV dysfunction ($15 > E/E' > 8$), it needs to be supplemented with other non-invasive investigations (blood-flow Doppler of mitral inflow, pulmonary venous flow, evidence of atrial fibrillation, BNP or NT-proBNP).

Assessment of hypertrophic myocardial function

Left ventricular hypertrophy may occur physiologically or pathologically (see Chapter 15). We need to be able to differentiate concentric hypertrophic cardiomyopathy without obstruction from "athlete's heart," a physiologic myocardium that presents with normal systolic and diastolic function although ventricular wall thickness is increased.

TDI velocities may be helpful in distinguishing myocardial hypertrophy seen in athletes' hearts from hypertrophic cardiomyopathy, where these velocities

are significantly decreased [27]. The best differentiation of pathologic from physiologic was provided by mean systolic annular velocity < 9 cm/s. Hypertrophic myocardium is also characterized by abnormal strain, presenting with regional differences in areas of localized hypertrophy. Results suggest that the greater the extent of segmental wall thickness, the greater the reduction in myocardial strain [28].

Transplant rejection

Early detection of organ rejection after heart transplant may also be aided by TDI, which may add information that can detect early changes in diastolic function as an indicator of rejection. Diastolic myocardial velocities may be reduced in heart transplant patients with rejection, and may return to normal after successful medical treatment [29].

Regional ventricular function

Regional myocardial velocities

Tissue Doppler technology has brought regional wall motion analysis to a more quantitative level. Since the sample volume can be placed in all of the segments, regional velocity mapping using PW-TDI was the first approach to assess regional ventricular function (Fig. 23.10).

CDMI may be more valuable. Since velocity data are available from every point of each wall, the sample volume can be placed wherever needed, and simultaneous data can be obtained from all three segments of each LV wall. With the simultaneous processing and curve display, regional mapping can easily be performed beat by beat.

However, regional ventricular function analysis based on velocity makes the direct comparison of absolute values difficult. The velocity of a segment can be the result of active contraction or passive motion – the "tethering effect," which can best be unmasked by deformation analysis.

Once regional ventricular function analysis is performed on local deformation, ε and SR data will overcome the limitations inherent in using regional velocity profiles.

Myocardial deformation, changes in contractility and perfusion deficits

Studies on the power of myocardial motion and deformation parameters have demonstrated myocardial velocity, ε, and SR to be sensitive to changes in contractility [30,31]. Strain data show characteristic changes related to changes in regional wall motion and occurrence of myocardial ischemia. Curve interpretation follows two principles:

- Normokinesia, hypokinesia, and akinesia are defined through their peak strain value (Fig. 23.21). Longitudinal deformation contraction presents with negative values. Dyskinesia is displayed through curves with either positive values or no clear direction (Fig. 23.22).
- Timing is critical for a proper curve interpretation. Normal systolic contraction ends with aortic valve closure (AVC); relaxation starts with mitral valve opening (MVO) and is displayed through a down-sloping strain curve. During ischemia, contraction is delayed and prolonged beyond AVC, with a characteristic postsystolic peak (Fig. 23.23).

Several studies have found that regional ischemia causes rapid, predictable, and reproducible changes in deformation. Induction of acute ischemia showed a gradual decrease in deformation and a concomitant appearance of postsystolic deformation [31–33]. The effect of ischemia on radial systolic and postsystolic thickening (PST) and the persistence of PST in early stages of reperfusion as a result of stunning have been described, including the passive nature of PST due to the contractile force of affected and non-affected neighboring segments [34].

Ischemia versus chronic infarction

The characteristic shapes of strain curves in ischemia and chronic infarction are easy to discriminate. A chronic transmural infarcted area will present with no systolic or postsystolic contraction, while acute ischemic myocardium will show delayed and reduced systolic contraction with postsystolic deformation (Fig. 23.24).

Diastolic changes during ischemia

Interpretation of diastolic function from regional velocity curves shows characteristic changes also: absolute velocities are reduced, early filling (E′) is even more reduced in relation to atrial filling (A′), and regional E′/A′ ratio is inverse [35]. These changes are apparent within seconds after onset of ischemia, and are reversible equally quickly with reperfusion.

Limitations of tissue Doppler imaging

In common with other Doppler modes, TDI is limited by angle dependency. Urheim et al. [36] demonstrated

that ε and SR curves are also affected by Doppler physics, and values may change substantially depending on the angle between the Doppler beam and the direction of myocardial deformation. Accurate TEE-based measurements of apical segments may not be possible in patients with a spherical LV.

Tethering effects represent another limitation, resulting in passively generated myocardial velocities of the ischemic segment.

One previous limitation of CDMI, its limited time resolution, has been resolved as processing power has increased substantially. By limiting the regions of interest, a frame rate of 200–300 frames per second is now possible.

Although these curves look "noisy," this is more of an advantage than a limitation. High temporal resolution means that the data contain information about brief events in the cardiac cycle, e.g. IVC. In order to analyze myocardial motion and deformation during IVC or IVR a minimum frame rate of 150 frames per second is needed.

Since blood-pool-derived measures of ventricular function are load-dependent, they may be significantly affected by changing preload or afterload conditions. Initially, TDI parameters were thought to be load-independent, but this view has had to be revised. Myocardial velocity data are less load-dependent than blood-pool-derived data, and deformation parameters are less affected than velocity data, but load effects are still significant, and need to be taken into account. Isovolumic phase indexes may give the best results, due to more stable loading conditions at that time.

Nonetheless, data indicate that SR will remain unchanged as long as increased LV dimensions and increased stroke volume stay balanced. Only when contractility drops will SR decrease as a result of the failing ventricle [37].

Speckle-tracking technique and two-dimensional strain (2D strain)

Significant efforts have been made to extract myocardial tissue information from the 2D image. Indeed, complex analysis of the speckles (acoustic markers within the myocardium) and their motion vectors during the cardiac cycle can now be analyzed to obtain velocity, strain, and strain rate.

The most recent development, speckle-tracking echocardiography (STE), is derived from the standard gray-scale image. STE may be the most versatile method to measure and display myocardial function.

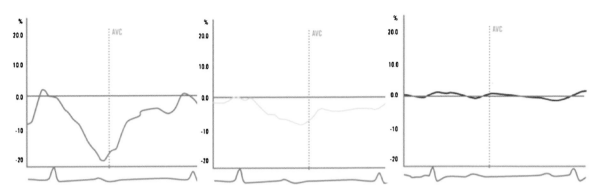

Figure 23.21. Characteristic curve presentation according to regional myocardial function: normokinesia (left), hypokinesia (middle), akinesia (right). AVC, aortic valve closure.

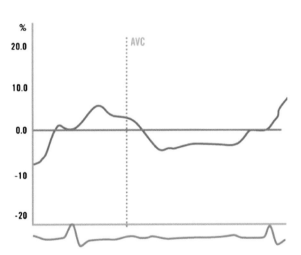

Figure 23.22. Dyskinesia with lengthening during systole.

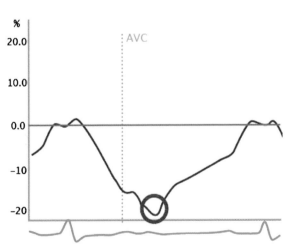

Figure 23.23. Postsystolic shortening, as indicated by a further increase of longitudinal strain after AVC closure.

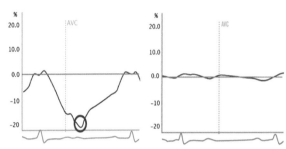

Figure 23.24. Strain curves of ischemic myocardium (left) and infarcted myocardium (right).

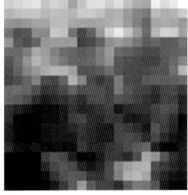

Figure 23.25. Speckle tracking is performed by tracking the unique pattern of a gray-scale image of 20 × 20 pixels. An example of such a "digital fingerprint" is shown.

Technology and limitations

The basic principle is to determine myocardial wall motion from the movement of specific speckles of the gray-scale image from the myocardial walls. The gray-scale information consists of speckles of different brightness and shape. By tracing these speckles in their movement throughout the cardiac cycle, they can be analyzed to derive their direction and velocity.

Current speckle-tracking techniques do not trace specific speckles but regions within the myocardium of the size of 20 × 20 pixels, generating a specific pattern of speckles – a "digital fingerprint" (Fig. 23.25).

Using cross-correlation this characteristic pattern can be traced frame by frame throughout a major part of the cycle (Fig. 23.26). Once a region of interest is defined – superimposed on the black-and-white B-mode – the software is able to automatically track its motion and deformation on subsequent frames.

To ensure adequate tracking, the deformation from frame to frame has to be small enough that the corresponding pattern can be found in each frame. Since the technique is 2D-based, tracking is difficult, especially when speckles move out of the plane due to motion of the myocardium.

To some extent, speckles that have moved out the scan plane can be replaced by their neighbor in order to continuously determine the velocity of the myocardial tissue on the scan plane (Fig. 23.27).

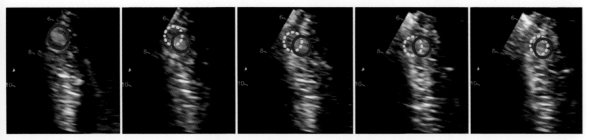

Figure 23.26. Tracing of a speckle (red dot) over the heart cycle frame by frame. Changes in the position of the speckle (blue circle previous position, yellow circle actual position) are analyzed to calculate direction and velocity.

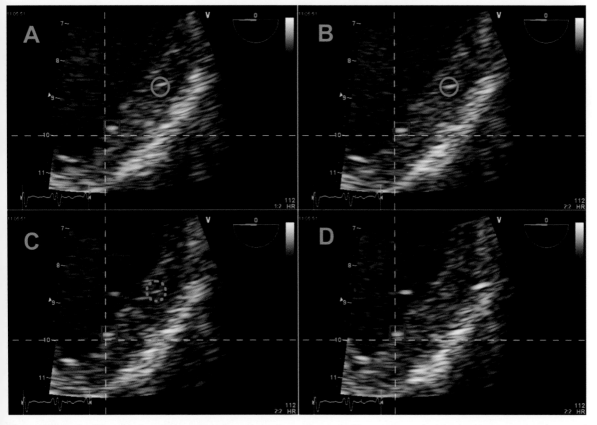

Figure 23.27. Speckle analysis: speckle tracking throughout the cardiac cycle. The pattern marked by the blue square can be traced throughout the cycle moving slightly down and leftward, while the pattern marked by the green circle fades in C and has disappeared in D.

383

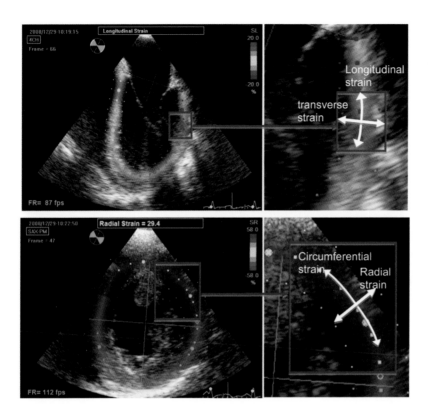

Figure 23.28. Different strain components to be analyzed in different planes. First row, ME four-chamber: longitudinal and transverse strain can be obtained. Second row, TG mid SAX: radial and circumferential strain can be obtained.

Speckle tracking at high frame rates is difficult, as the contours and delineation of speckles get lost. The optimal frame rate is in the range of 50–120 frames per second, although the technique is proven to be robust enough to handle low-frame-rate scans down to 30 frames per second.

Speckle tracking and transesophageal echocardiography

The great advantage of the technique is that angle dependency is no longer an issue, and the simultaneous analysis of motion vectors in all directions within the 2D plane can be performed.

Different strain components can be analyzed, depending on LV motion and their relation to the TEE probe. From the mid-esophageal level, longitudinal strain is shown in the apicobasal contraction, and transverse strain in thickening of the walls. In transgastric short-axis planes, radial strain can be seen in inward motion and wall thickening, while circumferential strain is expressed through circumferential shortening (Fig. 23.28). Since the different strain components are calculated simultaneously for the whole myocardium in a given plane, it is easy to switch between one and the other using the software.

Myocardial deformation analysis from TEE is no longer limited by a spherical apical region. Analysis of all segments is possible with reliable results.

Normal data, parameters, and curve interpretation

With TDI, strain, strain rate, and velocity can be measured. By contrast, the primarily calculated parameters in speckle-tracking analysis are deformation parameters, from which strain may be derived. Velocity may then be calculated from strain.

The presentation of the parameters is as follows:

1. The myocardial region of interest is superimposed on the black-and-white B-mode image (dots marking mid-myocardium and the borders), and the myocardium is then colorized according to the selected parameter. For an intuitive interpretation, the brightness of the color defines the amount of contraction (Fig. 23.29A).

2. Each analyzed LV wall in the mid-esophageal planes is divided into three segments, and the myocardium in TG SAX planes is divided into six segments, by the software. The calculated parameters are presented in graphic form, either

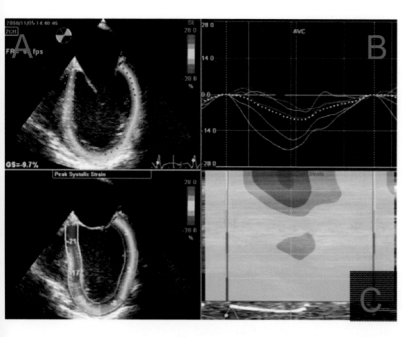

Figure 23.29. Two-dimensional strain parameter presentation: (A) parametric; (B) curve display; (C) curved M-mode.

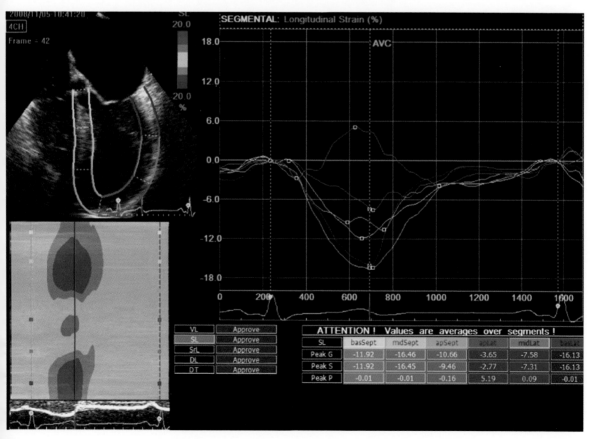

Figure 23.30. Two-dimensional strain analysis: numerical presentation of results.

simultaneously displayed as the average measure for each segment within one plane, or from every point within the myocardium (Fig. 23.29B).

3. A curved anatomical M-mode presents motion/deformation of all analyzed segments within a plane, plotted over time (Fig. 23.29C).

4. Calculated data can also be presented numerically in tabular form (Fig. 23.30).

Rotation, rotation rate, and torsion

Rotation and rotation rate are defined as the angular displacement and velocity, respectively, of the LV about its central axis in the short-axis image. They are stated in units of degrees (rotation) and degrees per second (rotation rate) (Figs. 23.31, 23.32). Counterclockwise LV rotation as viewed from apex is denoted as a positive value, clockwise rotation as a negative value.

Since the LV myocardium rotates clockwise in basal and counterclockwise in the apical segments, torsion is the net difference between apical and basal rotation, stated in units of degrees (Fig. 23.33). Because the degree of rotation for the same amount of LV torsion increases as the distance from the mid-ventricular level increases, LV torsion is expected to vary with the

distance between the planes at which basal and apical short-axis images are obtained. Therefore a torsion index can be calculated by dividing the torsion values by the torsion length (degrees/cm).

Validation of speckle-tracking technique

A number of studies have evaluated the feasibility and accuracy of speckle tracking [9,10,38].

Several manufacturers have developed quantification tools for myocardial deformation using speckle tracking, including automated function imaging (AFI: General Electric) and vector velocity imaging (VVI: Siemens), and these have been compared with magnetic resonance imaging (MRI) [39]. Both techniques underestimated longitudinal strain compared to MRI.

Clinical applications of speckle tracking and 2D strain

Speckle tracking and 2D strain have been shown to be extremely useful, especially in TEE, since they are not technically limited when applied to TEE-acquired images. Thus, they provide useful additional information

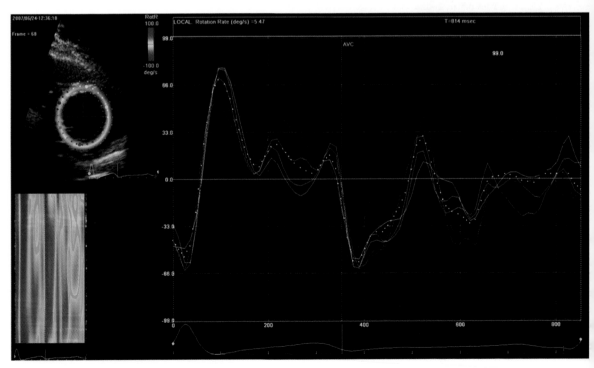

Figure 23.31. Rotation rate analysis.

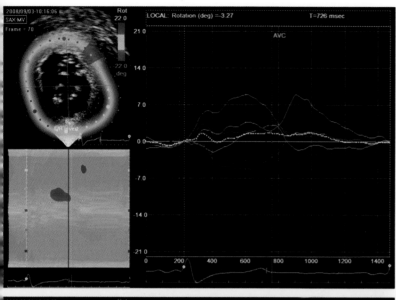

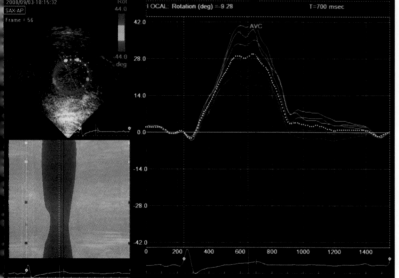

Figure 23.32. Rotation at the base (top) and at the apex (bottom).

on global and regional ventricular function based on myocardial deformation analysis.

Global and regional ventricular function

Differently oriented muscle fibers contribute to global LV contraction, and contraction of each of the three layers of the muscle band generates a deformation vector in either longitudinal, radial, or circumferential direction. Deformation during systole occurs as a counterclockwise rotation of the LV apex (as viewed from the apex), whereas the base rotates clockwise, creating a torsional deformation originating from the

dynamic interaction of oppositely twisted epicardial and endocardial myocardial fiber helices. The net result of this wringing contraction pattern is a shortening in longitudinal direction (Fig. 23.34).

Global longitudinal peak systolic strain

Since longitudinal shortening is a major determinant of systolic function, global longitudinal peak systolic strain (GLPSS) is a representative measure of LV systolic strain.

GLPSS is calculated from the average of the peak systolic values of all LV segments. The three mid-esophageal

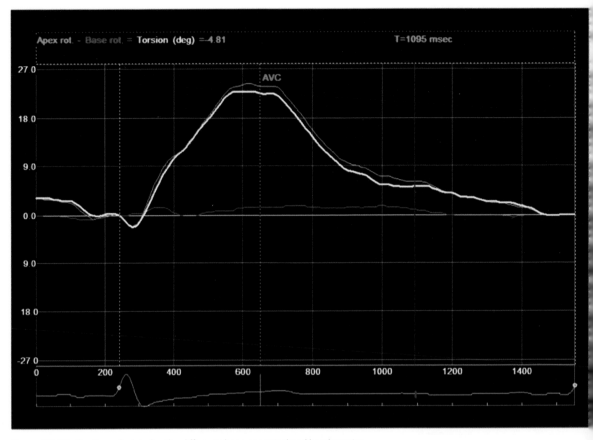

Figure 23.33. Torsion, calculated as the difference between apical and basal rotation.

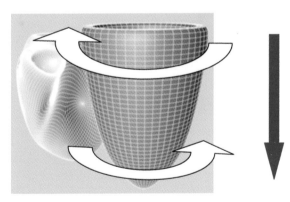

Figure 23.34. Longitudinal shortening of the LV as a result of LV torsion.

planes (ME four-chamber, ME two-chamber, ME LAX) have to be analyzed in order to calculate mean peak systolic strain for the whole U-shaped length of the ventricular walls in each plane (Fig. 23.35) [40]. Fast access to the regional distribution of peak systolic strain along the different segments of the LV gives the parametric visualization tool "bull's eye," with deformation displayed in colorized form over the schematic diagram of the LV (Fig. 23.36). It provides information about the magnitude of peak systolic strain in each segment and the distribution of regional peak systolic strain. Regional deformation abnormalities may be graphically displayed. Several studies have validated GLPSS in healthy volunteers and patients after myocardial infarction, LV hypertrophy, or hemodialysis [40–42].

Right ventricular systolic function is much more difficult to assess, because of the complex three-dimensional shape of the right ventricle. However, 2D strain allows us to measure mean peak systolic longitudinal strain from the U-shaped length of right ventricular free wall and septum (Fig. 23.37).

Longitudinal peak systolic strain and regional ventricular function

Speckle tracking overcomes most of the limitations of TDI, fulfilling almost all requirements on sensitivity

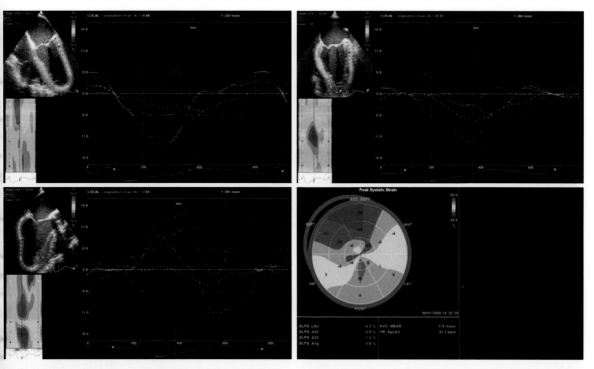

Figure 23.35. GLPSS analysis: mean LPSS obtained from ME four-chamber, ME two-chamber, ME LAX planes. GLPSS is the average of all three planes.

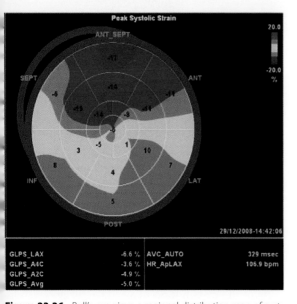

Figure 23.36. Bull's-eye view: a regional distribution map of systolic (postsystolic strain).

and specificity in the detection of ischemia, i.e. robustness and small inter-observer variability, semi-simultaneous analysis of all LV segments regardless of position or angulation, parametric imaging with quantification of regional wall motion, detection of postsystolic events, and regional distribution mapping.

Regional function analysis is performed following the principles of strain curve interpretation. Peak systolic strain values define normokinesia (at least 18–20%), hypokinesia (reduced deformation), or akinesia (no deformation) (Fig. 23.38A,B,C). Dyskinesia presents with positive values, since lengthening occurs during systole (Fig. 23.38D).

A major advantage over TDI is the way simultaneous strain curves can be obtained within one plane, and with only a short delay from all three planes. Therefore the information is more or less simultaneously displayed for all segments of the LV (Fig. 23.39).

Interpretations can be made either from the curves or from the bull's eye (BE) view. Systolic (or postsystolic) ε is displayed in a colorized manner according to its peak (post-)systolic value for all segments. Therefore, from the regional distribution of hypokinetic, akinetic, or dyskinetic areas it is easy to interpret ischemic or infarcted myocardium and the coronary artery territory involved (Fig. 23.40).

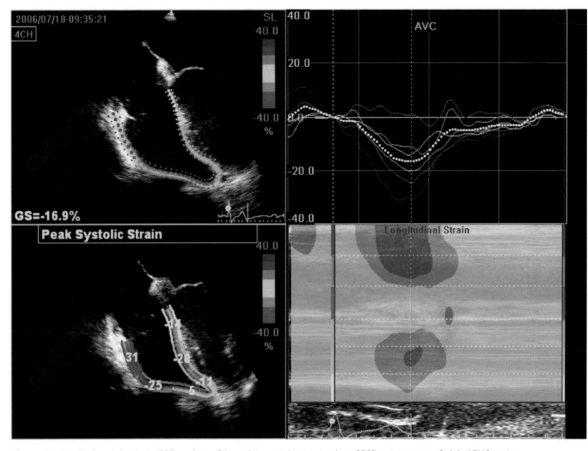

Figure 23.37. Peak systolic strain (PSS) analysis of the right ventricle: mean value of PSS as a measure of global RV function.

Postsystolic shortening, postsystolic index

Postsystolic shortening in the longitudinal direction (postsystolic thickening, PST, in the radial direction) has been shown to be a sensitive and specific marker for myocardial ischemia (Fig. 23.41). As with TDI, the fact that deformation occurs mostly after AVC (postsystolic) means that correct timing is essential.

Since acute ischemia induces a combination of decreased systolic deformation and increased postsystolic (early diastolic) deformation, peak systolic and postsystolic ε can be related. This postsystolic index (PSI) was first postulated by Kukulski et al. [43], who found PSI to be a highly sensitive and specific marker for ischemia with cutoff values for longitudinal PSI of 25% and radial PSI of 22%, with a sensitivity of 95% and 92% respectively, and a specificity of 89% for both longitudinal and radial.

PSI can also be displayed in the BE view, allowing the regional distribution of ischemic myocardium to be mapped for rapid interpretation and allocation to coronary perfusion territories (Fig. 23.42).

Since strain pathologies due to myocardial ischemia have an immediate onset and are rapidly reversible with reperfusion, STE and systolic/postsystolic strain analysis is an ideal tool to detect myocardial ischemia and monitor surgical or interventional treatment. Figure 23.43 shows a BE view of the distribution of systolic and postsystolic strain before and after revascularization, demonstrating a significant postoperative reduction in the affected area. Figure 23.44 shows rapid reversal of ischemia following intra-aortic balloon pump therapy.

When interpreting ε curves on postsystolic events one has to consider that delayed deformation may

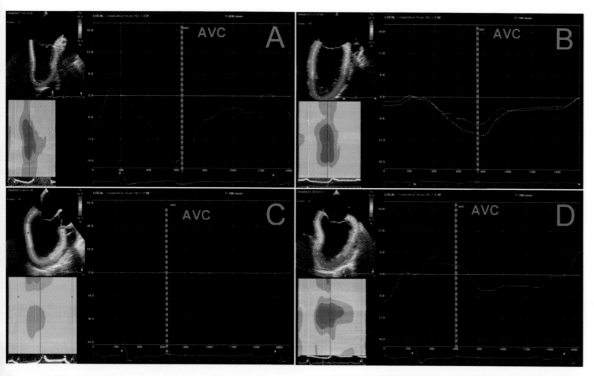

Figure 23.38. Characteristic curve shape according to regional myocardial function: (A) normokinesia; (B) hypokinesia; (C) akinesia; (D) dyskinesia.

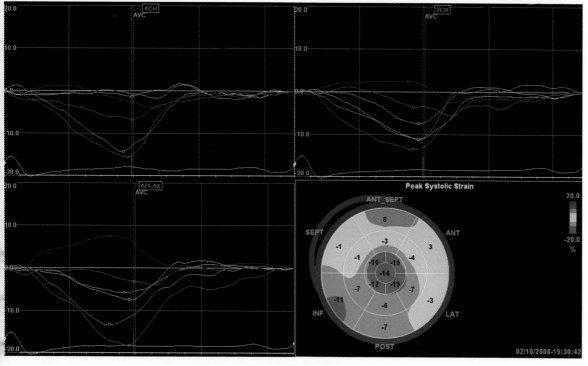

Figure 23.39. Bull's-eye and curve display: simultaneous acquisition and interpretation of all LV segments.

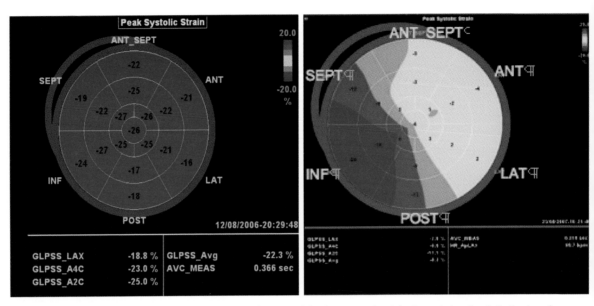

Figure 23.40. Peak systolic strain, bull's-eye view: on the left a normal distribution, on the right the typical regional distribution of an acute myocardial infarction in the LAD territory.

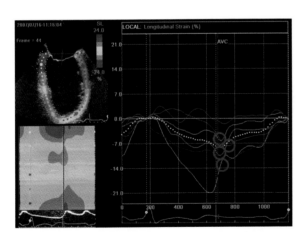

Figure 23.41. Acute ischemia and occurrence of postsystolic strain in the mid- and apical inferior, basal, and mid anterior wall. Apical anterior wall is dyskinetic.

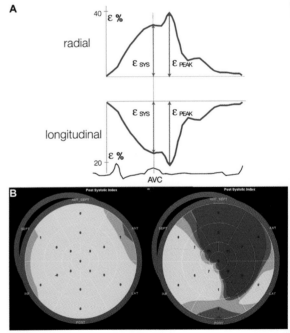

Figure 23.42. (A) Peak systolic and peak postsystolic strain in radial and longitudinal strain curves. (B) PSI in BE view: normal (left) versus acute ischemia with extended postsystolic strain regions in the LAD territory (right).

occur due to non-ischemic reasons such as left bundle branch block in cardiomyopathy.

Torsion and global ventricular function

Although the helical arrangement of myocardial fibers has been known for a long time, the importance of fiber orientation to LV torsion and thereby normal cardiac function has only recently been under-stood. The LV twisting motion is a consequence of orientation of the subendocardial and subepicardial fibers, representing two oppositely directed spirals.

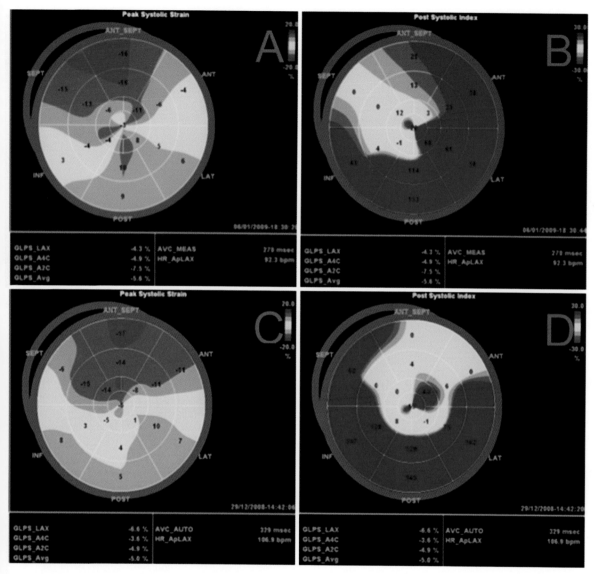

Figure 23.43. Case 1: LCX occlusion. (A,B) acute event; (C,D) postoperative day 1.

Since the magnitude of LV twist represents contractile force, "twist" during systole and "untwist" during diastole play an important role in both systolic and diastolic function. The measurement of such a fundamental determinant of ventricular motion could therefore provide a sensitive marker of LV function.

Initially LV torsion was investigated using MRI. However, the method is expensive, time-consuming, and not universally applicable, and has not become part of clinical routine. With STE, a relatively simple

technique, which has already been validated with tagged MRI, has been implemented for the measurement of torsion [44,45].

Studies on healthy subjects and patients with previous myocardial infarction demonstrated a substantial contribution of LV torsion and twist to the assessment of global and regional ventricular function. Impairment of LV torsion has been related to infarct size, indicating that LV torsion is a determinant of resting function [46]. Normal values of 3.16 ± 1.3 degrees/cm have been quoted for torsion in healthy subjects.

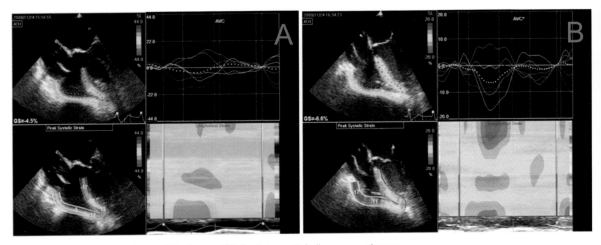

Figure 23.44. Case 2: RV ischemia, (A) before and (B) after intra-aortic balloon pump therapy.

Others have found that, compared to normals, LV torsion was significantly increased in mild diastolic dysfunction, normalizing again in the advanced stages of disorders of diastolic function [47].

Limitations

The major limitation of the STE technique is temporal resolution, and its contribution to the delineation of speckles. With increasing frame rate, speckles move a very short distance. Therefore it is difficult to analyze direction and distance of the individual speckles. A low frame rate helps to distinguish myocardial structure, but information about brief events in the cardiac cycle gets lost. Taking that into account, frame rates of 50–120 frames per second are ideal for analysis. It is not yet possible to analyze brief events – IVC and IVR, with a duration of 40–80 ms – in the cardiac cycle.

Conclusion

Accurate analysis of myocardial function is one of the most challenging aspects of modern echocardiography. The conventional techniques referred to elsewhere in this book are valuable and have stood the test of time. However, modern developments in Doppler imaging and myocardial velocity imaging, as described above, represent a major advance in our ability to understand and to quantify myocardial function. Coupled with advances in 3D technology, these techniques represent significant progress, and promise much for the future.

References

1. Isaaz K, Ethevenot G, Admant P, Brembilla B, Pernot C. A new Doppler method of assessing left ventricular ejection force in chronic congestive heart failure. *Am J Cardiol* 1989; **64**: 81–7.

2. Isaaz K, Thompson A, Ethevenot G, *et al.* Doppler echocardiographic measurement of low velocity motion of the left ventricular posterior wall. *Am J Cardiol* 1989; **64**: 66–75.

3. McDicken WN, Sutherland GR, Moran CM, Gordon LN. Colour Doppler velocity imaging of the myocardium. *Ultrasound Med Biol* 1992; **18**: 651–4.

4. Heimdal A, Stoylen A, Torp H, Skjaerpe T. Real-time strain rate imaging of the left ventricle by ultrasound. *J Am Soc Echocardiogr* 1998; **11**: 1013–19.

5. Brodin LA, van der Linden J, Olstad B. Echocardiographic functional images based on tissue velocity information. *Herz* 1998; **23**: 491–8.

6. Sutherland GR, Kukulski T, Voight JU, D'Hooge J. Tissue Doppler echocardiography: future developments. *Echocardiography* 1999; **16**: 509–20.

7. Hatle L, Sutherland GR. Regional myocardial function: a new approach. *Eur Heart J* 2000; **21**: 1337–57.

8. Kaluzynski K, Chen X, Emelianov SY, Skovoroda AR, O'Donnell M. Strain rate imaging using two-dimensional speckle tracking. *IEEE Trans Ultrason Ferroelectr Freq Control* 2001; **48**: 1111–23.

9. Rappaport D, Adam D, Lysyansky P, Riesner S. Assessment of myocardial regional strain and strain rate by tissue tracking in B-mode echocardiograms. *Ultrasound Med Biol* 2006; **32**: 1181–92.

10. Leitman M, Lysyansky P, Sidenko S, *et al.* Two-dimensional strain: a novel software for real-time quantitative echocardiographic assessment of myocardial function. *J Am Soc Echocardiogr* 2004; **17**: 1021–9.

11. Simmons LA, Weidemann F, Sutherland GR, *et al.* Doppler tissue velocity, strain, and strain rate imaging with transesophageal echocardiography in the operating room: a feasibility study. *J Am Soc Echocardiogr* 2002; **15**: 768–76.

12. Cheung MM, Li J, White PA, *et al.* Doppler tissue echocardiography: can transesophageal echocardiography be used to acquire functional data? *J Am Soc Echocardiogr* 2003; **16**: 732–7.

13. Skarvan K, Filipovic M, Wang J, Brett W, Seeberger M. Use of myocardial tissue Doppler imaging for intraoperative monitoring of left ventricular function. *Br J Anaesth* 2003; **91**: 473–80.

14. Norrild K, Pedersen TF, Sloth E. Transesophageal tissue Doppler echocardiography for evaluation of myocardial function during aortic valve replacement. *J Cardiothorac Vasc Anesth* 2007; **21**: 367–70.

15. Sanchez-Quintana D, Climent V, Ho SY, Anderson RH. Myoarchitecture and connective tissue in hearts with tricuspid atresia. *Heart* 1999; **81**: 182–91.

16. Vogel M, Schmidt MR, Kristiansen SB, *et al.* Validation of myocardial acceleration during isovolumic contraction as a novel noninvasive index of right ventricular contractility: comparison with ventricular pressure-volume relations in an animal model. *Circulation* 2002; **105**: 1693–9.

17. Vogel M, Cheung MM, Li J, *et al.* Noninvasive assessment of left ventricular force–frequency relationships using tissue Doppler-derived isovolumic acceleration: validation in an animal model. *Circulation* 2003; **107**: 1647–52.

18. Missant C, Rex S, Claus P, Mertens L, Wouters PF. Load-sensitivity of regional tissue deformation in the right ventricle: isovolumic versus ejection-phase indices of contractility. *Heart* 2008; **94**: e15.

19. Kukulski T, Hubbert L, Arnold M, *et al.* Normal regional right ventricular function and its change with age: a Doppler myocardial imaging study. *J Am Soc Echocardiogr* 2000; **13**: 194–204.

20. Kowalski M, Kukulski T, Jamal F, *et al.* Can natural strain and strain rate quantify regional myocardial deformation? A study in healthy subjects. *Ultrasound Med Biol* 2001; **27**: 1087–97.

21. Camici PG, Prasad SK, Rimoldi OE. Stunning, hibernation, and assessment of myocardial viability. *Circulation* 2008; **117**: 103–14.

22. Greenberg NL, Firstenberg MS, Castro PL, *et al.* Doppler-derived myocardial systolic strain rate is a strong index of left ventricular contractility. *Circulation* 2002; **105**: 99–105.

23. Nagueh SF, Middleton KJ, Kopelen HA, Zoghbi WA, Quiñones MA. Doppler tissue imaging: a noninvasive technique for evaluation of left ventricular relaxation and estimation of filling pressures. *J Am Coll Cardiol* 1997; **30**: 1527–33.

24. Hillis GS, Moller JE, Pellikka PA, *et al.* Noninvasive estimation of left ventricular filling pressure by E/e′ is a powerful predictor of survival after acute myocardial infarction. *J Am Coll Cardiol* 2004; **43**: 360–7.

25. Ommen SR, Nishimura RA, Appleton CP, *et al.* Clinical utility of Doppler echocardiography and tissue Doppler imaging in the estimation of left ventricular filling pressures: a comparative simultaneous Doppler-catheterization study. *Circulation* 2000; **102**: 1788–94.

26. Paulus WJ, Tschöpe C, Sanderson JE, *et al.* How to diagnose diastolic heart failure: a consensus statement on the diagnosis of heart failure with normal left ventricular ejection fraction by the Heart Failure and Echocardiography Associations of the European Society of Cardiology. *Eur Heart J* 2007; **28**: 2539–50.

27. Vinereanu D, Florescu N, Sculthorpe N, *et al.* Differentiation between pathologic and physiologic left ventricular hypertrophy by tissue Doppler assessment of long-axis function in patients with hypertrophic cardiomyopathy or systemic hypertension and in athletes. *Am J Cardiol* 2001; **88**: 53–8.

28. Yang H, Sun JP, Lever HM, *et al.* Use of strain imaging in detecting segmental dysfunction in patients with hypertrophic cardiomyopathy. *J Am Soc Echocardiogr* 2003; **16**: 233–9.

29. Sun JP, Abdalla IA, Asher CR, *et al.* Non-invasive evaluation of orthotopic heart transplant rejection by echocardiography. *J Heart Lung Transplant* 2005; **24**: 160–5.

30. Weidemann F, Kowalski M, D'hooge J, Bijnens B, Sutherland GR. Doppler myocardial imaging: a new tool to assess regional inhomogeneity in cardiac function. *Basic Res Cardiol* 2001; **96**: 595–605.

31. Weidemann F, Dommke C, Bijnens B, *et al.* Defining the transmurality of a chronic myocardial infarction by ultrasonic strain-rate imaging: implications for identifying intramural viability: an experimental study. *Circulation* 2003; **107**: 883–8.

32. Jamal F, Kukulski T, Strotmann J, *et al.* Quantification of the spectrum of changes in regional myocardial function during acute ischemia in closed chest pigs: an ultrasonic strain rate and strain study. *J Am Soc Echocardiogr* 2001; **14**: 874–84.

33. Jamal F, Szilard M, Kukulski T, *et al.* Changes in systolic and postsystolic wall thickening during acute coronary

occlusion and reperfusion in closed-chest pigs: Implications for the assessment of regional myocardial function. *J Am Soc Echocardiogr* 2001; **14**: 691–7.

34. Bijnens B, Claus P, Weidemann F, Strotmann J, Sutherland GR. Investigating cardiac function using motion and deformation analysis in the setting of coronary artery disease. *Circulation* 2007; **116**: 2453–64.

35. Garcia-Fernández MA, Azevedo J, Moreno M, *et al.* Regional diastolic function in ischaemic heart disease using pulsed wave Doppler tissue imaging. *Eur Heart J* 1999; **20**: 496–505.

36. Urheim S, Edvardsen T, Torp H, Angelsen B, Smiseth OA. Myocardial strain by Doppler echocardiography. Validation of a new method to quantify regional myocardial function. *Circulation* 2000; **102**: 1158–64.

37. Marciniak A, Claus P, Sutherland GR, *et al.* Changes in systolic left ventricular function in isolated mitral regurgitation: a strain rate imaging study. *Eur Heart J* 2007; **28**: 2627–36.

38. Serri K, Reant P, Lafitte M, *et al.* Global and regional myocardial function quantification by two-dimensional strain: application in hypertrophic cardiomyopathy. *J Am Coll Cardiol* 2006; **47**: 1175–81.

39. Bansal M, Cho GY, Chan J, *et al.* Feasibility and accuracy of different techniques of two-dimensional speckle based strain and validation with harmonic phase magnetic resonance imaging. *J Am Soc Echocardiogr* 2008; **21**: 1318–25.

40. Reisner SA, Lysyansky P, Agmon Y, *et al.* Global longitudinal strain: a novel index of left ventricular systolic function. *J Am Soc Echocardiogr* 2004; **17**: 630–3.

41. Choi JO, Shin DH, Cho SW, *et al.* Effect of preload on left ventricular longitudinal strain by 2D speckle tracking. *Echocardiography* 2008; **25**: 873–9.

42. Ng AC, Tran da T, Newman M, *et al.* Left ventricular longitudinal and radial synchrony and their determinants in healthy subjects. *J Am Soc Echocardiogr* 2008; **21**: 1042–8.

43. Kukulski T, Jamal F, Herbots L, *et al.* Identification of acutely ischemic myocardium using ultrasonic strain measurements: a clinical study in patients undergoing coronary angioplasty. *J Am Coll Cardiol* 2003; **41**: 810–19.

44. Notomi Y, Lysyansky P, Setser RM, *et al.* Measurement of ventricular torsion by two-dimensional ultrasound speckle tracking imaging. *J Am Coll Cardiol* 2005; **45**: 2034–41.

45. Helle-Valle T, Crosby J, Edvardsen T, *et al.* New noninvasive method for assessment of left ventricular rotation: speckle tracking echocardiography. *Circulation* 2005; **112**: 3149–56.

46. Bansal M, Leano RL, Marwick TH. Clinical assessment of left ventricular systolic torsion: effects of myocardial infarction and ischemia. *J Am Soc Echocardiogr* 2008; **21**: 887–94.

47. Park SJ, Miyazaki C, Bruce CJ, *et al.* Left ventricular torsion by two-dimensional speckle tracking echocardiography in patients with diastolic dysfunction and normal ejection fraction. *J Am Soc Echocardiogr* 2008; **21**: 1129–37.

24 Transesophageal echocardiography reporting

John Kneeshaw, Kamen Valchanov

Report (noun) – a story or piece of information that may or may not be true

Oxford English Dictionary

Introduction

Transesophageal echocardiography (TEE) is an imaging modality capable of providing valuable diagnostic information, and providing a full assessment of cardiac function. In common with other imaging modalities, every TEE examination should be accompanied by a properly constituted report. It would be inconceivable to perform CT or MRI without producing a full report of that event, and TEE should be treated similarly.

TEE examinations are performed by physicians from several disciplines. In cardiology, it has been recommended that TEE should follow a transthoracic examination, in which case a single report may be produced which encompasses both examinations [1].

From a worldwide perspective, anesthesiologists in the field of cardiac surgery are performing an increasing number of TEE examinations, and they may represent the largest group of TEE operators[2]. The practice of TEE, either as a stand-alone procedure or in association with transthoracic echocardiography (TTE), is also rapidly spreading into intensive care and emergency-room practice [3].

In many of these situations, TEE may be a stand-alone procedure. It may be that, in this setting, a TEE examination is regarded by some practitioners as a monitoring rather than diagnostic episode, and this may explain the reluctance of some operators to produce a formal report. However, the application of TEE to any clinical situation should generate a full report of the examination, and this report should automatically become a part of the permanent patient record.

What is the function of a TEE report?
Provision of information

An echo report primarily provides information to the referring physician or, in the case of intraoperative studies, to the operating surgeon. In either case the data will be used to help formulate a medical management plan, and later to inform the patient of the presence or absence of pathology. It is also important to note that the content of an echo report should be intelligible to the intended reader. This may not always be a physician with a good knowledge of cardiac anatomy or physiology. A concise summary of findings understandable to the non-echo practitioner should always be provided, as well as detailed data about cardiac dimensions, Doppler-derived data, and other echo-specific information.

Perioperative decision making

Perioperative examinations carried out in operating rooms pose a number of challenges. In order to maintain appropriate patient safety, care should be taken to ensure that the business of echocardiography does not distract the anesthesiologist from his or her primary duty of care to the anesthetized patient. The information from the TEE needs to be acquired and interpreted relatively quickly and incorporated with other data relating to the patient's hemodynamic state so that a surgical treatment plan can be formulated and followed. Commonly the surgical plan is merely confirmed and followed; however, in a number of cases echocardiographic findings will cause the plan to be changed [2,4]. Where TEE data lead directly to a change in surgical management it is even more important that the data, the conclusions drawn from those data, and the resulting change in plan are fully documented and permanently recorded.

Core Topics in Transesophageal Echocardiography, ed. Robert Feneck, John Kneeshaw, and Marco Ranucci.
Published by Cambridge University Press. © Cambridge University Press 2010.

Provision of a comparator for future studies

An echocardiography report leaves a permanent time-related record from the imaging episode that will allow future studies to follow the progression of a patient's disease, or the effect of therapy. For example a small echo-dense mass visible on a prosthetic mitral annuloplasty ring could be a benign finding (i.e. a piece of suture material), but if the mass were seen to increase in size in a follow-up study it may be a sign of developing prosthetic endocarditis.

Training and accreditation

The writing of an echocardiography report is as much a part of the TEE training process as is learning to manipulate a probe and acquire images. The presentation of echo reports is used to assess a trainee's ability to assimilate and interpret findings. It is also used to ensure that trainees have performed the required number of studies for accreditation in echocardiography. In Europe and in North America standard requirements for training accreditation and certification have been introduced that specify a number of echo reports to be submitted before accreditation can be granted [5,6].

Where a report of a TEE study is produced by a trainee as part of the training process it should be verified by a trained expert echocardiographer, to quality-assure the output of the echo service and to facilitate continuous assessment of the trainee's progress.

Medicolegal issues

Occasionally the treatment and investigation of a patient by a hospital or a doctor is subjected to legal scrutiny. This may be under the auspices of a coroner or in the civil or criminal jurisdictions. On such occasions the only reliable source of information about events that occurred in months or years past will be the patient's contemporaneously created medical notes. The presence in the notes of a full and comprehensive report of a TEE examination, and its findings, may provide data that explain a subsequent course of action. The failure to provide a report of a TEE examination, which may be documented by others as having occurred, may be treated at best as poor practice and at worst as negligence.

Audit

Echocardiography reporting facilitates audit. The number of reports produced by a doctor or by an echocardiography service provides evidence of activity. This information may be used to support requests for more staff, more training, or more equipment. It is difficult to plan and develop a service without knowing how much work is done, by whom, and when and where this activity takes place. Continuous audit of the content of echo reports also helps to drive and maintain good standards of clinical practice.

Research

A database of echocardiographic activity and findings in cohorts of patients can be a valuable research tool. TEE reports can and should contain numerical data which may be useful in both randomized controlled trials and large-scale observational studies and case series. Failure to record such data is a waste of a potentially valuable resource.

What form should a TEE report take?

A TEE examination report may be paper-based, electronically generated, or presented verbally.

Verbal reports

Verbal reporting is essential in perioperative and emergency echo. In these areas the communication of echo findings is time-sensitive. An operating surgeon approaching mitral valve repair surgery needs to be told the mechanism of the mitral lesion clearly and concisely at the start of the procedure, and also needs a clear description of the effectiveness of surgery at the end of cardiopulmonary bypass. The team managing an acutely ill patient in an intensive care unit also need immediate feedback of information that may change the patient's management. In these circumstances the report describes the state of the heart at a precise moment in time, with given loading conditions and contractility, both of which may be affected by a range of anesthetic or other hemodynamically active drugs. In some patients there may also be mechanical devices, such as an intra-aortic balloon pump, providing mechanical circulatory support.

Careful thought should be given to the way a verbal report is phrased. The report will be delivered once only, and it may have a profound impact on the way an individual patient is treated. Too much irrelevant information may confuse the situation, but sufficient data must be given to ensure that the listener understands the principal findings. For example, the primary finding may be severe prolapse of the P2 scallop of the mitral valve; supporting information may be the left atrial dimensions; and subsidiary but relevant information may be the presence of severe aortic atheromatous disease. It is also important that one communicates how certain one is of the findings.

This is particularly relevant when a specific question calling for a particular focus is asked: for example, "Is intracardiac thrombus present?" A positive "Yes" is clear. The negative response, however, should be considered, and "None seen" is usually preferable to a simple "No."

We strongly advocate that any verbal report should be followed by a permanent comprehensive report, which should be generated within a short time of the examination.

Written reporting

Perhaps the easiest approach to a written TEE report is the blank sheet of paper. This allows the echocardiographer total freedom to describe the findings, make deductions from those findings, and then summarize the event with a concluding statement. Paper reports of this type can be extremely effective, but they do require considerable discipline on the part of the reporter to ensure that all of the necessary information has been recorded.

For most operators, some form of standardized reporting system alleviates the problem of a lot of repetitive material, which of necessity is involved in echo reporting. Standardized systems can also contain useful information such as the normal range of values for cavity dimensions, wall thicknesses, pressure gradients, velocity–time integrals, valve areas, and any other variables that are frequently reported.

A standardized report form can also act as an aide-memoire, a reminder for example to look at the thoracic descending aorta or to check for pleural effusions.

There are a number of "check-box" type TEE report forms in use, which greatly simplify the recording of data [7]. These are particularly useful in perioperative echocardiography. An example of such a form produced by the Society of Cardiovascular Anesthesiologists (SCA) is shown in Figure 24.1, and an example from the UK is shown in Figure 24.2. The disadvantage of this sort of form is that it frequently does not allow the operator room to explain the data that led to a particular item being recorded. For example, a box indicating severe aortic stenosis may be ticked, but there may be no supporting data recorded. These check-box forms often have little scope for free text to explain conclusions or to summarize findings in patients where more than one pathological finding is present. Great care should be exercised when using such systems, and echocardiographers should avoid the submission of reports which only record conclusions, rather than showing how those conclusions were reached from raw data. This is particularly important where the intraoperative report identifies new findings, and where the intraoperative report results in a change in the planned surgery.

Computerized reports

A standardized written reporting system is relatively easy to adapt to computerized storage and recall. In some institutions echo data are collected onto standardized forms which can be entered into a database. The check-box type of form (see above) is particularly easy to use in this way. Most current echocardiography platforms contain some sort of reporting feature, and in the absence of any other institutional system these will provide acceptably formatted reports.

At the present time, when digital storage of data is relatively easy, many echocardiography departments have a policy of storing samples of moving and still images to demonstrate echo findings from an examination to complement the non-visual data. These electronic data are best managed by incorporating them into the hospital's electronic record system so that they are available to complement other diagnostic imaging data obtained from the patient.

Some computer based reporting systems have been available for some time, while newer more interactive systems are still under development [8].

What data should be recorded?

There is currently no defined and agreed minimum dataset for a TEE report. The following is our recommendation for safe and efficient practice.

1. **Patient demographics.** The name, date of birth, and hospital ID of the patient are absolute requirements. The age, height, and weight of the patient may guide the interpretation of certain data.
2. **Date, time and location of the study.**
3. **Name and grade of the operator.** It is important to document who performed a study, and who reported it.
4. **Name of the referring physician,** to whom a copy of the report should be sent.

399

Perioperative Echo Report

1. Demographic and Other Identifying Information

Name_____ Unit #_____DOB_____ M/F Date_____ Time_____
Location: ICU/OR/ER/PACU, Phys requesting Echo _____, Examiner_____
Indication_____ CPT Codes_____ ICD-9 codes_____
Intubated: Y/N, Sedated: Y/N, Insertion: Easy/Difficult /Failed Probe Type: pediatric/ biplane/multiplane/
epicardial/epiaortic Modalities: 2D/CFM/PWD/CWD/Contrast/Pharm/Stress Tape/OD #_____

2. Echocardiographic and Doppler Measurements

Aorta	Size	Diam (cm)	Dissection	Plaque thick (mm)	Plaque mobile
Ascending Ao	nl, dilated, aneur		y/n	0-3, >3	y/n
Ao Arch	nl, dilated, aneur		y/n	0-3, >3	y/n
Descending Ao	nl, dilated, aneur		y/n	0-3, >3	y/n

Valves	Annulus	Stenosis	Area/ Gradient	Regurg	Leaflet Morphology	Leaflet Motion
Aortic Valve	normal, dilated, calc, bioprosth, mechanical	No, mild, Mod, severe		0, 1+, 2+, 3+ 4+	Nl, Calc, Veg, Perf, Bicuspid Thickened,	Nl, Prolapse Flail, Restricted NCC/RCC/LCC
Mitral Valve	normal, dilated, calc, bioprosth, mechanical	No, mild, Mod, severe		0, 1+, 2+, 3+ 4+	Nl, Calc, Veg Perf, Myxom Thickened	Nl, Prolapse, Flail, SAM, Restricted P_1, P_2, P_3
Tricuspid	normal, dilated, calc, bioprosth, mechanical	No, mild, Mod, severe		0, 1+, 2+, 3+ 4+	Nl, Calc, Veg Perf, Myxom Thickened	Nl, Prolapse Flail, Restricted

Atria	Size	SEC (smoke)	Thrombus	Tumor	Device
Right atrium	normal, dilated	y/n	y/n	y/n	y/n
Left atrium	normal, dilated	y/n	y/n	y/n	y/n

Left atrial appendage:
Interatrial Septum: Morphology: Normal, Aneurysm Lipomatous Hypertrophy, PFO, ASD (Primum, Secundum, Sinus Venosus, AV Canal) Shunt: (r->l, l->r, bidirectional)
Interventricular Septum Morphology: Normal, Hypertrophy, Shift, Defect (membr, musc), Shunt: (r->l, l->r)

Ventricles	Cavity size	Cavity Dimension	Hypertrophy	Thrombus	Global FXN	EF
RV	normal, dilated		y/n	y/n	Nl, ↓, ↓↓,↓↓↓	
LV	normal, dilated		y/n	y/n	Nl, ↓, ↓↓,↓↓↓	

Regional Function: (1=normal, 2=hypokinetic, 3= akinetic, 4=dyskinetic)

Basal Segments	Mid Segments	Apical Segments
Anterior	Anterior	Anterior
Anteroseptal	Anteroseptal	Septal
Inferoseptal	Inferoseptal	Inferior
Inferior	Inferior	Lateral
Inferolateral	Inferolateral	True apex
Anterolateral	Anterolateral	

Pericardium: Normal, Thickened, Effusion: mild, moderate, severe, Tamponade **Pleura:** nl,effusion

Post Intervention Follow-up Study: See additional report, No Change, **Ventricular Fxn:** Global FXN: Improved, Decreased, Regional FXN: Improved, Decreased, **Valve FXN:** Native Valve: no change, improved, Normal Prosthetic Valve type_____ nl fxn?: Y/N, Valve repair: 0 leak, 1+,2+,3+, Valve area____

3. Comments: _____
_____

4. Summary: _____
_____

5. Complications: None,details:_____

Figure 24.1. Perioperative TEE report form designed by the Society of Cardiovascular Anesthesiologists (SCA) in North America.

Perioperative TOE Report

NHS

Date: Time:

Surgeon: Theatre/ICU:

Examiner(s):

Indication:

Insertion: Easy/Difficult/Failed

ADDRESSOGRAPH

Valves	Measurements	Stenosis	Area/Gradient	Regurg	Leaflet Morphology	Leaflet Motion
Aortic Valve	Annul ___ cm SV ___ cm STJ ___ cm	No Mild Mod Severe		No Mild Mod Severe	Normal Calc Veg Perf Bicuspid Thickened	Normal Prolapse Flail Restricted NCC/RCC/LCC
Mitral Valve	Annul ___ cm	No Mild Mod Severe		No Mild Mod Severe	Normal Calc Veg Perf Thickened	Normal Prolapse Flail SAM Restricted A1 A2 A3 P1 P2 P3
Tricuspid	Annul ___ cm	No Mild Mod Severe		No Mild Mod Severe	Normal Calc Veg Perf Thickened	Normal Prolapse Flail Restricted

Atria	Size	SEC (smoke)	Thrombus	Tumor	Device
Right atrium	normal, dilated	Y / N	Y / N	Y / N	Y / N
Left atrium	normal, dilated	Y / N	Y / N	Y / N	Y / N

<u>Interatrial Septum:</u>   ASD Y/N   Type: Shunt direction

Ventricles	Cavity size	Cavity Dimension	Hypertrophy	Thrombus	Global FXN
RV	normal, dilated		Y / N	Y / N	Good Mod Poor
LV	normal, dilated	LVEDD____ LVESD____ FS_____% EF_____%	Y / N	Y / N	Good Mod Poor

<u>Interventricular Septum:</u>   VSD Y/N   Type: Shunt direction

Regional Function: hypokinetic, akinetic, dyskinetic, normal (insert below)

SEPTAL	INFERIOR	POSTERIOR	LATERAL	ANTERIOR

Aorta	Diam	Dissection	Plaque thick	Plaque mobile
Ascending Ao	___ cm	Y / N	0-3, >3mm	Y / N
Ao Arch	___ cm	Y / N	0-3, >3mm	Y / N
Descending Ao	___ cm	Y / N	0-3, >3mm	Y / N

<u>Pericardium:</u>   Normal/ Thickened   Effusion: Y / N   Size_____ cm   Tamponade Y / N

<u>Pleural:</u>   Effusion Y / N   L / R

COMMENTS:

<u>Post Intervention:</u>

Ventricular Fxn: No change / Improve / Decreased   Regional FXN: Improved / Decreased
PROSTHETIC Valve: type_____   Perivalvular leak: Y / N
Valve repair: Regurg No / Mild / Mod / Severe   Stenosis: Y / N

Did TOE lead to a management change   Y / N
How?_____

Figure 24.2. Perioperative TEE report form in use in several UK hospitals.

5. **Equipment employed.** There is no doubt that technology is evolving rapidly and the use of more modern equipment is associated with better studies.

6. **Indications for performing the study.** Although we recommend the comprehensive approach to echocardiography, the indication for the study may place greater emphasis on some areas of structure and function than others.

7. **Quality of the study, difficulties, and complications.** There will be occasions when some echo windows are not available, and when some structures will not be interrogated. Such difficulties need to be indicated in the report. Any difficulties with probe insertion, physical trauma, or other complications should be recorded.

8. **Hemodynamic conditions.** Many features of the findings of a TEE examination are related to the hemodynamic state of the patient at the time of the examination. Heavy sedation, general anesthesia, and the supine position all have profound effects on preload, afterload, and contractility. Patients with regurgitant valve lesions will appear to have less severe lesions in the anesthetized, supine state than when awake. Estimates of ventricular function may be similarly affected.

9. **Specific findings.** This will form the body of the report and should include:

   Chambers
   left and right atrial dimensions
   spontaneous contrast, tumor, thrombus, and the presence of devices
   atrial septum: record morphology and the presence of defects and shunt direction/velocity
   ventricular systolic and diastolic cavity dimensions
   wall thickness, noting thinning or hypertrophy
   left ventricular segmental motion using the 17-segment model (see Chapter 4), noting movement and thickening
   ventricular septum
   left and right ventricular function: it is important to note the methodology used to measure function

   Valves
   dimensions, annular and other, e.g. sinus diameter, sinotubular junction diameter
   leaflet morphology
   leaflet motion
   degree of stenosis or regurgitation and supporting evidence; valve area
   it is important to state how valve function and dimensions were measured

   Vessels
   ascending, arch, and descending aorta, noting dimensions and pathology
   pulmonary arteries and venae cavae with dimensions and pathology

   Pericardium, noting effusions or thickening

   Pleurae, noting the presence of effusions

   Wherever possible the description of abnormal findings should be accompanied by the data which support those findings. These may be measurements from M-mode, a description of color-flow Doppler, VTIs or other velocity measurements from spectral Doppler, etc.

10. **Conclusions.** Although the concluding statement may be one of the last things that the echocardiographer writes in a report, it may well be the first or indeed the only part of the report that the referring physician reads. It should be a clear, concise, and logical summary of the findings of the examination. The pathology should be presented in order of severity and significance. Where there is more than one abnormal finding the conclusion should, if possible, link the findings in such a way as to make a coherent pathophysiological story. For example, "There is severe aortic stenosis (valve area 0.7 cm^2) and left ventricular hypertrophy (lateral wall thickness 14 mm) consistent with the valve lesion." Similarly, where there are apparently conflicting findings, this too should be highlighted. Less significant pathology should be mentioned later. For example "There is mild myxomatous degeneration of both mitral leaflets with trivial central regurgitation." The conclusion must be intelligible to a non-echo-trained physician.

11. **Therapeutic suggestions.** A physician trained and experienced in TEE may make therapeutic suggestions at the end of a study. Significant changes to therapy are usually best discussed with the referring physician or surgeon.

References

1. Nihoyannopoulos P, Fox K, Fraser A, Pinto F. EAE laboratory standards and accreditation. *Eur J Echocardiogr* 2007; **8**: 80–7.

2. Fox J, Glas K, Swaminathan M, Shernan S. The impact of intraoperative echocardiography on clinical outcomes following adult cardiac surgery. *Semin Cardiothorac Vasc Anesth* 2005; **9**: 25–40.

3. Price S, Via G, Sloth E, *et al.* Echocardiography practice, training and accreditation in the intensive care: document for the World Interactive Network Focused on Critical UltraSound (WINFOCUS). *Cardiovasc Ultrasound* 2008; **6**: 49.

4. Klein AA, Snell A, Nashef SAM, *et al.* The impact of intra-operative transoesophageal echocardiography on cardiac surgical practice. *Anaesthesia* 2009; **64**: 947–52.

5. Pearlman AS, Gardin JM, Martin RP, *et al.* Guidelines for physician training in transesophageal echocardiography: recommendations of the ASE Committee for Physician Training in Echocardiography. *J Am Soc Echocardiogr* 1992; **5**: 187–94.

6. Kneeshaw JD. Transoesophageal echocardiography (TOE) in the operating room. *Br J Anaesth* 2006; **97**: 77–84.

7. Savage R, Hillel Z, London M, *et al.* Recommendations for a standardized report for adult perioperative echocardiography from the Society of Cardiovascular Anesthesiologists/ American Society of Echocardiography Task Force for Standardized Perioperative Echocardiography Report. www.scahq.org/sca3/Report_of_Task_Force.pdf (accessed September 2009).

8. Pybus DA. A perioperative echocardiographic reporting and recording system. *Anesth Analg* 2004; **99**: 1326–9.

Index